Nephrotoxicity

In Vitro to *In Vivo*
Animals to Man

Nephrotoxicity

In Vitro to *In Vivo*
Animals to Man

Edited by
P. H. Bach

The Robens Institute of Industrial and Environmental Health and Safety
University of Surrey
Guildford, Surrey, United Kingdom

and
E. A. Lock

ICI Central Toxicology Laboratory
Macclesfield, Cheshire, United Kingdom

Plenum Press • New York and London

Library of Congress Cataloging in Publication Data

International Symposium on Nephrotoxicity (3rd: 1987: University of Surrey)
   Nephrotoxicity: *in vitro* to *in vivo:* animals to man / edited by P. H. Bach and E. A. Lock.
     p.   cm.
   "Proceedings of the Third International Symposium on Nephrotoxicity: Extrapolation from Animals to Man and *In Vitro* to *In Vivo,* held August 3–7, 1987, at the University of Surrey, Guildford, Surrey, United Kingdom" — T.p. verso.
   Includes bibliographies and indexes.
   ISBN 0-306-43153-X
   1. Kidneys — Pathophysiology — Congresses. 2. Toxicology — Animals models — Congresses. 3. Kidneys — Effect of drugs on — Congresses. 4. Kidneys — Effect of metals on — Congresses. I. Bach, P. H. (Peter H.) II. Lock, E. A. (Edward A.) III. Title.
RC903.I58   1987   89-3850
599'.02149 — dc19   CIP

Proceedings of the Third International Symposium on Nephrotoxicity:
Extrapolation from Animals to Man and *In Vitro* to *In Vivo,*
held August 3–7, 1987, at the University of Surrey,
Guildford, Surrey, United Kingdom

© 1989 Plenum Press, New York
A Division of Plenum Publishing Corporation
233 Spring Street, New York, N.Y. 10013

Printed in the United States of America

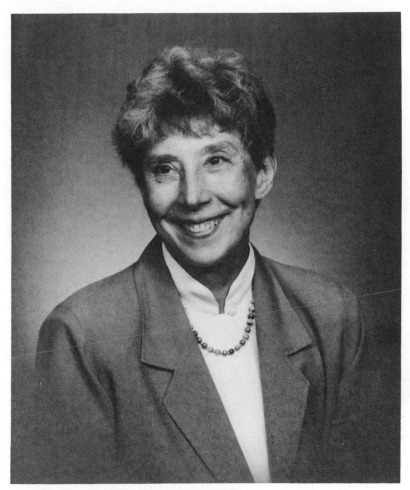

BODIL SCHMIDT-NIELSEN

BODIL SCHMIDT-NIELSEN

It is often difficult to be certain whether hereditary or environment contributes most to those who establish a long list of scientific achievement.   In the case of Bodil Schmidt-Nielsen both factors have contributed to make a very special person. As the daughter of August and Marie Krogh she inherited an enquiring mind and grew up in an environment where physiology and medicine were the day to day pulse.   Throughout the rest of her life it has been places and people that played a major role in shaping her contributions to science; in particular comparative renal physiology.

Bodil Schmidt-Nielsen's basic training at the University of Copenhagen was in dentistry.   She continued to complete a doctorate in odontology on the biochemistry of saliva, its formation and composition. These and other innovative studies resulted in her receiving an award from the King Christian 10th Fund for her work on the role of saliva in protection against carries.

She left her post as assistant professor at the University of Copenhagen and moved to the United States of America in 1946, where she became involved in studying excretory organs and particularly renal physiology.   Over a number of years as research associate, assistant professor or professor she worked at Stanford, the Kettering Institute Cincinnati, the Department of Zoology at Duke University, and the Department of Biology at Case Western Reserve, where she was chairman in 1970, and adjunct professor from 1971 to 1975.   Over these years her research interest had focused on fluid and electrolyte changes in species as varied as the amoeba, and fish, reptiles and the mammalian kidney.   Shortly after her arrival in the United States of America she was invited to undertake research at the Mount Desert Island Biological Laboratory, Salsbury Cove, in Maine.   It is here that the field of renal physiology and epithelial transport was associated with many of the giants amongst nephrophiles. These included Homer Smith, E.K. Marshal, Roy Foster and others.

In 1971 she moved to the idyllic area of Salsbury Cove to undertake research at the **Mount Desert Island Biological Laboratory,** first as research scientist, then as deputy director in 1979, vice-president in 1980 and president from 1981 to 1985.

The Mount Desert Island Laboratory was incorporated under the state laws of Maine as a non-profit scientific and educational institute. While its original purpose was to teach undergraduates marine biology it has always been the focus of a vibrant research interaction between large numbers of researchers who use this unique location to study aquatic and non-aquatic animals to probe the wonders of kidney function. While much of the research focus at Mount Desert Island has been on normal renal regulation and function, the problems of increasing marine pollution has necessitated an orientation towards studying the effects of chemicals on these processes and now toxicology is an integral part of the research programme.

It is in the area of urea handling and water metabolism, particularly its adaptation under extreme situations such as the arid conditions experienced by the Kangaroo rat and the camel, that Bodil achieved her worldwide renown. She was awarded the John Simon Guggenheim Memorial Fellowship in 1953 for her work on the water metabolism of camels in the Sahara Desert.

Her immense contribution to research has been recognised by her being an established investigator of the American Heart Association, and the principal investigator of NIH training and research awards throughout her career. She was also president of the American Physiological Society, Associated Editor of the American Journal of Physiology, Council Member of the Society for Experimental Biology and Medicine, Fellow of the New York Academy of Science, Fellow and Council Delegate of the American Association for the Advancement of Science, Fellow of the American Academy of Arts and Sciences and Trustee of the Mount Desert Island Biological Research Laboratory. Bodil has authored over 250 scientific contributions and trained scores of life scientists and physicians. Few people linked to renal physiology or nephrology have not been influenced by her research or teaching.

Bodil Schmidt-Nielsen stands foremost in using a comparative approach to combine the assessment of renal function and morphology in different species. This is vital for the area of nephrotoxicity, where due to the cascade of events following a primary injury the changes in function are very often followed by changes in morphology and vice versa. In addition, it is most important to choose an animal model with renal speciality or attributes that provide a research handle, instead of making use of whatever is available, but may be inappropriate.

The comment that Bodil is a "very special person" is also supported by the fact that she gave the first Bowditch lecture in 1956. She was the first (and so far only) female president of the American Physiological Society and president of the Mount Desert Island Biological Laboratory. In retirement she continues to serve as an active member of a number of learned societies, attends and participates in international scientific meetings, takes the responsibility in directing future planning as a member of several boards of trustees and puts energy into writing overviews and reviews. She is also writing a long overdue biography of August Krogh and his Nobel Prize winning research, not only as a loving daughter, but also as an equal international scientist who can place her father's valuable contributions in prospective.

She lives a warm relationship with her husband, Roger Chagnon, friends and children and continues her long-term passionate love for the outdoors, where she will "out-walk or swim" many younger people. Research associates, friends and family know her as an accomplished vegetable gardener, an excellent cook and she is renowned for baking one of the best home-made breads in the State of Maine and probably much beyond. A very special lady!

Hilmar Stolte,
Hannover,
Federal Republic of Germany

PREFACE

There has been a growing awareness that nephrotoxicity represents a key factor in human nephropathies, where, irrespective of the causative agent, only a few clinical end-effects are diagnosed. Thus nephropathies are generally classified as acute or chronic renal failure, malignancies or immunological changes. The weaknesses in diagnosing nephropathies arises because of the effective role the kidney plays in maintaining homeostasis, despite the fact that it has been extensively damaged.

The frequencies of some type of chemically-induced acute renal failure is well documented, but the causes of chronic renal failure, malignancy, and other nephropathies are far more difficult to associate with a chemical aetiology.

Many of the new therapeutic agents have important beneficial effects, but they are found to have marked nephrotoxic effects. Thus there is a growing urgency to increase the stringency of chemical safety evaluation for their potential nephrotoxic effects. This is strongly countered by the increased financial pressure to identify potentially nephrotoxic chemicals earlier in their development and humanitarian considerations to more closely relate animal test to the clinical situation. Part of the challenge may be achieved by the increasing use of in vitro techniques.

The objectives of this symposium have been to draw these central issues together and to try and establish where animal nephrotoxicity data is relevant to the clinical situation. If it is not, there is a need to define the factors that have to be considered to improve the validity of safety evaluation studies. Similarly, there is a need to define under what situation in vitro studies can effective mirror the normally functioning kidney and replace the use of animals. Where these techniques currently have limitations new and innovative approaches are needed to better define the mechanism of renal injury and relate this to risk-benefit considerations in developing novel chemicals or using established substances under a diverse set of circumstances.

The Symposium could not have been organized without the contribution of the Scientific Advisory Committee, the Sponsors, and the secretarial support of Lisa Breitner, Laura Mellor, Mimps E. van Ek, Janet Williams and Sally Basford. The index was prepared by Enoch Kwizera.

Peter Bach
Edward Lock

ACKNOWLEDGEMENTS

This Symposium was supported by

American Petroleum Institute
Bayer UK Ltd
Beecham Pharmaceuticals
The Boots Company plc
Ciba-Geigy Pharmaceuticals Ltd
ECETOC
Esse Petroleum Company Ltd
Fisons Pharmaceuticals
Glaxo Group Research Ltd
Huntingdon Research Centre
Imperial Chemical Industries plc
The Institute of Petroleum
Inveresk Research Foundation
Johnson Matthey
Johnson Wax
Merck Sharp & Dohme Ltd
E. Merck Ltd
Mobil Oil Corporation
Organon International BV
Pfizer Central Research
Richardson-Vicks Europe
RTZ Limited
Sandoz Pharmaceuticals
Shell UK
Smith Kline & French Research Ltd
Sterling Winthrop Group Europe

CONTENTS

NUCLEAR MAGNETIC RESONANCE

LIGHT HYDROCARBON NEPHROPATHY

HALOGENATED AND OTHER ORGANIC MOLECULES

NEW ASPECTS OF NEPHROTOXICITY

APPLICATION OF IMMUNOLOGICAL MARKERS

IN VITRO METHODS

SPECIES DIFFERENCES IN RENAL STRUCTURE AND FUNCTION - APPLICATIONS TO NEPHROTOXICITY IN MAN

Bodil Schmidt-Nielsen

Mount Desert Island Biological Laboratory, Salisbury Cove, Maine 04672, USA

INTRODUCTION

A classical example of how physiologists can take advantage of a specific renal adaptation is that of E.K. Marshall Jr. and the aglomerular goose fish (26). Marshall had shown that dog renal tubules accumulate the dye phenol red even when glomerular filtration was stopped by lowering the blood pressure. However, due to the belief held by most physiologists in the theory proposed by Cuhsny (that tubular secretion did not exist), the proofs presented by Marshall were not accepted. Then Marshall found from the literature that some fishes have renal tubules without glomeruli and therefore must form urine entirely by secretion. He came to Mount Desert Island Biological Laboratory in the summer of 1926 to work with the goose fish Lophius piscatorius. The work proved that not only is phenol red secreted by the renal tubules of the goose fish, but also a number of organic acids and bases as well as fluid and electrolytes (27). When these results were presented by Marshall his staunch opponent A.N. Richards was overheard saying: "at last Marshall has found one animal that fits his theories" (26).
There are two reasons why physiologist use a variety of vertebrates and invertebrates in experimental research. First, there is a desire to learn how the animals cope with their environments and how the organs have adapted to different physiological needs. Secondly, we try to find animals that are especially suited to solve certain problems, either because an organ has functional characteristics that make it amenable to study certain mechanisms or because in lower vertebrates certain structures are more available for experimental manipulation that they are in mammals. Both of these aspects will be discuss as they relate to how the kidneys of animals have accommodated to different life styles and how advantage can be taken of these specialized kidneys and other excretory organs in toxicological studies.

The ancestry, environment, and life style of an animal determines its kidney function. Mammals being primarily terrestrial animals have inherited the basic design of their kidneys from their aquatic ancestors the freshwater fishes. The mammalian renal tubules and vascular elements have been rearranged spatially in such a way that not only can the kidneys eliminate excess water efficiently, the kidney can also concentrate salt and urea while conserving water. Aquatic vertebrates, on the other hand, have modified the structure and function of renal tubules, bladders etc.

as their environment changed from freshwater to salt water and as other organs such as gills and salt glands took over essential excretory functions. Also, the nitrogenous end product of protein metabolism determines the kidney structure (31). All of these evolutionary modifications are useful in the search for animal models to study the mechanism of nephrotoxicity in the mammalian kidney. Even among mammals certain specializations of the kidney will decide the choice of mammal for different experimental studies.

THE FIRST FUNCTIONS OF THE KIDNEY

In its most primitive form the kidney was designed to excrete water and to regulate the volume of body fluids. The excretion of nitrogenous waste, acid-base regulation and excretion or uptake of monovalent ions was handled by the gills, salt glands or integuments (31). Even in many terrestrial vertebrates such as birds and reptiles excretion of monovalent ions is handled by specialized salt glands (34). However, in spite of the specialization of the mammalian kidney the basic functions of the glomerulus and the nephron segments are only modifications of the more primitive kidneys found in our freshwater ancestors (31).

Each environment places particular stresses or demands on the animal because the osmotic concentration and ionic composition of the environment may differ notably from those of the body fluids (Figure 1). All freshwater vertebrates have a higher osmotic concentration of the blood than that of their environment (they are hyper-osmoregulators). Thus, freshwater forms will tend to gain water and lose salts by diffusion. The kidneys therefore are designed to conserve salt and excrete the excess water.

Marine fishes, on the other hand, face different challenges. In the primitive hagfish (belonging to the class Agnatha) the extracellular fluids have the same osmolality and essentially the same ionic composition as as the sea water. Thus, being an osmo-conformer the hagfish does not lose salt or gain water from the environment unless the osmolality of the sea water decreases. If that happens the kidneys must serve in volume regulation excreting salt and water in the same osmotic concentration as the blood. Another class of marine fishes, Condrichtyes, to which the sharks, rays and rat fish belong, maintain a slightly higher osmolality than the sea water by maintaining a high concentration of urea and tri-methylamine oxide in the body fluids. They gain water and salt through the gills, since the plasma sodium and chloride concentrations are lower than in the sea water.
Their kidneys therefore, must be capable of excreting excess water and conserve urea and trimethylamine oxide. The marine teleost fishes (class Osteicthyes) maintain a lower osmolality of the body fluids than that of the sea. Therefore they tend to gain salt, (including divalent ions) and lose water. To compensate for the water lost they drink sea water and their kidneys must conserve water and excrete the divalent ions, while the excess sodium and chloride is excreted through gills (31).

THE VERTEBRATE KIDNEY

When vertebrates invaded the terrestrial environment they were faced with a new challenge, that of variable access to water and sometimes lack of water. The nitrogenous waste product ammonia which in the aquatic forms is excreted through gills or integuments is toxic and cannot be permitted to accumulate in the blood. Therefore, in terrestrial vertebrates, either urea, uric acid or both serve as end products of protein (Figure 1) metabolism and must be excreted through the kidneys (31). The kidneys must maintain the capacity to excrete excess water and must also be able

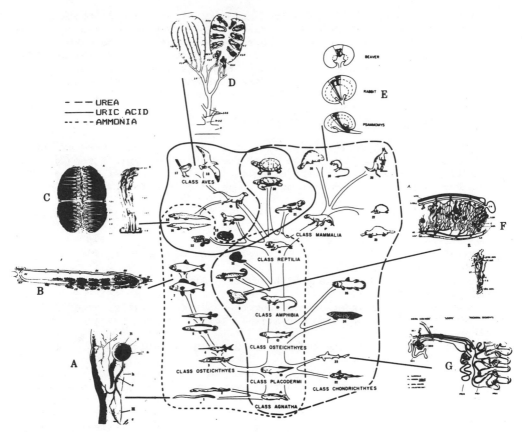

Figure 1. Types of vertebrate kidneys as related to phylogeny and nitrogen excretion solid and dashed lines enclose groups of vertebrates which predominantly excrete that type of nitrogenous waste product.

A. The hagfish in Class Agnatha has a atubular kidney.
B. Some marine teleost have aglomerular kidneys.
C. The crocodilians are aquatic, but they have retained the same kidney type as their terrestrial relatives. Their tubules secrete ammonia. Reptiles cannot produce an osmotically concentrated urine, but can concentrate uric acid as it precipitates out.
D. Birds have predominantly reptilian type nephrons, but have a limited countercurrent system with mammalian type nephrons.
E. All nephrons of mammalian kidneys all have loops of Henle, but some water loving mammals, with no need for water conservation, have only short loops and no inner zone of the medulla.
F. Frogs and other amphibians secrete urea into the tubules, but do not produce an osmotically concentrated urine.
G. Kidneys of marine sharks and rays conserve urea by tubular reabsorption in a special bundle region of their nephrons.

to conserve water and concentrate the nitrogenous waste and sometimes the salts in the urine. Reptiles and birds excrete uric acid which has a low solubility and precipitates out in the urine as water is reabsorbed from the tubular fluid. In marine reptiles and birds excess salt is excreted by extra-renal salt glands (34), consequently, reptiles have no need for producing an osmotically concentrated urine, while birds with their higher water loss, due to evaporation during flight, have the need and the ability to produce an osmotically concentrated urine. Mammals having the highly soluble urea as the nitrogenous end product and no extra-renal salt glands must be able to produce a concentrated urine when water conservation is essential and in mammals the highly efficient renal countercurrent system is developed to an extreme (31,32).

RENAL STRUCTURES TO MATCH THE CIRCUMSTANCES

These varied functions of the kidneys have been met during the evolution by ingenious modifications on the basic design of the typical nephron from freshwater fishes, which are the ancestors of all higher vertebrates. The typical freshwater teleost nephron is composed of the following regions:-

1) a renal corpuscle containing a well vascularized glomerulus with inconspicuous mesangium,
2) a ciliated neck region of variable length,
3) an initial proximal segment with prominent brushborder and numerous prominent lysosomes,
4) a second proximal segment with numerous mitochondria, but with less developed brush border,
5) a narrow ciliated intermediate segment which is variably present,
6) a distal segment with relatively clear cells with elongated mitochondria, and
7) a collecting duct system and usually a bladder (19).

Similar regions of the nephron are seen in the kidneys of amphibians, reptiles, and mammals. These regions are morphologically and physiologically similar, although not identical in all of these vertebrates. Functionally, these nephrons are designed for producing a large volume of dilute urine and excreting harmful organic substances and excess divalent ions. The ultrafiltrate of the blood formed in the glomeruli is modified in the initial proximal segment by the reabsorption of valuable molecules such as protein, glucose and amino acids. The primary functions of the second part of the proximal tubule are secretory. In this region, organic acids and bases are secreted, such as uraemic substances, uric acid p-aminohippurate, phenol red and many drugs and their metabolites. It is also in this segment that fluid secretion takes place in aglomerular as well as glomerular fishes and that divalent ions are secreted (2,11,27,35). The intermediate segment serves various functions which are not so well understood. The distal tubule is the diluting segment with a low permeability to water. Here sodium and chloride are reabsorbed leaving a dilute tubular fluid behind. There are two ways in which this basic tubule has been modified to meet the environmental requirements: one is through the loss of one or several segment of the nephron; the other is through a spatial rearrangement of the tubules. As pointed out by Marshall parts of the nephron have become lost or underveloped in several fishes (25). In the osmo-conformer the hagfish the filtration apparatus is large but the kidney is atubular. In marine fishes (hypo-osmoregulators) the distal tubule, diluting segment of the nephron, is lost and in the aglomerular fishes also the first part of the proximal tubule is lost (Figure 2). In Marshall's time the significance of the spatial countercurrent arrangements of the nephrons was not yet recognized and therefore he presented the tubules as straight.

The spatial rearrangement of the tubules is seen in the urea conserving (sharks and rays) elasmobranchs which exhibit a peculiar countercurrent system the bundle region of each tubule (Figure 1 G). The physiological significance of this arrangement is not yet fully understood, but it appears to serve in reducing the urea concentration in the urine (18). The

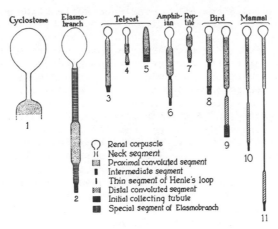

Figure 2. Schematic representation of nephrons of different vertebrates reprinted from Marshall (25).

true countercurrent system where some or all of the nephrons work together to produce a concentrated urine is found in the birds and mammals, respectively (Figure 1 D and E).

RENAL SPECIES DIFFERENCES IN PHYSIOLOGICAL TERMS

The various types of kidneys and extra-renal salt excreting structures can or have been used as models for specific segments of the mammalian nephron. They are used in vivo and in vitro, as isolated tubules, as cell cultures and as vesicles of apical and basolatereral membranes.

Glomeruli. For the study of glomerular function Richards and his co-workers used salamanders and frogs (30). The reason for choosing amphibians rather than mammals was that the glomeruli are accessible on the surface of the kidney, which made it possible to perform the first glomerular micropuncture studies in history. As is well known these studies proved that the fluid entering the renal tubule is an ultrafiltrate of the blood. Since that time a special strain of rats the Munich Wistar rats have been found to have glomeruli accessible on the surface of the kidney. But nature has also designed a fish that is particularly useful for studies of glomerular function. The hagfish, the osmo-conformer, has 30 to 35 very large paired glomeruli (0.68-1.02 mm in diameter) on each side of the spine (19). It has no renal tubules, instead the filtered fluid drains into the Archinephric duct which modifies the fluid only slightly. The body fluids of the hagfish are isosmotic with the sea water and the fish apparently uses its kidneys primarily for volume regulation (36). Stolte and his collaborators have taken advantage of this specialization and have worked extensively with the hagfish to study the haemodynamics of glomerular function (36).

In the hagfish as in other marine fishes the mesangial cells of Bowman's capsule have have processes which often completely embrace the capillary lumen, whereas in freshwater teleost they do not (19). The functional significance of this is not known; but the difference in structure may lend itself to further studies of toxic effect on the mesangium.

Proximal tubules. In mammals at least two functionally different segments of the proximal tubule are recognized; the pars convoluta and the

5

pars recta.   These segments correspond to the first and second segment of
the proximal tubule of glomerular fishes.

For toxicological studies of the second segment the aglomerular fishes are
ideally suited.   Due to the lack of other nephron segments renal studies
performed on the intact animal specifically illucidate the function of
this segment as shown by extensive studies by Marshall, Forster and their
colleagues (2,11,27).   In whole animal studies such as these it is also
possible to take advantage of the the renal portal system which is present
in all lower vertebrates (with the exception of the lamprey) by perfusing
the tubules of one of the kidneys through the renal portal vein, while the
other kidney serves as a control (11).   Fish tubules can also be studied
in vitro using the technique pioneered by Forster (12). The mechanisms of
secretion of dyes (organic acids and bases) across the basolateral
membranes and across the apical membranes were studied by Forster using a
simple method of placing the teased out fish tubules in an oxygenated
solution in a petri dish.   The tubules automatically seal at the ends and
the intra-cellular and intra-tubular dye concentrations could be estimated
visually (12,13).   These studies which required freshly caught flounders
necessitated that part of the workday was spent in a boat on the bay
fishing for flounders and researcher adopting this technique were the envy
of other workers at Mount Desert Island Biological Laboratory.   The
technique for estimating dye concentrations were later refined by Kinter
(23).   Isolated proximal fish tubules can also be studied by microperfusion in vitro (3).   Beyenback using this technique was able to show
that fluid secretion into the flounder tubules is hyper-osmotic and is
driven by NaCl secretion into the tubule.   In his experiments the tubule
is closed in one end and fluid is collected through a micropipette in the
other end (3).   The isolated tubular preparations have many advantages in
the studies of transport across tubular epithelium.   However, they do not
readily lend themselves to the more exact electro-physiological studies
that can be performed on epithelial membranes such as frog skins and toad
bladders.

Recently, a promising new preparation of proximal tubular cells from
flounders has been developed by Dickman and Renfro (7).   The principle of
their technique is that a primary cell culture of flounder proximal
tubules forms a continuous sheet of polarized cells when grown on a
collagen gel from rat tail tendons.   Transport across these sheets can
then be studied in Ussing-chambers.   Finally, the technique pioneered by
Kinne (29) of studying transport across basolateral and apical membrane
vesicles has been extensively used in the study of ion co-transport,
transport of organic substances and the effect of hormones.   The technique
has already been used in toxicological studies.

Distal tubule.   The diluting segment of the kidney is present in freshwater forms of almost all vertebrates as well as invertebrates.   It is
also present in all terrestrial vertebrates including mammals.   The
function of the diluting segment can be studied in the whole animal and in
isolated perfused distal tubules.   The primary function which is an active
chloride transport across the tubular epithelium has, however, been found
to be shared by a number of other salt transporting epithelia.   As
mentioned earlier, marine teleost fishes reabsorb NaCl and water from the
intestine and excrete the NaCl not through the kidneys but through
specialized salt secreting cells in the gills (chloride cells).
Elasmobranchs excrete salt through rectal glands.   Salt excreting organs
are also found in marine and terrestrial reptiles and in oceanic birds
(34).   The salt transporting organs that are useful as model systems are
primarily the teleost intestine and gills, and the rectal gland in
elasmobranchs.   In gills and rectal glands the transport of NaCl is from
the serosal to mucosal side of the cells.   This is the opposite direction

of NaCl transport in the thick ascending limb of the loop of Henle in mammals and in fish intestine. In spite of this difference the transport characteristics have been found to be very similar (8,9,14-16). In teleost gills and in the rectal gland the transport consists of a NaCl-KCl co-transport into the cells across the basolateral membrane, with a passive entry of Na and and active transport of K. 2Cl- diffuse down the concentration gradient across the apical membrane while 2Na+ move down the electrochemical gradient through the para cellular pathway. In the thick ascending limb of mammalian kidneys the co-transport is on the apical side and the passive chloride movement is across the basolateral membrane (8). Transport by the chloride cells of the gills can be studied in an isolated perfused fish head (5). In recent years, however, another very useful preparation has been developed. Karnaky discovered that the opercular skin of sea water adapted kilifish is particularly rich in chloride cells (20,21). Since the opercular membrane can be removed an studied as an epithelial membrane in an Ussing chamber this tissue is useful for the study of chloride cell function (6). The function of the rectal gland of the dogfish shark was first discovered by Burger who working with intact dogfish discovered that the rectal gland secretes an almost pure NaCl solution (4). Later isolated perfused rectal glands were studied (17). Then a technique was developed to separate the secretory tubules and work with the isolated perfused tubules (10). Recently, primary cell cultures of rectal glands have been developed (37) and vesicle preparations of plasma membranes have been intensively studied (29).

MAMMALIAN KIDNEYS OF DIFFERENT TYPES AS MODELS FOR NEPHROTOXICITY STUDIES.

Mammalian kidneys differ in several significant respects. These differences include variations in length of the inner medulla, number of nephrons, relative number of short and long looped nephrons, nephron heterogeneity, vascular bundles in the inner stripe, differences in renal pelvic extensions etc. (1). The thickness of the inner medulla vary with the need and ability of the mammals to conserve water (1,32). Desert rodents with the highest possible urinary concentrating ability have the longest renal papilla (1,32), while water loving mammals have no inner medulla of the kidney no vascular bundles and no long looped nephrons (Figure 1 E). To these belong the beaver Castor canadensis and the mountain beaver Aplodontia rufa (32,33). Species differences are also found in the epithelium of the renal tubules (24). For example the thin limbs of long loops differ significantly both anatomically and functionally in rabbit and rat (24). Profound differences are found in the vascular bundles in the inner stripe of the outer medulla, some of which incorporate the thin limb of descending short loops of Henle (1,24). Species differences have also been found in the effect of hormones on the various segments of the renal tubule (28).

In conclusion, nature has provided a wide range of vertebrate kidneys, each adapted to fulfil a series of functional roles that provides a series tool with which to understand the complexities of the kidney. Many of these have been well documented by physiological and anatomical research. Nephrotoxicity studies represents a new and exciting discipline, where the appropriate choice of a species can offer unique renal characteristics that can be exploited to study the effects of chemicals on the key processes that are the basis of nephropathies. This diversity of structure and function still needs to be adopted as a tool to investigate the many problems relating to the adverse effects of drugs and chemicals on the kidney that are under investigation.

REFERENCES

1. L. Bankir and C. de Rouffignac, 1985, Urinary concentrating ability:

insights from comparative anatomy, Am. J. Physiol., 249:R643.

2. F. Berglund and R.P. Forster, 1958, Renal tubular transport of inorganic divalent ions by the aglomreular marine teleost Lophius americanus, J. Gen. Physiol., 41:429.

3. K.W. Beyenbach, 1982, Direct demonstration of fluid secretion by glomerular renal tubules in a marine teleost, Nature., 299:54.

4. J.W. Burger and W.N. Hess, 1960, Function of the rectal gland in spiny dogfish, Science, 131:670.

5. J.B. Claiborne and D.H. Evans, 1980, The isolated perfused head of the marine teleost fish, Myoxocephalus octodecimspinosus: Hemodynamic effects of epinephrins, J. Comp. Physiol., 138:79.

6. K.J. Degan, K.J. Karnaky, Jr. and J.A. Zadunaisky, 1977, Active chloride transport in the in vitro opercular skin of a teleost (Funduslus hetroclitus), a gill-like epithelium rich in chloride cells, J. Physiol., 271:155.

7. K.G. Dickman and J.L. Renfro, 1986, Primary culture of flounder renal tubule cells: transepithelial transport, Am. J. Physiol., 251:F424.

8. F.H. Epstein and P. Silva, 1985, Na-K-Cl Cotransport in chloride-transporting epithelial in: Membrane Transport driven by Ion Gradients. Ann. N. Y. Acad. Sci., 456:187.

9. J.M. Eveloff, M. Field, R. Kinne and H. Murer, 1980, Sodium-cotransport systems in intestine and kidney of the winter flounder, J. Comp. Physiol., 135:175.

10. J.N. Forrest, Jr., F. Wong and K. Beyenbach, 1983, Perfusion of isolated tubules of the shark rectal gland: electrical characteristics and response to hormones, J. Clin. Invest., 72:1163.

11. R.P. Forster, 1973, Comparative vertebrate physiology and renal concepts, In: Handbook of Physiology - Renal Physiology, Am. Physiol. Soc. Washington D.C., 161.

12. R.P. Forster, 1948, Use of thin kidney slices and isolated renal tubules for direct study of cellular transport kinetics, Science, 108:65.

13. R.P. Forster and S. Hong, 1958, In vitro transport of dyes by isolated renal tubules of the flounder as disclosed by direct visualization. Intracellular accumulation and transcellular movement, J. Cell. Comp. Physiol., 51:259.

14. R.A. Frizzell, P.L. Smith and M. Field, 1981, Sodium chloride absorption by flounder intestine: a model for the thick renal ascending limb, Membrane Biophysics: Structure and function in epithelia. Alan R. Liss, Inc. New York, 67.

15. R. Gregor and E. Schlatter, 1984, Mechanism of NaCl secretion in the rectal gland of spiny dogfish (Squalus acanthias). I. Experiments in isolated perfused rectal gland tubules, Pfluegers Arch., 402:63.

16. J.A. Hannafin and R. Kinne, 1985, Active chloride transport in rabbit thick ascending limb of Henle's loop and elasmobranch rectal gland: chloride fluxed in isolated plasma membranes, J. Comp. Physiol. B, 155:415.

8

17. J.D. Hayslett, D. Schon, M. Epstein and C.A.M. Hogben, 1974, In vitro perfusion of the dogfish rectal gland, Am. J. Physiol., 226:1188.

18. H. Hentschel, M. Elger and B. Schmidt-Nielsen, 1986, Chemical and morphological differences in the kidney zones of the elasmobranch, Raja erinacea MITCH, Comp. Biochem. Physiol., 84A:553.

19. C.P. Hickman, Jr. and B.F. Trump, 1969, The Kidney in: Fish Physiology. Vol. 1. Hoar and Randall, eds. Academic Press, New York, 91.

20. K.J. Karnaky, Jr., 1980, Ion-secreting epithelia: chloride cells in the head region of Fundulus hetroclitus, Am. J. Physiol., 238:R185.

21. K.J. Karnaky, Jr., K.J. Degnan and J.A. Zadunaisky, 1977, Chloride transport across isolated opercular epithelium of killifish: A membrane rich in chloride cells, Science, 195:203.

22. R. Kinne, B. Koenig, J. Hannafin, E. Kinne-Saffran, D.M. Scott and K. Zierold, 1985, The use of membrane vesicles to study the NaCl/KCl cotransporter involved in active transepithelial chloride transport, Pfluegers Arch., 405:S101.

23. W.B. Kinter, 1975, Structure and function of renal tubules isolated from fish tubules, Fortschritte der Zoologie, 23:223.

24. W. Kirz, 1981, Structural Organization of the renal medulla, Am. J. Physiol., 241:R3.

25. E.K. Marshall, Jr., 1934, The comparative physiology of the kidney in relation to theories of renal secretion, Physiol. Rev., 14:133.

26. E.K. Marshall, Jr., 1966, Two lectures on renal physiology, Physiologist, 99:367.

27. E.K. Marshall, Jr., A.L. Graflin and L. Vickers, 1928, The structure and function of the kidney of Lophius piscatorius, Bull. Johns Hopkins Hosp., 43:205.

28. F. Morel, M. Imbert-Teboul and D. Chabardes, 1987, Receptors to vasopressin and other hormones in the mammalian kidney, Kidney Inter., 31:512.

29. H. Murer and R. Kinne, 1980, The use of isolated membrane vesicles to study epithelial transport processes, J. Membrane Biol., 35:81.

30. A.N. Richards and A.M. Walker, 1937, Methods of collecting fluid from known regions of the renal tubules of amphibia and of perfusing the lumen of a single tubule, Am. J. Physiol., 118:111.

31. B. Schmidt-Nielsen and W.C. Mackay, 1972, Comparative physiology of electrolyte and water regulation with emphasis on sodium, potassium, urea, and osmotic pressure, In: Clinical Disorders of Fluid and Electrolyte Metabolism. Maxwell and Kleeman. eds. McGraw-Hill Second Edition, New York, 45.

32. B. Schmidt-Nielsen and R. O'Dell, 1961, Structure and concentrating mechanism in the mammalian kidney, Am. J. Physiol, 200:1119.

33. B. Schmidt-Nielsen and W.E. Pfeiffer, 1970, Urea and urinary concentrating ability in the mountain beaver, Aplodontia rufa, Am. J. Physiol., 218:1370.

34. K. Schmidt-Nielsen, 1960, The salt secreting gland of marine birds, *Circulation*, 21:955.

35. H. Stolte, R.G. Galaske, F.M. Eisenbach, C. Lechene, B. Schmidt-Nielsen and J.W. Boylan, 1977, Renal tubule ion transport and collecting duct function in the elasmobranch little skate, *Raja erinaecea*, *J. Exp. Zool.*, 199:403.

36. H. Stolte and K.H. Neumann, 1982, Hochdruck und renale Volumenregulation-Untersuchungen an *Myxine glutinosa* (Schleimaal), *In*: Essential Hypertonie. D. Vaits, Ed. Springer, Berlin, Heidelberg, 21.

37. J.D. Valentich and J.N. Forrest, 1986, Cell physiology of cultured *Squalas acanthias* rectal gland epithelium, *Bull. Mount Desert Island Biol. Lab.*, 26:91.

LEAD INDUCED NEPHROTOXICITY: KIDNEY CALCIUM AS AN INDICATOR OF TUBULAR INJURY.

R.A. Goyer (1), C.R. Weinberg (2), W.M. Victery (3) and C.R. Miller (2)

(1) Department of Pathology, University of Western Ontario, Canada, (2) The National Institute of Environmental Health Sciences, and (3) The Environmental Protection Agency, Research Triangle Park, N.C., U.S.A.

INTRODUCTION

Chronic nephropathy is one of the oldest recognized health effects of lead; yet less is known about dose and renal effects than for any of the other major health effects of lead. Some of the reason for this is that chronic renal disease from lead exposure does not become evident until late in life and usually after many years of excessive exposure. At that time exposure information may not be available. In fact, the role of lead may not be recognized since the pathological changes in the late stages are not specific so that it is difficult to differentiate lead nephropathy from any other form of chronic renal failure. The succession of morphological and functional changes characteristic of renal effects of lead have been determined from studies of animal models and workmen exposed to lead. In this brief review a sequence of pathological changes is described comparing similarities and differences in experimental models and man. Current studies to identify biologic markers or diagnostic criteria for the early recognition of lead nephropathy are also reviewed. Finally, results of recent studies in animals will be presented that suggest that there is a threshold level of lead exposure for the onset of acute renal tubular cell effects to occur and that these observations are consistent with the few reported observations of minimal renal lead effects in humans.

PROGRESSION OF LEAD NEPHROPATHY

The progression of lead nephropathy, acute to chronic renal disease, is shown in Figure 1. The process is divided into three stages, Stage I, acute or reversible nephropathy; Stage II, chronic nephropathy which is not reversible and Stage III, renal tubular cell neoplasia or adeno-carcinoma.

Stage I is the period of acute effects and is limited to functional and morphological changes in proximal tubular cells. Two changes are important. There is impairment of mitochondrial function with decrease in energy dependent transport functions including aminoaciduria, glycosuria, and changes in specific ion transport. Another early change is the appearance of inclusion bodies, or lead protein complexes in nuclei and sometimes in cytoplasm of affected cells. These changes as they relate to assessment and pathogenesis considerable more detail elsewhere [1]. The

11

```
                    Rat                                              Man

     STAGE I    Acute nephropathy                      Oral or inhalation
                lead in diet                           exposure
                20 weeks


                              Similarities

                        Swollen proximal tubular lining cells
                        Inclusion bodies
                        Tubular dysfunction


  R
  E        Differences                              Differences
  V
  E          Impaired oxid/phos                       Not studied
  R          Reversible? (not studied)                Reversible
  S          Progresses to chronic                    Progression to chronic
  I           nephropathy                             nephropathy - not
  B                                                   demonstrated
  L
  E

     STAGE II   Chronic nephropathy


                              Similarities

                        Some inclusion bodies
                        Tubular atrophy and dilitation
                        Interstitial fibrosis
                        Renal failure
                        Hyperuricemia (inconsistent)


  I
  R
  R        Differences                              Differences
  E
  V          High incidence                           Rare renal tumors
  E          Renal tumors
  R
  S
  I
  B
  L
  E
```

Figure 1. Comparison of Pathogenesis of Lead Nephropathy in Man and Rat

changes are reversible following treatment with EDTA [2].

Stage I changes have been better studied in experimental models than in
man, but effects in animals, morphological and functional, seem identical.
The functional changes characteristic of Stage I are more conspicuous in
children than adults or experimental models.   Early ultrastructural
changes with occupational exposure in workers are, however, identical to
those occurring in the early stages of lead exposure in the rat.

As lead nephropathy progresses to an irreversible form of chronic renal
disease, **Stage II,** pathological and clinical changes are more difficult to
compare between experimental models and man. Progression in man is usually
over several years and the clinical manifestations are similar to that for
any form of chronic nephropathy. Although a late effect is increase in
blood urea nitrogen (BUN) or creatinine and reduced glomerular filtration
rate, the glomerulus does not seem to be a primary target of lead
toxicity. Glomerular injury probably only occurs secondary to tubular
atrophy, interstitial nephropathy and nephron loss.   In this later stage
there are fewer nuclear inclusion bodies in human biopsy material than
found in rats but this difference may be explained by level of lead
exposure [3].   Without recent exposure or following treatment with
chelating agents inclusion bodies may be completely absent so that there
may be no morphological features to identify the nephropathy as being
related to lead exposure [2]. Increase in serum uric acid and clinical
gout may be associated effects.

Hyperplasia, cytomegaly and dysplastic cellular changes in proximal tubular lining cells are common to man and experimental animals in **Stage III**. These changes are associated with renal adenocarcinoma in a high percentage of lead exposed rats [5] but have only been reported a couple of times in man [6,7]. A recent study of mortality among a large number of employees of lead battery plants and lead-producing plants, 1947-1980 showed a significant number of excess deaths from malignant neoplasms, and nephritis but no increase in renal tumours [8]. There was an increase in lung and gastric cancers but the excess was not statistically significant. The reason for the difference in organ specificity between rodents and people isn't known but it may be related to differences in route of exposure. Rats in experimental studies are exposed to large doses of lead in drinking water and hence the large renal exposure and urinary excretion. Workers in lead battery plants and lead producing plants are exposed by inhalation and some secondary ingestion, but this is speculation. Both have an excess of nephritis or chronic lead nephropathy so people are similar to rodents in this regard. In terms of the level of exposure as measured by blood lead levels it is not possible to make meaningful comparisons. There are few blood lead level measurements for lead exposed rats on carcinogen studies, but they must be high because of the high level of lead exposure. The workers in the Cooper study were also heavily exposed. The mean blood lead concentration of 1326 battery plant workers with three or more analyses was 62.7 ug/100g (3.0 uMol/l), 404 had means of 70 ug or more (3.4 uMol/l), 24 of which had means over 100 ug/100g (4.8 uMol/l). For the lead production workers in four plants the mean for 537 men was 79.7 ug/100g (3.9 uMol/l). These populations of workers were therefore exposed to lead in amounts far exceeding the present workplace standards.

The most important current issue, for recognition of lead effect on the kidney is the need for a biological indicator or early marker. For effects of lead on the nervous system, there is now available a battery of cognitive and behavioural tests, and there are tests to evaluate motor function [9]. Changes in haem metabolism and haem enzymes are both sensitive and specific indicators of lead effect [10]. But, for the kidney, the only guide to a renal effect is evidence of reduced glomerular filtration rate as measured by increase in blood urea nitrogen or creatinine. When these changes are evident, a chronic interstitial nephropathy is present which is irreversible and in most instances is probably progressive.

A list of various biologic parameters that might be considered as potential early indicators of lead nephropathy are listed in Table 1. Lead nephropathy does not have a specific proteinuria. This seems difficult to rationalize in view of the nature of toxicity of lead on proximal tubular cells much in the way that cadmium, chromium or even uranium does. These metals induce a tubular proteinuria with excretion of low molecular weight proteins like beta-2-microglobulinuria and retinal binding protein, but this has not been observed in either experimental or clinical lead toxicity.

Table 1.   Potential Early Indicators of Lead Nephropathy

Decreased GFR	Proteinuria
Aminoaciduria	Enzymuria (NAG)
Urine zinc and/or calcium	Increase in renal calcium

Also one might expect to be able to identify inclusion body protein in the urine. Inclusion bodies in tubular cells are an early pathological change

[11] and can be found microscopically in urine sediment in epithelial cells that have been shed from renal tubules but there are so few of them that it is not possible to recognize them chemically [12]. However, efforts to enhance the excretion of this protein with EDTA have not been successful. If a monoclonal antibody can be developed to the protein it might have the necessary sensitivity and specificity. Excretion of high molecular weight proteins or albuminuria with reduction in GFR is usually a sign of chronic interstitial nephropathy and is not an early indication of lead effect. Other signs of proximal tubular dysfunction such as aminoaciduria are inconsistent and are more often found in children than adults even in the earliest stages of excess occupational exposure to lead [3].

Urinary excretion of the lysosomal enzyme N-acetyl-D-glucosaminidase (NAG) has been found to be a sensitive indicator of renal tubular cell damage due to injury by a variety of toxins including the heavy metal mercury [13]. Increase in NAG in urine serves as a good prognostic indicator of renal transplant rejection and it is increased in experimental animals and workers exposed to a number of nephrotoxins but observations of excretion following lead exposure have been inconsistent [14]. Ong and co-workers [15] measured the excretion of NAG in over 200 low to moderate lead exposed workers with blood lead ranging from 10 to 80 ug/dl and found a highly significant correlation between lead in urine and NAG in urine. NAG has been found to be increased in other studies of lead exposed workers as well, but we have not been able to repeat these finding in lead exposed rats. In the Ong [15] study there was poor association between lead in blood and NAG in urine and it was thought therefore that NAG was a poor reflector of lead in the kidney. Thus at this time we are uncertain of the significance of NAG in the urine of lead workers. To be clinically useful and to provide a basis for risk assessment a biologic indicator must be related to lead dose, and blood lead is presently the best measure of lead dose.

In recent studies in our laboratory we have shown that acute exposure to lead alters urinary excretion of essential trace metals including zinc and calcium [16,17]. In these studies lead acetate was added to drinking water. Four different levels of lead, 0, 200, 500 and 1,000 ppm were given to rats for three different periods of time; 4, 8 and 12 weeks. The mineral content of the diet was close to the recommended dietary allowance of 5.0g of calcium and 0.012g zinc/kg diet. Two hundred ppm of lead was chosen as the lowest dose of lead because in previous experiments this had been determined to be the minimally toxic dose with this level of calcium in the diet. There were significant reductions in body weight at 4 and 8 weeks at the 200 ppm level; kidney weight/body weight ratios increased for all groups. This parameter had been shown previously to be one of the most sensitive indices of lead effect. The 200 ppm groups have blood lead levels in the range of 40 to 60 ug/dl, but the groups are very high. The experiment could be repeated with at least one or two lower doses to obtain blood lead levels in the range we are presently concerned with, but when we identified 200 ppm as the minimally toxic dose we were concerned with blood lead in the 40 ug/dl range and this is the level present occupational health standards in the United States are designed to prevent. We collected urine from each group before killing the animals at 4, 8 and 12 weeks and measured urinary lead, zinc and calcium. Figure 2 shows the correlation between urinary zinc and lead.

A best-fit curve was drawn through all the points; at 4-week lead exposure all rats had zinc excretion greater than control. The increase in zinc excretion closely parallels lead excretion rising rapidly at low-lead excretion rate and reaching a plateau at higher levels. These results

14

suggest that zinc excretion is an indicator of increased lead exposure at low levels of exposure. The correlation between lead and zinc excretion suggests that these two cations may compete for a common reabsorptive or secretory pathway in the renal tubule and the fact that zinc excretion does not increase above 25 ug/day suggests that there is a maximum level of zinc transport which is not subject to further increase by lead. It has been previously shown that urinary excretion of zinc is a tightly regulated excretory pathway and is affected by starvation, infection, diabetes, glucagon and insulin levels [16,17]. In dogs, renal tubular reabsorption sites for zinc and lead were shown in both the proximal and distal nephron [18].

The increase in urine zinc with lead exposure, although a renal phenomenon, is not really useful as an early indicator of renal effect because the effect is probably more physiological than pathological and that values from individuals would be more difficult to interpret than for the mean of a group.

Another point of interest is whether chronic lead exposure can result in zinc deficiency. It is very difficult to assess zinc status in an individual by measuring zinc levels in accessible tissues. Zinc levels were measured in several tissues after 12 weeks. Although plasma zinc tended to be lower, it was not statistically significant. Kidney, liver and erythrocyte zinc was not affected but brain, testis and bone were all decreased. Zinc in pancreas was increased. Of course, it is well-known

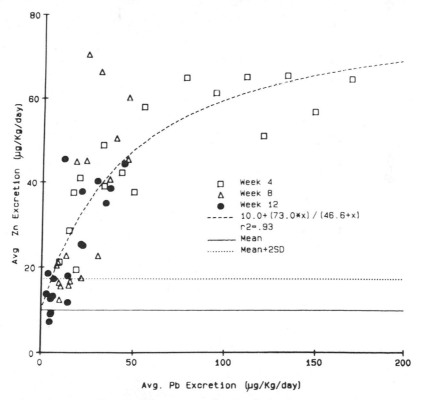

Figure 2. Correlation of average daily urine zinc excretion with average daily lead excretion. Mean and mean±2SD for control animals shown by solid and dotted line respectively. Equation of best fit line drawn on graph given in legend. (Reproduced from Ref. 17 with permission of publisher.)

that lead exposure reduces the activity of several zinc-dependent enzymes such as delta-aminolaevulinic acid dehydratase [19].

The relationship between urine and kidney lead and calcium was also studied. Although there is a positive correlation between lead and calcium excretion for the group, values from individual animals did not show any consistent relationship so these parameters would not be useful indicators of renal effect of lead. However, if kidney calcium is plotted with kidney lead, an interesting relationship does appear (Figure 3). Values for the control mean±2SD, is shown by the solid and dotted lines. The control mean, plus two standard deviations, is 90.1 ug kidney calcium. Kidney calcium does not exceed the upper normal limit until kidney lead reaches a particular level that might be interpreted as a threshold level. This suggests that at this particular concentration of kidney lead there may be loss of calcium homeostasis in the kidney.

Normally intracellular calcium is less than 1 uM and is tightly regulated by cation pumps which are dependent on mitochondrial ATP generation. With any of a number of forms of cell injury such as hypoxia and/or toxins like lead that impair sodium potassium ATP'ase there is loss of energy dependent cation and water regulation. This explains the cellular swelling and mitochondrial changes that are seen early in lead toxicity [20]. If the injury is prolonged, or more severe, it becomes irreversible with disruption of cell membranes and cell death. The initial changes, however, are reversible with influx into the cell of water and cations, particularly calcium [21,22] and is reflected by increase in kidney weight and increase in kidney calcium.

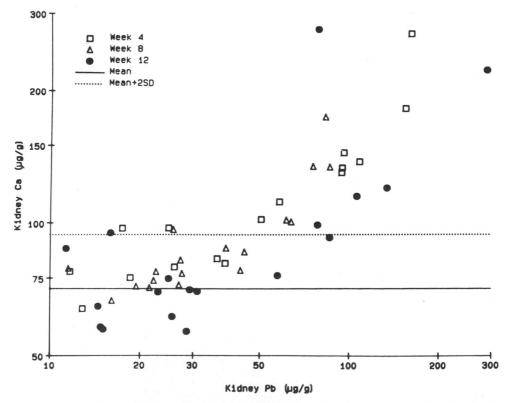

Figure 3. Correlation of kidney calcium and lead concentration in lead-exposed rats. Values for control mean±2 SD are shown by the solid and dotted lines. (Reproduced from Ref. 17 with permission of publisher.)

16

The kidney lead/kidney calcium relationship is a potential marker of early onset of renal tubular cell injury but neither parameter is measurable in vivo so that the question was asked whether blood lead might be substituted for kidney lead. The blood lead level at which the change in kidney calcium is likely to occur was estimated by maximum likelihood, using the GLIM statistical system published by Baker and Nelder [23]. The statistical methodology is described in the appendix of this paper. Figure 4 shows a fitted curve corresponding to a 4-parameter logistic model relating blood lead level to the probability that kidney calcium exceeds 90.1 ug/g, the upper limit of normal from the control animals. From this model it is suggested that a blood lead level of 60 ug/dl is the upper threshold for onset of acute renal tubular cell injury to lead.

As expected, if kidney lead per se is used to calculate the threshold a much better fit is obtained and the rise begins with a kidney lead at 45 ug/g with a 95% confidence interval of 17.4-61.5 ug/g. Blood lead does not improve the fit once kidney lead has been put in the model. Thus, the biologically important exposure is how much lead is in the kidney and blood lead represents a weak but perhaps useful surrogate.

To confirm the relationship between increase in renal calcium and mito-chondrial injury ultrastructure from 8 rats with high kidney lead were studied. Four of the kidneys had kidney calcium greater than 90.1 ug/g; 4 had normal calcium. Two blocks of embedded tissue were examined from each kidney. Three of the four kidneys with elevated calcium contained cells with swollen mitochondria; the fourth was ambiguous. These changes are therefore consistent with hypothesis that kidneys with elevated calcium show early and probably reversible cell injury. The proposed threshold of 60 ug/dl of blood lead is also consistent with the few reported observations of kidney effect or absence of kidney effect in humans. For example, Buchet and co-workers [24] reported that workers who do not have a recorded blood Pb level over 62 or 63 dl for up to 12 years do not have lead nephropathy. On the other hand, from the Cooper studies, where an increase in lead nephropathy was found, the mean blood lead was greater than 62 uq/dl with many values considerably higher.

The proposed threshold 60 ug/dl for renal effects of lead is a higher blood lead level than effects on other organs occur such as the nervous system and haematopoietic system. Also, these observations are in rats. Although there are reasons to be confident about the similarities in pathogenesis or mechanisms responsible for lead nephropathy in man and rats, there is little data to support extrapolation of dose-response relationships.

CONCLUSIONS

Blood lead level of 60 ug/dl is the threshold for renal cell injury as reflected by the point at which tubular cellular cells lose their ability to maintain homeostatic mechanism for maintaining intracellular water and cation balance. A threshold for renal cell injury at blood lead level of 60 ug/dl lead is consistent with the few observations available in man.

The kidney is not the critical organ in lead toxicity, particularly in children where nervous system effects are known to occur at considerably lower levels (about 15-20 ug/dl) and for which, in fact, there may be no threshold.

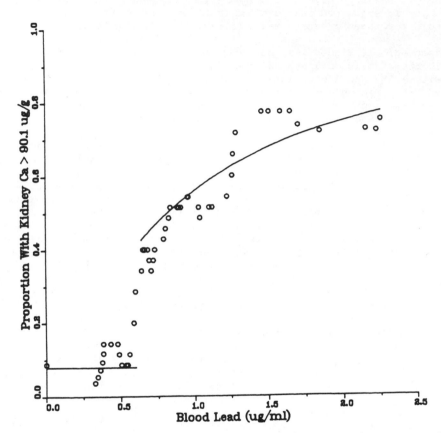

Figure 4.   The open circles correspond to a weighted moving average based
on the data,   (used an eleven-point window with a weighting scheme: 1, 2,
3,   4, 5, 5, 5, 4, 3, 2, 1). The plot shows a breakpoint or jump increment
in blood lead in the region of 60 to 64 ug/dl blood lead.   From this model
it is suggested that a blood lead level of 60 ug/dl is the upper threshold
for onset of acute renal tubular cell injury to lead.

Finally, the rat model does serve to provide some understanding of the mechanisms of the pathogenesis of lead exposure in humans. Quantitative extrapolation from rat to man must be validated. Perhaps most importantly, there is need for a reliable indicator or biological marker of lead effect on the kidney that can be applied to human populations.

APPENDIX

The probability that kidney Ca exceeds 90.1 ug/g (based on mean±2 SD for controls) was modelled as a function of blood Pb by a 4-parameter logistic regression model which incorporated a (possibly discontinuous) threshold effect as follows:

$$\ln \left[\frac{P}{1-p} \right] = \begin{cases} C \text{ for blood Pb } < T \\ \\ C + D + E \ln \text{ (blood Pb) for blood Pb } \geq T \end{cases}$$

where P denotes the probability that kidney Ca > 90.1.

The parameters were fitted by the method of maximum likelihood, using the GLIM (23) statistical system. The resulting fitted curve is shown in Figure 4.

REFERENCES

1. R.A. Goyer, The nephrotoxic effects of lead In: "Nephrotoxicity, Assessment and Pathogenesis", P.H. Bach, F.W. Bonner, J.W. Bridges, and E.A. Lock, eds. John Wiley and Sons, New York (1982).

2. R.A. Goyer, and M.H. Wilson, Lead-induced inclusion bodies: results of EDTA treatment, Lab. Invest. 32:149 (1975).

3. K. Cramer, R.A. Goyer, O.R. Jagenburg, and M.H. Wilson, Renal ultra-structure, renal function and parameters of lead toxicity in workers with different lengths of lead exposure, Brit. J. Indust. Med. 31:113 (1974).

4. V. Batuman, J.K. Maesala, B. Haddad, E. Tepper, E. Landry and R. Wedeen, The role of lead in gout nephropathy, N. Engl. J. Med. 304:520 (1981).

5. P. Mao, and J.J. Molnar, The fine structure and histochemistry of lead-induced renal tumors in rats, Am. J. Pathol. 50:571 (1967).

6. E.L. Baker, R.A. Goyer, B.A. Fowler, U. Khettry, O.B. Bernard, S. Adler, R. White, R. Babayan and R.G. Feldman, Occupational lead exposure, nephropathy and renal cancer, Am. J. Indust. Med. 1:139 (1980).

7. R. Lilis, Long-term occupational lead exposure: Chronic nephropathy and renal cancer: a case report, Am. J. Indust. Med. 2:293 (1981).

8. W.C. Cooper, O. Wong, L. Kheifets, Mortality among employees of lead battery plants and lead producing plants, 1947-1980, Scand. J. Work. Environ. Health. 11:331 (1985).

9. M. Rutter, Low level lead exposure: sources, effects and implications, In: "Lead versus Health", (M. Rutter, and R. Russell Jones, eds. John Wiley and Sons, New York (1983).

10. M.R. Moore, and A. Goldberg, Health implications of the hematopoietic effects of lead. In: "Dietary and Environmental Lead: Human Health Effects", K.R. Mahaffey, ed. Elsevier, Amsterdam (1985).

11. R.A. Goyer, D.L. Leonard, J.F. Moore, B. Rhyne, and M.R. Krigman, Lead dosage and the role of the intranuclear inclusion body, Arch. Environ. Health. 20:705, (1970).

12. G.B. Schumann, S.I. Lerner, M.A. Weiss, L. Gawronski, and G.K. Lohiya, Inclusion bearing cells in industrial workers exposed to lead, Am. J. Clin. Pathol. 74:192 (1980).

13. R.G. Price, J. Halman, and C.T. Yuen, Urinary enzymes as early indicators of renal changes, In: "Occupational and Environmental Chemical Hazards", V. Foa, E.A. Emmett, M. Maroni, and A. Colombi, eds. Ellis Horwood, Chichester (1987).

14. B.R. Meyer, A. Fischbein, K. Rosenman, Y. Lerman, D.E. Drayer, and M.M. Reidenberg, Increased urinary enzyme excretion in workers exposed to nephrotoxic chemicals, Am. J. Med. 76:989 (1984).

15. C.N. Ong, G. Endo, K.S. Chia, W.O. Phoon, H.Y. Ong, Evaluation of renal function in workers with low blood lead levels, In: "Occupational and Environmental Chemical Hazards", V. Foa, E.A. Emmett, M. Maroni, and A. Colombi, eds. Ellis Horwood, Chichester, England (1987).

16. W.M. Victery, C.R. Miller and R.A. Goyer, Essential trace metal excretion from rats with lead exposure and during chelation therapy, J. Lab. Clin. Med. 107:129 (1986).

17. W.M. Victery, C.R. Miller, S. Zhu and R.A. Goyer, Effect of different levels and periods of lead exposure on tissue levels and excretion of lead zinc and calcium in the rat, Fund. Appl. Toxicol. 8:506 (1987).

18. W.M. Victery, J.M. Smith, and A.J. Wander, Renal tubular handling of zinc in the dog, Amer. J. Physiol. 241:F532-539 (1981).

19. V.N. Finelli, Lead, zinc, and delta-aminolevulinate, In: "Biochemical Effects of Environmental Pollutants", S.D. Lee, ed. Ann Arbor Science, Ann Arbor (1977).

20. R.A. Goyer, The renal tubule in lead poisoning. I. Mitochondrial swelling and aminoaciduria, Lab. Invest. 19:71 (1968).

21. J.L. Farber, Membrane injury and calcium homeostasis in pathogenesis of coagulative necrosis, Lab. Invest. 47:114 (1982).

22. J.G. Pounds, Effect of lead intoxication on calcium homeostasis and calcium-mediated cell function: a review, Neurotox. 5:295 (1984).

23. R.J. Baker, and J.A. Nelder, "The GLIM System, Release 3, Manual", Oxford: Numerical Algorithms Group (1978).

24. J.P. Buchet, H. Roels, A. Bernard, and R. Lauwerys, Assessment of renal function of workers exposed to inorganic lead, cadmium or mercury vapor, J. Occup. Med. 22:741 (1980).

PREDICTING THE KIDNEY BURDEN OF TOXIC METALS

Gary L. Diamond, Thomas W. Clarkson, John B. Hursh and M. George Cherian *

Environmental Health Science Center, University of Rochester Rochester, New York 14642, USA and * Department of Pathology, Pharmacology and Toxicology, University of Western Ontario London, Ontario, Canada

INTRODUCTION

The accurate assessment of risk associated with exposures to nephrotoxic metals demands an explicit understanding of relationships between level of exposure, the resulting dose to the kidney and effects on kidney function. Development of methods for directly measuring or predicting kidney burden of metals in humans is a central component of this problem. Experiments in laboratory animals allow a rigorous exploration of the biokinetics of metals in kidney and can lead to development of models relating level of exposure to kidney metal burden, and the latter to other biological indices of kidney burden (e.g. Urinary metal) and nephrotoxicity (e.g, proteinuria). However, extrapolation of these models to humans can not be made with certainty, unless they can be validated with quantitative assessments in humans. Methods for in vivo measurement or estimation of metals in kidney can be used to test models that are based on laboratory animal data, and thus, potentially, can lead to a greatly improved under- standing of exposure-effect relationships for nephrotoxic metals in humans.

Recent progress in the field of in vivo trace metal analysis has led to development of nuclear-based techniques for measuring many different metals in bone and superficial body tissues (1,2). The use of X-ray fluorescence (XRF) for measurement of bone lead and neutron activation analysis (NAA) for measurement of bone aluminium are two examples of this approach (3,4). Nuclear-based techniques that could be applied to in vivo analysis of deep visceral organs, such as kidney, are being vigorously explored. Substantial progress has been achieved in applications of NAA for quantifying renal cadmium (5-7). Improvements in NAA and XRF technologies have increased the sensitivity of these methods for mercury to the point where in vivo measurements of renal mercury may be feasible in the future (8,9).

Although great success has been achieved with NAA for cadmium, application of nuclear-based techniques for direct in vivo measurement of other important nephrotoxic metals in kidney, including mercury and lead, is not currently practical. Several different strategies for indirect in vivo prediction of metals in kidney are currently being explored with respect to applications in laboratory animals and humans. These include methods based on the isotope dilution principal and use of complexing agents for displacing metals from kidney into urine. Recent developments concerning application of these techniques to the problem of in vivo prediction of kidney burden of toxic metals are discussed below, with emphasis on mercury.

IN VIVO ESTIMATION OF KIDNEY BURDEN OF MERCURY BY ISOTOPE DILUTION

A method that is based on the isotope dilution principle is currently being explored as a means for quantifying kidney mercury burdens in humans (10). Unlike nuclear-based techniques, isotope dilution does not provide a direct measurement of mercury in kidney. Nevertheless, it can provide a reliable estimate of the size of the exchangeable mercury compartment in kidney, and when certain implicit assumptions are satisfied, an estimate of kidney mercury burden.

The basic protocol for the isotope dilution method consists of administering a tracer dose of radioactive mercury to the subject by injection, and after allowing a period for equilibration of the injected isotope with the renal mercury pool, renal mercury burden is estimated from the specific activity of the mercury excreted in the urine. The validity of the isotope dilution technique is based on two assumptions:-

1) that the pool of mercury in kidney can be labelled with a known amount of injected radioactive mercury, and

2) that the specific activity of mercury in urine and kidney are the same. If these assumptions hold, then kidney mercury burden (Hg_K) can be estimated as follows:

$$Hg_K = Hg^*_K/saHg_U$$

where Hg_K represents kidney mercury burden (mg), Hg^*_K represents the amount of injected radioactive mercury in kidney (Ci) and $saHg_U$ is the specific activity of mercury in urine (Ci/mg).

It has been possible to test these assumptions in laboratory animals, and to a limited extent, determine the feasibility of isotope dilution for estimating kidney mercury burden in humans after exposure to inorganic mercury. For the purpose of satisfying assumption 1) a known amount of radioactive inorganic mercury (e.g. mercuric chloride) must be injected into the subject. Two radioactive isotopes of mercury are available for this purpose, 203-Hg (half-line 46.6 day) and 197-Hg (half-life 64.1 hr). 197-Hg is preferred for human studies because of its relatively short radioactive half-life, which reduces the internal radiation dose that is required for accurate measurements of the $saHg_U$ (10).

Assumption 1 also demands that the value for Hg^*_K known with certainty. However, Hg^*_K cannot be measured directly in humans with current available technologies, and thus, must be estimated from biokinetic models. The results of numerous kinetic studies indicate that prompt uptake of 203-Hg administered by intravenous or intramuscular injection as Hg++ by inhalation as Hg^o is relatively constant for many different mammalian species; approximately 30% of the administered dose is taken up in kidney (Table 1). In the absence similar data for humans, a value of 30% is the best available estimate of uptake of injected radioactive inorganic mercury and has been used to estimate Hg^*_K (10). Selection of the most appropriate value for percent renal uptake of injected radioactive tracer is crucial to the accuracy of the isotope dilution method. The value for renal mercury burden will be underestimated if renal uptake of mercury actually exceeds the predicted 30% of the injected dose, and conversely, will be overestimated if uptake is less than the predicted value.

The second assumption has been tested directly in laboratory animals (10). Rats received i.v. injections of $HgCl_2$ and 12 days later, received intravenous injections of 203-$HgCl_2$. One group of rats received 5 i.p. injections of the metal complexing agent 2,3-dimercaptopropane-1-sulphonate (DMPS). Specific activities of mercury in kidney and urine were nearly identical 3-5 days after injection of radioactive mercury (Table 2). Similar results were obtained a group of dogs that were exposed to Hg^o, insufflated into the lungs, and subsequently received i.v. injections of 203-HgCl (Table 3). In both the rat and dog experimental models, estimates of kidney mercury burden, based on isotope dilution, agreed closely with measured values (Table 4).

Table 1. Prompt uptake of 203-Hg in kidney after injection or inhalation

Species		Route	Time (days)	Hg in Kidney (as % dose)	Reference
Rat	(n = 2)	i.v.	1	33	(11)
Rat	(n = 2)	i.v.	2	40	(11)
Rat	(n = 2)	i.v.	1	37	(12)
Rat	(n = 2)	i.v.	4	20	(12)
Dog	(n = 3)	i.v.	3-5	27 ± 1.3	(10)
Rat	(n = 10)	i.v.	3	31 ± 1.1	(10)
Rat	(n = 10)	i.v.	3	30 ± 1.2	(10)
Rat	(n = 2)	inh.	1	38	(12)
Rat	(n = 2)	inh.	4	33	(12)
Rat	(n = 8)	inh.	3	24 ± 1.6	(13)
Mice	(n = 9)	inh.	3	24 ± 0.4	(13)
Rat	(n = 6)	i.m.	1	34	(14)
Rat	(n = 2)	i.m.	3	49	(14)

203-Hg was in the form of $HgCl_2$ when given by injection and in the form of Hg^o when given by inhalation. Table is adapted from reference (10).

Table 2. Specific activity of mercury in urine and kidney of rats pretreated with $HgCl_2$ followed by 203-Hg

	Specific Activity (nCi 203-Hg x 10^{-3}/ng Hg)	
	Urine	Kidney
Control rat (n = 10)	5.72 ± 0.21	6.36 ± 0.34
DMPS-treated rat (n = 10)	7.29 ± 0.50	7.82 ± 0.31

Rats (n = 20) received i.v. injections of $HgCl_2$ (100 ug Hg). A subgroup (n = 10) received daily i.p. injection of DMPS (3 mg/kg) on days 6-10 after injection of $HgCl_2$. On day 12 all rats received i.v. injections of 203-Hg (200 nCi). Values are shown as mean $\pm$ S.E. for specific activities of urine collected 40-72 hr after injection of 203-Hg, and for kidney collected 72 hr after injection of 203-Hg. Table is adapted from reference (10).

Data from the isotope dilution experiments also provide some insight about the source of urinary mercury in the dogs. Conceivably, urinary mercury could be derived from two distinct sources; the plasma mercury pool, by glomerular filtration of mercury in plasma or the kidney mercury pool by secretion of mercury from kidney directly into urine. Since plasma and kidney mercury pools have different specific activities (Table 3), it is possible to estimate the relative contribution of each to urinary mercury. The maximum value possible for the specific activity of urinary mercury is that of plasma. This would occur if all urinary mercury was derived from plasma without having first mixed with the renal mercury pool. The minimum value possible for the specific activity of urinary mercury would be that of the kidney mercury pool, and would occur if all urinary mercury was derived from kidney. Assuming steady-state conditions, in which specific activities of plasma, kidney and urinary mercury pools remain constant during the observation period, the fraction of the total urinary mercury derived from kidney, exclusive of that derived from plasma, can be estimated from the specific activity difference ratio (17) as follows:

$$\text{Kidney fraction} = (saHg_p - saHg_U)/(saHg_p - saHg_K)$$

The estimated value for the kidney fraction for dogs reported in Table 3 was 1.019 ± 0.042, indicating that most if not all mercury in urine was derived from kidney. Thus, if glomerular filtration of mercury occurs to any extent, its contribution to mercury excretion, relative to other mechanisms, appears to be relatively minor. Similar conclusions were reached for humans (18) and rabbits (19). Furthermore, uptake of filtered mercury into the renal mercury pool would be expected, based on results of intratubular microinjection studies (20).

Table 3. Specific activity of mercury in urine, kidney and plasma of dogs pretreated with intratrachael instillations of liquid mercury

Specific Activity
(nCi 203-Hg x 10^{-3}/ng Hg)

	Urine	Kidney	Plasma
Dog 1	1.38	1.34	2.78
Dog 2	1.42	1.35	5.79
Dog 3	2.50	2.63	3.90

Dogs received 7-15g of liquid mercury by intratrachael instillation, followed by an i.v. dose of 203-Hg (4-5 uCi) 8 days (dog 1) or 53 days (dogs 2 and 3) later. Shown are values for specific activity 3 days (dog 1) or 5 days (dogs 2 and 3) after injection of 203-Hg. Adapted from reference (10).

Table 4. Ratios of predicted and measured kidney mercury burden in dogs and rats pretreated with inorganic mercury

	Kidney Hg Burden (Predicted/Measured)	
	Mean$\pm$S.E.	Range
Dog (n = 3)	1.10 ± 0.07	0.96-1.18
Rat (n = 20)	1.09 ± 0.03	0.79-1.32

Kidney mercury burden was predicted by isotope dilution and measured by cold vapor atomic absorption (15,16). See Table 2 and 3 legends for description of mercury pretreatment. Adapted from reference (10).

An opportunity to explore use of the isotope dilution technique to estimate kidney mercury burden in a human being occurred when a 61 year-old ruptured a liquid mercury-containing bag by coughing as an intestinal tube was being passed down her throat, with the result that she aspirated a substantial fraction of the mercury released. After remaining symptom-free for a period of 6 months, she developed a mild proteinuria, at which time, the consensus of medical opinion was that it would be valuable to determine the kidney burden of mercury and to take steps to reduce renal mercury burden, if possible, by administering a complexing agent. The patient was administered two intravenous doses of 197-HgCl$_2$ (1 uCi; sp. act. 0.1 - 2.9 uCi/ug); one before and one after oral administration of DMPS (300 mg/day for 6 days). Distribution of injected radioactive mercury to the kidney was examined by external gamma counting of the kidney region after each dose of 197-HgCl and was found to be unaffected by DMPS treatment. Values for the estimated kidney mercury burden, as determined by isotope dilution, were 28.1 mg prior to treatment with DMPS and 19.6 after treatment. Thus, DMPS treatment resulted in net removal of approximately 8.8 mg mercury from the kidney. Data on excretion of mercury in urine and mercury concentration in blood and plasma of the same patient are shown in Figure 1. Cumulative urinary loss of mercury during the DMPS treatment amounted to 19.8 mg. Assuming a kidney weight of 275 g for the 52.8 kg patient, the predicted concentration of mercury before treatment with DMPS was 104 ug/g kidney.

Although the above observations are limited to only one individual, they provide some insight into dose-effect relationships for mercury in humans. The patient displayed mild but significant proteinuria (3 g/day) which persisted for three years after the exposure and subsequently disappeared. Thus, data obtained with the isotope dilution method support a minimum value of 104 ug Hg/g kidney for the renal threshold for nephrotoxicity in the human after exposure to Hg$^{\circ}$. This is consistent with other known cases of poisoning due to mercuric salts, in which values between 10 and 70 ug Hg/g kidney for the concentration of mercury in kidney have been reported, based on analyses of renal biopsy specimens (21).

ESTIMATION OF KIDNEY METAL BURDEN WITH COMPLEXING AGENTS

The use of the chelating agent, EDTA, to estimate body burden of lead was proposed by Chisolm and has since become a standard for diagnosis of lead exposure (22). Metal complexing agents may provide another viable approach for estimating renal burdens of lead and mercury, and perhaps other metals as well. Several new, water soluble complexing agents have been described that promote displacement of lead and mercury from the kidney into urine (23). These agents can be used to enrich urine with metal derived from kidney, to the extent that estimates of kidney metal burden may be obtained (24). More recently, the possibility of using complexing agents to estimate kidney burdens of metals has been explored in connection with the water soluble complexing agent DMPS. This agent has been shown to be effective for decreasing the retention of mercury and lead in humans, when it is given orally (10,25,26). Although the clinical future of DMPS is still in question, studies on the pharmacology of DMPS have provided important insight about the potential for using water soluble agents for predicting kidney metal burdens. These findings may have relevance to other agents, including 2,3-dimercaptopsuccinic acid (DMSA).

In theory, a complexing agent could be used for estimating kidney metal burden, if at a given dose of the agent, a constant fraction of the renal

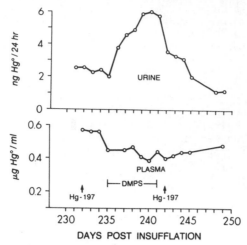

Fig. 1. Urinary excretion of mercury and concentration of mercury in plasma in a human patient during the 230 and 250 day period following accidental insufflation of Hg^o. DMPS was administered as an oral dose of 300 mg/day for 6 days. (Adapted from reference 10).

metal burden is excreted in a readily sampled excretory compartment. The results of numerous in vivo studies have confirmed that administration of DMPS to laboratory animals that have been exposed to inorganic lead, inorganic mercury or methyl mercury results in net transfer of these metals from kidney into urine (24,27-29). In rats exposed to inorganic mercury, the amount of mercury excreted in the urine in response to DMPS is proportional and nearly equivalent to the net loss of mercury from the kidney (Figure 2). Thus, under certain conditions, DMPS appears to exert a complexing activity that is highly specific for kidney.

Studies performed in vivo and in isolated perfused rat kidneys (IPRK) have provided some insight about mechanisms for the direct effects of DMPS on the retention and excretion of renal mercury. A saturable tubular secretory mechanism for DMPS has been identified in the chicken. The secretory mechanism is inhibited by other organic anions, including some, but not all, alkane sulphonates (30). A similar excretory mechanism for DMPS appears to exist in rat kidney. In the IPRK, secretion of DMPS is saturable and can be blocked by other organic anions (Figure 3), suggesting the existence of a carrier mediated secretory mechanism for DMPS.

When kidneys from rats that have been exposed to $HgCl_2$, are perfused in the presence of DMPS, mercury is excreted from renal cortex and outer medulla, into urine and venous perfusate. Urinary excretion of mercury that is induced by DMPS is completely inhibited by concentrations of PRB that completely inhibit net tubular secretion of DMPS. Dose-effect relationships and effects of PRB are illustrated in Figures 4 and 5.

These results show that DMPS can decrease retention of mercury in kidney by inducing net transfer of mercury from kidney into urine. The ability of the kidney to transport DMPS by a carrier mediated mechanism may explain the apparent selectivity of DMPS for metals in kidney. It is possible that a transport requirement confers selectivity of the complexing activity to kidney and other tissues capable of transporting DMPS. Conceivably, this

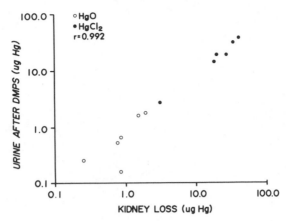

Fig. 2. Urinary excretion of mercury induced by treatment with DMPS plotted against kidney mercury burden at the time of treatment. Animals were exposed for 60 min to mercury vapour (0.5, 1.0, or 2.0 mg Hg/m^3) or given an i.p. dose of HgCl$_2$ (0.1, 0.5 or 1.0 mg Hg/kg), DMPS was administered (1 mmole/kg, i.p.) between 7 to 11 days after exposure to mercury (Cherian et al., submitted).

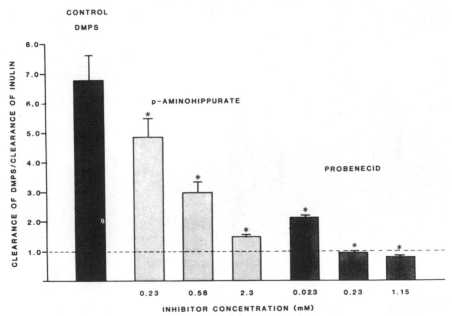

Fig. 3. Effects of p-aminohippurate and probenecid on the tubular secretion of DMPS in the IPRK. Kidneys were perfused for 60 min with DMPS (4.3 ug/l) and inulin (0.8 mg/l) and with or without p-aminohippurate or probenecid in the arterial perfusate at the concentrations indicated.

Values shown are mean±S.E. for 3 to 5 kidneys (Klotzbach and Diamond, submitted).

27

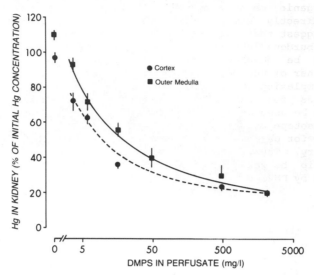

Fig. 4. Effects of DMPS on retention of mercury in, renal cortex and outer medulla. Rats received single injections of $HgCl_2$ (0.5 umol/kg, i.p.) and, 48 hr later, kidneys were isolated and perfused for 60 min. DMPS was present in perfusate for 30 min. Shown are concentrations of mercury in cortex (circles) and outer medulla (squares) at the end of perfusion, expressed as a percent of initial mercury concentration (nmol/g dry tissue). Values are mean for±S.E. for 3 to 5 kidneys (Klotzbach and Diamond, submitted).

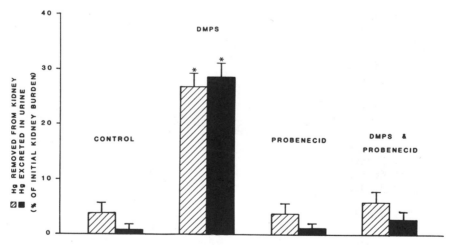

Fig. 5. Effects of probenecid on DMPS-induced excretion of mercury. Rats were treated with $HgCl_2$ and kidneys were perfused as described in legend for Figure 4. Kidneys were perfused with and without DMPS (5.3 mg/l) and with or without probenecid (0.23 mM) in arterial perfusate. Values are mean±S.E. for 3 or 4 kidneys and * indicates significantly different from controls ($p < 0.05$) (Klotzbach and Diamond, submitted).

specificity could be exploited for estimating renal mercury burden, if a quantitative relationship existed between the kidney burden and the amount of metal excreted in response to administration of DMPS.

28

Relationships of this kind have been established for both inorganic lead (24) and inorganic mercury in the rat (Figure 2). Although it is not possible to directly extrapolate these results to humans, the above observations suggest that application of complexing agents for estimating kidney metal burdens in humans may be promising. However, before such procedures can be developed for practical use, it is necessary to establish whether or not quantitative relationships between kidney metal burden and complexing activity of a given agent exist in humans. This requires methods for estimation or direct measurement of kidney metal burden that can be used in conjunction with the complexing agent. Results obtained with isotope dilution, described above, suggest that this method may be useful for calibrating the effects of DMPS in humans exposed to inorganic mercury. Thus, it may be feasible to begin to probe in humans the relationship between kidney mercury burden and urinary excretion of mercury induced by DMPS or other complexing agents, such as DMSA.

CONCLUSIONS

Developments in the area of nuclear-based in vivo measurements of metals in kidney have led to substantial improvement of our current understanding of the dose-effect relationships for cadmium in humans. These techniques may soon be extended to studies of other important nephrotoxic metals. Until such methods can be made practical for studies of lead and mercury, indirect in vivo methods for estimating renal burdens of these metals are being examined. Methods based on the isotope dilution principle have been shown to be feasible for studies in humans exposed to inorganic mercury. The development of new complexing agents, such as DMPS, that show greater specificity for metals in kidney may offer another viable approach for predicting metal burdens of lead and mercury in addition to their use as therapeutic agents. Further development of the use of these agents will be facilitated by development of alternative methods for measuring kidney metal burden in vivo which can be used to calibrate effects of complexing agents on kidney-metal burden.

REFERENCES

1. D.R. Chettle and J.H. Fremlin, Techniques for in vivo neutron activation analysis, Phys. Med. Biol. 29:1011-1042 (1984).

2. S.H. Cohn and R.M. Parr, Nuclear-based techniques for the in vivo study of human composition, Clin. Phys. Physiol. Meas. 6:275-301 (1985),

3. L. Wielopolski, K.J. Ellis, A.N. Vaswani, S.H. Cohn, A. Greenberg, J.B. Puschett, D.K. Parkinson, D.E. Fetterolf and P.J. Landrigan, In vivo bone lead measurements: A rapid monitoring method for cumulative lead exposure, Am. J. Ind. Med. 9:221-226 (1986).

4. K.J. Ellis and S.P. Kelleher, In vivo bone aluminum measurement in patients with renal disease, In: "In Vivo Body Composition Studies," K.J. Ellis, S. Yasamura, and W.D. Morgan, eds., Institute of Physical Science and Medicine, London (1987).

5. H.A. Roels, R.R. Lauwerys, J. Buchet, A. Bernard, D.R. Chettle, T.C. Harvey and I.K. Al-Haddad: In vivo measurement of liver and kidney cadmium in workers exposed to this metal: Its significance with respect to cadmium in blood and urine, Environ. Res. 26:217-240 (1986).

6. K,J. Ellis, W.D. Morgan, I. Zanzi, S. Yasumura, D. Vartsky amd S.H. Cohn, Critical concentrations of cadmium in human renal cortex: Dose-effect studies in cadmium smelter workers, J. Toxicol. Environ. Health 7:691-703 (1981).

7. K.J. Ellis and S.H. Cohn, Cadmium inhalation exposure estimates: Their significance with respect to kidney and liver cadmium burden, J. Toxicol. Environ. Health 15:173-187 (1985).

8. J.R.H. Smith, S.S. Athwal, D.R. Chettle and M.C. Scott, On the in vivo measurement of mercury using neutron capture and X-ray fluorescence, Int. J. Appl. Rad. Isotop. 33:557-651 (1982).

9. K.J. Ellis, D. Vartsky and S.H. Cohn, In vivo monitoring of metals in man: Cadmium and mercury, Neurotoxicology 4:164-168 (1983).

10. J.B. Hursh, T.W. Clarkson, T.V. Nowak, R.C. Pabico, B.A. McKenna, E. Miles and F.R. Gibb, Prediction of kidney mercury content by isotope techniques, Kidney Int. 27:898-907 (1985).

11. A. Rothstein and A.D. Hayes, The metabolism of mercury in the rat studied by isotope techniques, J. Pharmacol. Exp. Ther. 130:166-176 (1960).

12. M. Berlin, J. Fazacherleyand G. Nordberg, The uptake of mercury in the brains of mamlnals exposed to mercury vapor and to mercuric salts, Arch. Environ. Health 18:719-729 (1969).

13. J.B. Hursh, M.R. Greenwood, T.W. Clarkson, J. Allen and S. Demuth, The effect of ethanol on the fate of mercury inhaled by man, J. Pharmacol. Exp. Ther. 214:420-427 (1980).

14. T.W. Clarkson and L. Magos, Effect of 2,4-dinitrophenol and other metabolic inhibitors on the renal disposition and excretion of mercury, Biochem. Pharmacol. 19:3029-3037 (1970).

15. L. Magos and T.W. Clarkson, Atomic absorption determination of total, inorganic and organic mercury in blood, J. Assoc. Off. Anal Chem. 55:966-971 (1972).

16. H. Satoh, J.B. Hursh and T.W. Clarkson, Selective determinations of elemental mercury in blood and urine exposed to mercury vapor in vitro, Appl. Toxicol. 1:177-181 (1968).

17. G.L. Diamond and A.J. Quebbemann, In vivo quantification of renal sulfate and glucuronide conjugation in the chicken, Drug Metab. Dispos. 9:402-409 (1981).

18. M.G. Cherian, J.B. Hursh, T.W. Clarkson and J. Allen, Radioactive mercury distribution in biological fluids and excretion in human subjects after inhalation of mercury vapor, Arch. Environ. Health 33:109-114 (1978).

19. M. Berlin and S. Gibson, Renal uptake, retention and excretion of mercury, Arch. Environ. Health 6:617-625 (1963).

20. M. Cirkrt and J. Heller, Renal tubular handling of $^{203}Hg^{++}$ in the dog: A microinjection study, Environ. Res. 21:308-313 (1980).

21. M. Berlin, Dose-response relationships and diagnostic indices of mercury and mercurials, In: Effects and Dose-Response Relationships of Toxic Metals, G.G. Nordberg, ed., Elsevier Scientific Publishing Co., Amsterdam (1976).

22. J.J. Chisolm, Poisoning due to heavy metals, Pediatr. Clin. North Am. 17:591-615 (1970).

23. H.V. Aposhian, DMSA and DMPS-water soluble antidotes for heavy metal poisoning, _Ann. Rev. Pharmacol. Toxicol_. 23:193-2215 (1983).

24. T. Twarog and M.G. Cherian, Chelation of load by dimercaptopropane sulfonate and a possible diagnostic use, _Toxicol. Appl. Pharmacol_. 72:550-556 (1984).

25. T.W. Clarkson, L. Magos, C. Cox, M.R. Greenwood, L. Amin-Zaki, M.A. Majeed and S.F. Al-Damluji, Tests of efficacy of antidotes for removal of methylmercury in human poisoning during the Iraqui outbreak, _J. Pharmacol. Exp. Therp_ 218:74-83 (1981).

26. J.J. Chisolm and D.J. Thomas, Use of 2,3-dimercaptopropane-1-sulfonate in treatment of lead poisoning in children, _J. Pharmacol. Exp. Ther_. 235:605-624 (1985).

27. B. Gabard, The excretion and distribution of inorganic mercury in the rat as influenced by several chelating agents, _Arch. Toxicol_. 35:15-24 (1978).

28. B. Gabard, Treatment of methylmercury poisoning in the rat with sodium 2,3-dimercaptopropane-1-sulfonate, _Toxicol. Appl. Pharmacol_. 38:416-424 (1976).

29. F. Planas-Bohne, The effect of 2,3-dimercaptopropane-1-sulfonate and dimercaptosuccinic acid on the distribution and excretion of mercuric chloride in rats, _Toxicol_. 19:275-278 (1981).

30. J.R. Stewart and G.L. Diamond, Renal tubular secretion of the alkane-sulfonate 2,3-dimercapto-1-propanesulfonate, _Am. J. Physiol_. 252:F800-F810 (1987).

A PROSPECTIVE STUDY OF PROTEINURIA IN CADMIUM WORKERS

Harry Roels, Robert Lauwerys, Jean-Pierre Buchet, Alfred Bernard, Alfons Vos, and Maurice Oversteyns

Unite de Toxicologie lndustrielle et Medecine du Travail, Universite Catholique de Louvain, Clos Chapelle-aux-Champs 30.54, B-1200 Brussels, Belgium

INTRODUCTION

In man, the kidney is the critical organ following chronic exposure to Cd. An increased urinary excretion of plasma proteins usually represents the earliest biological sign of Cd interference with kidney function. Cadmium can decrease the tubular reabsorption of low molecular weight proteins (< 40,000 dalton), such as ß2-m and RBP, and it can also enhance the glomerular filtration of high molecular weight proteins (> 40,000 dalton), such as albumin, representing also an early manifestation of excessive cadmium exposure (Lauwerys et al., 1974 and 1984). The health significance of an increased urinary excretion of specific plasma proteins (e.g. ß2-m, RBP, albumin) without clinical proteinuria which may be found in workers chronically exposed to Cd, remains a matter of controversy (Lauwerys and Bernard, 1986). We have followed up 23 male workers with such renal changes at the time of their removal from exposure to Cd in order to assess whether these early toxic effects of exposure to Cd were predictive of an accelerated decline in renal function.

SUBJECTS AND METHODS

The Cd workers had been exposed previously to Cd oxide dust and fume in two Belgian non-ferrous smelters for nearly 25 years on average. About three years prior to the present study, the Cd body burden in 21 of these workers had been assessed by measuring the levels of Cd in liver and kidney using neutron activation analysis: the Cd concentrations (wg/g wet weight) in liver and kidney cortex ranged from 24 to 158 (mean 61) and from 133 to 355 (mean 231), respectively. They had been removed from exposure because enhanced urinary excretion of ß2-m (> 250 ug/g creatinine; n = 18) and/or RBP (> 250 ug/g creatinine; n = 17) and/or albumin (> 15 mg/g creatinine; n = 8) had been detected. However, the levels of serum creatinine were still normal (< 13 mg/l) in 18 subjects and marginally increased in 3 subjects (13 - 14 mg/l); only 2 subjects had significantly elevated serum creatinine levels at the time of removal from cadmium (20 and 22 mg/l). These 23 subjects have been examined once a year for 5 years consecutively. Their first follow-up examination took place when they had been removed from Cd exposure for 6 years on average and at that time their age ranged from 45 to 68 yr (mean 58.6 yr). Examination of the past medical records and the medical questionnaires collected at the start of the study did not reveal previous or current diseases, or drug consumption habits which might interfere with renal function. At each survey, the examination took place between 9 and 12 a.m., the subjects having had a light breakfast, and samples of venous blood and urine were collected. The following biological analyses were made (Roels et al., 1982; Bernard and Lauwerys, 1983): Cd in blood and urine, total proteins and amino acids in urine, ß2-m in serum and urine, RBP and albumin in urine, and creatinine in serum and urine.

RESULTS AND COMMENTS

Figure 1 shows for the 5-year follow-up period the average change (expressed as percentage of the 1st survey values) of Cd in blood and urine, and that of serum creatinine and serum ß2-m. The Cd concentration in blood and urine decreased significantly ($p < 0.001$) with time, whereas the levels of ß2-m and creatinine in serum significantly ($p < 0.001$) increased with time. The other parameters did not exhibit a statistically significant time-trend.

Their geometric group mean values (range) were at the start of the study: total proteinuria 179 mg/g creatinine (55-843); aminoaciduria 134 mg.Á-N/g creatinine (94-247); ß2-microglobulinuria 1400 ug/g creatinine (22-41,800); RBP in urine 1240 ug/g creatinine (77-48,200); and albuminuria 18 mg/g creatinine (2.2-373). None of the individual values of urinary ß2-m, RBP, and albumin which were significantly enhanced at the time of the 1st survey, returned to normal level 5 years later. This confirmed our previous conclusion based on a retrospective study (Roels et al., 1982), that Cd-induced proteinuria is not reversible. Over the 5-year study period, the prevalence of elevated values for urinary parameters did not vary significantly as shown by the results obtained at the first and last surveys: total proteins (> 150 mg/g creatinine) 48 vs 57 %, amino acids (> 150mg alpha-N/g creatinine) 30 vs 43 %, ß2-m (> 250 ug/g creatinine) 78 vs 78 %, RBP (> 250 ug/g creatinine) 74 vs 78 %, and albumin (> 15 mg/g creatinine) 35 vs 43 %. On the contrary, the prevalence of elevated values increased significantly between the first and fifth survey for serum creatinine (> 13 mg/l) 30 vs 52% ($p < 0.05$) and for serum ß2-m (> 2 mg/l) 30 vs 74 % ($p < 0.01$).

The increase with time of serum creatinine and serum ß2-m observed in the present prospective study clearly indicates a progressive reduction of the GFR despite removal from exposure to Cd. Using the serum levels of ß2-m to estimate the GFR (Wibell et al., 1973), all the examined Cd workers showed at the end of the observation period a decrease of the GFR, which varied from 9 to 78 ml/min/1.73 m^2 (on average 31 ml/min/1.73 m^2). The expected age-related decline of the GFR in the age range 45-75 years (Lindeman, 1981) would normally not exceed 6.5 ml/min/1.73 m over 5 years. All the Cd workers exhibited at the 5th survey a decrease of their GFR which is greater (on average about 5 times) than that value. This decrease was, however, not more pronounced in workers with impaired renal function at the start of the study (GFR < 80 ml/min/1.73 m^2; serum creatinine > 13 mg/l) than in those presenting only with subclinical signs of renal damage.

Furthermore, it should be recognized that in Cd workers the presence of a microalbuminuria is not a prerequisite for predicting a loss of glomerular function because (a) a significant reduction of the GFR (> 30 ml/min/1.73m^2) during the 5-year observation period was also found in workers who had only an increased urinary excretion of low molecular weight proteins, and (b) the decrease of the GFR was not significantly different in workers with or without increased albuminuria at the first survey.

34

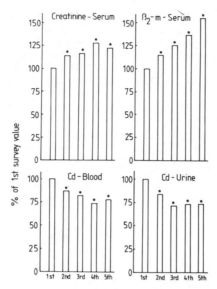

Fig. 1. Time course of cadmium in blood and urine, and creatinine and ß2-microglobulin (ß2-m) in serum expressed as percentage of 1st survey values (mean of 23 subjects). The 5 consecutive surveys were performed 6, 7.1, 8.6, 9.6, and 10.7 years (average) after removal from exposure to cadmium. Mean values at the first survey: Cd-blood 14.3 ug/l; Cd-urine 16.2 ug/g creatinine; creatinine-serum 12.0 mg/l; ß2-m-serum 1.9 mg/l. Asterisks: mean values (%) significantly different from 1st survey value. Workers removed from Cd exposure.

This study indicates that the early renal effects of Cd, i.e. the increased urinary excretion of low and/or high molecular weight plasma proteins, may be followed up by an exacerbation of the age-related decline of the GFR despite removal from exposure. Therefore, they should be regarded as adverse effects. in addition to the measurement of the urinary excretion of specific plasma proteins such as RBP and albumin, it might be useful to include the determination of serum ß2-m in the health surveillance programme of Cd workers in order to detect a reduction in GFR as early as possible.

REFERENCES

Bernard, A., and Lauwerys, R., 1983, Continuous-flow system for the automation of latex immunoassay, Clin. Chem., 29:1007.

Lauwerys, R., Buchet, J.P., Roels, H., Brouwers, J., and Stanescu, D., 1974, Epidemiologlcal survey of workers exposed to cadmium: effect on lung, kidney and several biological indices, Arch. Environ. Health, 28:145.

Lauwerys, R., Bernard, A., Roels, H.A., Buchet, J.P., and Viau, C., 1984, Characterization of cadmium proteinuria in man and rat, Environ. Health Perspect., 54:147.

Lauwerys, R.R., and Bernard, A.M., 1986, Cadmium and the kidney, Brit. J. Ind. Med., 43:433.

Lindeman, R.D., 1981, Kidney: Kidney and Body Fluids, In: "Handbook of

Physiology in Aging", E.J. Masoro, ed., CRC Press lnc., Boca Raton, Florida.

Roels, H., Djubgang, J., Buchet, J.P., Bernard, A., and Lauwerys, R., 1982, Evolution of cadmium-induced renal dysfunction in workers removed from cadmium exposure, Scand. J. Work Environ. Health, 8:191.

Wibell, L., Evrin, P.E., and Berggard, 1., 1973, Serum ß2-microglobulin in renal disease, Nephron, 10:320.

RED BLOOD CELL NEGATIVE CHARGES AS AN INDEX OF THE GLOMERULAR POLYANION IN CHRONIC CADMIUM POISONING

Alfred Bernard, Ali Ouled Amor, Harry Roels and Robert Lauwerys

Unite de Toxicologie lndustrielle et Medecine du Travail, Universite Catholique de Louvain, Clos Chapelle-aux-Champs 30.54, B-1200 Brussels, Belgium

INTRODUCTION

Fixed negative charges on the glomerular capillary wall (glomerular polyanion) provide an electrostatic barrier to the filtration of anionic macromolecules such as albumin (1). Loss of glomerular polyanion in clinical or experimental renal diseases is associated with an enhanced excretion of anionic molecules. Evidence has been presented by recent studies (2,3) that the negative charges of the red blood cells (RBCs) membrane, as determined by the binding of the cationic dye Alcian blue (AB) might reflect the charges of the glomerular polyanion. Applying this AB binding test to RBCs from cadmium (Cd)-exposed workers and to both RBCs and isolated glomeruli from Cd-treated rats, we demonstrate here that, at an early stage of the intoxication, Cd can decrease negative charges of RBCs membrane and that this phenomenon reflects a concomitant loss of the charge selectivity of the glomerular basement membrane.

MATERIALS AND METHODS

Sprague-Dawley female rats given 100 ppm Cd (as $CdCl_2$) in drinking water for up to 10 months Renal glomeruli and tubules were isolated by a graded sieving technique. The AB binding was determined either to membranes of tubules or glomeruli homogenates (1200 g x 10 min pellet) or to glomerular basement membranes prepared according to the method of Meezan et al (5). The 4% sodium desoxycholate treatment (the last step of the procedure) was not performed so that the GBM preparation was partially purified and still contained cell and intracellular membranes.

For measuring the AB binding, we have slightly modified the method described by Levin et al (2). Immediately before use the AB solution (Alcian Blue 8GX, Sigma St. Louis) was prepared as follows: the dye was dissolved (4 mg AB/ml) in a solution containing 25 mmol $MgCl_2$ and 0.15 mol NaCl per litre. This solution was vigorously vortex mixed fo 10 min., then centrifuged (2000 g x 10 min.) and filtered through Whatman no. 1 in order to remove undissolved dye. The AB concentration was determined from the extinction coefficient. The results presented here were obtained with a saturating AB concentration of about 1.5 mg/ml. The incubation of AB with RBCs or tissues membranes and the reading was then performed as described by Levin et al (2). The protein concentration in the tissue homogenates was determined by the biuret method. RBCs were counted with a Technicon Autocounter.

Three groups of male workers chronically exposed to Cd were examined: 26 workers aged 20-55 years and moderately exposed to Cd on the average for 8 years (group I); 11 workers (ages 34-61 years) high exposure to Cd on the average for 6.6 years (group II) and 12 workers (ages 51 to 72 years) who had been exposed to Cd for 28 years on the average, but who were removed from Cd exposure since 6 to 14 years (group III). Two groups of 10 subjects each, matched for age with the Cd-workers, were used as controls. The exposure parameters of these groups are presented in Table 1.

The concentrations of albumin, ß2-microglobulin (ß2-m), retinol-binding (RBP) in human or rat urine were determined by latex immunoassay (6). Standard methods were used for the other parameters. Differences between control and exposed groups were ascertained by the Student's t-test, applied in most cases to log transformed data. All the results presented here are expressed as the mean $\pm$ SD.

RESULTS

The ß-microglobulin excretion of rats given 100 ppm Cd in drinking water started to increase significantly from the 8th month of treatment, at a stage at which the critical level of 200 ppm Cd in renal cortex was reached. The albuminuria rose significantly from the 2nd month of Cd treatment and continued to increase up to the 10th month. Between months 2 and 8 Cd-treated rats presented thus with an isolated increase of the albuminuria (results not shown).

At month 4, we found that the albuminuria of Cd-treated rats was associated with a significant reduction of AB binding to membranes of glomeruli homogenates (18 $\pm$ 3 vs 27 $\pm$ 2.5 mg/mg protein, n = 6) and to RBCs (118 $\pm$ 10 NS 133 $\pm$ 22 ng/10^6 RBCs, n = 6). The albuminuria was negatively correlated with RBCs charges (r = -0.77, p < 0.005, n = 11) and glomerular charges (r = -0.51, n = 11). These results were confirmed by reexamining the animals 6 months later i.e. at the 10th month of Cd treatment. At that stage, the AB binding test was applied to partially purified GBM. Negative charges of the GBM preparation were significantly decreased in Cd-treated rats and, as depicted in Fig. 1A, showed a close negative correlation with the albumin excretion, which indicates that Cd enhances the albumin excretion by reducing the glomerular polyanion charges. This loss of charge selectivity induced by Cd can be predicted by measuring membrane negative charges of RBCs which, as shown by Fig. 1B, were also negatively correlated with the albumin excretion.

The effect of Cd on RBCs and glomerular negative charges cannot be interpreted as a simple masking by the Cd cation since it cannot be reproduced in vitro. in addition, the AB binding to liver and renal tubular membranes was not affected which suggests that the phenomenon might be confined to the vascular compartment (results not shown).

Compared to age-matched controls, workers currently exposed to Cd (groups I and II) exhibited a significant reduction of RBCs charges (Table 1). This loss of RBCs charges paralleled the internal dose of Cd as evidenced by the highly significant correlations between RBCs charges and the log of Cd concentration in urine (r = -0.83, p < 0.001) and in blood (r = -0.76, p < 0.005). None of these Cd workers had a dipstick detectable proteinuria. However, subjects with an albuminuria > 10 or between 5 and 10 mg/g creatinine had on the average significantly lower RBCs charges than those with an albuminuria below 5 mg/g creatinine. This type of relationship was not observed when workers were classified according to the level of ß2-m or RBP in urine (results not shown).

Table 1. Biological indices of Cd exposure and RBCs membrane negative charges

Cd workers	n	Cadmium in urine (Ìg/g creatinine)	Cadmium in blood (Ìg/l)	AB bound to RCs (ng/10^6 RBCs)
Group I	26	4.6±4.2	5.9±3.4	187±27*
Group II	11	60.9±40	33±13.7	146±23*
Group III	12	12.9±4.5	10.3±3.9	180±29*
Control				
Group I[a]	10	0.4±0.1	1.8±0.4	240±29*
Group II[b]	10	1.6±0.9	1.5±0.6	231±28*

a control group age-matched with group I and II of Cd workers
b control group age-matched with group III of Cd workers
* value significantly different from that of age-matched controls

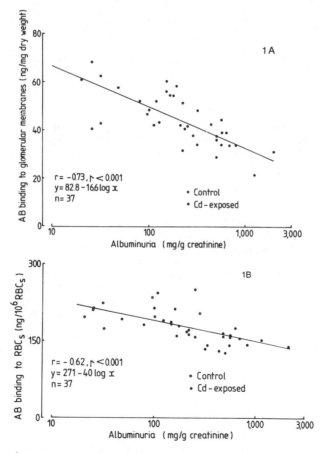

Fig 1. Correlation between glomerular (Fig. 1A) or RBCs (Fig. 1B) membrane negative charges as assayed by the Alcian Blue binding test and the albuminuria in rat given 100 ppm Cd in drinking water for 10 months and in their controls.

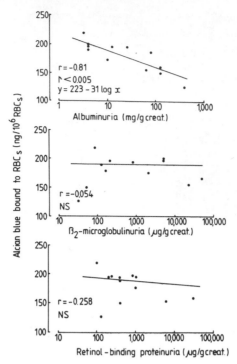

Fig. 2. Correlations between RBCs membrane negative charges and the urinary excretion of albumin, ß2-microglobulin or retinol-binding protein in 12 workers removed from Cd exposure.

Workers removed from Cd exposure (group III) also showed a significant reduction of RBCs charges (Table 1). The RBCs charges of these workers were negatively correlated with the urinary output of albumin, but not with that of ß2-m or RBP (Fig. 2).

CONCLUSION

Altogether the present experimental and human data provide strong evidence that Cd can enhance the glomerular permeability to proteins by reducing the glomerular polyanion charge. This phenomenon is irreversible and precedes the classical tubular dysfunction induced by this metal. It offers an explanation to the occurrence of a glomerular or mixed type proteinuria in Cd exposed workers (7). The present study also demonstrates that RBC membrane negative charges as assayed by the AB binding test reliably mirror the loss of charge selectivity of the glomerular filter induced by chronic Cd exposure.

ACKNOWLEDGEMENTS

X. Dumont, T. Seminck, M. Dasnoy are gratefully thanked for their technical assistance. A. Bernard is Research Associate of the Belgian Fund for Scientific Research.

REFERENCES

1. W.J. Deen, M.P. Bohrer, C.R. Robertson and B.M. Brenner, Determinants of the transglomerular passage of macromolecules, Fed. Proc. 36:2614 (1977).

2. M. Levin, C. Smith, M.P.S. Walter, P. Gascoine and T.M. Barratt, Steroid-responsive nephrotic syndrome: a generalised disorder of membrane negative charges, _Lancet_ 2:239 (1985).

3. J.M. Boulton-Jones, G. McWilliams, and L. Chandrachad, Variation in charge on red cells of patients with different nephropathies, _Lancet_ 2:186 (1986).

4. J.I. Kreisberg, R. L. Hoover and M.Y. Karnovsky, Isolation and characterization of rat glomerular epithelial cells in vitro, _Kidney Int_. 14:21 (1978).

5. E. Meezan, J.T. Hjelle, K. Brendel and E.C. Carlson, A single, versatile, nondisruptive method for the isolation of morphologically and chemically pure basement membranes from several tissues, _Life Sciences_ 17:1721 (1976).

6. A.M. Bernard and R.R. Lauwerys, Continuous flow system for automation of latex immunoassay. _Clin. Chem_. 29, 1007 (1983).

7. A.M. Bernard, J.P. Buchet, H. Roels, P. Masson and R. Lauwerys, Renal excretion of proteins and enzymes in workers exposed to cadmium. _Eur. J. Clin. Invest_. 9:11 (1979).

SOME CONSIDERATIONS ON CRITICAL CONCENTRATION OF CADMIUM FOR RENAL TOXICITY IN RATS

Chiharu Tohyama, Naoko Sugihira, Kazuo T. Suzuki, Masataka Murakami and Hiroshi Saito*

Environmental Health Sciences Division, National Institute for Environmental Studies, Onogawa, Yatabe-machi, Tsukuba, Ibaraki 305, Japan * Present address: Department of Preventive Medicine and Community Health, Nagasaki University School of Medicine, Nagasaki 852: Japan

INTRODUCTION

Cadmium (Cd) is a widespread toxic environmental pollutant. Environmental and occupational exposure results in the accumulation of this metal particularly in the liver and kidney and during the life-long exposure a renal Cd concentration becomes higher than a hepatic Cd concentration, which often causes renal tubular dysfunction (Friberg et al., 1985). Thus, we need to know the critical concentration of Cd to obtain information on the safety margin of exposure to this metal and the allowable daily intake levels.

The purpose of the present paper is two-fold: (i) to briefly review the studies on the critical concentration of Cd for the renal toxicity in man and experimental animals, and (ii) to discuss, among several aspects of studies on the critical concentration, the possible contribution of Cd-metallothionein and hepatic damage to the onset of renal damage in rats with special reference to the critical concentration. The critical concentration of a metal was defined by the Subcommittee on the Toxicology of Metals of the Permanent Commission and International Association on Occupational Health as follows (Task Group on Metal Toxicity, 1976): mean concentration of a metal in the organ at the time adverse functional changes, reversible or irreversible, occur in the cell.

To determine the critical concentration, one has to choose indicators of critical effects of Cd. From a historical point of view, Friberg et al., (1974) proposed the critical concentration in Cd-exposed industrial workers based on pathological observations of a few autopsy and biopsy samples and also the presence of total proteinuria. The group estimated the critical concentration value as 100-300 ug Cd/g renal cortex, or an average of 200 ug Cd/g renal cortex. Later on, compiling the result of other workers' studies (Ellis et al., 1981: Roels et al., 1981) where a new indicator, ß2-microglobulinuria and hepatic and renal Cd levels determined by in vivo neutron activation analysis were used, the same research group (Kjellstram et al., 1984) proposed a new concept of "population concentration 10", which is defined as 10% of the target population has ß2-microglobulinuria. According to their calculation, the value turned out to be 180-220 ug/g renal cortex, which is identical with the earlier value based on the pathological observation and total proteinuria. Nevertheless, it may be important to point out that although the values obtained by the two studies are similar, the later study may have detected more subtle change of renal dysfunction.

In animal studies on the critical renal effects of Cd the indicators such as pathological observation, proteinuria (total protein, amino acids, enzymes), glucosuria and Cd have been utilized (Nomiyama, 1981; Suzuki and Yoshikawa, 1981). In Cd-treated rats the critical concentration was incidentally about 200 ug Cd/g kidney, and this value has been used as supporting evidence of the critical concentration in man. Our recent studies (Sugihira et al., 1986; Tohyama et al., 1987a) have provided clear-cut data on drastic increases in urinary levels of total protein, metallothionein, lactate dehydrogenase, N-acetyl-ß-D-glucosaminidase, Cd, copper and zinc when renal Cd concentration reaches 100-200 ug/g kidney. In addition, a Cd concentration in the renal cortex was estimated to be 1.5 times higher than that in the whole kidney (Friberg et al., 1974), but the factor was reassessed to be 1.25 in the more resent study (Friberg et al., 1985).

The critical concentration of Cd for renal toxicity has been suggested to be affected by several factors such as species, dose, route of exposure, sex, ageing, ambient temperature, concomitant treatment of drugs and "active" forms of cadmium (Nomiyama, 1981; Lauwerys and Bernard, 1986). Among these factors recent research interest may be associated with ageing, "active" forms of Cd and another factor, involvement of Cd-metallothionein in the manifestation of renal toxicity. Ageing apparently results in the decrease of the critical concentration of Cd for renal toxicity by developing the tubular injury (Nomiyama et al., 1980), which may be related to possible decrease in the capacity of synthesis of metallothionein in the kidney cells. Recent studies revealed that when Cd is administered either as a complex with cysteine or with mercaptoethanol, it causes nephrotoxicity at a renal Cd level of approximately 10 ug/g tissue (Maitani et al., 1985; Nomiyama and Nomiyama, 1986). From these studies Cd in the sediment fraction and also Cd bound to high molecular weight fractions (Maitani et al., 1985) or "unbound" (ionic) Cd (Nomiyama and Nomiyama, 1986) were considered to be a candidate for toxic forms of Cd. Although these studies provide novel experimental models for the investigations on mechanism of Cd toxicity, further studies are needed to assess the extent of possible contribution of the toxic forms of Cd to the manifestation of the renal toxicity in actual Cd poisoning in man.

Compared to a large number of studies on the effect of Cd on the kidney, not much attention has been paid to the liver. Because dose used in experimental studies is often much higher than the exposure level to Cd in man, and Cd is often administered by injections, liver could accumulate higher concentrations of Cd than kidney and is more likely to be affected. The presence of hepatic damage caused by Cd or the release of Cd-metallothionein from the liver should be considered to be another factor that may alter the critical concentration.

The earlier study (Tohyama et al., 1981) revealed that urinary metallothionein level gradually increases with the elevation of renal Cd level, followed by a drastic increase in the urinary metallothionein at a renal Cd level of approximately 200 mg/g renal cortex in Cd-treated rats (Figure 1). In contrast, the same study demonstrated that no such a drastic increase was found in Cd-smelter workers whose renal Cd levels reached this level that modifying factors that were described earlier, dose and route of exposure as well as species difference were considered to be major differences between the Cd-treated rats and smelter workers.

Metallothionein, a cysteine-rich low molecular weight protein, is induced upon exposure to Cd and plays a protective role against the toxicity of Cd

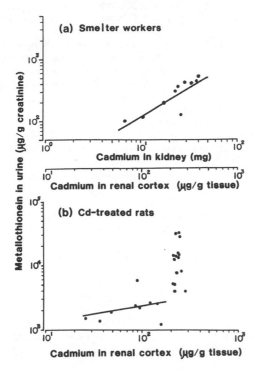

(a) Smelter workers

Metallothionein in urine (μg/g creatinine)

Cadmium in kidney (mg)

Cadmium in renal cortex (μg/g tissue)

(b) Cd-treated rats

Cadmium in renal cortex (μg/g tissue)

Figure 1. The relationship between urinary metallothionein and renal cadmium in (a) smelter workers and (b) cadmium-injected rats. Least-squares lines predicting urinary metallothionein concentrations from tissue cadmium levels are drawn. (Modified from Tohyama C. et al., 1981. With permission).

by binding it whereas this protein is also known to have apparently an opposite toxic effect on the kidney once it exists in the circulation as a form of Cd-metallothionein (Kagi and Nordberg, 1979; Webb, 1979). Earlier studies (Cherian and Shaikh, 1975; Cherian et al., 1976; Nordberg et al., 1975; Tanaka et al., 1975) showed that Cd-metallothionein infused in the circulation is selectively taken up by the kidney and exerts severe renal damage. It has been considered that Cd-metallothionein released from damaged hepatic cells may be involved in the onset of renal damage in Cd-treated rats (Suzuki, 1982) and we have tried to elucidate the apparent discrepancy observed in the Cd-treated rats and smelter workers in terms of the involvement of Cd-metallothionein released from the damaged hepatic cells.

RESULTS AND DISCUSSION

When male Wistar rats were injected subcutaneously with $CdCl_2$ at a dose level of 0.5 mg Cd/kg body weight, 5 days a week, for up to 10 weeks, both hepatic and renal cortex Cd concentrations reached maxima at Cd concentrations of 444 ug/g liver at week 13 and 240 ug/g kidney at week 9, respectively (Tohyama and Shaikh, 1981). A plasma metallothionein level increased with duration of Cd treatment and reached a plateau at week 6. Apparently the plasma metallothionein level drastically increases once hepatic and/or renal Cd level(s) reach(es) a certain level. It is considered that the elevation of the plasma metallothionein level may originate from the liver rather than kidney (Goyer et al., 1984) because earlier studies (Bernard et al., 1981; Tanaka et al., 1981) indicated that Cd accumulated in the liver was liberated and transferred to the kidney through the circulation once Cd-loaded rats were treated with carbon tetrachloride.

The presence of severe hepatic damage in rats exposed continuously to Cd was demonstrated by Dudley et al. (1985). In their study a renal Cd level reached a plateau at approximately 150 ug/g kidney. At week 10 serum enzymes, such as aspartate aminotransferase, alanine aminotransferase and succinate dehydrogenase, that are indicators of hepatic damage, drastically increased. A plasma metallothionein level showed a concomitant increase with these serum enzymes at week 10 and levelled off thereafter. Urinary excretion of total protein and Cd also showed a marked increase at the same time as those of serum enzymes and metallothionein. It should be pointed out here that proteinuria and elevated excretion of Cd persisted throughout the study period of 26 weeks.

To examine the possible involvement of Cd-metallothionein in the manifestation of renal damage and to evaluate it with regard to the critical concentration, we have selected a dosing condition under which the renal Cd level reaches 200 ug/g kidney and the hepatic damage could be minimal. Thus, female wistar rats were subcutaneously injected with $CdCl_2$ at a dose of 1.5 mg Cd/kg body weight, 4 times a week, for the first 6 weeks and left without the Cd treatment for further 15 weeks (Tohyama et al., 1987b). Cadmium accumulated in the liver, reached a maximum at approximately 600 ug/g liver at week 6 and decreased with time. On the other hand, a Cd concentration in the kidney reached a plateau of about 200 ug Cd/g kidney at week 7 and levelled off thereafter despite the cessation of Cd injections.

During the Cd treatment for the first 6 weeks, urinary excretion of total protein, glucose and enzymes such as lactate dehydrogenase, N-acetyl-ß-D-glucosaminidase and alkaline phosphatase tended to increase but then decreased after the cessation of Cd treatment. As a rebound phenomenon, there observed the second peaks in the case of these enzymes at week 12. It should be emphasized that no severe proteinuria and glucosuria were observed despite the retention of Cd at about 200 ug/g kidney throughout the study. It has been suggested that proteinuria caused by Cd exposure is usually irreversible in man (Roels et al., 1982; Elinder et al., 1985), thus it may be important to determine if minor renal dysfunction caused by Cd in rats could be cured. It was also found that the urinary excretion of metallothionein, Cd, copper and zinc increased during the Cd administration but did not level off despite the retention of Cd at 200 ug/g kidney. Second peaks of urinary excretion of metallothionein, Cd and copper were also observed at week 12.

As to indicators of hepatic damage, serum levels of aspartate aminotransferase and alanine aminotransferase continued to increase until week 10 and then decreased. Serum alkaline phosphatase increased during Cd treatment, followed by a decrease. The decrease of these serum enzyme levels may reflect, to a certain extent, the recovery from liver damage after the cessation of Cd treatment. This idea is also supported by the recovery of serum cholinesterase level just after the cessation of Cd treatment. Serum Cd and metallothionein levels also increased during the Cd treatment and decreased after the cessation of the Cd treatment. This decrease may reflect the decreased levels of Cd and metallothionein in the liver. It is reasonable to assume that severe proteinuria and glucosuria did not take place because of the decreased level of Cd-metallothionein in the circulation after week 6. However, the amount of Cd-metallothionein taken up by the kidney may be still large enough to cause renal damage, thus causing the second peaks of urinary enzymes, metallothionein and heavy metals.

In summary, rats could be used for an excellent experimental model to study the mechanism of some aspects of renal toxicity of Cd in man. At the same time, there are some limitations for the extrapolation of animal data to man. In rats chronically treated with Cd the metal is predominantly sequestered in the liver and kidney and Cd-metallothionein released from damaged hepatic cells may play an important role in the manifestation of the nephrotoxicity. In contrast, although people who are environmentally or occupationally exposed to Cd for a relatively long time and whose renal Cd level reaches about 200 ug/g renal cortex may have developed renal dysfunction, the occurrence of hepatic damage due to Cd exposure has not been reported in the human population. Thus, the difference in the urinary excretion of various substances between Cd-treated rats and Cd-exposed people may depend on the presence of hepatic damage, or possibly the release of Cd-metallothionein from damaged hepatic cells. It is suggested that one should be careful enough to adopt the critical concentration value itself obtained in such animal experiments to substantiate the critical concentration in man because almost no hepatic damage by Cd has been reported and the contribution of Cd-metallothionein released from the liver is considered less in man.

REFERENCES

Bernard, A. and Lauwerys, R.R., 1981, The effects of sodium chromate and carbon tetrachloride on the urinary excretion and tissue distribution of cadmium in cadmium-pretreated rats, Toxicol. Appl. Pharmacol., 57:30.

Cherian, M.G. and Shaikh, Z.A., 1975, Metabolism of intravenously injected cadmium-binding protein, Biochem. Biophys. Res. Commun., 65:863.

Cherian, M.G., Goyer, R.A. and Delaquerriere-Richardson, L., 1976, Cadmium-metallothionein-induced nephropathy, Toxicol. Appl. Pharmacol., 38: 399.

Dudley, E.R., Gammal, M.L. and Klaassen, C.D., 1985, Cadmium-induced hepatic and renal injury in chronically exposed rats: likely role of hepatic cadmium-metallothionein in nephrotoxicity, Toxicol. Appl. Pharmacol., 77: 414.

Elinder, C.-G., Edling, C., Lindberg, E., Kagedal, B. and Vesterberg, O., 1985, ß2-Microglobulinuria among workers previously exposed to Cd: follow-up and dose-response analysis, Am. J. Ind. Med., 8:553.

Ellis, K.J., Morgan, W.D., Zanzi, I., Yasumura, S., Vartsky, D. and Cohn, S.H., 1981, Critical concentration of cadmium in human renal cortex: dose-effect studies in cadmium smelter workers, J. Toxicol. Environ. Health, 7:691.

Friberg, L., Piscator, M., Nordberg, G.F. and Kjellstram, T., 1974, Cadmium in the Environment, 2nd ed., CRC, Cleveland.

Friberg, L., Elinder, C.-G., Kjellstrom and Nordberg, G.F., Editors, 1985, "Cadmium and Health: A Toxicologixcal and Epidemiological Appraisal," CRC press, Boca Raton.

Goyer, R.A., Cherian, M.G., and Delaquerriere-Richardson, L, 1984, Correlation of parameters of cadmium exposure with onset of cadmium-induced nephropathy in rats, JEPTO, 5:89.

Kagi, J.H.R. and Nordberg, M., 1979, Metallothionein, Birkhauser Verlag, Basel.

Kjellstrom, T.; Elinder, C.-G. and Friberg, L., 1984, Conceptual problems in establishing the critical concentration of cadmium in human kidney cortex, Environ. Res., 33:284.

Lauwerys, R.R. and Bernard, A.M., 1986, Cadmium and the kidney, Brit. J. Ind. Med., 43:433.

Maitani, T., Saito, Y. and Suzuki, K.T., 1985, Cadmium found in non-soluble fraction of kidney homogenates and its relation to renal dysfunction after cadmium-cysteine administration, Toxicology, 37:27.

Nomiyama, K., 1981, Renal effects of cadmium, In: "Cadmium in the Environment, " J.O. Nriagu ed., John Wiley & Sons, New York.

Nomiyama, K. and Nomiyama, H., 1986, Critical concentration of "unbound" cadmium in the rabbit renal cortex, Experientia, 42:149.

Nomiyama, K., Nomiyama, H. and Yotoriyama, M., 1980, Ageing, a factor aggravating chronic toxicity of Cd, Toxicol. Lett., 6:225.

Nordberg, G.F., Goyer R.A. and Nordberg, M., 1975, comparative toxicity of cadmium-metallothionein and cadmium chloride on mouse kidney, Arch. Pathol., 99:192.

Roels, H.A., Lauwerys, R.R., Buchet, J.-P., Bernard, A., Chettle, D.R., Harvey. T.C. and Al-Haddad, I.K., 1981, In vivo measurement of liver and kidney cadmium in workers exposed to this metal: its significance with respect to cadmium in blood and urine, Environ. Res., 26:217.

Roels, H., Djubgang, J., Buchet, J. P., Bernard, A. and Lauwerys, R., 1982, Evolution of cadmium-induced renal dysfunction in workers removed from exposure, Sand J. Work Environ. Health, 8:191.

Sugihira, N., Tohyama C., Murakami, M. and Saito, H., 1986, significance of increase in urinary metallothionein of rats repeatedly exposed to cadmium, Toxicology, 41:1.

Suzuki, K.T., 1982, Induction and degradation of metallothionein and their relation to the toxicity of cadmium, In: Biological Roles of Metallothionein, E.C. Foulkes, ed., Elsevier North-Holland, Amsterdam.

Suzuki, Y. and Yoshikawa, H., 1981, Cadmium, copper and zinc excretion and their binding to metallothionein in urine of cadmium-exposed rats, J. Toxicol. Environ. Health, 8:479.

Tanaka, K., Sueda, K., Onosaka, S. and Okahara, K., 1975, Fate of 109 Cd-labelled metallothionein in rats, Toxicol. Appl. Pharmacol., 33:258.

Tanaka, K., Nomura, H., Onosaka, S. and Min, K.-S., 1981, Release of hepatic cadmium by carbon tetrachloride treatment, Toxicol. Appl. Pharmacol., 59:535.

Task Group on Metal Toxicity, 1976, Conceptual considerations: critical organ, critical concentration in cells and organs, critical effect, subcritical effect, dose-effect and dose-response relationships, In: "Effects and Dose-response Relationships of Toxic Metals," G.F. Nordberg, ed., Elsevier / North-Holland, Amsterdam.

Tohyama, C. and Shaikh, Z.A., 1981, Metallothionein in plasma and urine of cadmium-exposed rats determined by a single-antibody radioimmunoassay, Fundam. Appl. Toxicol., 1:1.

Tohyama, C., Shaikh, Z.A., Ellis, K.J. and Cohn, S.M., 1981, Metallothionein excretion in urine upon cadmium exposure: its relationship with liver and kidney cadmium, Toxicology, 22:181.

Tohyama, C., Sugihira, N. and Saito, H., 1987a, Critical concentration of cadmium for renal toxicity in rats, J. Toxicol. Environ. Health, 22: (in press).

Tohyama, C., Ishida, M., Sugihira, N. and Suzuki, K.T., 1987b, Metallo-thionein in the tissues and, body fluids in Cd-injected rats, In: "Toxicology of Metals; clinical and experimental research," S.S. Brown and Y. Kodama, ed., Ellis Horwood, Chichester.

Webb, M., 1979, The metallothioneins, In: The Chemistry, Biochemistry and Biology of Cadmium, M. Webb, ed., Elsevier / North-Holland, Amsterdam.

HISTORICAL PERSPECTIVE ON CADMIUM-INDUCED NEPHROTOXICITY

Vera R. Porter and Dora B. Weiner

Department of Psychiatry and Behavioral Sciences, School of Medicine, University of California, Los Angeles, California 90024, USA

Cadmium is a critical element for advancement of our industrial society, where it is used in alkaline batteries, alloys, paints, plastics, photographic supplies, antiseptics and other products (9,25). By recognizing the toxicity of cadmium it has been possible to limit exposure to this element while benefiting from its many products. This paper will trace the history of the predominant toxic manifestation of cadmium exposure, i.e. nephrotoxicity, as a model for understanding how its pathology and aetiology were recognized. It will become apparent that our understanding of a comparatively "modern" disease can shed light on prior observations of the pathological processes of nephrotoxicity.

The history of cadmium-induced nephrotoxicity is also the history of the search for the cause and effect relationship between a toxic element and its pathology on a selected organ system. Cadmium was not identified as an element until 1817 (38). The metal is found in nature in association with zinc. Hence, cadmium, which is now known to be potentially toxic for humans and animals, has managed to make its place in history with its antithesis, zinc, an element essential to life.

Cadmium is now known to produce symptoms of nephrotoxicity in humans when inhaled or ingested (4,18,23,24,40). There are several limitations in searching early historical records for reports including symptoms of nephrotoxicity related to cadmium exposure. The modern tools of biochemistry and pathology for the diagnosis of nephrotoxic symptoms were not available, and thus a search of medical reports must be confined to symptoms such as anuria or enlarged kidneys at autopsy (21,29,39). Any search through records prior to the discovery of cadmium that time must be directed at reports of those substances which can retrospect be seen to contain this element. The search of early reports must take into consideration the current information on processes, e.g. heating of ores, which release cadmium. Since cadmium rarely is found free in nature, but usually in association with other metals, primarily zinc and sometimes copper and lead (10,25), any toxic reactions occurring as a result of exposure to cadmium mixed with these other elements could be due to one or more components.

THE EARLY HISTORY OF CADMIUM

One of the first descriptions of a substance which may have contained cadmium was attributed to Aristotle in his book, On Marvels (320 B.C.), in which there is an account of the manufacture of bronze at Mossynoecia, near the Black Sea, from which an earth-like substance of a glossy, bright yellow appearance was extracted (27). From Greek and Roman times, brass was made by cementing zinc ore with copper. Analysis of a large brass object of the Cassia family of 20 B.C. was found to contain zinc (1). The zinc mineral substance, which likely was present in the bronze, was termed "cadmia" by Dioscorides and Pliny in the first century A.D. (1,27) The name was thought to be derived from Cadmos, son of Agenor, king of Phoenicia, who was the first to introduce the use of zinciferous earth at Thebes in Greece (27). Since we now know that zinc and cadmium coexist in nature, it is likely that early bronze and brass contained small amounts of cadmium.

"Cadmia" is a term which can be used to trace the history of cadmium if one is cautious. "Cadmia" should be regarded as a mineral mixture which probably contained zinc, cobalt, arsenic and possibly copper (1,8). In different references, the combinations of minerals vary, but the common element in most of the mixtures appears to be zinc. Hoover and Hoover (1) trace the history of the terminology and components of the substances termed "cadmia fossilis," "cadmia metallica," and "cadmia fornacis" in some detail. A careful examination of their work would lead one to believe that most, if not all, of these "cadmias" contained zinc and hence, one could assume, some cadmium. The "cadmias" were produced in processes of heating the ores in furnaces or in the mine shafts (1,8,31).

Another probe to use in searching history is the terms used to describe zinc itself. About 2000 years ago, zinc was termed "false silver." The oldest known object made of zinc is an idol, found among prehistoric ruins in Romania, which contained 87% zinc. Zinc-filled bracelets, dating to 500 B.C., were found on the island of Rhodes. Roman coins were made with a zinc alloy. Zinc appears to have been used in India about 1000 to 1300 A.D. and the Chinese were aware of it even before that time (7). Paracelsus, in the sixteenth century, was the first to describe physical properties of zinc (1,26). Zinc was imported from Asia to Europe in the sixteenth and seventeenth centuries under the name "spelter". It is important to note that the technology of smelting was brought to Europe from China about 1730 (7). This is the process which now is known to release cadmium in toxic quantities. Prior to this time, a process of heating and burning ores, as described by Agricola (1) was used. Two other terms are also useful in tracing cadmium's history. "Pompholyx" and "spodos" were soot-like materials found in the furnaces used to burn ores. Hoover and Hoover (1) identify them as impure protoxides of zinc.

Cadmia was referred to by several different writers in the sixteenth and seventeenth centuries. Jerome Cardin, a physician and mathematician, identified cadmia as a "semi-metal" in 1562. Other references to cadmia were made by Mathesius, a Lutheran pastor, in 1571; by Libavius, a physician who used chemical remedies, in 1611; by Louis Savot, a physician to King Louis XIII, in 1612; and Canepario professor of medicine in Venice, in 1619 (26). These references were to cadmia as used in the production of inks, brass, or as a residue in the heating of ores.

The discovery of cadmium as an element was made in 1817 by Stronmeyer, professor of metallurgy at Gottingen. He described a yellow tinge in a sample of iron-free zinc carbonate from Salzgitter, Germany, and attributed the yellow colour to a new element. Stronmeyer introduced the name "cadmium" after "cadmia" (Latin) and "kadmeia" (Greek), the ancient name for calamine, zinc carbonate (27,38). Another German chemist, Hermann, precipitated the element in 1818 (25,27). Cadmium was confirmed by Meissner and Karsten in 1819. Cadmium and several of its compounds were indexed in the Illustrated Encyclopedia Medical Dictionary (11).

HISTORY OF THE RECOGNITION OF TOXICITY OF CADMIUM

One of the earliest works which described the relationship between exposure to metals and the associated medical conditions was the treatise De Re Metallica (1556) by Georg Bauer, more commonly known after the Latinized version of his name, Agricola (1). Agricola was a physician and the author of this first complete treatise on mining. He wrote: "At Altenberg in Meissen there is found in the mines black pompholyx, which eats wounds and ulcers to the bone; this also corrodes iron, for which reason their sheds are made of wood. Further, there is a certain kind of cadmia which eats away the feet of the workmen when they have become wet and similarly their hands, and injures their lungs and eyes (p. 214)."

Hoover and Hoover (1) and Rosen (31) interpret these reactions to be due to the arsenic component which they assumed would be in the cadmia or pompholyx. However, Nriagu (25) in a brief introduction to the toxic properties of cadmium, cites this passage in Agricola as an example that the toxic properties of cadmium were well known to miners long before the metal was identified as an element. It is likely that the cadmia of Agricola was a mixture of elements which included zinc, cobalt, arsenic, and possibly copper. It is certainly reasonable to assume that cadmium would also be included in the mixture.

Hoover and Hoover (1) cite a passage from Dioscorides in which he refers to a light blue pompholyx which is made from cadmia by continually blowing with bellows. It is interesting that cadmium is described as a light blue metal in several references (15,25,38). While the exact chemical identity of the pompholyx and cadmia of Agricola cannot be established with certainty, it is apparent that the furnaces used to refine the ores and the mine shafts, in which minerals were extracted with heat, contained minerals highly toxic for the miners.

THE FIRST CASE STUDY OF CADMIUM POISONING IN HUMANS

The first reported case of poisoning of a human with a compound known to contain cadmium as the only metallic element occurred in 1858 (32). This case report is of special historical significance because it contains the results of a chemical analysis of the offending substance and a listing of symptoms appearing in the three people exposed.

The account describes a servant who was polishing silverware with cadmium carbonate. The servant brushed off the residue and created a dust which he inhaled. Towards evening the servant began to feel a dryness in the throat and a tightness in the chest. The next day he was joined by two other servants in the task. After a few hours all began to show symptoms of dizziness, vomiting, diarrhoea, and shortness of breath. The first servant went on to develop pallor, cold extremities, prostration, cramps, constriction of the throat and thorax, nausea, vomiting, colic, and, of particular interest for this report, anuria and "tenesmus" of the bladder. The servant died a few days later. The other two servants recovered. The physician at first thought that he was dealing with a case of mercury poisoning, but sent the material for analysis by a pharmacist. The material was assayed as cadmium carbonate free of mercury, lead, copper, zinc, or tin. Hence, one could conclude that this was the first reported case of nephrotoxicity caused by cadmium poisoning in a human.

CONTINUING EVIDENCE OF TOXICITY OF CADMIUM

The toxicity of cadmium was established again in 1862 when Van Hasselt described an experiment by Burdach where vomiting had been induced with a grain (1 grain = 64.797 mg) of cadmium sulphate. As cited by Prodan (27), Van Hasselt thought that the chemical and toxicological properties of cadmium resembled those of zinc. In 1980, Prasad (28) noted that many of the toxic effects attributed to zinc in the past may actually have been due to other contaminating elements such as cadmium, lead or arsenic.

Reports of toxic symptoms in miners were frequent throughout the 1800's (20,30,31), but the relationship between cadmium exposure in the workplace and development of nephrotoxicity remained tenuous until Stephens, in 1920 (33), reported chronic interstitial nephritis, at autopsy, in a 67-year old person who had worked in a zinc smelter. Chemical analysis of the liver showed no traces of lead, but traces of copper, 0.91 grain of cadmium per pound, and 0.77 grain of zinc per pound. Stephens believed that this was a case of poisoning by cadmium and zinc. During a period of six years he found eight similar workers with liver cadmium levels from 0.094 to 0.91 grain per pound and zinc levels from 0.03 to 0.77 grain per pound (27).

In 1867, Marme published results of experiments, summarized by Prodan (27), in which cats, dogs, pigeons and rabbits were injected with or fed cadmium salts in high doses. A wide variety of toxic symptoms resulted which included diffuse inflammation of the kidneys. This was followed by a report (27), in 1896 by Severi, in which he induced lesions in kidneys of dogs and rabbits injected subcutaneously daily and then every other day with 10 mg of cadmium per kg. This report included a description of microscopic findings at autopsy which showed intense necrosis of tubules, but little alteration of the glomeruli and collecting tubules. This work marked the beginning of an era of experimental nephrotoxicity in which cadmium was recognized as the casual agent in the development of toxicity.

Legge, in 1923, reported cadmium poisoning in a worker in a paint factory in which cadmium ingots were melted. On autopsy the worker in charge of the melting operation had acute inflammation of the kidneys (27). In the 1920's cadmium salts were used in the treatment of syphilis, malaria, and tuberculosis. Patients treated showed transient albuminuria in some cases. Prodan (27) reviewed several reports of uses of cadmium salts and concluded that "...cadmium stored up in the liver and kidneys during such treatment may seriously damage these organs."

A classic case of cadmium poisoning in human beings occurred in Japan beginning as early as 1906 (35,36). Osteomalacia and concurrent kidney disease occurred in farmers suffering long-term exposure to cadmium in the rice fields. Irrigation water in the rice paddies had been contaminated by a nearby zinc mine and factory. Women working in the fields showed symptoms of painful joints, waddling gait, and glucose and protein in the urine. Their bones showed decalcification and deformities. Pain was so intense that the disease became known as Itai-Itai (Ouch-ouch). Examination of the sediment of the river bed near the rice paddies showed 3.8 to 5.6 ppm cadmium upstream from the factory and 89.9 to 160 ppm downstream. At the site of the factory, the concentrations were incriminatingly high -- 363 to 832 ppm. This is to be compared to the United States drinking water standard at that time of 0.01 ppm cadmium. The cases of the disease were all in women who were at least in their forties and who had borne children (35,36). Friberg notes that, as of 1985, the casual role of cadmium in the aetiology of Itai-Itai had not been unequivocally recognized (14). However, the disease was included in almost all of the major works on cadmium poisoning.

In 1948 (12) and 1950 (13) Friberg reported on the prevalence of lung emphysema, kidney dysfunction, and proteinuria in factory workers. In a group of 43 workers who had been exposed to cadmium from 9 to 34 years, proteinuria was present in 65% using the nitric acid test and in 81% using a trichloroacetic acid test. In 15 workers who had been exposed to cadmium oxide for only 1 to 4 years, no positive reactions for proteinuria were seen. Shortly after this report, a series of observations from several different groups confirmed that exposure to cadmium induced renal damage in human beings. Throughout these observations, it should be noted that the nature of exposure to cadmium plays a role in the reaction in the kidney. Acute cadmium poisoning in human beings is rare and is associated with such generalized toxaemia that it is difficult to sort out primary and secondary effects of the exposure.

It has been shown (16) that when cadmium is ingested or inhaled, the first effect seen is slight renal tubular damage. In long-term animal studies, renal effects have preceded or occurred simultaneously with other effects. In studies of long-term exposure to cadmium in human workers, respiratory effects without renal effects have seldom been reported.

Clinically, the first detectable signs of proteinuria following occupational poisoning with cadmium do not appear until 9 to 25 years after the initial exposure. Proteinuria is usually of tubular origin and may persist for several years after the initial exposure has ceased. Furthermore, the effects of cadmium on bone in humans rarely occur in the absence of renal tubular damage. In animal studies, dietary deficiencies of calcium and protein appear to affect the severity of the bone disease resulting from cadmium poisoning (6).

After the publication of reports of Itai-Itai disease (17,22,35,36) there was a developing awareness of the risks of cadmium exposure in areas distant from operations which involved known industrial exposure. There are still reports of environmental contamination with cadmium resulting from mining operations years ago (34). From 1700 to 1850, zinc was mined at Shipham, England and used with copper to make brass. The ore was washed in ponds in the area. Garden soils in the area are still rich in cadmium, and there is evidence that the residents of Shipham have slightly higher cadmium levels than do persons in uncontaminated areas. In a health survey of residents in the Shipham area, there was no correlation between the cadmium content of diets or garden soils and the laboratory indices of exposure or effect (3). It has been postulated (34) that other beneficial metal ions, such as zinc and calcium, in the environment were affording some protection against the effects of cadmium, perhaps by saturating some exchange sites on plant roots and on animal tissues.

Currently, the exposure of workers to cadmium is controlled by means of safety regulations (2,5,19,37) which limit the levels permissible in workplaces, foods, and water. Thus, the stage of unwitting exposure of humans to this toxic element has been passed and man now has an awareness of the methods to safely coexistence with this element. There is little doubt that the needs for cadmium in our society will increase, and appropriate safety regulations offer the means to reduce the hazards so that we may derive its benefits.

ACKNOWLEDGEMENT

The authors express appreciation to Leon G. Fine, M.D., Chief of the Division of Nephrology, UCLA School of Medicine, for his advice and counsel throughout the preparation of this paper.

REFERENCES

1. Agricola G, De Re Metallica, 1556, English trans. by HC Hoover and LH

Hoover, The Mining Magazine, Salisbury House, London, 1912.

2.   Asami T, in Changing Metal Cycles and Human Health (JO Nriagu, ed)
Dahlem Konferenzen Springer-Verlag, New York, pp. 95-111, 1984.

3.   Barltrop D and Strehlow CD, Lancet, 2:1394-95, 1982.

4.   Bonner FW and Carter BA, In: Nephrotoxicity, Assessment and
Pathogenesis, (PH Bach, FW Bonner, JW Bridges and EA Lock, eds) John Wiley
and Sons, New York, pp. 310-319, 1982.

5.   Brakhnova IT, Environmental Hazards of Metals, Russian trans. by JH
Slep, Consultants Bureau, New York, 1975.

6.   Brewer ED, In: Renal Tubular Disorders. Pathophysiology, Diagnosis,
and Management (HC Gonick and V Buckalew, Jr, eds) Marcel Dekker, New
York, pp. 475-544.

7.   Cammarota VA, Jr, In: Zinc in the Environment, Part I. Ecological
Cycling (JO Nriagu, ed) John Wiley and Sons, New York, pp. 1-38, 1980.

8.   Dibner B, Agricola on Metals, Burndy Library, Connecticut, 1958.

9.   Elinder CG, In: Cadmium and Health: A Toxicological and
Epidemiological Appraisal, Vol. I. Exposure, Dose and Metabolism, CRC
Press, Boca Raton, Florida, pp. 23-63, 1985.

10.   Fassett DW, In: Metals in the Environment (HA Waldron, ed) Academic
Press, New York, pp. 61-110, 1980.

11.   Foster FP, Illustrated Encyclopedia Medical Dictionary, Part 4,
Daniel Appleton and Co., New York, pp. 745-755, 1892.

12.   Friberg L, J Indust Hyg Toxicol 30:32-36, 1948.

13.   Friberg L, Acta Med Scand 138 (Suppl. 240):1-124, 1950.

14.   Friberg L, In: Cadmium and Health: A Toxicological and
Epidemiological Appraisal. Vol. I. Exposure, Dose and Metabolism, CRC
Press, Boca Raton, Florida, pp. 1-6, 1985.

15.   Ingalls WR, The Metallurgy of Zinc and Cadmium, 2nd ed, The
Engineering and Mining Journal, New York, 1906.

16.   Kjellstrom T, In: Cadmium and Health: A Toxicological and
Epidemiological Appraisal, Vol. II. Effects and Response (L Friberg, CG
Elinder, T Kjellstrom, and GF Nordberg, eds) CRC Press, Boca Raton,
Florida, pp. 231-246, 1986.

17.   Kjellstrom T, In: Cadmium and Health: A Toxicological and
Epidemiological Appraisal, Vol. II. Effects and Response (L Friberg, et
al. eds) CRC Press, Boca Raton, Florida, pp. 257-290, 1986.

18.   Kjellstrom T, In: Cadmium and Health: A Toxicological and
Epidemiological Appraisal, Vol. II. Effects and Response (L Friberg, et
al. eds) CRC Press, Boca Raton, Florida, pp. 21-109, 1986.

19.   Martin MH and Coughtrey PJ, Biological Monitoring of Heavy Metal
Pollution: Land and Air, Applied Science Publ., New York, 1982.

20.   Meiklejohn A, The Life, Work and Times of Charles Turner Thackrah,

Surgeon and Apothecary of Leeds (1795-1833), E and S Livingstone, Ltd., Edinburgh and London, 1957.

21. Murphy JT, The History of Urology, Charles C. Thomas, Springfield, Illinois, 1972.

22. Nogawa K, In: Cadmium in the Environment, Part II. Health Effects (JO Nriagu, ed) John Wiley and Sons, New York, pp. 2-37, 1981.

23. Nogawa K, In: Changing Metal Cycles and Human Health (JO Nriagu, ed) Dahlem Konferenzen Springer-Verlag, New York, pp. 275-284, 1984.

24. Nomiyama K, In: Cadmium in the Environment, Part II. Health Effects (JO Nriagu, ed) John Wiley and Sons, New York, pp. 644-689, 1981.

25. Nriagu JO, In: Cadmium in the Environment, Part I. Ecological Cycling (JO Nriagu, ed) John Wiley and Sons, New York, pp. 36-70, 1980.

26. Partington JR, A History of Chemistry, Vol 2, Macmillan and Co., New York, 1961.

27. Prodan L, J Indust Hyg 14:132-155, 1932.

28. Prasad AS, In: Zinc in the Environment, Part II. Health Effects (JO Nriagu, ed) John Wiley and Sons, New York, pp. 29-59, 1980.

29. Ramachandra K, History of Medicine Relating to Kidney and Disorders of the Urinary Tract, University of Madras, Madras, 1973.

30. Ramazzini B, Diseases of Workers, English trans. from the Latin text, De Morbis Artificum, of 1713 by Wilmer Cave Wright, Hafner Publ. Co., New York, 1964.

31. Rosen G, The History of Miners' Diseases, Schuman's, New York, 1943.

32. Sovet, La Presse Medicale, Belge. 10:69-70, 1858.

33. Stephens GA, J Indust Hyg 2:129, 1920-1921.

34. Thornton I and Abrahams P, In: Changing Metal Cycles and Human Health (JO Nriagu, ed) Dahlem Konferenzen, Springer-Verlag, New York, pp. 7-25, 1984.

35. Tsuchiya K, Keio J Med 18:181-194, 1969.

36. Tsuchiya K, Keio J Med 18:195-211, 1969.

37. US Dept Health and Human Services, Fourth Annual Report on Carcinogens, 1985, National Toxicology Program Publication 85-002, pp. 48-50.

38. Weast, RC, ed, CRC Handbook of Chemistry and Physics, 65th Ed, CRC Press, Boca Raton, Florida, pp. 8-11, 1984.

39. Wershub, LP, Urology from Antiquity to the 20th Century, Warren H. Green, Inc., St. Louis, Missouri, 1970.

40. Yasumura S, Vartsky D, Ellis KJ and SH Cohn, In: Cadmium in the Environment, Part I. Ecological Cycling, John Wiley and Sons, New York, pp. 12-34, 1980.

CADMIUM MAY PREDISPOSE MICE TO IMMUNE COMPLEX-MEDIATED RENAL INJURY: ANOTHER POSSIBLE MECHANISM FOR CADMIUM-INDUCED NEPHROTOXICITY

Donna L. Vredevoe, Louis Levy and David W. Knutson*

Schools of Nursing and Medicine, University of California, Los Angeles, 90024, USA   *Present address: Chief, Division of Nephrology, Dept. of Medicine, Milton S. Hershey Medical Center of the Pennsylvania State University, Hershey, PA 17033, USA

INTRODUCTION

There is strong evidence that chronic ingestion of cadmium results in tubulointerstitial nephritis with a Fanconi-type syndrome in both humans and animals (2,4). There are fewer reports of glomerulonephritis associated with cadmium exposure (1-4). Those reports that mention glomerular damage usually attribute it to autoantibody production against tissue damaged by cadmium (1,2,4). Our laboratory has accumulated evidence that chronic cadmium ingestion can inhibit clearance of immune complexes by the mononuclear phagocytic system of mice. Such abnormalities may allow the persistence of soluble antigen antibody complexes in the circulation which in turn might lead to greater deposition of the complexes in the glomeruli of the kidney and possibly other sites potentially injurious to organ function.

Data which indicate an increase in deposition of immune-type complexes in the kidney of mice chronically ingesting cadmium are the focus of this report. These data will be placed in context regarding the effects of chronic cadmium exposure on the phagocytic system. An hypothesis to explain immune complex-mediated nephrotoxicity in mice chronically exposed to cadmium will be developed.

THE EXPERIMENTAL SYSTEM

Inbred male CBA/H mice were used for all experiments. Animals were 2-3 months of age at the initiation of experimentation. Cadmium chloride was available ad libitum in drinking water in concentrations ranging from 10 ppm to 300 ppm. Mice were fed a pelleted laboratory diet which was assayed to contain less than 0.3 ppm cadmium. All mice given increased concentrations of oral cadmium grew normally and showed no gross organ abnormalities when sacrificed. However, body weight for the mice on 300 ppm cadmium was slightly less than that of mice fed only 10 ppm or no cadmium chloride.

Aggregated immunoglobulin (A-IgG) was used as a model of immune complexes. IgG was isolated from Swiss-Webster mice normal sera. Human serum albumin (HSA), 5 times crystallized, was purchased (Miles Laboratories, Elkhart, Indiana). Aggregations were performed by heating. Soluble aggregates of molecules of approximately 5 to 50 x 10^6 molecular weight were separated by ultracentrifugation. The HSA was used as a molecule of similar size, but lacking Fc regions to A-IgG. Aggregates labelled with ^{125}I were injected intravenously into mice. Animals were bled at times ranging from 1 to 15 min after injection. Samples were measured for radioactivity and the level of cadmium in organs was measured by atomic absorption spectrophotometry using the methods described by Knutson (5).

RESULTS

Accumulation of cadmium in the kidney. Less than 0.5% of the total ingested cadmium accumulated in the kidney. After 3 months of cadmium ingestion the kidney accumulated significant (p < 0.001) amounts of cadmium (2.95 ug $\pm$ 0.21 compared to controls of 0.37 ug $\pm$ 0.05 at 10 ppm cadmium, and 31.4 ug $\pm$ 2.31 compared to 0.37 ug $\pm$ 0.05 at 300 ppm cadmium). These accumulated concentrations in the kidney were comparable to those in the liver on a per gram basis (5).

Blood clearance of A-IgG and A-HSA. The disappearance rates (T1/2) of A-IgG and HSA were plotted at various times from 5 to 260 days after introduction of 300 ppm cadmium in the drinking water (Figure 1). It can be seen that significant differences in T1/2 for A-IgG occurred by 90 days and differences between the cadmium-bearing and control animals were apparent as early as 35 days. The clearance times for A-IgG were significantly longer for the cadmium-bearing compared to controls. When similar experiments were performed using A-HSA, there was no statistical difference between its blood clearance in cadmium-fed as compared to control mice.

Thus, the significant reduction in clearance of A-IgG from the blood of cadmium-fed mice appeared to be specific to that molecule. Other work, reported previously, indicated that T1/2 of monomeric IgG and carbon black were not affected in the cadmium-fed animals (5).

Localization of A-IgG and A-HSA in organs. After obtaining blood samples for disappearance rates as described above, the animals were sacrificed. The organs were removed, weighed and measured for radioactivity. Organ weights were not significantly different for the cadmium-bearing and control mice. Organ localization of A-IgG-^{125}I was corrected for the ^{125}I counts present in the blood contained within the organ by the method described by Knutson, et al. (5).

Treatment of animals with A-HSA was identical to that for A-IgG. Figures 2 and 3 shows that as liver localization decreased due to increased cadmium load, A-IgG accumulation increased in the kidney and lung. The greatest increase in percentage concentration occurred in the kidney. This effect was specific to A-IgG, since only a slight shift to increased localization in the kidney occurred when A-HSA was used as the test molecule. Data which indicated that this defect in clearance of A-IgG was specific to the IgG molecule, and is not due to non-specific liver damage, have been presented previously.

DISCUSSION

Previous data from this laboratory have indicated that cadmium, available orally in drinking water, is able to cause a delay in the removal from the blood of particulate and soluble material bearing Fc fragments. This inhibition is reversible upon removal of cadmium exposure (8). The phagocytic system totally recovers within 2 weeks after the cessation of cadmium dosage, as measured by the uptake of sheep red blood cells coated with IgG. However, the organ concentration of cadmium did not change (7,8). This is interpreted to mean that only free cadmium is effective in

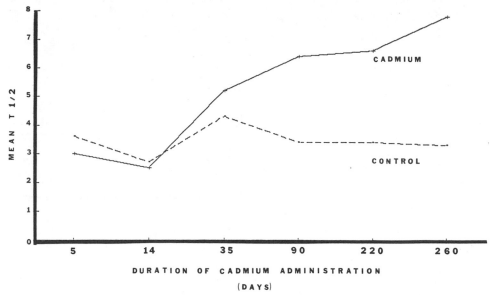

Figure 1. Half-life of A-IgG versus duration of the administration of 300 ppm cadmium chloride in drinking water.

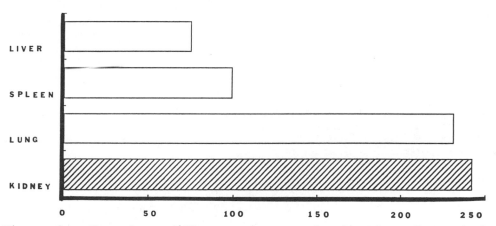

Figure 2. Percentage difference in organ localization of A-IgG in CBA/H mice recieving 100 ppm Cd for 8 months compared to controls.

inhibiting phagocytosis, while bound cadmium is inert. Hence, the two pools of cadmium, one bound and one unbound, are postulated.

This phagocytic inhibition was studied in vitro to identify the mechanism of the inhibition. The binding and ingestion of sheep red blood cells treated with IgG, for measurement of Fc receptor activity, or IgM and complement (C), for measurement of C receptor activity, by mouse peritoneal macrophages was studied. It was found that exposure to cadmium did not alter the binding of Fc or C-bearing erythrocytes. However, the ingestion of erythrocytes coated with Fc or C was significantly inhibited by the presence of cadmium. Cadmium did not appear to alter the expression of migration of Fc or C receptors on macrophages (6).

61

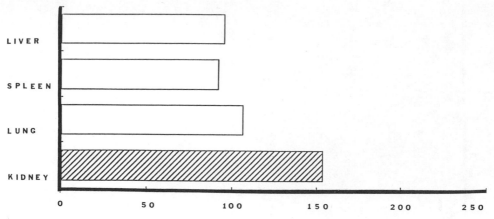

Figure 3. Percentage difference in organ localization of A-HSA in CBA/H mice recieving 300 ppm Cd in drinking water for 8 months vs controls.

Studies analysed here provide another interpretation to previously reported work. Evidence is presented which indicates that, as the ability of the liver to clear circulating immune complexes (tested by A-IgG as a model of immune complexes) is compromised, the complexes are deposited in significantly increasing amounts in the kidney and lung. The organ showing the greatest percentage increase in complex deposition or binding is the kidney. The effect appears to be specific to Fc-bearing material.

Data on increased localization of immune complexes in the kidney of cadmium-fed mice reported here and elsewhere (refs) suggest that the following series of events resulting in nephrotoxicity:

Based on the organ accumulation and reversibility it appears that, as the exposure to cadmium increases, the rate of tissue handling of immune complexes decreases. Two pools of cadmium were postulated, an unbound circulating and a storage pool. At some level of cadmium exposure, the unbound cadmium pool reaches concentrations which are capable of inhibiting the phagocytosis of immune complexes in the liver, the site of the largest portion of phagocytic activity of immune complexes. This inhibition is the result of the unbound cadmium acting to affect the Fc and C receptors on the surface of the phagocytic cells. If cadmium is removed from the diet, the unbound cadmium pool is rapidly depleted and clearance of immune complexes returns to normal despite a large storage pool of cadmium in the body. If the cadmium continues in the diet, the clearance of immune complexes from the blood stream is inhibited progressively due to a cadmium-mediated alteration in the Fc and C receptors of phagocytic tissue in the liver. Decreased clearance in the liver allows the complexes, which would normally be removed by the liver, to remain in the blood stream. The immune complexes then are accumulated in the lung and especially the kidney. Although there is no direct data to support it, immune complexes could be deposited in the glomeruli and capillaries and, to a lesser extent, the tubulointerstitial spaces in the kidney causing the release of inflammatory response mediators. These would contribute to degenerative changes in the kidney.

The results reported here offer a hypothesis for further experimental testing that suggests a role for the deposition of immune complexes to exogenous antigens in cadmium nephrotoxicity as a secondary effect of damage to the liver.

ACKNOWLEDGEMENT

This study was supported by research grant ES-02410 from the National Institute of Environmental Health Sciences, USPHS.

REFERENCES

1. P. Druet, A. Bernard, F. Hirsch, J.J. Weening, P. Gengoux, P. Mahieu and S. Birkeland, Immunologically mediated glomerulonephritis induced by heavy metals, <u>Arch. Toxicol</u>. 50:187 (1982).

2. H.C. Gonick and H.J. Kramer, Pathogenesis of the Fanconi Syndrome, <u>In</u>: "Renal Tubular Disorders. Pathophysiology, Diagnosis, and Management." H. C. Gonick and V. M. Buckalew, Jr., eds., Marcel Dekker, New York (1985), pp. 545-607.

3. B.C. Joshi, C. Dwivedi, A. Powell and M. Holscher, Immune complex nephritis in rats induced by long-term oral exposure to cadmium, <u>J. Comp</u>. <u>Pathol</u>. 91:11 (1981).

4. T. Kjellstrom, Renal effects, <u>In</u>: "Cadmium and Health: A Toxicological and Epidemiological Appraisal, Vol. II, Effects and Response." L. Friberg, C.G. Elinder, T. Kjellstrom, and G.F. Nordberg, eds., CRC Press, Boca Raton, Florida (1986), pp. 21-109

5. D.W. Knutson, D.L. Vredevoe, K.R. Aoki, E.F. Hays and L. Levy, Cadmium and the reticuloendothelial system (RES). A specific defect in blood clearance of soluble aggregates of IgG by the liver in mice given cadmium. <u>Immunology</u> 40:17 (1980).

6. L. Levy, D.L. Vredevoe and G. Cook, In vitro reversibility of cadmium-induced inhibition of phagocytosis. <u>Environ. Res</u>. 41:361 (1986).

7. D.L. Vredevoe and L. Levy, Organ-selective impairment of phagocytosis by cadmium, <u>In</u>: "Microenvironments in the Lymphoid System" G.G.B. Klaus, ed., Plenum Publ. Corp. (1985), pp. 749-755.

8. D.L. Vredevoe, L. Levy, D. Knutson, G. Cook and P. Cohen, Recovery of the murine mononuclear phagocytic system following chronic exposure to cadmium, <u>Environ. Res</u>. 37:373 (1985).

NEPHROTOXICITY OF CADMIUM IN CHICKENS

R.O. Blackburn*, D.N. Prashad and C. Whitehead

Life Science Department, Goldsmiths' College, University of London, Creek Road, London SE8 3BU*; School of Biological Sciences and Environmental Health, Thames Polytechnic, Wellington Street, London, SE18 6PF

INTRODUCTION

Many investigators have described the effects of accidental or experimental Cd^{2+} intoxication in a wide range of mammalian systems (for reviews see Samarawickrama, 1979; Webb, 1979). There are various common features such as bone demineralisation, hypercalcaemia, anaemia, hypertension, and accumulation of Cd^{2+} in the liver, then in other tissue, predominantly the kidney. Among the consequences of Cd^{2+} nephrotoxicity are various cellular and biochemical effects, proteinuria, glucosuria, hypercalciuria and aminoaciduria (Piscator, 1986; Samarawickrama, 1979). On administration, Cd^{2+} is bound to thionein, a low molecular weight protein synthesised in the liver. The resulting metallothionein builds up, and is slowly released by the liver. In the kidney it can pass through the glomeruli and be reabsorbed. At a certain total level of the metal, some Cd^{2+} will not be bound in metallothionein and can therefore exert a toxic effect (Piscator, 1986).

In the domestic fowl, there is a very high rate of calcium turnover in early growth and at maturity associated with egg laying activity. A drain on body calcium or disruption of calcium metabolism resulting from Cd^{2+} intoxication could therefore have profound consequences on growth and reproduction. This preliminary study was concerned with the effects of Cd^{2+} on growth rate and renal ultrastructure of young pullets over a 21 day period, and in evaluating the ability to two chelates, ferric and magnesium salts of EDTA (Fe and MgEDTA) in protecting the animals from the toxic insult.

MATERIAL AND METHODS

Twenty eight six week old Rhode Island Red cross Light Sussex pullets were maintained on a high calcium commercial diet containing 4.1% calcium and 0.9% phosphorous. They were randomly separated into six groups, each bird being given intramuscular injections at 48 hour intervals. Group 1 was given 0.5ml isotonic saline, groups 2 and 3, 0.5ml 1% FeEDTA and 1% MgEDTA respectively and group 4, 0.5ml $CdCl_2$ (total Cd^{2+} 3.07mg/injection). Groups 5 and 6 were given identical amounts of cadmium, but were additionally administered with FeEDTA and MgEDTA respectively, in concentrations identical to those given in groups 2 and 3. Where two

65

substances were administered, they were given in separate injections, and the total injection volume was kept constant.

All animals were weighed at regular intervals, and were sacrificed at day 21, their internal anatomy being examined at autopsy. The kidneys were flooded with 2.5% glutaraldehyde in cacodylate/sucrose buffer and the cranial divisions rapidly removed, from which 1mm cube blocks were cut. Postfixation was in 1% osmium tetroxide, after which the specimens were processes for electron microscopy.

RESULTS

Pullets treated with isotonic saline or with either chelate alone (groups 1, 2 and 3) showed no reduction in food and water intake, and gross internal anatomy was normal. Growth rates in groups 1, 2 and 3 indicated a progressive change in weight of 95 ± 2.0, 116 ± 3.5 and 123 ± 4.5 respectively. No significant differences between saline treated birds and those given either chelate alone were observed, the implication being that in isolation, neither chelate markedly affected the growth rate.

In birds treated with cadmium alone, however, there were increasing signs of ill health. Food and water intake were reduced, and fluid had accumulated in the thoracic and abdominal cavities. The kidneys were highly lobulated, with white superficial markings suggestive of renal necrosis or deposition of insoluble urate or calcium salts in the renal parenchyma. The adrenal glands were enlarged, and white blotches were seen on one or more lobes of the livers.

These abnormalities were not seen in those birds given cadmium in conjunction with either chelate, indicating that the chelates provided a notable level of protection in these respects.

Growth rates of pullets treated with cadmium alone were highly significantly reduced ($p < 0.001$), by about 60% of that observed in groups 1, 2 and 3. Those birds given cadmium in conjunction with either chelate, however, were unaffected, and there was no significant differences between their growth rates and those of animals given chelate alone. The implication is that the chelates protected the animals from the decrease in growth rate induced by cadmium intoxication.

Although glomerular morphology was found to be essentially normal in all groups, a highly significant increase in thickness of glomerular basement membrane was observed, from 168 ± 4nm in saline treated birds to 210 ± 5nm in birds treated with cadmium alone. No such increase was seen in any other group, indicating that the chelates protected the animals from this thickening.

Normal morphology was observed in proximal tubule cells of birds treated with saline (Fig. 1) or either chelate in isolation, indicating that the chelates did not themselves affect ultrastructural morphology. In birds given cadmium alone, however, considerable disorganization was seen (Fig. 2). The cytosol was highly vacuolated, and endoplasmic reticulum (ER) was dilated. Numbers of mitochondria were highly significantly reduced ($p < 0.001$), as indexed by mitochondrial cytoplasmic ratios (MCRs), which were 1:2.8 in saline, and 1:4.7 in cadmium alone treated birds. In animals given either chelate in conjunction with cadmium, cellular disorganization was not seen, and MCRs were not significantly different from those in the saline or chelate alone treated birds (MCRs; FeEDTA alone, 1:2.2; MgEDTA alone, 1:2.3). Mitochondrial structure was considerably disrupted in animals given cadmium alone, showing swelling, cavitation of the matrix and occasional rupture of the outer membrane. In addition, small intra-

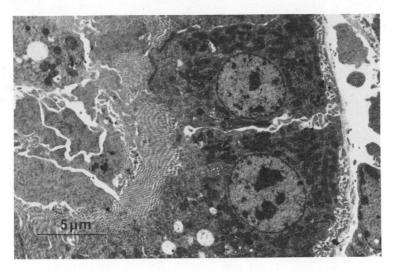

Fig. 1. TEM of proximal tubular cells derived from saline-treated (normal) bird.

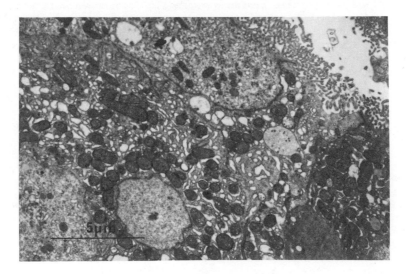

Fig. 2. TEM of proximal tubular cells derived from cadmium-treated bird.

mitochondrial granules were seen in this group. In animals given saline or either chelate alone, and in groups given cadmium in conjunction with either chelate these mitochondrial abnormalities were absent. Evidently the chelates had provided protection against the effects of cadmium intoxication.

Similar results were obtained for distal and collecting duct cells, but the vacuolation, dilatation of ER and reductions in mitochondrial numbers were rather less marked.

DISCUSSION

The reduced growth rate seen in cadmium intoxicated birds may be attributed, at least in part, to the decreased food intake. This has been seen in mammals, but the mode of action of this, and of the protection afforded by the chelates remains unclear. Interference with the absorption at cellular level, or subsequent utilisation of food material might also have contributed to this effect.

Hypertension has previously been observed to be associated with glomerular basement membrane thickening (Ghadially, 1982) and also with cadmium induced intoxication in mammals (Schroeder, 1964; Jenis and Lowenthal, 1977). In the present study, the thickening observed may act to reduce the glomerular filtration rate (GFR), and indeed Prashad et al (1986) have shown that cadmium causes a 40% reduction in GFR in birds. This being so, oedema might follow, and in these experiments cadmium treated birds were found to be somewhat oedematous, as shown by fluid accumulation in body cavities and intracellularly. In addition, this might also contribute to retention of cadmium and other toxic filtrands.

It has been noted that over 80% of the renal cell burden of cadmium is present in the cytosol and about 7% in the mitochondria (Webb, 1979). It is therefore not surprising that there are pronounced effects on the physiology and morphology of these cells. The swelling and cavitation seen in the mitochondria of proximal cells derived from cadmium alone treated birds would have profound metabolic consequences, and indeed, cadmium is known to disrupt mitochondrial metabolism, for example keto acid dehydrogenases are particularly susceptible (Sanadi et al, 1959; Webb, 1964), and Mustapha and Cross (1971) noted that mitochondrial electron transport was inhibited, presumably due to binding of Cd^{2+} to certain components. These workers also reported interference with the activity of ATPase, and inhibition of ATP hydrolysis as a result of cadmium treatment. Possibly, the mitochondrial damage observed leads to failure of ion-pumping which in turn could cause flooding of the cell with water (Ghadially, 1982). This may partly explain the evidence of the ingress of water seen in animals treated with cadmium alone. Certainly, ultra-structural damage to mitochondria and other organelles has been previously noted in cases of cadmium intoxication (Hoffman et al, 1975; Faeder et al, 1977).

Electron dense granules seen in matrices of mitochondria have been said to be more prominent in tissues transporting large amounts of ions or water (Peachey, 1964). They contain calcium, magnesium, phosphorous and organic material, predominantly lipid (Matthews et al, 1971) and are strongly osmophilic (Barnard and Afzelius, 1972). Peachey (1964) has hypothesised that divalent cations may be retained in the mitochondria either organically bound to pre-existing granules or as an inorganic precipitate, and that they occur more frequently when these ions are present in unusual concentrations. It seems possible, therefore, that the granules seen in the current study represent an increase in the level of calcium retention. Indeed, studies by Duffy et al (1971) have shown that calcium nephropathy results in similar ultrastructural changes to those observed in the current experiments. These workers also suggested that the consequences of hypercalcaemia would be the same, irrespective of the hypercalcaemic agent used. It may be, therefore, that cadmium acts not only as a toxic agent directly, but also indirectly, by inducing hypercalcaemia.

The dilatation of ER noted in the current work has also been observed in mammals treated with cadmium (Hoffman et al 1975); this would of course have additional consequences for cell metabolism.

The dilatation of ER noted in the current work has also been observed in mammals treated with cadmium (Hoffman et al 1975); this would of course have additional consequences for cell metabolism.

Both chelates used in these experiments appeared to exert notable protective effects from toxic insult by cadmium. It may be that they provided sites for the attachment of Cd^{2+} ions, thereby eliminating the metal from interactions with endogenous components of the cell. Conceivably cadmium might displace iron from the FeEDTA, providing a small 'pool' of iron which could contribute to the prevention of the anaemia known to occur in cadmium intoxicated birds (Sturkie, 1973), and perhaps supplement iron-requiring systems in cellular metabolism. Birds treated with cadmium are known to suffer from myocardial infarction, and low magnesium is associated with infarction. It may be that additional magnesium, supplied by the MgEDTA, assists in the prevention of this effect.

The use of electron probe microanalysis may well provide more information about the composition of the granules seen in the mitochondria, and it is hoped that these studies will be extended to this, and to the mode of action of these and other chelates in nephrotoxicity of metals.

REFERENCES

Barnard, T. and Afzelius, B.A., 1972. The matrix granules of mitochondria: a review, Sub-Cell, Biochem. 1:373.

Duffy, J.L., Suzuki, Y. and Churg, J., 1971. Acute calcium nephropathy. Early proximal tubule changes in the rat kidney, Arch. Pathol., 91:340.

Faeder, E.J., Chaney, S.Q., King, I.C., Hinners, T.A., Bruce, R. and Fowler, B.A., 1977. Biochemical and ultrastructural changes in livers of cadmium-treated rats, Toxicol. Appl. Pharmacol., 39:472.

Ghadially, F.N., 1982. "Ultrastructural Pathology of the Cell and Matrix," 2nd ed., Butterworths, London.

Hoffman, E.O., Cook, J.A., DiLuzio, N.R. and Coover, J.A., 1975. The effects of acute cadmium administration in the liver and kidney of the rat, Lab. Invest., 32:655.

Jenis, E.H. and Lowenthal, D.T., 1977. "Kidney Biopsy Interpretation," F.A. Davis, Philadelphia.

Matthews, J.L., Martin, J.H., Arsenis, C., Einstein, R. and Kuettner, K., 1971. The role of mitochondria in intracellular regulation, In: "Cellular Mechanisms for Calcium Transfer and Homeostasis," G. Nichols and R.H. Wasserman, eds., Academic Press, New York.

Mustapha, M.G. and Cross, C.E., 1971. Pulmonary alveolar macrophage. Oxidative metabolism of isolated cells and mitochondria and effect of cadmium ion on electron- and energy-transfer reactions. Biochemistry, 10:4176.

Peachey, L.D., 1964. Electron microscopic observations on the accumulation of divalent cations in intramitochondrial granules, J. Cell Biol., 20:95.

Piscator, M., 1986. The nephropathy of chronic cadmium poisoning, In: "Cadmium," Handbook Experimental Pharmamacology, 80, E.C. Foulkes, ed., Springer-Verlag, Berlin.

Prashad, D.N., Hawkins, E.A., Blackburn, R. and Haslam, J., 1986. Cadmium induced changes of renal haemodynamics in the domestic fowl, _Experientia_, 42:389.

Samarawickrama, G.P., 1979. Biological effects of cadmium in mammals, _In_: "The Chemistry, Biochemistry and Biology of Cadmium," M. Webb, ed., North Holland, Amsterdam.

Sanadi, D.R., Langley, M. and White, F., 1959. Ketoglutaric dehydrogenase VII. The role of thioctic acid, _J. Biol. Chem._, 234:183.

Schroeder, H.A., 1964. Cadmium hypertension in rats, _Am. J. Physiol._, 207:62.

Sturkie, P.D., 1973. Effects of cadmium on electrocardiogram, blood pressure and haematocrit of chickens, _Avian Dis._, 17:106.

Webb, M., 1964. The biological action of cobalt and other metals IV. Inhibition of alpha-oxoglutarate dehydrogenase, _Biochem, Biophys. Acta_, 89:431.

Webb, M., 1979. Interactions of cadmium and cellular components, _In_: "The Chemistry, Biochemistry and Biology of Cadmium," M. Webb, ed., North Holland, Amsterdam.

DIFFERENTIAL EFFECTS OF CADMIUM AND MERCURY ON LYSOSOMAL ENZYMES IN THE KIDNEY OF MYXINE GLUTINOSA

E. Elger, R. Sievers, B. Elger, C.J. Olbricht and H. Stolte

Med. Hochschule Hannover, Abt. Nephrologie, D-3000 Hannover 61, FRG and Mount Desert Island Biology Laboratory, Salsbury Cove, Maine 04672, USA

INTRODUCTION

In man and most animals the exposure to the environmental pollutants cadmium and mercury results in accumulation of these heavy metals especially in the kidneys and the liver. At the cellular level protein-bound heavy metals are enriched in the lysosomal system after pinocytotic uptake.

The aim of the present study was to show:

a) the validity of hagfish (Myxine glutinosa) as an animal model for the investigation of renal lysosomal enzymes. The archinephric duct of Myxine is comparable in ultrastructure to the first segment of the proximal tubule in mammals and also capable for extensive uptake of macromolecules from the luminal fluid (Ericsson and Seljelid, 1968),

b) the effects of cadmium and mercury on acid phosphatase (AcPase) and proteinases cathepsins B and L in lysosomes of kidney cells.

METHODS

Studies on renal AcPase and cathepsins were performed on hagfish (body weight 31-71g) which had been caught at the coast of Maine (USA) and the Oslo Fjord (Norway), respectively. Kidney tissue (Archinephric duct) was excised from anaesthetized animals (propylenphenoxetol, 2 ml/l seawater) after pressure controlled perfusion with Ringer's solution to remove the blood. The activities of AcPase and cathepsins were measured by fluorometric ultramicroassays utilizing 4-methylumbelliferylphosphate, Z-phenylalanyl-arginine-7-amido-4-methylcoumarine and N-CBZ-L-arginyl-arginine-7-amido-4-methylcoumarine, respectively, as the substrates (Olbricht et al. 1984, 1986). Test substances were added directly into the reaction mixture.

RESULTS

Characterization of cathepsins B, L in the kidney of Myxine

1. No enzyme degradation occurs at the incubation temperature of 37.5 ^{o}C which is unphysiological for the hagfish, but comparable to studies on

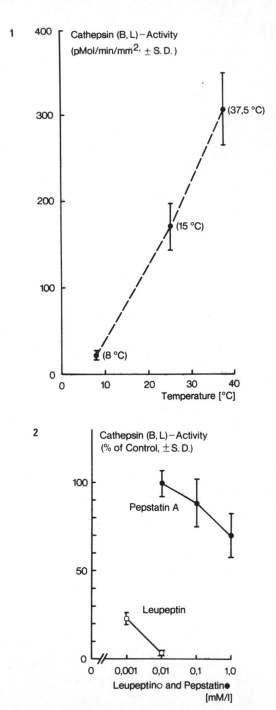

Figures 1 and 2. Effects of incubation temperature and inhibitors on the activity of cathepsins B, L.

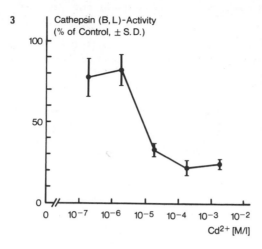

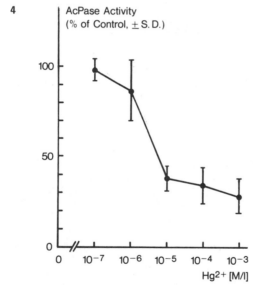

Figures 3 and 4. Dose response relationships of heavy metals and activities of lysosomal enzymes

mammalian cathepsins (the temperature in the natural marine habitat of the hagfish is 6-10°C).

2. The apparent K'_m determined by Lineweaver-Burk plots corresponds well with values obtained in mammals.

3. Iodoacetate (inhibitor for thiol proteinases but not serine proteinases) causes 100% inhibition of cathepsins B, L at concentrations above 0.05 mM/l.

4. Leupeptin is a specific inhibitor of cathepsins B, L but not of cathepsin H.

5. Pepstatin (inhibitor of cathepsin D and carboxyl proteases) does not inhibit cathepsins B, L at concentrations up to 0.01 mM/l.

Effects of cadmium and mercury on renal AcPase and cathepsins B, L in Myxine

1. Cadmium inhibits cathepsins B, L by more than 60% at 10^{-5} to 10^{-2} M/l.
2. Cadmium has inconsistent effects on AcPase activity leading on the average to no significant change.
3. Mercury inhibits AcPase by more than 60% at 10^{-5} to 10^{-3} M/l.

Table 1. K'_m values of cathepsins as determined from Lineweaver-Burk plots in different species.

Species	Cathepsins B and L	Cathepsin B	Authors
	K'_m	(mMol/l)	
Myxine	0.61	0.205	Elger (this study)
Rat	0.63	0.232	Olbricht (1986)
Rabbit	-	0.23	Madsen and Park (1986)
Pig	-	0.225	Takahashi (1982)

CONCLUSIONS

A) In comparison to renal cathepsins B, L in mammals the cathepsins of Myxine showed the same K'_m and the same response to a variety of specific inhibitors. Thus, Myxine is suited as an animal model to study basic mechanisms of the vertebrate renal lysosomal system.

B) Cathepsins B, L and AcPase respond different to cadmium and mercury. Moreover, the effects of cadmium and mercury are different within each group of enzymes and therefore, different molecular mechanisms have to be assumed.

ACKNOWLEDGEMENTS

This study was supported by DFG grant (SFB 146) and NIEHS grant (1P30 ES03828-01), and in part by the European Commission Biotechnology Action Programme on In Vitro Toxicology.

REFERENCES

1.   Ericsson J.L.E., R. Seljelid (1968), Z. Zellforsch., 90, 263-272.

2.   Madsen K.M., C.H. Par (1986), personal communication.

3.   Olbricht C.J., L.C. Garg, J.K. Cannon, C.C. Tisher (1984), Am. J. Physiol., 247, F252-F259.

4.   Olbricht C.J., J.K. Cannon, L.C. Garg, C.C. Tisher (1986), Am. J. Physiol., 250, F1055-F1062.

5.   Takahashi S., K. Murakami, Y. Miyake (1981), J. Biochem., 90, 1677-1684.

THE EFFECTS OF CADMIUM AND ADRIAMYCIN ON THE ISOLATED PERFUSED GLOMERULUS OF MYXINE GLUTINOSA (CYCLOSTOMATA)

L.M. Fels[1,3], M.-M. Barbey[1,3], B. Elger[1,3], J. Abel[2], and H. Stolte[1,3]

Division of Nephrology, Hannover Medical School, 3000 Hannover 61 FRG[1], Medical Institute for Environment Hygiene, 4000 Dusseldorf, FRG[2] and Mount Desert Island Biological Laboratory, Salsbury Cove, Maine 04672, USA[3]

INTRODUCTION

The severity and mechanisms of action of environmental and drug nephro-toxicity needs to be evaluated. While impaired renal function has often been based on chronic exposure studies, little attention has been paid to acute effects, especially renal dysfunction that occurs shortly after exposure to heavy metals or drugs. It may be difficult to define such changes in the whole animal, but in vitro techniques offer a simpler solution to assessing such changes.

Hagfish (Myxine glutinosa, Cyclostomata), are vertebrates with a kidney that consists of about 70 segmentally arranged glomeruli which are drained over a short neck segment directly into two parallel collecting ducts archinephric ducts. Because of this arrangement plus a morphology and fine structure that is similar to those of higher vertebrates (6,7), the animal lends itself to studies of glomerular processes.

The model of the isolated perfused single glomerulus (IPSG) of Myxine glutinosa has already been applied to study the effects of vasoactive substances (catecholamines) on single glomeruli (1). The technique can also be applied to study the acute effects of toxic substances on the glomerular apparatus. The IPSG allows the study of a variety of renal parameters, among which are changes of permeability for serum proteins, of charge of filtration barrier, and of the filtration coefficient.

The distribution of cadmium in the body, the uptake into the tissue, and the effects of a single injection of $CdCl_2$ on glomerular protein permeability were investigated to study the acute effect of cadmium. An increased excretion of proteins after cadmium treatment is usually attributed to tubular dysfunction (tubular-interstitial nephrosis). Low level cadmium exposure in rats causes profound histopathological changes not only at the tubular, but also at the glomerular level (2). The glomeruli showed fusion and withdrawal of epithelial foot processes and a thickening of the capillary endothelium. An increased cellular appearance and swelling of some glomeruli was caused by glomerular fibrosis and cell hypertrophy. In combination with these morphological changes, an increased urinary excretion of high molecular weight proteins (HMW) has been observed.

The effects of adriamycin (ADR) has also been assessed on the IPSG based on the fact that this anti tumour drug cause glomerular damages (increased protein permeability and reduced glomerular filtration rate) 5 days after 7.5 mg/kg in rats (3,4). Preliminary experiments have shown that the sieving coefficient for albumin in the model of the ISPG is unaltered 10 days after the injection of ADR. The involvement of reactive oxygen radicals, generated by ADR semiquinone radicals, is suggested to damage the cells (5). It was therefore investigated whether ADR alters protein permeability and whether it affects filtration rate (SNGFR) under conditions with a high oxygen pressure.

METHODS

A double barrelled perfusion cannula was inserted into the dorsal aorta and catheters in the archinephric duct using a pressure controlled microperfusion of single isolated glomeruli based on the method described (1) and shown below (Fig. 1). Perfusate was a hagfish Ringer's solution (8) containing 0.75% bovine serum albumin (BSA, MW 69,000). Perfusion pressure was held within a physiological range of 6 to 12 mm Hg.

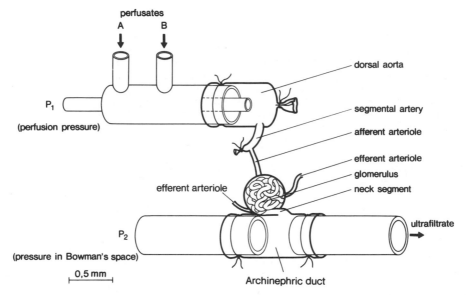

Fig. 1 Arrangements of glomerulus, perfusion cannula and catheters for _in vitro_ perfusion of single isolated glomeruli of Myxine glutinosa.

Cadmium. The animals were given a single injection of Cd at concentrations of 1 mg/kg (group 1) or 10 mg/kg (group 2) into the caudal blood sinus seven days prior to the experiments. A third group served as control. Cd concentrations in plasma and tissue were determined with an atomic absorption spectrophotometer.

Adriamycin. After the injection of ADR (5 mg/kg into the caudal blood sinus) the experimental animals were exposed to an artificial atmosphere of 80% O_2/20% N_2 for 48 hr and kept under normal O_2 conditions for further 8 days. Controls received O_2 in a corresponding manner. Single nephron glomerular filtration rate was calculated from the advance of fluid in the catheter and gravimetric measurement of the volume of the catheter. Analysis of albumin in perfusate and filtrate was undertaken using immunoelectrophoresis at pH 8.6 on 1% agarose gels (Gelbond Film, LKB, containing antibody from the rabbit, Dakopatts Hamburg) according to Laurell (9). Values are given as means±S.D.

RESULTS

The IPSG. The SNGFR ranged from 18.6 to 54.2 nl/min and was, due to the oncotic pressure of the BSA in the perfusate, lower than the mean SNGFR reported for experiments with colloid free perfusate (1). The sieving coefficient for BSA was 0.07 ± 0.05 (n = 11).

Cadmium. The SNFR of $CdCl_2$ - treated animals did not differ significantly from the one of controls, the values for group 1 and group 2 ranged from 11.4 to 56.5 nl/min. However the sieving coefficient for bovine serum albumin was significantly increased in group 2 (0.43 ± 0.3, n = 5) ($p < 0.05$, Student's t-test). The sieving coefficient of group 1 remained unchanged (0.07 ± 0.09, n = 6). One week after injection of $CdCl_2$ the plasma levels were still elevated. The heavy metal was mainly accumulated in the kidney and in the liver (Table 1). A 10-fold increase of the dose resulted in an increase of tissue content by about the factor 10.

Table 1. Cd-content of plasma and tissue after a single injection of $CdCl_2$

	plasma (ug/ml)	kidney (ug/g)	liver (ug/g)	muscle (ug/g)
Control	0.5x10-3 (5)	0.21±0.3 (5)	0.23±0.2 (5)	0.03 (5)
1 mg Cd/kg	2.60±1.4 (6)	2.32±1.4 (6)	3.04±0.5 (5)	0.48±0.1 (6)
10 mg Cd/kg	52.92±16.4 (6)	28.64±7.1 (6)	33.84±7.1 (6)	8.16±2.9 (6)

x ± S.D., (n)

Adriamycin. Control animals showed a sieving coefficient of 0.012 ± 0.002 (n = 6). The sieving coefficient of 0.054 ± 0.046 (n = 9) was significantly higher ($p < 0.05$, Student's t-test) 10 days after injection of 5 mg/kg (Fig. 2). SNGFR was unaffected.

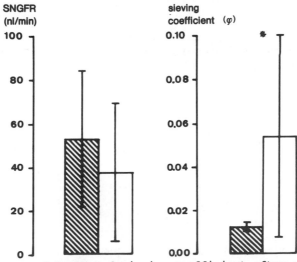

Fig. 2. Changes of SNGFR and sieving coefficient after an injection of ADR. Hatched bars: Controls. White bars: ADR-treated. *p < 0.05.

DISCUSSION

The ISPG. The model of the IPSG lacks a tubular apparatus, therefore alterations in excretion can only be attributed to glomerular effects of the applied substances. The results demonstrate the suitability of the model to study pathophysiological and toxicological effects with reference and in comparison to mammalian species. It allows utilization of knowledge that can be gained by in vitro studies on aquatic animals for a better understanding of glomerular process, especially glomerular permeability and vascular haemodynamic changes.

The sieving coefficient for the control groups of both studies are higher than under in vivo conditions. An explanation for generally increased permeability for serum proteins under in vitro conditions cannot be given yet. It should be noted that haemodynamic characteristics (e.g., filtration coefficient) of the experimental animal are well within the range of values found for higher vertebrates in in vitro experiments (1).

Cadmium. Epithelial transport and vascular haemodynamics are the two known sites of action of cadmium (10). The data of these preliminary experiments let it seem possible that there is an effect of Cd on the filtration barrier. No obvious changes in haemodynamics could be demonstrated.

In earlier studies protein permeability was found to increase with decreasing SNGFR in hagfish (11) as well as in mammals (12). The 7-fold increase in the sieving coefficient from the control group to group 2 can not be explained with a reduced SNGFR, because the filtration rates of all groups were within the same range. Minor changes of the SNGFR cannot account for a 7-fold alteration of the permeability.

The amount of Cd in renal tissue required to produce nephropathy in vivo is uncertain and appears to depend on the form of cadmium given and the dosage schedule (13). In this study a dose dependent accumulation of injected Cd, mainly into liver and kidney could be demonstrated. Between 10 and 200 ug Cd/g wet weight are associated with renal tubular damages in experimental animals (14). Based on these earlier data and on the assumption that glomeruli are sensitive to similar concentrations as tubules, an increased sieving coefficient with a tissue content of 2.32 ug/g wet weight (group 1) was unlikely. As 10 mg $CdCl_2$/kg body weight resulted in tissue levels around 30 ug/g wet weight, damages are more likely to occur.

Adriamycin. The results presented here are comparable with the effects of ADR on mammals, that is an unchanged glomerular water permeability, but increased protein permeability (3). Oxidative stress on membrane compounds mediated by ADR semiquinone radicals seems to be the most likely primary mechanism of ADR-toxicity.

ACKNOWLEDGEMENTS This work was supported by DFG (SFB-146A), NIEHS (EHS 1-P-30-ES-03828) to Center of Membrane Toxicity Studies, and Biotechnology Action Programme of the EC (BAP-0283).

REFERENCES

1. Fels, L.M., Elger, B. Stolte, H. (1987). Function of single isolated glomeruli of *Myxine glutinosa* and effects of catecholamines: In vitro microperfusion studies. *Pflugers Archiv*, submitted.

2.   Aughey,   E.,   Fell,   G.S.,   Scott,   R.,   and Black,   M.   (1984).
Histopathology of early effects of oral cadmium in the rat kidney.
Environ. Health Persp.   54: 153-161.

3.   O'Donnel, M.P., Michels, L., Kasiske, B., Raij, L., and Keane, W.F.
(1985).   Adriamycin-induced chronic proteinuria: A structural and
functional study.   J. Lab. Clin. Med.   106: 62-67.

4.   Bertani, T., Poggi, A., Pozzoni, R., Delaine, F., Sacchi, G., Thoua,
Y.,   Mecca, G., Remuzzi, G., and Donati, M.B.   (1982).   Adriamycin-induced
nephrotic syndrome in rats.   Sequence in pathologic events.   Lab. Invest.
46: 16-23.

5.   Mimnaugh, E.G., Trush, M.A., Gram, T.E. (1986).   A possible role for
membrane lipid peroxidation in anthracycline nephrotoxicity.   Biochem.
Pharm. 35: 4327-4335.

6.   Heath-Eves, M.J., McMillan, D.B.   (1974).   The morphology of the
kidney of the Atlantic hagfish,   Myxine glutinosa (L.).   Am. J. Physiol.
139: 309-334.

7.   Kuhn,   K.,   Stolte, H., and Reale, E. (1979).   The fine structure of
the kidney of the hagfish (Myxine glutinosa L.).   A thin section and
freeze fracture study.   Cell Tissue Res.   164: 201-213.

8.   Riegel,   J.A.   (1978).   Factors affecting glomerular function in the
Pacific hagfish,   Eptatretus stouti (Lockington).   J. Exp. Biol. 73: 261-
277.

9.   Laurell,   C.B.   (1966).   Quantitative estimation of proteins by
electrophoresis in agarose gel containing antibodies. Anal. Biochem.   15:
45.

10.   Samarawickram,   G.B.   (1979).   In: The chemistry, biochemistry and
biology of cadmium.   M.   Webb,   Ed. Elsevier/North Holland, Amsterdam, pp.
341-421.

11.   Rost, B., Schurek, H.J., Neumann, K.H., Stolte, H. (1983).   Perfusion
studies on single glomeruli of the Atlantic hagfish,   Myxine glutinosa
(L.). Bull. Mt. Desert Isl. Bio. Lab. 23 : 63-65.

12.   Stolte,   H.,   Neumann,   K.H.,   Reale, E., Alt, J., and Schurek, H.J.
(1981).   Renal handling of serum proteins as studied by micropuncture
study techniques.   Contr. Nephrol. 26:23-30.

13.   Diamond,   G.L., Cohen, J.J., Weinstein, S.L. (1986).   Renal handling
of cadmium in perfused rat kidneys and effect on renal function and tissue
composition.   Am. J. Physiol. 251 : F784-F794.

14.   Nordberg, M. (1984).   General aspects of cadmium: Transport, uptake
and metabolism by the kidney.   Environ. Health Persp.   54: 13-20.

PROTECTIVE EFFECT OF LOW CONCENTRATIONS OF MERCURY AGAINST $HgCl_2$-INDUCED NEPHROTOXICITY

J.C. Cal*, F. Larue*, P. Dormmua**, and J. Cambar*

* Groupe d'Etude de Physiologie et Physiopathologie Renales, Faculte de Pharmacie, Bordeaux, and ** Laboratoire Homeopathique Dolisos, Paris, France

INTRODUCTION

The reduction of $HgCl_2$-induced nephrotoxicity has been achieved by several factors affecting either the renal haemodynamics or the organ and/or subcellular distribution or excretion of mercury. Six main overlapping classes of compounds have been used to protect against mercury nephrotoxicity, these including beta-blocking agents, diuretics, chelators, substances that induce metallothioneins, agents involving a competition with mercury for the same binding sites or various nephrotoxicants. Among these, the pretreatment with small doses of Hg is of special interest because it provides a protection against nephrotoxic doses of $HgCl_2$ by a mechanism which seems to be ubiquitous in all metal nephrotoxicology since the same holds true for Ag, As, Cd, etc (Yoshikawa, 1970). Against this background, the present work was undertaken to determine whether a pretreatment with low concentrations of mercury, the so-called "Mercurius corrosivus" also protects against lethal doses of $HgCl_2$.

MATERIALS AND METHODS

Female Swiss mice (18-20g) were housed by 15 in a standardized room (12 hr light) and fed ad libitum. Two series of experiments were conducted so as to test the influence of a pretreatment with high dilutions of mercury on $HgCl_2$-induced mortality in mice and also to determine whether this effect is reproducible.

Low concentrations of Hg prepared by Dolisos laboratories from a mother solution (1g Hg/l in distilled water) i.e. Mercurius corrosivus 3d, diluted 1:9 to get Mercurius corrosivus 2c (0.1g Hg/l) and then potentized to Mercurius corrosivus 9c (10^{-3} pg/l) or 15c (theoretical concentration: 10^{-15} pg/l) by serial centesimal dilutions 1:99 and automated succession (100 impacts) at each step of dilution.

During the first study, after a 10-day standardization period: mice received a daily i.p. injection of 0.5 ml of Mercurius corrosivus 9c or 15c (pretreated groups) or of succussed distilled water (control groups) throughout a 7-day period. On the 7th day, one hour after the last preventive injection, they were given a single i.p. dose of 5, 6 or 7 mg Hg/kg of $HgCl_2$. All along the second series of experiments, 265 mice were pretreated with Mercurius corrosivus 15c according to the previous protocol and dosed with 5 mg Hg/kg of $HgCl_2$ at 5 months of the year. Mortality was recorded ten days after intoxication. The statistical analysis was undertaken using both frequency comparison tests and the single cosinor method.

RESULTS

The results of the first study indicate that Mercurius corrosivus can provide an important reduction of the lethal toxicity of $HgCl_2$, especially when the challenging dose is as close as possible to the LD50 value. Indeed, when mice received 5 mg Hg/kg, 73.4% died in the control group whereas only 50% and 26.7% (p < 0.01) died in groups pretreated respectively by Mercurius corrosivus 9c or 15c. Similarly, when mice were given 6 mg Hg/kg, 78.5% of control ones died while 66.7% of Mercurius corrosivus 9c pretreated ones and only 35.7% of Mercurius corrosivus 15c pretreated ones (p < 0.01) did so. This protective effect was lessened with the highest challenging dose (7 mg Hg/kg) since mortality rates were 93.3%, 73.4% and 78.5% when mice were pretreated respectively with distilled water, Mercurius corrosivus 9c or 15c. Such clear-cut an effect appears to be very reproducible in the second series of experiments as shown by the protection index i.e. the ratio of the difference in mortality rates between pretreated and control groups to control mortality rate. This index was, indeed, 63.6% in October, 26.15% in December, 11.15% in February, 49.9% in April and 75% in May. The effectiveness of Mercurius corrosivus against $HgCl_2$-induced mortality was thus demonstrated and moreover exhibited a circannual rhythm (p = 0.0113). The cosinor analysis permitted to locate the maximum of this rhythm in the efficacy of Mercurius corrosivus 15c in August and determine its mean value, 57.8 $\pm$ 2.06% and amplitude, 46.34 $\pm$ 2.17%.

DISCUSSION

The findings of this study demonstrating the protective effect of high dilutions of mercury against $HgCl_2$ toxicity are consistent with Magos and Webb (1979) who stated that any interaction with Hg can only lead to an antagonism of its toxic effects. The data presented here also agree with those of Yoshikawa (1970) who highlighted a beneficial effect of a pretreatment with small doses of Hg ranging from 0.04 to 0.8 mg Hg/kg i.e. dilutions close to Mercurius corrosivus 3c.

The mechanism of this protective effect of Mercurius corrosivus, in view of the high dilution of Hg, could be similar to selenium, which acts at low concentrations. The molecular basis could, therefore, be thst each molecule of Hg might induce the formation of a large protein complex which in turn would bind to more molecules of challenging Hg than the low molecular weight proteins (Chang, 1979). By this mechanism, a higher level of challenging Hg could therefore be trapped on inactivated by a lower concentration of metal in the pretreatment protocol. Never-the-less, these findings lead to a previously unrecognized role for high dilutions of mercury as one of the most effective methods to protect against $HgCl_2$-induced nephrotoxicity since the mean level observed along the one-year study was about 58%.

Though much work remains to be undertaken in order to maximize the potential preventive therapeutic applications of Mercurius corrosivus these data suggest an application in occupational medicine.

ACKNOWLEDGEMENTS

This research was supported by grant no. 84C1156 from the French Ministry of Research and Technology and by Dolisos laboratories, Paris, France.

REFERENCES

Chang, L.W., 1979, Pathological effects of mercury poisoning, <u>In</u>: "The biogeochemistry of mercury in the environment", J.O. Nriagu, ed., Elsevier, New-York, 519.

Magos, L., and Webb, M., 1979, Synergism and antagonism in the toxicology of mercury, <u>In</u>: "The biogeochemistry of mercury in the environment", J.O. Nriagu, ed., Elsevier, New-York, 581.

Yoshikawa, H., 1970, Preventive effect of pretreatment with low dose of metals on the acute toxicity of metals in mice, <u>Indus. Health</u>, 8, 184.

INDUCTION OF ANTINUCLEAR ANTIBODIES BY MERCURIC CHLORIDE IN MICE

P. Hultman and S. Enestrom

Department of Pathology I, University of Linköping, Sweden

INTRODUCTION

Reports suggest that exposure to low doses of mercury or mercuric compounds in man could lead to proteinuria or nephrotic syndrome (Kazantzis, 1962; Belghiti et al, 1986). Immunologically mediated glomerulonephritis (GN) of IC type has been described in such patients (Gaultier et al, 1968; Tubbs et al, 1982). The closer mechanism of action in human mercury-induced glomerular disease remains unknown, but there is evidence that mercury can modify the immunoregulation (Charpentier et al, 1981).

Bariety et al (1971) described the induction of immune-mediated membranous GN by mercury in Wistar rats. Brown-Norway (BN) rats develop anti-glomerular basement membrane (anti-GBM) disease after exposure to mercurials by different routes (Sapin et al, 1977; Bernaudin et al, 1981). Circulating immune complexes develop, and granular IC deposits replace the linear anti-GBM antibodies (Druet et al, 1978; Bellon et al, 1982). A possible pathogenetic mechanism in BN rats could be T-cell dependent polyclonal B-cell activation (Hirsch et al, 1982) with antibodies to single-stranded DNA (SS-DNA)(Bellon et al, 1982). Such antibodies have also been found in other inbreed rat strains susceptible to induction of GN by mercuric chloride (Druet et al, 1982), and antibodies to DNA-associated proteins occur in both serum and renal immune deposit (Weening et al, 1978; Weening et al, 1980)

Exposure to inorganic mercury causes mesangial IC-GN in certain mouse strains (Enestrom and Hultman, 1984), whereas other strains are resistant (Hultman and Enestrom, 1987). The susceptible strains develop systemic IC deposits and raised serum immunoglobulin concentrations with an isotype pattern dependent on the strain and any immunopotentiation used (Hultman and Enestrom, 1987). Antinuclear serum antibodies without IC deposits have been described in mice (Robinson et al, 1984). The present study was undertaken to characterize the autoantibodies, and to study the relation between these antibodies and the renal IC deposits.

MATERIAL AND METHODS

Experimental Procedure. Twenty two female SJL mice aged 8-10 weeks were given subcutaneous injections of 1.6 mg $HgCl_2$/kg body weight at 3-day intervals over a period of 2, 4, or 12 weeks. The same number of controls received 0.1 ml of a sterile 0.9% NaCl solution.

Serum Autoantibody Test.   Serum obtained at the end of the   experimental
period was tested by indirect immunofluorescence using normal and mercury
treated mouse kidney and HEp-2 cells as substrates (Enestrom and Hultman,
1984).   Anti-native DNA anti-bodies were studied by the Crithidia luciliae
assay (Aarden et al, 1973).   Acid extraction was performed on HEp-2 slides
and cryostat sections of acetone-fixed mouse kidney by incubation in
acetate buffer (Weening et al, 1980) or 0.1-N HCl (Tan et al, 1976).   For
histone reconstitution calf thymus histones were freshly prepared in a
0.01-M PBS solution (pH 7.2) in a concentration of 25 ug/ml,   and the acid
eluted slides were immersed in this solution for 60 min.   Sera were
absorbed with calf thymus double- or single-stranded DNA, histones, calf
liver ribonucleic acid (Sigma Chemical Co), 5S- and 16S/23S RNA from E
coli (Boehringer Mannheim GmbH), whole chicken-erythrocyte nuclei, and
purified chromatin (Sung et al, 1977).   The absorbents were always used in
excess, and were incubated with the sera for 1 h at 37°C and then; at 4 $^{\circ}$C
overnight.   Sera were analysed by double immunodiffusion for the presence
of antibodies to the non-histone nuclear antigens Sm, ribonucleoprotein
(RNP), SS-A: and SS-B.   The antigens were obtained by saline extraction of
calf thymus using a modified version of the method described by Sharp et
al (1972), and standard sera containing antibodies were included as
reference agents.

Kidney studies.   Direct immunofluorescence was performed on cryostat
sections of kidney blocks using antibodies to IgG and C3c, and the
deposits were titrated as described elsewhere (Hultman and Enestrom,
1987).   Light- and electron microscopy studies were performed as described
elsewhere (Enestrom and Hultman, 1984).   Kidneys from mercury treated and
control SJL mice and female MRL mice were acid eluted by Bartolotti's
method (1977).

RESULTS

Serum Autoantibodies.   A strong nucleolar (Fig. 1a) and a weaker
homogeneous (Fig. 1b) ANA pattern with strongly stained chromosome regions
in metaphase cells (Fig. 1c) were found after 4 and 12 weeks' mercury
treatment.   No autoantibodies to mouse kidney structures apart from ANA
could be demonstrated.   Acid extraction resulted in weakening of the
homogeneous staining (Fig. 2b), which was not restored after
reconstitution with histones (Fig. 2c).   Absorption with whole chicken-
erythrocyte nuclei (Fig. 2e) or purified chromatin (Fig. 2f) abolished the
homogeneous staining, leaving only the nucleolar fluorescence.   The other
absorbents caused no reduction in the homogeneous or the nucleolar
staining.   No precipitating antibodies to the tested antigens were found.

Kidney studies.   Mercury treatment for 4 weeks or longer resulted in
significantly increased deposition of IgG and C3c in the glomerular
mesangial regions (Fig. 3a) and in the walls of the interlobular arteries
and arterioles.   A slight increase in endocapillary cells and a widening
of the mesangial zones took place after mercury treatment.   Electron dense
deposits were found in the mesangium (Fig. 3b) and vessel walls. Eluates
of kidneys from mice treated with mercury for 4 weeks showed a strictly
nucleolar ANA pattern (Fig. 3c); no homogeneous staining was detected.
The eluate from control mice showed no staining, and the eluate from MRL
mice gave strong homogeneous staining.

DISCUSSION

Mercury induced a polyclonal autoantibody response in mercury treated SJL
mice, with two main ANA patterns, homogeneous and nucleolar.   The

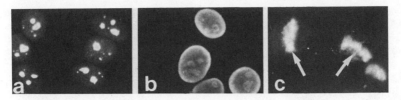

Fig. 1.   Indirect IF.   Sera from SJL mice treated with mercury for 4 weeks, incubated on HEp-2 cells x 600.

a)   Strong nucleolar pattern, weaker homogeneous pattern;

b)   Strong homogeneous pattern, weaker nucleolar pattern;

c)   Staining of chromosome regions of metaphase cells.

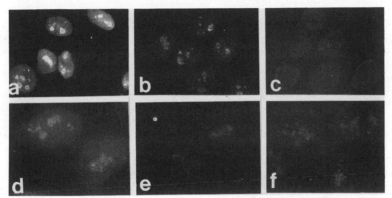

Fig. 2.   Indirect IF.   Serum from an SJL mouse treated with, mercury for 4 weeks, incubated on HEp-2 cells.

a)   Untreated cells;

b) Treatment with acid acetate buffer. Weakening of the homogeneous staining;

c) Reconstitution with histones of the acid-treated section. Further weakening of the staining. x 500;

d)   Control absorption with buffer;

e) Absorption with whole chicken-erythrocyte nuclei. Abolishment of homogeneous staining

f)   Absorption with purified chromatin, staining as in e. x 900.

homogeneous pattern was associated with strongly staining chromosome regions of metaphase cells, indicating that the antibodies were directed against a chromatin antigen; this was further supported by the absorption of the anti-bodies with purified chromatin.   The main groups of chromatin antigens include DNA, histones, and non-histone proteins (Nakamura and Tan, 1986).   The antibodies in our study were not absorbed by single- or double-stranded DNA, and the Crithidia luciliae test was negative, making DNA an unlikely antigen.   The lack of absorption with histones and the

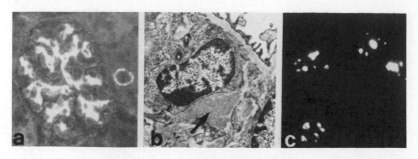

Fig. 3.

a) FITC-conjugated goat-antimouse IgG antibodies incubated on cryostat
section   of kidney of mercury-treated SJL mouse.   Deposits of IgG in the
mesangium and in the walls of an arteriole x 450;

b) Electron microgram of a mercury-treated mouse, showing electron-dense
deposits in the mesangium x 8900;

c) Indirect IF.   Eluate of kidneys of mercury-treated SJL mice, incubated
on HEp-2 cells.   Strictly nucleolar and nucleolar dot staining x 700.

failure   to   restore   the   staining by   histone   reconstitution   of   acid-
extracted sections are strong evidence against histones as the responsible
antigens (Fritzler and Tan, 1978).   By exclusion, then, the only remaining
group of chromatin antigens are the non-histones.   Antibodies to some of
the known antigens in this group were.   Searched for by immunodiffusion,
but   none were found.   Autoantibodies with a nucleolar ANA pattern have
been   discovered   in   patients with   autoimmune   disease.   The   following
underlying antigens have been reported: RNA (Pinnas et al, 1973): U3RNA-
protein complex (Nakamura and Tan, 1986), RNA polymerase I (Stetler et al,
1985),   and   several other nucleolar proteins such as fibrillarin (Ochs et
al, 1985).

Progressive systemic sclerosis (PSS) is the connective tissue disease most
commonly associated with a nucleolar ANA pattern, being present in 43-48S
(Bernstein et al, 1982; Riboldi et al, 1985) of the patients, often in
association with other ANA patterns.   Some of the nucleolar ANA patterns
described in patients with PSS (Bernstein et al, 1982) closely resemble
those   found in mercury-treated SJL mice, suggesting that the underlying
antigen or antigens might be identical.   It is therefore of interest that
renal IC deposits in the mesangium and vessels walls have been reported in
kidneys from PSS patients (Geber, 1975; McCoy et al, 1976).   Moreover,
antibodies   giving   nucleolar staining have been eluted from such kidneys
(McCoy et al, 1976), further mimicking the findings in mercury-treated SJL
mice.   The   IC   deposits   in   PSS patients might   have   a   role   in   the
pathogenesis of the renal arterial lesions (Heptinstall, 1983); however,
we found no such lesions in SJL mice.   Furthermore, the mercury treated
mice did not develop the widespread fibrotic changes which are a hallmark
of PSS (Haynes and Gershwin, 1982).

It is not known whether PSS and the mercury-induced autoimmune disease in
SJL mice have anything more in common than antinucleolar antibodies with a
very similar ANA pattern.   A great number of humoral and cellular immune
aberrations have been described in patients with PSS (Haynes and Gershwin,
1982; Jimenes, 1983), but the underlying regulatory defect remains
obscure.   No significant alterations have been found in regulatory T-cell

subsets in mercury-treated SJL mice (Hultman and Enestrom, unpublished observations), but SJL mice are unable to suppress an induced autoantibody response (Cooke and Hutchings, 1984).

REFERENCES

Aarden, L.A., de Groot, E.R., and Feltkamp, T.E.W., 1975, Immunology of DNA. III. Crithidia luciliae, a simple substrate for the determination of anti-dsDNA, with the immunofluorescent technique, Ann N.Y. Acad Sci., 245:505.

Bariety, J., Druet, F., Laliberte, F., and Sapin, C., 1971, Glomerulo-nephritis with gamma- and ßIC globulin deposits induced in rats by mercuric chloride, Am J Pathol., 65:293.

Bartolotti, S.R., 1977, Quantitative elution studies in experimental immune complex and nephrotoxic nephritis, Clin Exp Immunol., 29:334.

Belghiti, D., Patey, O., Berry, J.P., Antelin, C., Hirbec, G., and Lagrue, G., 1986, Nephrose lipoidique d'origine "toxique" Deux cas, Presse M'edicale, 15:1953.

Bernaudin, J.F., Druet, E., Druet, P., and Masse, R., 1981, Inhalation or ingestion of organic or inorganic mercurials produces autoimmune disease in rats, Clin Immunol Immunopathol., 20:129.

Bellon, B., Capron, M., Druet, E., Verroust, P., Vial, M-C., Sapin, C., Girard, J.F., Foidart, J.M., Mahieu, P., and Druet, P., 1982, Mercuric chloride induced autoimmune disease in Brown-Norway rats: sequential search for anti-basement membrane antibodies and circulating immune complexes, Eur J Clin Invest., 12:127.

Cooke, A., and Hutchings, P., 1983, Defective regulation of erythrocyte autoantibodies in SJL mice, Immunology., 51:489.

Bernstein, R.M., Steigewald, J.C., and Tan, E.M., 1982, Association of antinuclear and antinucleolar antibodies in progressive systemic sclerosis, Clin Exp Immunol., 48:43.

Charpentier, B., Moullot, Ph., Faux, N., Manigand, G., and Fries, D., 1981, Functions lymphocytaires T au cours d'une glomerulonephrite extra-membraneuse induite par une intoxication chronique au mercure, N'ephrologie, 2:153.

Druet, E., Sapin, C., Fournie, G., Mandet, C., Gnther, E., and Druet, P., 1982, Genetic control of susceptibility to mercury-induced immune nephritis in various strains of rat, Clin Immunol Immunopathol., 25:203.

Druet, P., Druet, E., Potdevin, F., and Sapin, C., 1978, Immune type glomerulonephritis induced by $HgCl_2$ in the Brown Norway rat, Ann Immunol., 129:777.

Enestrom, S., and Hultman, P., 1984, Immune-mediated glomerulonephritis induced by mercuric chloride in mice, Experientia, 40:1234.

Fritzler, M.J., and Tan, E.M., 1978, Antibodies to histones in drug-induced and idiopathic lupus erythematosus, J Clin Invest., 62:560.

Gaultier, M., Fournier, E., Gervais, P., Morel-Maroger, L., Bismuth, C., and Rain, J.-D., 1968 Deux cas de syndrome nephrotique dans une fabrique de thermometres, Soc Med Hopit Paris, 119:47.

Gerber, M.A., 1975, Immunohistochemical findings in the renal vascular lesions of progressive systemic sclerosis, Hum Pathol., 6:343.

Haynes, D.C., and Gershwin, M.E., 1982, The immunopathology of progressive systemic sclerosis (PSS), Semin Arthr Rheumat., 11:331.

Heptinstall, R.H., 1983, Hemolytic uremic syndrome, thrombotic thrombocytopenic purpura, and systemic scleroderma (progressive systemic sclerosis), In: "Pathology of the Kidney", Little Brown and Company, Boston and Toronto.

Hirsch, F., Couderc, J., Sapin, S., Fournie, G., and Druet, P., 1982, Polyclonal effect of $HgCl_2$ in the rat, its possible role in an experimental autoimmune disease, Eur J Immunol., 12:620.

Hultman, P., and Enestrom., 1987, The induction of immune complex deposits in mice by peroral and parenteral administration of mercuric chloride: strain dependent susceptibility, Clin Exp Immunol., 67:283.

Jimenez, S.A., 1983, Cellular Immune dysfunction and the pathogenesis of scleroderma, Semin Arthr Rheumat., 13:104.

Kazantzis, G., Schiller, K.F.R., Asscher, A.W., and Drew, R.G., 1961, Albuminuria and the nephrotic syndrome following exposure to mercury and its compounds, Q J Med., 124:403.

McCoy, R.C., Tisher, C.C., Pepe, P.F., and Cleveland, L.A., 1976, The kidney in progressive systemic sclerosis. Immunohistochemical and antibody elution studies, Lab Invest., 35:124.

Nakamura, R.M., Tan,.E.M., 1986, Recent advances in laboratory tests and the significance of autoantibodies to nuclear antigens in systemic rheumatic diseases, Clin. Lab. Med., 6:41..

Ochs, R.L., Lischwe, M.A., Spohn, W.H., and Busch, H., 1985, Fibrillarin: a new protein of the nucleolus identified by autoimmune sera, Biol Cell., 54:123.

Pinnas, J.L., Northway, J.D., and Tan, E.M., 1973, Antinucleolar antibodies in human sera, J Immunol., 3:996.

Riboldi, P., Asero, R., Origgi, L., Crespi, S., Meroni, P.L., Sguotti, C., and Sabbadini, M.G., 1985, Antinuclear antibodies in progressive systemic sclerosis, Clin Exp Rheumatol., 3:205.

Robinson, C.J.G., Abraham, A.A., and Balazs, T., 1984, Induction of antinuclear antibodies by mercuric chloride in mice, Clin Exp Immunol., 58:300.

Sapin, C., Druet, E., and Druet, P., 1977, Induction of anti-glomerular basement membrane antibodies in the Brown-Norway rat by mercuric chloride, Clin Exp Immunol., 28:173.

Sharp, G.C., Irvin, W.S., Tan, E.M., Gould, R.G., and Holman, H.R., 1972, Mixed connective tissue disease - an apparently distinct rheumatic disease syndrome associated with a specific antibody to an extractable nuclear antigen (ENA), Am J Med., 52:148.

Stetler, D.A., Sipes, D.E., and Jacob, S.T., 1985, Anti-RNA polymerase I antibodies in sera of MRL lpr/lpr and MRL +/+ autoimmune mice. Correlation of antibody production with delayed onset of lupus-like disease in MRL +/+ mice, J Exp Med., 162:1760.

Sung, M.T., Harford, J., Bundman, M., and Vidalakas, G., 1977, Metabolism of histones in avian erythroid cells, Biochemistry, 16:279.

Tan, E.M., Robinson, J., and Robitaille, P., 1976, Studies on antibodies to histones by immunofluorescence, Scand J Immunol., 5:811.

Tubbs, R.R., Gephardt, G.N., McMahon, J.T., Pohl, M.C., Vidt, D.G., Barenberg, S.A., and Valenzuela, R., 1982, Membranous glomerulonephritis associated with industrial mercury exposure, Am J Clin Pathol., 1982:409.

Weening, J.J., Fleuren, G.J., and Hoedemaeker, Ph.J., 1978, Demonstration of antinuclear antibodies in mercuric chloride-induced glomerulopathy in the rat, Lab Invest., 39:405.

Weening, J.J., Grond, J., van der Top, D., and Hoedemaeker, Ph.J., 1980, Identification of the nuclear antigen involved in mercury-induced glomerulopathy in the rat, Invest Cell Pathol., 3:129.

ANALYSIS OF UNSCHEDULED DNA SYNTHESIS AND S-PHASE SYNTHESIS IN F344 RAT KIDNEY AFTER IN VIVO TREATMENT WITH MERCURIC CHLORIDE

K. Steinmetz, C. Hamilton, J. Bakke, M. Ramsey, and J. Mirsalis

SRI International, 333 Ravenswood Ave., Menlo Park, California, 94025, USA

A variety of short-term test have been developed to predict the outcome of carcinogenicity bioassays. Unfortunately, the majority of these do not address the issue of tissue-specificity. Tests that focus on tissue-specific responses such as the in vivo - in vitro unscheduled DNA synthesis (UDS) and S-phase synthesis (SPS) assays (Mirsalis, et al., 1985; Mirsalis, 1987) have been reasonably successful in the prediction of hepatocarcinogenic potential. The most widely used system employs hepatocyte cultures derived from animals treated in vivo (Mirsalis and Butterworth, 1980); however, systems for the kidney (Tyson and Mirsalis, 1985; Loury et al., 1987), pancreas (Steinmetz and Mirsalis, 1984), trachea (Doolittle and Butterworth, 1984), stomach (Furihata et al., 1984), and spermatocytes (Working and Butterworth, 1984) have recently been developed.

The kidney UDS assay developed by Tyson and Mirsalis (1985) was used to detect genotoxic carcinogens in male Fischer-344 (F344) rat proximal tubule epithelial cells. Not all renal carcinogens tested yield positive results in this assay. This may be because some compounds exert their carcinogenic effect via a nongenotoxic mechanism. Loury et al. (1987) utilized a similar cell isolation technique and measured UDS and SPS, an indicator of cell proliferation. They evaluated the genotoxic and cell proliferative abilities of chemicals following in vivo exposure to male and female F344 rat proximal tubule epithelial cells.

Measurement of SPS in hepatocytes, an indication of liver hyperplasia, has been shown to correlate well with chemicals which may act via a nongenotoxic mechanism (Mirsalis, 1987). It has been shown that chemicals such as carbon tetrachloride (Loury et al, 1986) and methapyrilene (Steinmetz, et al., in prep) induce SPS as a result of toxicity resulting in necrosis. There are also a few chemicals such as di(2-ethylhexyl)phthalate which induce hyperplasia in the absence of toxicity (Butterworth, et al., 1983). Loury et al. (1986) demonstrated that the treatment of rats with unleaded gasoline (UG) resulted in an increase in SPS in male rat kidney only, which correlated with the renal carcinogenicity of UG.

We selected mercuric chloride (MC), a known nephrotoxin (Hook and Dixon, 1981), to systematically evaluate the effects of SPS induction in the kidney. MC has never been tested for rodent carcinogenicity, therefore, we cannot correlate our results with carcinogenicity data, and most studies examining MC nephrotoxicity have been performed in male rats only or other species (Ware et al., 1975; Ellis et al., 1973). In this study, we have compared the differences in MC-induced SPS in male and female rat kidney.

METHODS

Chemicals. Mercuric chloride (MC) was purchased from Sigma Chemical Company (St. Louis, MO). Streptozotocin (STZ) was purchased from The Upjohn Company (Kalamazoo, MI). STZ has been shown to induce UDS in the rat kidney following in vivo treatment (Tyson and Mirsalis, 1985).

Animals. Male and female Fischer-344 (F344) rats (weights: males-190 to 380 g; females-160 to 235 g) were purchased from Harlan Sprague-Dawley (Indianapolis, IN). Rats were quarantined for one week. Animals were randomized and ear punched at this time. Rats were housed in a environmentally-controlled room, with 3 rats per polypropylene cage and using hardwood chip bedding. Rats received Purina Rodent Chow #5002 and tap water ad libitum. The light cycle was maintained at 12 hr light:12 hr dark.

Rats were treated by oral gavage with either MC or water or by i.p. injection with STZ 16 or 96 hr prior to sacrifice. A volume of 5 ml/kg body weight (BW) was administered for all dosing solutions.

Kidney cell isolation. Rats were anaesthetized with sodium pentobarbital (0.2 ml/100 g body weight). The kidneys were removed, trimmed of fat and extraneous tissue, rinsed in Williams' medium E (WME), and minced into a solution of collagenase Type I (Sigma) and trypsin (Sigma) as described (Tyson and Mirsalis, 1985). Kidney cells were isolated by dissociation for 45 to 60 min. Cells were washed with WME and viability was determined using Trypan blue exclusion. Cell viability for control animals was routinely >90 %. Approximately 2×10^5 and 4×10^5 cells were inoculated into 6-well culture dishes containing Thermanox coverslips and WME supplemented with foetal bovine serum (20 %) and containing 10 uCi/ml ^{3}H-methyl-thymidine (specific activity 60 to 80 Ci/mmol).

Cell Fixation and Autoradiography. Following incubation for 21 to 23 hr in 5% CO_2:95% air at 37°C, cultures were washed with WME, swelled with 1% sodium citrate, fixed with 1:3 acetic acid:ethanol, and washed with deionized water. Dried coverslips were mounted with Permount to glass slides. Slides were dipped in Kodak NTB-2 nuclear track photographic emulsion and exposed at -20°C for 7 (SPS) or 14 (UDS) days. Slides were developed in Kodak D-19 developer, fixer, washed in water for 25 min, then stained with 1% methyl-green pyronin Y.

UDS and SPS Evaluation. Following autoradiographic procedures, slides were scored for UDS as previously described by Mitchell and Mirsalis (1984). Thirty, randomly-selected, morphologically-unaltered cells were scored from each of 3 slides/animal. The net grains/nucleus (NG) was calculated as the grains over the nucleus minus the highest of the grain counts over two adjacent, nuclear-sized areas over the cytoplasm. The percentage of cells in repair (%IR) was calculated as the percentage of cells with at least 3 NG. UDS data are presented as the means and standard errors (SE) for each treatment group.

Approximately 3000 cells/animal were scored for SPS as described previously (Mirsalis et al., 1985). Cells undergoing SPS are easily distinguished from UDS-positive cells. SPS data are presented as the mean and SE for each treatment group.

RESULTS

Rats treated with 25 mg/kg MC or the control vehicle at 16 hr yielded < 0 net grains/nucleus (NG) compared to 11.4 NG for male rats and 4.7 NG for female rats treated with STZ (Table 1). Control animals evaluated for SPS yielded < 0.60%S. Male rats sacrificed at 16, 24, 48, 96, 120 or 168 hr posttreatment with 25 mg/kg MC yielded 0.47, 0.53, 5.67, 12.14, 5.08 or 2.38 %S, respectively (Fig. 1). Female rats treated with 25 mg/kg MC and sacrificed at 16, 24, 96, 120 or 168 hr yielded 0.08, 0.47, 3.30, 6.16 and 1.95 %S. Male rats treated at 96 hr with 2, 5, or 10 mg/kg MC yielded 0.46, 2.33 and 10.81 %S, respectively (Fig. 2). Female rats treated at 96 hr with 2, 5, 10 and 50 mg/kg MC yielded 0.37, 0.13, 0.13 and 12.54 %S, respectively. Three male rats treated with 50 mg/kg MC (96 hr) died before scheduled sacrifice. Kidneys from the female rats treated with 50 mg/kg MC (96 hr) were sliced cross sectionally at which time tan cortices were observed. Tissue in the centre of the sections was a dark red colour. Digestion of the entire kidneys yielded viable cultures for SPS evaluation.

Table 1. INDUCTION OF UNSCHEDULED DNA SYNTHESIS IN RAT KIDNEY CELLS FOLLOWING IN VIVO EXPOSURE TO MERCURIC CHLORIDE

Chemical	Dose mg/kg	Time hr	Male NG ± SE	%IR	Female NG ± SE	%IR
Control/water	0	16	-4.6 ± 0.9	6	-4.5 ± 0.2	2
Streptozotocin	250	16	11.4 ± 1.6	79	4.7 ± 1.0	58
Mercuric Chloride	25	16	-3.3 ± 0.6	3	-3.5 ± 0.2	0

NG = Net grains/nucleus; SE = Standard errors between animals; % IR = Percent of cells with greater than 3 NG; three animals were used for each time point.

DISCUSSION

We studied the effects of MC exposure on male and female F344 rat kidney cells by using the in vivo - in vitro kidney UDS and SPS assays. From the data presented here, we conclude that although MC does not induce UDS, it does induce SPS, an indicator of cell proliferation, in male and female rats. At 10 mg/kg, male rats yield 10.81 %S compared to 0.13 %S in females. SPS induction by MC is therefore much greater in male rats than in female rats. There was a 24-hr delay in the peak induction time for female rats as compared to the male rats (Fig. 1).

Similar sex differences have been observed in the kidney SPS assay following exposure to p-dichlorobenzene (PDCB; Steinmetz et al., 1988) and unleaded gasoline (UG; Loury et al., 1986). In the cases of PDCB and UG, the sex differences correspond with the sex differences observed in the carcinogenicity data of these compounds (National Toxicology Program, 1987; MacFarland, 1982). PDCB and UG produce a significant elevation in male rat kidney tumours, but with a lack of these tumours observed in female rats. Since a bioassay has not been performed on MC, correlations to carcinogenicity are not possible. From this study we conclude that MC is a potent SPS inducer and should be a model compound for examining the effects of regenerative hyperplasia in the kidney.

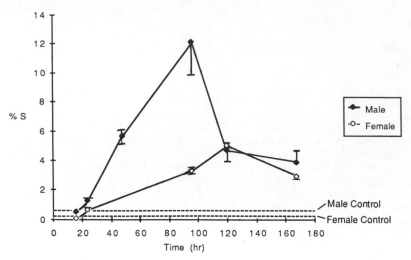

Fig 1.   Induction of S-phase synthesis in male and female F-344 rats treated by gavage with 25 mg/kg mercuric chloride at selected time points prior to sacrifice.   %S = Percent of cells in S-phase synthesis.

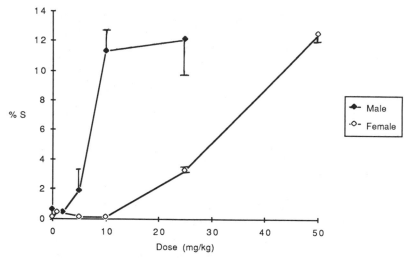

Fig 2.   Induction of S-Phase synthesis following exposure to mercuric chloride at selected doses in male and female F344 rats.   Rats were treated by gavage with selected doses of MC 96 hr prior to sacrifice. Three male rats treated at 50 mg/kg MC died prior to scheduled sacrifice. %S = Percent of cells in S-phase synthesis.

REFERENCES

Butterworth, B.E., Bermudez, E., Smith-Oliver, T., Earle, L., Cattley, R., Martin, J., Popp, J.A., Strom, S., Jirtle, R., and Michalopoulos, G., 1984, Lack of genotoxic activity of di(2-ethylhexyl)phthalate (DEHP) in rat and human hepatocytes, Carcinogenesis, 5:1329-1335.

Doolittle, D.J., and Butterworth, B.E., 1984, Assessment of chemically-induced DNA repair in rat tracheal epithelial cells, Carcinogenesis, 5:773-779.

Ellis, B.G., Price, R.G., and Topham, J.C., 1973, The effects of tubular damage my mercuric chloride on kidney function and some urinary enzymes in the dog, Chem. Biol. Interact., 7:101-113.

Furihata, C., Yamawaki, Y., Jin, S.S., Moriya, H., Kodama, K., Matsushima, T., Ishikawa, T., Takayama, S., and Nakadate, M., 1984, Induction of unscheduled DNA synthesis in rat stomach mucosa by glandular stomach carcinogens, JNCI, 72:1327-1333.

Loury, D.J., Smith-Oliver, T., Strom, S., Jirtle, R., Michalopoulos, G., and Butterworth, B.E., 1986, Assessment of unscheduled and replicative DNA synthesis in hepatocytes treated in vitro and in vivo with unleaded gasoline or 2,2,4-trimethylpentane, Toxicol. Appl. Pharmacol., 85:11-23.

Loury, D.J., Smith-Oliver, T., and Butterworth, B.E., 1986, Assessment of unscheduled DNA synthesis in rat kidney cells exposed in vitro or in vivo to unleaded gasoline, Toxicol. Appl. Pharmacol., 87:127-140.

MacFarland, H.N., 1982, Chronic gasoline toxicity, In: "Proceedings of the Symposium. The Toxicology of Petroleum Hydrocarbons," H.N. MacFarland, C.E. Holdsworth, J.A. MacGregor, R.W. Call, and M.L. Kane, eds., American Petroleum Institute, Washington, D.C.

Mirsalis, J.C., Tyson, C.K., and Butterworth, B.E., 1982, Detection of genotoxic carcinogens in the in vivo-in vitro hepatocyte DNA repair assay, Environ. Mutagen., 4:553-562.

Mirsalis, J.C., Tyson, C.K., Loh, E.N., Steinmetz, K.L., Bakke, J.P., Hamilton, C.M., Spak, D.K., and Spalding, J.W., 1985, Induction of hepatic cell proliferation and unscheduled DNA synthesis in mouse hepatocytes following in vivo treatment, Carcinogenesis, 6:1521-1524.

Mirsalis, J.C., 1987, In vivo measurement of unscheduled DNA synthesis and S-phase synthesis as an indicator of hepatocarcinogenesis in rodents, Cell. Biol. Toxicol., 3:165-173.

Mitchell A.D., and Mirsalis, J.C., 1984, Unscheduled DNA synthesis as an indicator of genotoxic exposure, In: "Single-Cell Mutation Monitoring Systems, " A.A. Ansari and F.J.DeSerres, eds., Plenum Publishing Corp.,New York (1984).

National Toxicology Program, 1987, Toxicology and carcinogenesis studies of 1,4-dichlorobenzene in F344/N rats and B6C3F1 mice, Technical Report Series No. 319.

Steinmetz, K.L., Tyson, C.K., Meierhenry, E.F., Spalding, J.W., and Mirsalis, J.C., 1986, Examination of genotoxicity, toxicity, and morphologic alterations in hepatocytes following in vivo or in vitro exposure to methapyrilene, in preparation.

Tyson, C.K., and Mirsalis, J.C. 1985, Measurement of unscheduled DNA synthesis in rat kidney cells following in vivo treatment with genotoxic agents, Environ. Mutagen., 7:889-899.

Ware, R.A., Burkholder, P.M., and Chang, L.W., 1975, Ultrastructural changes in renal proximal tubules after chronic organic and inorganic mercury intoxication, Environ. Res., 10:121-140.

Working, P.K., and Butterworth, B.E., 1984, An assay to detect chemically induced DNA repair in rat spermatocytes, Environ. Mutagen., 6:273-286.

IN VITRO AND IN VIVO HgCl$_2$-INDUCED NEPHROTOXICITY ASSESSED BY TUBULAR ENZYMES RELEASE

J.C. Cal, D. Nerlet and J. Cambar

Groupe d'Etude de Physiologie et Physiopathologie Renales Faculté de Pharmacie, Bordeaux, France

INTRODUCTION

The assessment of the nephrotoxicity in clinical practice, as in experimental setting, was based largely on the determination of changes in haemodynamic parameters and electrolytes excretion. However, the acute tubular necrosis involved in many forms of toxic nephropathy is frequently detected and quantified by the evaluation of the urinary activity of marker enzymes form various segments of the nephron. Enzymuria has been shown to be an early and are much a more sensitive index of tubular damage than haemodynamic or electrolyte changes (Price, 1982).

Similarly, the rapid development of renal cell cultures can be used to better defined morphological and biochemical aspects of nephrotoxicity, and offers the potential to study the mechanisms of chemically related injury in target cell in vitro (Bach et al., 1985). Extrapolation between animals and man, and from the in vitro to in vivo has still not been adequately defined in terms of the renal response to a nephrotoxicant in these different systems. We have assessed the release of marker enzymes for the proximal tubule in urine of rats given a sublethal dose of mercuric chloride and in the culture medium of human renal cells exposed to HgCl$_2$ as the first part of investigation into multi-species and in vivo - in vitro comparisons.

MATERIALS AND METHODS

For in vivo studies, 24 male Wistar rats (200-220g) were housed in individual metabolism cages in a sound-attenuated, temperature and light controlled room (12 hr light:dark cycle) and fed ad libitum. After a 10-day standardization period, they were given a single i.p. injection of 1, 2 or 3 mg Hg/kg of HgCl$_2$ or of distilled water. The urines were collected at 6-hr intervals during 5 consecutive days, 3 days before and 2 days after intoxication. So as to assess renal function, sodium, potassium, urea and creatinine were assayed by conventional methods. Gamma-glutamyltransferase (GGT) and alkaline phosphatase (AlP), two brush border marker enzymes, and N-acetyl-ß-D-glucosaminidase (NAG), a lysosomal marker, were assayed by colourimetric procedures using Boerhinger Nannheim kits.

For in vitro studies, fresh human cortical tissue (morphologically normal portions from cancer kidneys) was cut into 1 mm and digested with collagenase for 1 hr at $37^{\circ}c$ with stirring agitation. Proximal tubular cells were harvested from sequential filtering through a series of steel meshes. They were collected on the 25 Ìm mesh, resuspended in Hank's solution and plated in culture flasks (10^6 cells/ml), and grown in a mixture of Dulbecco's modified Eagle's medium and Ham's F12 (1:1) medium supplemented with insulin (1 U/ml), penicillin (100 U/ml), streptomycin (100 ug/ml), 5% foetal calf serum, and HEPES buffer (10 mM). Confluent monolayers were exposed to 5, 10, 20 or 50 ug Hg/ml as $HgCl_2$ for 6 or 24 hr. At the end of the exposure period GGT and AlP were assayed in the culture medium, as indicated previously. Enzyme activities were calculated as nmoles of substrate hydrolysed per minute and per mg of total intracellular proteins. Proteins were assayed by Lowry's method. Statistical analysis was carried out using a multivariate analysis (in vivo) or a two way analysis of variance (in vitro) and Newman-Keuls multiple range test for group comparisons.

RESULTS AND DISCUSSION

The dose-effect relationship in $HgCl_2$-induced renal cell injury was demonstrated both in vivo and in vitro. Indeed, enzymuria in rat greatly increased whatever the marker enzyme, up to 25-fold the control values for GGT after 1 mg Hg/kg (Hotelling-Lawley trace: 5.188; $F_{(4,28)} = 18.16$; $p < 0.001$). The classical renal. function tests confirmed these findings, but only from 18 hr after $HgCl_2$ dosing (these changes included a decrease in the urinary excretion of creatinine, urea, etc.). In vitro, though the enzyme release was less important than in vivo, the loss of brush border enzymes in the culture medium was statistically significant. Enzyme activity was highest for GGT (up to 4-fold the physiological release when cells were exposed to 5 ug/ml for 24 hours - Fig. 1). In both in vivo and in vitro systems GGT appeared to be the most sensitive of the assayed marker enzymes. This very good correlation is consistent with the fact that the main proximal tubular segment affected by $HgCl_2$ is the pars recta which is the richest in GGT (Guder and Ross, 1984). Similarly, with regard to the dose-effect relationship in both models, it is of interest to note that the lowest toxic dose involved the highest increase in enzymes release whatever the marker enzyme. Never-the-less, during the first hours after intoxication, in vivo, or during the smaller exposure period (6-hr) in vitro, the highest loss of enzymes occurred in groups given the intermediate toxic doses: 10 ug/ml for GGT and AlP, in vitro; 2 mg/kg in vivo as shown by the kinetics of excretion of GGT (Fig. 2). These findings are in accordance with our knowledge of $HgCl_2$ nephrotoxicity since the sublethal doses are known to induce a focal necrosis with tubular obstruction and tubuloglomerular feedback leading to oligo-anuria (see 3mg/kg, Fig. 2) and death. Cell necrosis is accompanied by a protein synthesis inhibition and thus by the observed decrease in enzyme release in vitro (Fig. 1). Though the tubular obstruction induced by the highest doses of $HgCl_2$, in vivo, is a limitation in our attempt to correlate in vivo and in vitro observations in enzymes leakage from the renal epithelium, the findings of this study show that in vitro results compare very favourably with in vivo ones. Finally, certain points warrant emphasis:-

a) This comparative study between cytotoxicity of mercuric chloride in vivo and in vitro has been made possible by the culture of proximal tubular cells having retained many differentiated and specific functions as shown by the special increase in GGT release following cells exposure to $HgCl_2$.

b) The dynamics of the toxic processes should reveal very similar mechanisms of toxicity in the cell culture system and in the rat kidney.

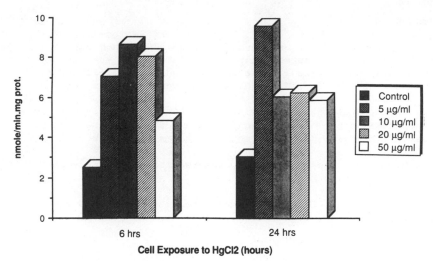

Fig. 1. GGT activity in human cell culture medium at the end of a 6-hr or a 24-hr exposure span to HgCl$_2$.

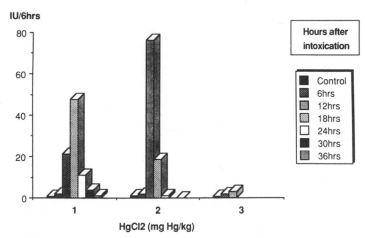

Fig. 2. GGT activity per 6-hr sample in Wistar rat urine after a single ip injection of HgCl$_2$.

c) In emphasizing the extrapolation of the information gained in our in vitro model to in vivo setting, one should notice the absence of significant interspecies differences since the response of human renal tubular cells to HgCl$_2$ was very similar to that of whole rat kidney.

d) An important limitation of the culture model should be, however, pointed out even if it was unclear in our studies i.e. the lack of contribution of the other systems of the live animal to the development of the renal resistance to toxic injury and, among these, the hormonal system or the liver.

e) Such good a correlation between in vitro and in vivo results in metal nephrotoxicity is in agreement with recent report by Batzer and Aggarwal (1986) on the platinum derivatives toxicity.

REFERENCES

Bach, P.H., Ketley, C.P., Benns, S.E., Ahmed, I., and Dixit, M., 1985, The use of isolated and cultured cells in nephrotoxicity - Practice, potential and problems, In: "Renal Heterogeneity and Target Cell Toxicity", P.H. Bach and E.A. Lock, eds., J. Wiley & Sons, New York, pp. 505.

Batzer, M.A., and Aggarwal, S.K. , 1986, An in vitro screening system for the nephrotoxicity of various platinum coordination complexes. A cytochemical study. Cancer Chemother. Pharmacol., 17:209.

Guder, W.G., and Ross, B.D., 1984, Enzyme distribution along the nephron, Kidney Int., 26:101.

Price, R.G., 1982, Urinary enzymes, nephrotoxicity and renal disease, Toxicology, 23:99.

PREVENTION AND REVERSAL OF MERCURIC CHLORIDE-INDUCED INCREASES IN RENAL VASCULAR RESISTANCE BY CAPTOPRIL

Z.H. Endre, L.G. Nicholls, P.J. Ratcliffe and J.G.G. Ledingham

Nuffield Department of Clinical Medicine, University of Oxford, John Radcliffe Hospital, Oxford, UK

INTRODUCTION

By inducing ischaemia, changes in renal vascular resistance (RVR) may contribute substantially to the extent of nephrotoxic injury. The in vitro perfused rat kidney (IPRK) allows changes in RVR to be monitored precisely following nephrotoxin exposure. Mercuric chloride causes dose-dependent increases in RVR in filtering perfused rat kidneys (1). We have examined the prevention and/or reversibility of these alterations in RVR by hydralazine, verapamil and captopril.

METHODS

Right kidneys from Wistar rats (300-400 g) were perfused at $37^{\circ}C$ at a cannula tip pressure of 85-110 mm Hg with Krebs bicarbonate buffer supplemented with amino acids, 5 mmol/l glucose and 6.7 g/dl albumin (1). Perfusate flow rate (F) and tip pressure (P) were monitored throughout and RVR (mm $Hg.min.ml^{-1}$) measurements calculated from P/F. Renal function was monitored from ^{14}C inulin clearance and urinary Na and K excretion. At the end of each experiment, kidneys were fixed for morphological examination by perfusion with 2.5% glutaraldehyde.

Mercuric chloride dissolved in Krebs buffer, 0.22 um filtered and warmed to $37^{\circ}C$, was added to the perfusion circuit after 60 min of baseline perfusion. In experiments using hydralazine, verapamil or captopril, these were added to a given concentration at 60 min and mercuric chloride was added at 75 min. The perfusion was then continued for a total of 180 min.

RESULTS

The addition of 2 mg/dl (final concentration) mercuric chloride caused a slow progressive increase in RVR over the following 120 min of perfusion. RVR increased by an average of 25% from an initial value of 2.0 ± 0.6 (SD) mm $Hg.min.ml^{-1}$ (Fig. 1). The overall increase in RVR averaged 300%, 120 min following 8 mg/dl mercuric chloride. However, at this higher dose there was an acute transient increase in RVR of much larger magnitude (Fig. 2). A typical experiment showing changes in perfusion flow rate and mean perfusion pressure following 8 mg/dl chloride is illustrated in Fig. 3. In this experiment, perfusion pressure was increased progressively from 85 mm Hg to 170 mm Hg following mercuric chloride in order to restore

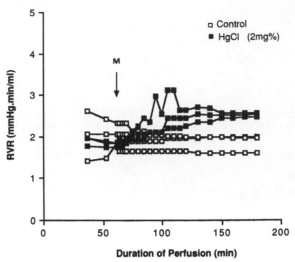

Fig. 1. Effect of $HgCl_2$ on renal vascular resistance (mm $Hg.min.ml^{-1}$) following low dose (2 mg/dl) mercuric chloride.

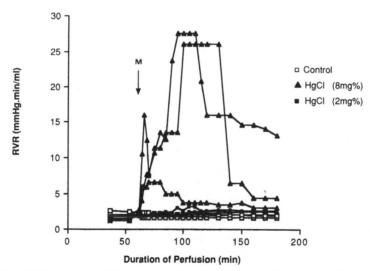

Fig. 2. Effect of $HgCl_2$ on renal vascular resistance following high dose (8 mg/dl) mercuric chloride. (NB. Figure actually shows both 2 and 8 mg/dl).

flow. Additional spontaneous recovery of perfusate flow occurred while holding the perfusion pressure constant at the higher level.

Preperfusion with 1 mg/ml captopril completely prevented the acute rise in RVR following high dose mercuric chloride and reduced the final extent of increase in RVR at 120 min to 160% of the baseline value (Fig. 4). When given 10 min after 8 mg/dl mercuric chloride, captopril rapidly reversed the acute rise in RVR. Neither acute nor progressive changes in RVR following 8 mg/dl mercuric chloride were prevented by either verapamil (7 mg/dl) or hydralazine (44 mg/dl).

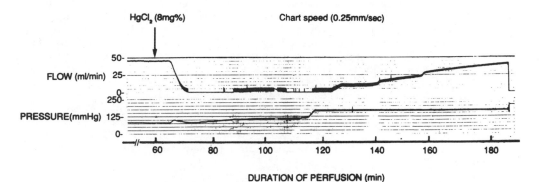

Fig. 3. Typical IPRK experiments following addition of 8 mg/dl mercuric chloride (at 60 min). perfusion flow rate is recorded in The upper panel and mean perfusion pressure measured at the cannula tip is recorded in the lower panel. Perfusion pressure was held constant by a servo control mechanism. The pressure was increased manually from 85 mm Hg in the interval between 75 and 115 min and then held constant at 170 mm Hg.

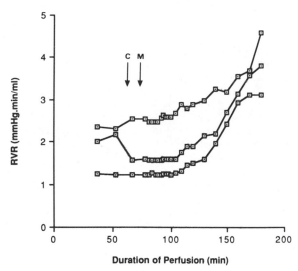

Fig. 4. Prevention of acute increase in RVR by captopril (100% mg) followed by HgCl$_2$ (8 mg%). Note that while the acute rise is completely abolished, the slow progressive background increase in RVR remains.

DISCUSSION

Mercuric chloride appears to cause two distinct patterns of increase in RVR. Both high (8 mg/dl) and low (2 mg/dl) doses produce an irreversible and progressive "background" increase of limited magnitude. High doses (8 mg/dl) result in more elevated RVR after 120 min of perfusion than the lower dose. However, in addition, high doses produce a transient and very large increase in RVR which is both preventable and reversible by captopril but not the other vasoactive drugs tested. Experiments in the non-filtering kidney exclude a direct vascular effect of the mercuric chloride (2).

The dose of captopril required to prevent the acute rise in RVR (1 mg/ml) is well above the dose required to block circulating angiotensin converting enzyme (10 ug/ml). Other experiments have demonstrated that enalaprilat (1 mg/ml) does not prevent the acute rise, while addition of glutathione to the perfusion medium has a protective effect similar to captopril.

These results suggest that captopril prevents the acute rise in RVR following high dose mercuric chloride by direct binding of mercuric ions through its free SH group. These experiments suggest a possible role for captopril as an excretable ligand and as a sulphydryl group donor during heavy metal intoxication.

Circulating mercuric ions bound to captopril or glutathione do not promote the acute increase in RVR. The mechanism of this acute reversible increase in RVR is not known. However, irrespective of the actual mechanism (eg tubuloglomerular feedback), these experiments suggest that it is triggered by the reversible binding of renal tubular sulphydryl groups at the luminal cell surface.

REFERENCES

1. Z.H. Endre, P.J. Ratcliffe, L.G. Nicholls, J.G.G. Ledingham, J.D. Tange and G.K. Radda, ^{31}P NMR studies of mercuric chloride nephrotoxicity in the in vitro perfused rat kidney, (this Symposium).

2. P.J. Ratcliffe, Z.H. Endre, L.G. Nicholls, J.D. Tange and J.G.G. Ledingham, The isolated perfused rat kidney: filtering and non-filtering models in the assessment of altered renal vascular resistance in nephrotoxicity, (this Symposium).

REGIOSELECTIVE ACUTE TUBULAR NECROSIS IN RENAL CORTICAL SLICES FOLLOWING

$HgCl_2$ and $K_2Cr_2O_7$: LOCALIZATION AND TRANSPORT STUDIES

C.E. Ruegg, A. J. Gandolfi and K. Brendel

Department of Pharmacology and Toxicology, University of Arizona, Tucson, AZ 85724 USA

INTRODUCTION

Recently, the selective necrosis of renal convoluted (CPT) and straight proximal tubules (SPT) following administration of $K_2Cr_2O_7$ and $HgCl_2$, respectively, has been reproduced in renal cortical slices (Ruegg et al, 1987a). This demonstrates that the toxicity of these two metals results from the innate sensitivity of these segments of the nephron to the specific metal and is not a result of altered blood flow or feed-back mechanisms. The question remains as to why these nephron segments are specifically intoxicated. Is it the result of a specific uptake and localization of the metals in the intoxicated cells?

The idea of determining the localization and specific transport of these two metals is not new. Autoradiographic studies have shown that radio-labelled $HgCl_2$ is localized at the cortical medullary junction (Berlin and Ullberg, 1963) and the renal concentration and toxicity of $HgCl_2$ is linked to glutathione levels (Berndt et al, 1985). While there are no published localization studies following $K_2Cr_2O_7$ intoxication, Berndt (1976) determined that the accumulation of chromate within the kidney occurred by an active transport process but did not identify the carrier.

The positional cortical slices offer a system where the in vivo toxicity of these metals can be reproduced and specific cells or cell groups examined. Hence, localization and transport studies were undertaken to determine if the metals are specifically transported and concentrated within the injured cell types.

METHODS

$HgCl_2$ and $K_2Cr_2O_7$ (analytical grade) were obtained from Sigma Chemical Company, St Louis, MA). Precision-cut, positional cortical slices were prepared from NZW rabbits (Ruegg et al, 1987b). Slices were incubated in a Krebs-Ringers-HEPES buffer in an open slice support system gassed with O_2/CO_2 (95:5) at room temperature. The decrease in intracellular K^+ was used as an indicator of toxicity (Ruegg et al, 1987a). The tissue distribution of free sulphydryls was examined using a modified methyl orange thiol stain (Mescon and Flesch, 1952). The cellular localization of Hg ion was detected using the silver amplification of mercury-selenide complexes (Danscher and Moller-Madsen, 1985). Chromium localization within

thin sections from slices incubated with $K_2Cr_2O_7$, was detected using electron probe elemental analysis on a Jeol JEM-100CX II transmission electron microscope (Moreton, 1981).

The effect of $HgCl_2$ and $K_2Cr_2O_7$ on steady state accumulation (40 min) of organic acid (^{14}C-PAH) and organic base (^{14}C-TEA) after exposure to the metals was performed as previously described (Hassall et al, 1983). To identify if $K_2Cr_2O_7$ was gaining access to the cell via the organic acid or base transport system, slices were incubated in the presence of increasing concentrations of $K_2Cr_2O_7$ and a fixed concentration of either ^{14}C-PAH or ^{14}C-TEA and the kinetic uptake of PAH or TEA measured (Ruegg et al, 1987c). Probenecid and quinine were used as positive controls to indicate the inhibition of PAH and TEA transport, respectively. Since $K_2Cr_2O_7$ exists mainly as CrO_4^{2-} at physiological pH, the effect of increasing concentrations of structurally similar anions, PO_4^{2-} and SO_4^{2-}, on $K_2Cr_2O_7$-induced positional renal slice toxicity (intracellular K^+) was examined. The effect of increasing concentrations of $K_2Cr_2O_7$ on the uptake of SO_4^{2-} or PO_4^{2-}, into the renal slices was used as an indicator of common uptake mechanism via either of these transport processes (Ruegg et al., 1987c). The uptake of $HgCl_2$ before or after complexing with either cysteine or glutathione was monitored using gamma counting.

Data gathered from different experiments under the same conditions were pooled and compared to concurrent control values by analysis of variance (ANOVA) for statistical differences ($p < 0.05$).

RESULTS

Localization: The selective SPT and CPT injury induced by $HgCl_2$ and $K_2Cr_2O_7$, respectively, could be a result of selective uptake mechanisms for these metals by the respective cell types. Although, an even staining with methyl orange was observed throughout the cells of the slices, indicating a uniform distribution of tissue sulphydryl groups, positional cortical slices exposed to 100 uM $HgCl_2$ for 8 hr had Hg ion localized in the SPT segments (mostly in the nuclei) as detected by the silver deposits of the mercury-selenium complexes. The CPT, collecting ducts, and ascending thick limbs had only background levels (Figure 1). Chromium was detected within the nuclei of the CPT by electron probe microanalysis. Chromium was not detected within the cytoplasmic compartment of CPT or within nuclei of collecting ducts.

Effect of $HgCl_2$ and $K_2Cr_2O_7$ on PAH/TEA Transport: Steady state accumulations of PAH and TEA were inhibited by both $HgCl_2$ and $K_2Cr_2O_7$ in a time and dose-dependent manner (Figure 2). To investigate whether $HgCl_2$ or $K_2Cr_2O_7$ gained access to the renal tubules via the PAH or TEA transport systems, competition for the uptake rate of the organic acid/base was examined (Table 1). The results indicate that the metals did not use these transport systems since accumulation factors did not decrease in the presence of increasing metal concentrations.

Transport of $HgCl_2$ by Sulphydryl Complexes: The presence of nonprotein sulphydryl compounds, cysteine and glutathione, in varying concentrations had no effect on the rate of uptake of $HgCl_2$ (Table 2), indicating that $HgCl_2$ gains access to the SPT independent of the glutathione or cysteine carrier systems.

Effect of SO_4^{2-} and PO_4^{2-} on $K_2Cr_2O_7$, Toxicity and Transport: At physiological pH $K_2Cr_2O_7$, exists as CrO_4^{2-} (Berndt, 1976), which is structurally similar to SO_4^{2-} and PO_4^{2-}. Hence competition studies were performed to determine if either SO_4^{2-} or PO_4^{2-} could alter the toxicity or uptake of $K_2Cr_2O_7$. Neither a 100-fold excess of SO_4^{2-} or 1000-fold

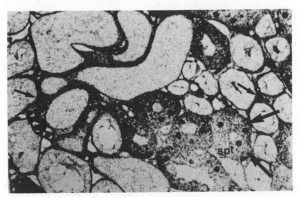

Figure 1. Silver amplification of mercury-selenide complexes in renal cortical slices following in vitro exposure to 100 uM $HgCl_2$ for 8 hr. Note selective accumulation of silver within the SPT and interstitial spaces (arrows).

Table 1. Effect of $HgCl_2$ and $K_2Cr_2O_7$ on the Kinetic Accumulation of PAH and TEA in Positional Renal Cortical Slices.

	Accumulation Factor Slice ^{14}C substrates: Medium ^{14}C substrates			
	Slice H_2O		Medium H_2O	
	PAH	TEA	PAH	TEA
Control	3.90±0.63	4.56±1.16		
Probenecid (200 uM)	0.88	3.85		
Quinine (1 mM)	1.83	0.82		
$HgCl_2$ or $K_2Cr_2O_7$	($HgCl_2$)		($K_2Cr_2O_7$)	
0.1 uM	3.30	3.70	3.42	5.60
1 uM	3.86	3.98	4.69	5.31
10 uM	4.01	5.97	5.16	5.16
100 uM	6.88	3.33	4.57	4.60

Values represent the accumulation factor of the organic substrate (at 10 uM) measured at 20 min. Values represent the mean of 2 slices from two independent experiments except the controls which are the mean±SD for 4 slices.

Table 2. Effect of Glutathione and Cysteine on the Uptake of $HgCl_2$ into Positional Renal Cortical Slices.

	$HgCl_2$ Accumulation Factor at Sulphydryl Concentrations (uM) [a]			
Sulphydryl Compound	0	1	10	100
Cysteine	10.5	11.5	8.1	8.5
Glutathione	10.8	11.3	8.0	6.4
SH/$HgCl_2$ Ratio		1:10	1:1	10:1

a $HgCl_2$ concentration was 10 uM. Incubations were for 40 min. Each value represents the mean of two slices from a single experiment.

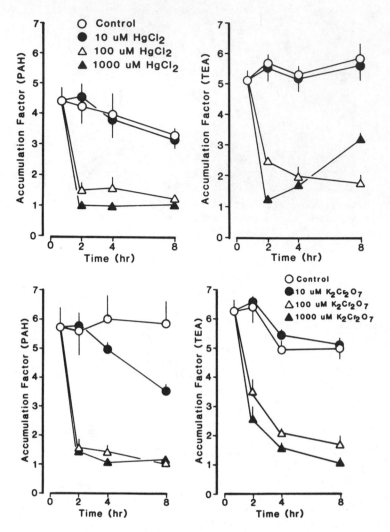

Figure 2. Inhibition of PAH and TEA transport in renal cortical slices following in vitro exposure to $HgCl_2$ and $K_2Cr_2O_7$. Each point represents the mean±SD of 4 slices.

excess of $PO_4{}^{2-}$ altered the decrease in intracellular K^+ caused by 100 uM $K_2Cr_2O_7$ (Table 3). However, the toxicity was examined over a 4 hr incubation and may be the result of an early accumulation of $K_2Cr_2O_7$. Therefore, short-term accumulation studies of $SO_4{}^{2-}$ and $PO_4{}^{2-}$ were undertaken. Increasing concentrations of $K_2Cr_2O_7$ inhibited the accumulation of $SO_4{}^{2-}$ dramatically (Figure 3), while having much less of an effect on the uptake of $PO_4{}^{2-}$.

DISCUSSION

These studies indicate that there is a selective accumulation of the metals in the nephron segments that they intoxicate. Mercuric ion was only found in the straight proximal tubule even though there is a rather uniform distribution of the sulphydryl content throughout the positional cortical slice. Detectable chromium accumulation was only found in the

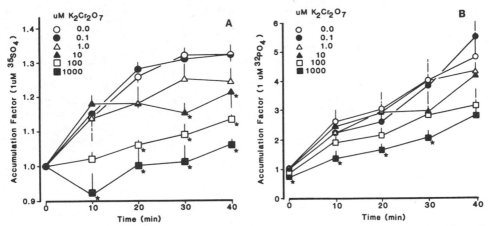

Figure 3. Effect of increasing $K_2Cr_2O_7$ concentrations on the kinetic uptake of SO_4^{2-} (A) and PO_4^{2-} (B) into positional cortical slices. Each point represents the mean±SD of 4 slices from two independent experiments.

Table 3. Effect of Sulphate and Phosphate on the Toxicity of Chromate in Positional Renal Cortical Slices

	K^+/DNA (nmol/ug) [a]	
Additions	Control	plus 0.1 mM $K_2Cr_2O_7$
Sulphate		
0.02 mM	27±3	14±1
0.5 mM	33±5	18±2
10 mM	42±1	16±4
Phosphate		
0.01 mM	35±3	13±2
1.0 mM	36±1	17±1
100 mM	34±2	12±1

a = Determined 4 hr after incubation. Values are the mean±SE (n = 4).

nuclei of the convoluted proximal tubules. The rationale for the high concentration in the nuclei remains to be established.

Although both $HgCl_2$ and $K_2Cr_2O_7$ inhibited the steady state accumulation of PAH and TEA, neither compound appeared to be taken up by these transport processes. Therefore other mechanisms of uptake were examined. Since the addition of exogenous non-protein sulphydryls can mediate the renal toxicity of $HgCl_2$ and decrease the renal Hg content (Berndt, 1985), the effect of adding sulphydryl compounds was tested in the positional slice system. excessive amounts of either cysteine or glutathione did not alter the uptake of Hg into the slices indicating that Hg-sulphydryl complexes do not facilitate transport. Thus the selective uptake mechanism of Hg ion into the SPT remains unknown. Since $K_2Cr_2O_7$ exists primarily as CrO_4^{2-} at physiological pH, the possible transport of this ion via systems with similar structures, SO_4^{2-} and PO_4^{2-}, was examined. Although increasing concentrations of either SO_4^{2-} or PO_4^{2-} did not protect against the loss of intracellular K^+ following exposure to 100 uM $K_2Cr_2O_7$, kinetic accumulation of SO_4^{2-} was reduced in a dose-dependent manner by increasing concentrations of $K_2Cr_2O_7$ while PO_4^{2-} was less effected. The observation that sulphate uptake plateaued by 30 min may indicate that $K_2Cr_2O_7$ accumulates quickly within the slice, which may explain why the toxicity of $K_2Cr_2O_7$ could not be blocked by excess SO_4^{2-} over an extended time course. To our knowledge, this is the first experimental evidence for the interactions of CrO_4^{2-}, SO_4^{2-} and PO_4^{2-} in the kidney.

This research demonstrates that the injury to specific regions of the proximal tubules relates to an innate susceptibility of the intoxicated cell type to accumulate the toxicant, independent of physiological feedback or blood delivery patterns proposed as mechanisms of selective injury from in vivo studies.

ACKNOWLEDGEMENTS

Supported by Johns Hopkins CAAT and NIH GM 328290.

REFERENCES

Berlin M and Ullberg S. Accumulation and retention of mercury in the mouse. I. An autoradiographic study after a single intravenous injection of mercuric chloride. Arch Environ Health 6:589-601, 1963.

Berndt WO. Renal chromium accumulation and its relationship to chromium-induced nephrotoxicity. J Toxicol Environ Health 1:449-459, 1976.

Berndt WO, Baggett JM, Blacker A and House M. Renal glutathione and mercury uptake by kidney. Fund Appl Toxicol 5:832-839, 1985.

Danscher G and Moller-Madsen B. Silver amplification of mercury sulfide and selenide: A histochemical method for light and electron microscopic localization of mercury in tissue. J Histochem Cytochem 33:219-228, 1985.

Hassall CD, Gandolfi AJ, Brendel K. Effect of halogenated vinyl cysteine conjugates on renal tubular active transport. Toxicology 26:285-294, 1983.

Mescon H and Flesch P. Modification of Bennett's method for the histochemical demonstration of free sulfhydryl groups in skin. J Invest Dermatology 17:261-266, 1952.

Moreton RB. Electron-probe x-ray microanalysis: Techniques and recent applications in biology. Biol Rev 56:409-461, 1981.

Ruegg CE, Gandolfi AJ, Brendel K, Nagle FB. Differential Patterns of injury to the proximal tubule of renal cortical slices following in vitro exposure to mercuric chloride, potassium dichromate, or hypoxic conditions. Toxicol Appl Pharmacol, in press, 1987a.

Ruegg CE, Gandolfi AJ, Brendel K, Nagle RB, and Krumdieck CL. Preparation of positional renal slices for study of site-specific toxicity. J Pharm Methods 17:111-123, 1987b.

Ruegg CE. Mechanisms underlying regioselective acute tubular necrosis of renal proximal tubular segments. Doctoral Thesis, University of Arizona, 1987c.

IN-VIVO BONE LEAD MEASUREMENTS AND RENAL EFFECTS

H.J. Mason*, L.J. Somervaille+, D.R. Tennant*, D.R. Chettle+, M.C. Scott+

*Health and Safety Executive, London, and +Department of Physics, University of Birmingham, Birmingham, U.K.

INTRODUCTION

Reports that both chronic and acute exposure to lead (Pb) could cause nephropathy were first published in the middle of the last century. Recent epidemiological, clinical and biochemical studies still suggest that excessive Pb uptake can be related to renal disease or dysfunction (1,2). The ubiquitous nature of Pb in the modern environment and the number of workers occupationally exposed to the metal suggest that an understanding of the dose-effect relationships is important. However the relationships between various parameters of functional or morphological changes in the kidney, the development of clinical renal disease and estimates of the Pb dose still remain unclear.

A number of studies have used blood Pb measurements or the EDTA mobilization test as indices of dose. Blood Pb levels reflect recent or current exposure and therefore a single measurement is of little value in assessing chronic or cumulative Pb uptake. The EDTA mobilization test has been shown to provide an index of the mobile, and possibly more toxicologically active, portion of total Pb body burden. However the various inputs from body compartments (soft-tissue, bone etc.) to the measured chelated urine lead are ill-defined. Furthermore this test, which involves intramuscular injection of EDTA and collection of timed urine samples, is invasive and requires medical facilities. An alternative index of Pb burden is the concentration of Pb in bone since skeletal Pb constitutes over 90% of Pb in the body and has a long half-life. This can be measured by in-vivo X-ray fluorescence (IVXRF) of the tibia (3) and has been shown to correlate closely with cumulative Pb exposure (4). The use of a transportable IVXRF system allows comparatively rapid, non-invasive measurements of Pb dose to be made with minimum inconvenience to the subjects.

We have presently made over 200 in-vivo bone lead measurements of occupationally Pb exposed subjects in the UK together with an assessment of blood lead levels and a range of biochemical markers of various organ systems. Preliminary analysis of the data has allowed identification of four subgroups of male workers. These have been selected to reflect differences in either chronic exposure or recent exposure to Pb as defined by tibia and blood Pb levels respectively. We report here results of a range of renal function parameters within subgroups.

POPULATION AND METHODS

Seventy-two occupationally Pb exposed males, between the ages of 21 and 65 were stratified into four subgroups according to their tibia and blood Pb levels (i.e. high or low tibia Pb, and high or low blood Pb). A few individuals are common between high Pb subgroups and similarly between the two low Pb subgroups. The subjects were selected so that age distributions in subgroups (A) and (B) in subgroups (C) and (D) were similar.
Thus:-

Subgroup A: High tibia Pb, mean 103 ug/g mineral bone   n = 21
Subgroup B: Low tibia Pb, mean   20 ug/g mineral bone   n = 21
Subgroup C: High blood Pb, mean 61 ug/dl   n = 26
Subgroup D: Low blood Pb, mean   26 ug/dl   n = 26

Subgroup A: mean age = 48;   Subgroup B: mean age = 47;   Subgroup C: mean age = 41;   Subgroup D: mean age = 40.

The in-vivo measurement technique uses a Cd-109 gamma ray source to fluorescence K-shell X-rays from Pb in the cortical mid-shaft of the tibia. The measurement is self-normalising for overlying tissue and bone geometry by using coherently scattered gamma rays from the calcium and phosphate of the bone itself. The measurement sensitivity for tibia Pb is approximately 18 ug/g bone mineral for a very small radiation dose of 100 uSV (10 mrem) to a 1.5 kg section of the leg. The whole body dose equivalent of this irradiation is about 3 uSV (0.3 mrem). In-vitro comparisons with the atomic absorption spectrometry have shown it to be accurate to about 1 ug/g bone mineral.

Blood samples and a spot urine sample were taken from each subject on the same day as in-vivo tibia measurements were made, and a detailed health questionnaire completed.

Blood and urine lead concentrations were measured by atomic absorption spectrometry using electrothermal atomization. Measurements of aminolaevulinic acid (ALA), free erythrocyte protoporphyrin (FEP), phosphate, calcium, urate, total protein (TP), albumin (ALBU), retinol binding protein (RBP) and creatinine were performed using our routine laboratory methods. Urinary kallikrein levels were measured using D-valyl-cyclohexylalanyl-arginine-4-nitroanilide as substrate in phosphate buffer pH 9.1. 1,25-Dihydroxyvitamin D was measured using a commercially available assay system (Immuno Inc., USA).

Urine results were expressed per mmol of creatinine, to reduce the effect of renal diuresis on measured analyte concentrations. Fractional excretion indices of calcium and urate were calculated as the ratio of analyte clearance to creatinine clearance. A Phosphate Excretion Index (PEI) was calculated according to the formula of Fraser and McIntyre (5).

RESULTS AND DISCUSSION

Means for the measured variables within the four subgroups are shown in Table 1. Levels of significance for differences between subgroups (A) and (B) and between subgroups (C) and (D) are indicated.

Two variables often used to monitor the haemopoetic effect of Pb, FEP in blood and urinary ALA, showed expected significant increases in both the high tibia lead (A) and high blood lead (C) subgroups compared to their respective low exposure subgroups (B) and (D).

No increase in total proteinuria or in the excretion of the specific proteins (albumin and retinol binding protein) was detected in either the high chronic Pb exposure subgroup (A) or high recent exposure subgroup (C) relative to their corresponding low exposure subgroups (B) and (D). There was no evidence of a deleterious effect on glomerular filtration rate, as estimated by plasma creatinine, as a result of higher chronic or acute Pb exposure. Similarly the renal tubular handling of calcium and phosphate did not appear to be altered in the subgroups with increased blood Pb levels (C) or high tibia Pb burden (A).

The fractional excretion of urate was significantly decreased in high blood Pb subgroup (C) relative to (D) suggesting an inverse relationship between blood Pb and the fractional excretion of urate. The significant negative correlation found between fractional excretion of urate and blood Pb ($r = -0.261$, $p = 0.028$) in all 72 subjects substantiates this. Interestingly this decrease in the renal clearance of urate relative to creatinine clearance was not reflected in significantly higher serum urate levels in subgroup (C). However in subgroup (A) serum urate levels were significantly increased compared to the low tibia subgroup (B) but differences in the fractional excretion of urate failed to reach statistical significance between these subgroups. Again there was a significant correlation between serum urate and tibia Pb ($r = 0.264$, $p = 0.025$) in all 72 workers. Pb-induced decreases in uric acid excretion, either as a result of decreased tubular secretion or increased reabsorption, have been reported previously by Emmerson (6). It has also been reported that Pb increases uric acid production (7). Data from this study appears to support the concept that Pb may affect both urate synthesis and renal handling and that this may depend on the chronic or current nature of the Pb exposure.

Renal kallikrein is excreted in the distal tubules. It appears to be involved in the regulation of water and electrolyte transport by the distal nephron although its definitive role in the regulation of blood pressure or in the pathogenesis of hypertension is unclear. Several reports have suggested a decreased urinary excretion of kallikrein in subjects occupationally exposed to Pb. Our data confirm these findings but only in those workers with high chronic exposure (subgroup A), however there is no difference between groups (C) and (D) despite the difference in tibia lead levels. Thus further study of renal kallikrein and prostaglandin synthesis in chronic Pb exposure may be important (8).

The hormone 1,25-dihydroxyvitamin D, which is centrally involved in the regulation of calcium homeostasis, is synthesised from 25-hydroxyvitamin D by the activity of a renal mitochondrial hydroxylase enzyme. Significant increases in serum 1,25-dihydroxyvitamin D were found in both the subgroups with high tibia and high blood Pb (Table 1). These findings are substantiated by the significant positive correlations between the circulating hormone levels and both blood Pb ($r = 0.443$, $p = 0.0006$) and tibia Pb ($r = 0.379$, $p = 0.004$) (Figure 1). This appears to contrast with the recent occupational study of Greenberg et al (9) who found no effect of Pb on 1,25-dihydroxyvitamin D and the work of Rosen et al (10) who found a negative correlation between Pb and this hormone in children. However the latter may be due to the increased susceptibility of children to the toxic effect of Pb, proximal tubular dysfunction being more common in Pb intoxicated children than in adults. It is difficult to compare the degree of lead body burden in Greenberg's 38 subjects to this population, although a similar tibia Pb X-ray fluorescence technique was used. Tibia Pb levels were greater than 30 ug/g wet weight (equivalent to 54 mg/g bone mineral) with a mean blood Pb of 32 14 ug/dl in 58% of his study group.

TABLE 1. COMPARISON OF GROUP MEANS

	GROUP A High Tibia Pb		GROUP B Low Tibia Pb		GROUP C High Blood Pb		GROUP D Low Blood Pb	
	n	mean	n	mean	n	mean	n	mean
Glucose (U) (umol/mmol creatinine)	21	30.0	21	33.1	26	84.4	26	28.0
Creatinine (S) (umol/l)	21	102.1	21	103.8	26	100.3	26	106.5*
Urate (S) (umol/l)	21	378.4	21	334.6**	26	356.8	26	345.7
Phosphate (S) (umol/l)	20	1.19	18	1.17	23	1.19	23	1.22
TP (U) + (mg/mmol creatinine)	21	3.5	21	3.3	26	4.4	26	3.1
ALBU (U) + (mg/mmol creatinine)	21	0.49	21	0.51	26	0.67	26	0.50
RBP (U) + (ug/mmol creatinine)	19	5	20	7	19	6	20	6
Fract. Excr. Urate	21	8.38	21	9.60	26	7.61	25	9.79**
Fract. Excr. Calcium	21	1.81	21	1.47	26	1.60	25	1.89
Phosphate excretion index	17	0.034	18	0.0067	19	0.015	22	0.039
1,25 Vitamin D (ng/l)	16	44.9	17	34.3**	20	44.3	20	35.0**
Kallikrein (U) (IU/mmol creatinine)	16	0.076	19	0.115**	19	0.10	24	0.09
Haemopoetic/Lead Exposure Indices								
Tibia Pb (ug/g bone mineral)	21	103.3	21	19.8**	26	75.8	26	20.4**
Blood Pb (ug/dl)	21	57.7	21	32.1**	26	61.2	26	26.1**
Urine Pb (ug/mmol creatinine)	21	10.7	21	3.8**	26	10.7	26	2.7**
Haemoglobin (g/dl)	21	14.7	20	15.3	26	15.0	23	14.9
FEP + (ug/dl)	21	106	20	14.0**	26	122.0	23	15.0**
ALA + umol/mmol creatinine)	20	4.7	21	2.0**	25	4.8	26	2.2**

* significant at 5% level.
** significant at 1% level.

(U) = Urine; (S) = Serum
+ = Log transformed variable, geometric mean shown

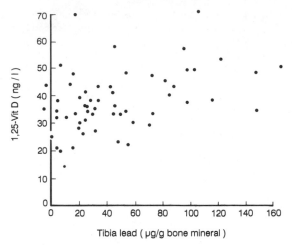

Fig. 1.   Correlation between 1,25-dihydroxyvitamin D and tibia lead

Thus it is feasible that a proportion of our study population had higher
recent and/or long-term exposure.

Although Pb nephropathy has been recognized for many years in those with
high exposure, it is apparent that changes in renal function can be
detected at the modest exposure levels currently experienced in the
occupational field.   The use of in-vivo bone lead measurements will allow
description of dose-effect models related to low level chronic
accumulation;   such data may not be obtainable using other indicators of
Pb dose or from animal studies.

REFERENCES

1.   W.M. Bennett, Lead nephropathy, <u>Kid. Int</u>., 28:212 (1985)

2.   W.C. Cooper, O. Wong and L. Kheifets, Mortality among employees of
battery plants and lead producing plants 1947-1980, <u>Scand. J. Work
Environ. Health</u>, 11:331 (1985).

3.   L.J. Somervaille, D.R. Chettle and M.C. Scott, In-vivo measurement of
lead in bone using X-ray fluorescence, <u>Phys. Med. Biol</u>., 30:929 (1985).

4.   L.J. Somervaille, D.R. Chettle, M.C. Scott, D.R. Tennant, M.J.
McKiernan, A. Skilbeck and W.N. Trethowan, In-vivo tibia lead measurements
as an index of cumulative exposure in occupationally exposed subjects,
<u>Brit. J. Ind. Med</u>., In press, (1987).

5.   R. Fraser and I. MacIntrye, Disorders of bone and calcium metabolism,
<u>In</u>: "Biochemical disorder in human disease", R.H. Thompson, I.D. Wootton,
ed. Churchill, London (1970).

6.   B.T. Emerson, W. Mirosch and J.B. Douglas, The relative contribution
of tubular reabsorption and secretion of urate excretion in lead
nephropathy, <u>N. Z. J. Med</u>. 4:353 (1971).

7.   J.L. Granick, S. Sassas and A. Kappas, Some and clinical aspects of
lead intoxication, <u>Adv. Clin. Chem</u>., 20:289 (1978).

8.   R.   Lauwerys,   A.   Bernard, Early detection of nephrotoxic effects of industrial chemicals: state of the art and future prospects, <u>Am. J. Ind</u>. <u>Med</u>., 11:275 (1987).

9.   A.   Greenberg,   D.K.   Parkinson,   D.E. Fetterolf, J.B. Puschett, K.J. Ellis, L. Wielopolski, A.N. Vaswani, S.H. Cohn and P.J. Landrigan, Effects of elevated lead and cadmium burdens on renal function and calcium metabolism, <u>Arch. Environ. Health</u>, 41:69 (1986).

10.   J.F.   Rosen,   R.W.   Chesney,   A.J.   Hamstra,   H.F.   DeLuca, and K.R. Mahffey,   Reduction in 1,25-dihydroxyvitamin D in children with increased lead absorption, <u>N. Eng. J. Med</u>., 302:112 (1980).

EARLY INDICATORS OF LEAD NEPHROPATHY

F. Khalil-Manesh,* H. C. Gonick,* E. Weiler,* V. Rosen,* L. Roche,* A. Mutti,** E. Bergamaschi,** R. Alinovi,** and I. Franchi**

Departments of Medicine/Nephrology*, Trace Elements Lab., Cedars-Sinai Med. Center and UCLA School of Medicine, Los Angeles, CA, USA, and Universita degli Studi di Parma**, Italy

INTRODUCTION

Detection of early lead nephropathy in industrial workers has been difficult, particularly as albuminuria is absent until late stages of the disease (1). Changes in serum creatinine and blood urea nitrogen (BUN) have proved to be relatively insensitive indices of renal impairment in individual workers, although epidemiological studies in large numbers of workers have indicated a statistically significant increase in both parameters with length of exposure to lead, even when corrected for age (2). Furthermore, Wedeen (1) demonstrated that lead workers with normal serum creatinine and BUN values may have subtle renal impairment, as indicated by a reduction in glomerular filtration rate (GFR) and abnormal renal biopsies.

It was the purpose of the present study to determine in an animal model of lead toxicity whether selected urinary enzymes and/or immuno-assayable brush border antigen might serve as early indicators of lead nephrotoxicity. Several urinary enzymes, derived from renal tubular cytoplasm, or proximal tubular brush border, have been proposed as markers of tubular injury. Of these substances, the lysosomal enzyme, N-acetyl-ß-D-glucosaminidase (NAG), has been successfully employed in several clinical situations (e.g., acute renal failure, renal transplant rejection) (3). Glutathione-S-transferase (GST), a component of ligandin also appears in the urine following tubular injury, but selectively reflects chemical injury rather than ischaemic injury (4). Renal shedding of proximal tubular brush border antigen (BBA) measured by specific monoclonal antibodies in an ELISA assay, has already proved to be a useful marker of tubular injury in groups of subjects exposed to or treated with cadmium, cisplatin, chromium, mercury, and hydrocarbons (5).

The animal model of lead nephrotoxicity has been based on prior studies by Goyer et al (6,7), in which animals were given 1% lead acetate in drinking water. The principal modifications were a reduction in lead concentration to 0.5% and the use of a semi-purified diet, shown to enhance the sensitivity of the rat to lead intoxication (8). At different time intervals after exposure, urinary excretion of NAG, GST and BBA in experimental animals and pair-fed controls were correlated with whole blood, plasma, and urinary lead values, true serum creatinine chromogen, iothalamate clearance (as an index of GFR) and renal pathology.

METHODS

<u>Animals:</u>   Male Sprague-Dawley rats were fed a semi-purified diet (ICN Pharmaceuticals, Ohio) and given 0.5% lead acetate in their drinking water beginning at eight weeks of age.   Experimental animals were pair-fed with their counterpart controls. Four groups of animals (n = 11 in each group) were studied: I) one month control (C1);   II) one month experimental (EC1);   III) three month control (C3);   IV) three month experimental (EC3).

<u>Pathology:</u>   Kidneys were excised, blot dried, weighed and 1-2 mm slices were dissected out and fixed for electron and light microscopy.   Electron microscopy staining was performed with uranyl acetate and lead citrate; light microscopy sections cut thin (3um) and stained with hematoxylin and eosin.

<u>Determination of Glomerular Filtration Rate:</u>   GFR was assessed indirectly by measurement of serum true creatinine chromagen according to the method of Polar and Metcoff (9).   A more precise measure of GFR was afforded by employing the single injection iothalamate clearance technique (10). Clearances are expressed as ml/min/100 g body weight.

<u>Urine Collection and Analysis:</u>   Urine samples were collected in chilled containers and aliquots removed and frozen until required.   Urinary creatinine and NAG activity were measured colourimetrically (11, 12) and GST was determined by the method of Feinfeld et al (4).   Enzyme activity for all procedures was expressed per g creatinine.   Appearance of brush border membranes in urine was determined by ELISA as described by Mutti et al (13).

<u>Ultrafiltration of Plasma</u>   Plasma samples were filtered through Amicon membranes with molecular weight exclusion of 50 K daltons. Filtrates were collected in plastic tubes and their lead contents were determined.

<u>Determination of Lead in Blood and Urine:</u>   Lead determinations were performed in duplicate on whole blood, urine, and plasma, using an atomic absorption spectrophotometer (Perkin Elmer, Model #305, with graphite furnace).

<u>Statistical Analysis:</u>   Comparisons between experimental and control groups were performed by unpaired t-test. Correlations were calculated by method of least squares.

RESULTS

<u>Pathology</u>   EC1 kidneys showed no differences from control animals except for the appearance of some nuclear inclusion bodies in both the proximal convoluted tubules and pars recta.   EC3 kidneys demonstrated enlargement of proximal convoluted tubules with nucleomegaly (Fig. 1).   Nuclear inclusion bodies were wide-spread.   Tubules were irregularly dilated with spotty and patchy atrophy.   Glomeruli appeared relatively normal with the exception of mesangial thickening in some glomeruli of EC3 animals.

When compared to control rats (Fig. 1C), proximal tubules of EC1 kidneys revealed nucleomegaly, with nuclei containing dense small frequently lobulated inclusion bodies exhibiting peripherally radiating spikes (Fig. 1A).   There were some dilated cisterns of endoplasmic reticulum and increased lysosomes, with associated crowding of mitochondria away from the base of the cell toward the nucleus.   Mitochondria were rounded and showed irregular and angular arrangement of cristae.   Occasional cells

120

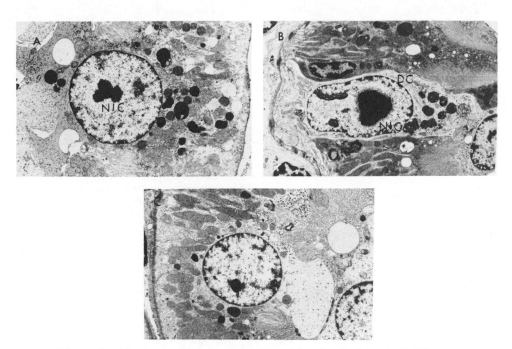

Fig. 1 Electron microscopy of proximal tubules (X 5400)
A. EC1 lead-exposed; B. EC3 lead-exposed and C. C3 control

NIC=Nuclear inclusion body DC=Degenerated cell without brush border
between two relatively normal cells.

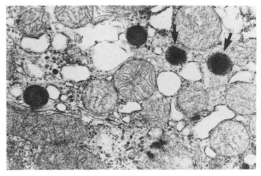

Fig. 2 Electron microscopy of proximal tubules of ECI lead exposed
animals (X 28,500). Arrows point to intracytoplasmic inclusion bodies.
Note rounded mitochondria with irregular cristae.

exhibited centrally dense, peripherally fuzzy bodies, consistent with
cytoplasmic lead inclusions (Fig. 2). Proximal tubules of EC3 animals
demonstrated extremely large nuclear inclusion bodies within large oval
nuclei, interspersed necrotic cells with pyknotic nuclei and loss of brush
borders (Fig. 1B). Mitochondria showed increased density as compared to
EC1 kidneys; changes in the cristae were similar to EC1.

Glomerular filtration rate Differences in GFR between experimental and
control groups were not statistically significant but there was a trend

121

toward increased GFR in EC3 (1.00 ± 0.14 ml/min/100 g body weight in EC3 vs. 0.83 ± 0.26 in C3; p = 0.054). A relative increase in GFR in the EC3 rats was supported by parallel decreases in serum creatinine in EC3 as compared to C3 (1.05 ± 0.16 mg/dl in EC3, vs. 1.24 ± 0.26 in C3; p = 0.031). A positive correlation was also noted between blood lead and GFR in the experimental animals (Fig. 3).

Blood and Urine Analyses   Plasma lead ranged between 1.0 and 4.1 ug/dl in EC1 and EC3, with no differences between groups, and was below the limits of detection in C1 and C3. The ultrafilterable plasma lead was less than 10% of total plasma lead in EC1 and EC3. Lead concentration in blood and urine of both the EC1 and EC3 animals were significantly increased as compared to their respective control groups (Fig. 4), with higher values noted in EC3 than EC1 animals.

Urinary NAG and GST enzyme activities and BBA excretion are shown in Fig. 5. Urinary enzymes and BBA values were not increased in EC1 as compared to C1. However, all three parameters increased significantly in EC3 animals (NAG 191 ± 87 um MNP/h/g creatinine in EC3 vs. 75 ± 24 in C3, p < 0.001; GST, 5.05 ± 4.92 units/g creatinine in EC3 vs. 1.31 ± 0.21 in C3, p = 0.027; BBA, 0.321 ± 0.293 OD/g creatinine in EC3 vs. 0.116 ± 0.024 in C3, p = 0.032).

When urine lead was plotted against urinary NAG in both experimental groups (Fig. 6), there was a significant positive correlation (r = 0.834, p < 0.001). Similar correlations were also observed between urine lead and GST (r = 0.832, p < 0.001).

DISCUSSION

There are several stages in the development of lead nephropathy in rats fed lead in their drinking water. Goyer et al (6,7) found that when rats were given 1% lead acetate in drinking water the earliest evidence of lead effect was the formation of nuclear inclusion bodies in the proximal tubules. Within the first 20 weeks the animals developed aminoaciduria associated with swollen proximal tubule lining cells and alterations in mitochondrial structure and function. Later there was a diminution in the number of proximal tubular inclusion bodies in association with tubular dilatation and atrophy and interstitial fibrosis. These observations in experimental animals were paralleled by the findings in renal biopsy samples from industrial workers exposed to lead for variable time periods. Cramer et al (14) showed that of five biopsied workers, with industrial exposure between 6 weeks to 20 years, two individuals with exposure less than one year had nuclear inclusion bodies and abnormal appearing mitochondria on electron microscopy, but relatively normal light microscopy appearance. Biopsies from the other three workers with exposure of 4, 10 and 20 years did not have nuclear inclusion bodies, but showed significant peritubular and interstitial fibrosis.

Goyer and coworkers (6,7) demonstrated that the nuclear inclusion bodies are composed of lead bound to a 28 K dalton protein, postulating that the nuclear inclusion bodies segregate lead in a non-toxic form with the net effect of maintaining a relatively low and thus less toxic cytoplasmic concentration of lead. Other investigators have demonstrated the presence of three classes of lead-binding proteins (11.5 K daltons, 63 K daltons, and > 200 K daltons) in the rat kidney cytosol (15-17).

A number of investigators have indicated that albuminuria and/or low molecular weight proteinuria and glycosuria are not seen in the early stages of lead nephropathy, although accurate measurements of GFR may reveal abnormally low values (1,13). It is, therefore, essential to

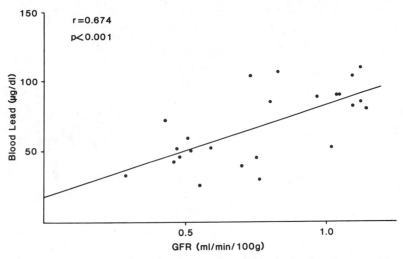

Fig. 3 Correlation of blood lead level and GFR in lead-exposed animals

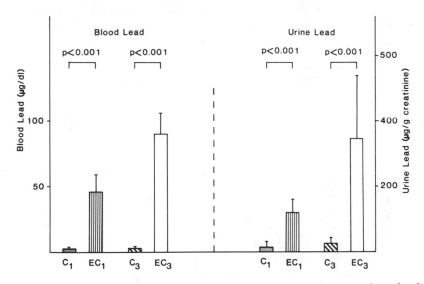

Fig. 4 Blood and urine lead in lead-exposed and control animals

develop alternative, sensitive indices of early tubular injury that might be applicable to a nephrotoxin such as lead. In the present study, GFR did not change in the EC1 animals, but there was a trend toward an increase in the EC3 animals; the change in GFR was found to correlate positively with blood lead values. Kidneys from these animals were also hypertrophied and some glomeruli demonstrated thickening of the mesangium. These findings parallel observations in two other experimental models of nephropathy, namely diabetic nephropathy (18) and the subtotal nephrectomized model (19), in which glomerular hyperfiltration has been postulated as the initiating event in the production of both glomerular and tubular damage.

Proximal tubules of kidneys from both EC1 and EC3 experimental animals showed an abundance of nuclear inclusion bodies, increasing in size and

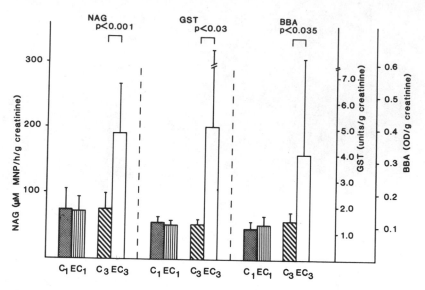

Fig. 5 NAG, GST and BBA in lead-exposed and control animals.

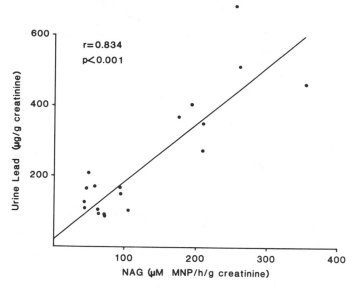

Fig. 6 Correlation of urinary lead and NAG in lead-exposed animals.

number with duration of exposure. Although these large numbers of nuclear inclusion bodies would be anticipated to store lead in a non-toxic form (6,7,15-17), perhaps accounting for the relative paucity of tubular degenerative changes, there were some proximal tubules in EC3 which showed necrotic changes with loss of brush border. These early alterations in tubular morphology were reflected by increased urinary NAG and GST activities in combination with shedding of BBA into the urine. Changes in enzymes or BBA excretion were not found in the EC1 animals, whose proximal tubules were virtually intact. Of major interest was the observation that urinary lead excretion correlated positively with these markers of tubular injury. It is unlikely that the increased urinary lead excretion in

experimental animals reflected increased glomerular filtration of lead as
the majority of plasma lead (> 90%) was found to be non-filterable (i.e.,
bound to proteins > 50 K daltons), and there was relatively little
variation in total plasma lead among the experimental groups. These data
suggest that urinary lead may also serve as a sensitive index of early
tubular injury rather than providing information about total body burden
of lead. Whether urinary lead represents the shedding of lead-containing
tubular debris or an alteration in renal tubular handling of lead remains
to be demonstrated.

ACKNOWLEDGEMENTS

The authors gratefully acknowledge the secretarial assistance of Beverly
Gil and Ruby McCarty, and the technical assistance of Cathy Agness and
Michael Paya. This work was supported by a generous grant-in-aid from
the International Lead Zinc Research Organization.

REFERENCES

1. B. P. Wedeen, D. K. Mallik, and V. Batuman, Detection and treatment
of occupational lead nephropathy, Arch. Int. Med. 139:53 (1979).

2. R. Lilis, J. Valcinkas, A. Fishbein, et al, Renal function impairment
in secondary lead smelter workers: Correlations with zinc protoporphyrins
and blood lead levels, J. Environ. Pathol. Toxicol. 2:1447 (1979).

3. J. M. Wellwood, B. G. Ellis, R. G. Price, et al, Urinary N-acetyl-ß-
D-glucosaminidase activities in patients with renal disease, Br. Med. J.
3:408 (1975).

4. D. A. Feinfeld, J. J. Bourgoignie, G. Fleischner, et al, Ligandinuria
in nephrotoxic acute tubular necrosis, Kidney Int. 12:387 (1977).

5. A. Mutti, S. Lucertini, P. P. Valcari, et al, Urinary excretion of
brush-border antigen: early indicator of toxic nephropathy, Lancet
8461:914 (1985).

6. R. A. Goyer, The renal tubule in lead poisoning. I. Mitochondrial
swelling and aminoaciduria, Lab. Invest. 19:71 (1968).

7. R. A. Goyer, Lead and the kidney, Curr. Top. Pathol. 55:147 (1971).

8. A. A. Mylorie, L. Moore, B. Olyai, et al, Increased susceptibility to
lead toxicity in rats fed simplified diets, Environ. Research 15:57
(1978).

9. E. Polar, and J. Metcalf, True creatinine chromagen determination in
serum and urine by semi-automated analysis, Clin. Chem. 11:713 (1965).

10. C. W. Bryan, R. C. Jarchow, and J. Maher, Measurement of glomerular
filtration rate in small animals without urine collection, J. Lab. Clin.
Med. 89:845 (1972).

11. R. W. Bosnes and H. H. Tanssky, On the colorimetric determination of
creatinine by the Jaffe Procedure, J. Biol. Chem. 158:581 (1945).

12. C. T. Yuen, P. R. Kind, R. G. Price, et al, Colorimetric assay for N-
acetyl-glucosaminadase in pathological urine using the W-nitristyoyl
substrate, Ann. Clin. Biochem. 21:295 (1984).

13. A. Mutti, S. Lucertini, M. Farnari, et al, Urinary excretion of

brush-border antigen revealed by monoclonal antibodies in subjects occupationally exposed to heavy metals, Proc. Intern. Conf. on Heavy Metals in the Environment, 1:565 (1985).

14. K. Cramer, R. A. Goyer, R. Jagenburg, et al, Renal ultrastructure, renal function, and parameters of lead toxicity in workers with different periods of lead exposure, Br. J. Indust. Med. 31:113 (1974).

15. A. Oskarsson, K. S. Sqiubb, and B. A. Fowler, Intracellular binding of lead in the kidney: The partial isolation and characterization of post-mitochondrial lead binding components, Biochem. Biophys. Res. Commun. 104:290 (1982).

16. P. L. Goering and B. A. Fowler, Regulation of lead inhibition of delta-aminolevulinic and acid dehydratase by a low molecular weight, high affinity renal lead-binding protein, J. Pharmacol. Exper. Ther. 231:66 (1984).

17. P. Mistry, G. W. Lucier, and B. A. Fowler, High affinity lead-binding proteins in rat kidney cytosol mediate cell-free nuclear translocation of lead, J. Pharmacol. Exp. Ther. 232:462 (1985).

18. T. H. Hostetter, H. G. Rennke, B. M. Brenner, The case for intrarenal hypertension in the initiation and progression of diabetic and other glomerulopathies, Am. J. Med. 72:375 (1982).

19. T. H. Hostetter, J. L. Olson, H. G. Rennke, et al, Hyperfiltration in remnant nephrons: A potentially adverse response to renal ablation, Am. J. Physiol. 241:F85 (1981).

NEPHROTOXICITY OF URANYL FLUORIDE AND REVERSIBILITY OF RENAL INJURY IN THE RAT

G.L. Diamond, P.E. Morrow, B.J. Panner, R.M. Gelein, and R.B. Baggs

Environmental Health Science Center, University of Rochester, Rochester, New York 14642, U.S.A.

INTRODUCTION

Recent accidental exposures of workers and members of the public to uranium hexafluoride (UF_6) releases have reinforced interest in the nephrotoxic properties of uranium compounds (1). Additionally, a large industrial work force is engaged in several types of uranium production operations in which intermittent exposures frequently occur. Despite recent improvements in our understanding of the toxicology and biokinetics of uranium, there remain several important issues for which there are virtually no occupational or experimental data. Foremost of these issues is the time course and extent to which nephrotoxic actions of uranyl uranium are reversible, particularly after exposures at or near the so-called threshold for injury of 3 ug U/g kidney (2-5). More-over, better procedures for detecting uranium-induced renal injury need to be identified, particularly for injury associated with exposure to occupationally relevant uranium compounds. The objective of the present study was to examine severity and duration of renal injury produced in the rat from exposures to low levels of uranyl fluoride (UO_2F_2).

METHODS

Animals. Specific pathogen- and viral antibody-free male rats (Crl:LE-BR, SPF-VAF) weighing 120 g were obtained from Charles River Portage Facility (Portage, MO). Rats were housed individually in stainless steel metabolic cages located within a barrier facility. A total of 71 rats were randomly assigned to an euthanasia schedule within a control group (n = 18), a low dose group (n = 18), a high dose group (n = 18) or health surveillance group (n = 17).

Uranium Injections. Sterile (ultrafiltered) solutions of UO_2F_2 (4) were prepared in isotonic sodium chloride (60 and 120 ug. U/ml). Rats in the low dose group received five injections at a dose level of 60 ug U/kg body wt, followed by three injections at a dose level of 120 ug U/kg body weight. The high dose group received five injections of 120 ug U/kg, followed by three injections of 240 ug U/kg (Figure 1).

Observation Protocols. Observations of rats in the control, low dose and high dose groups began 9 days prior to the first injection of UO_2F_2 and continued for 110 days. Rats from the health surveillance, control, low

127

dose and high dose groups (n = 2) were euthanized at selected times during the observation period for histopathology and determination of uranium in kidney. Rats in the surveillance group were subjected to a complete necropsy, including routine histologic examination of lung, liver, heart, kidney, adrenal, gastrointestinal tract, pancreas, brain, thymus, lymph nodes, salivary gland and spleen. Tracheal washing was performed using aseptic technique for isolation of respiratory bacterial pathogens (i.e. S. pneumonia, C. kutscheri, P. pneumotropica, Mycoplasma sp.). Faecal specimen was examined for ova and parasites, pelt was examined for ectoparasites and serum was tested for viral antibodies (Microbiological Associates, Rodent Screen).

Analytical. Uranium in injection solutions and in kidney was quantified by plasma emission spectroscopy. Concentrations of uranium above 0.05 İg/ml (0.5 ug U/g dry kidney) were reliably measured. Urinary enzymes (LDH, lactate dehydrogenase; AST, aspartate aminotransferase; NAG, N-acetyl-ß-D-glucosaminidase; GGT, gamma-glutamyltransferase; AP, alkaline phosphatase0 and protein, and plasma and urinary osmolality, creatinine, glucose and alpha-amino nitrogen were determined as previously described (6).

RESULTS

Kidney Uranium Burden. Mean uranium content of the kidney is shown in Figure 1 as a function of time during and after administration of UO_2F_2. The highest uranium burden was observed 3 days after the last injection of UO_2F_2' thereafter, renal uranium declined to less than 10% of observed peak levels within 21 days after the last uranium injection (day 54 of the experiment). The decline in uranium levels in kidney involved at least two distinct first order kinetic components. A rapid component occurred with a T1/2 of 1.5-2.5 days and a slow component, involving approximately 10% of the renal burden, occurred with T1/2 of 50-60 days. Uranium was not detected in kidneys of the control group.

Kidney Function and Urine Composition. Total solute content of the urine, as reflected by urine osmolality, was relatively constant during and after exposure to UO_2F_2. However, output of certain specific solutes was transiently elevated. This is illustrated for glucose (Figure 2) and LDH (Figure 3) which showed the greatest magnitude of response of solutes that were examined (Table 1). Fractional excretion of glucose and alpha-amino nitrogen was substantially elevated in high dose rats, reaching highest values 7 days after exposure to UO_2F_2. Creatinine clearance and plasma concentrations of glucose and alpha-amino nitrogen in exposed rats were not different from controls, confirming impairment of tubular reabsorption of these solutes. Urinary excretion of total protein and albumin was elevated in the high dose group during and after exposure to UO_2F_2 (Table 1). Excretion of brush border enzymes, GGT and AP appeared to decrease in the high dose group relative to the control group (Table 1).

Histopathology. Histology of kidneys from control rats at every sacrifice was normal as assessed by light microscopy. Kidneys from both low and high dose groups showed slight but definite histological changes at day 19, 3 days after the third injection of UO_2F_2. At this time, changes consisted of vacuolization of distal S2 and S3 segments of the pars recta of proximal tubule, and occurrence of apoptotic cells and apical cellular sloughing in these same segments. Changes were focal and scattered in low dose and more severe in high dose rats. Coinciding with tubular epithelial changes was focal loss of PAS staining of brush borders.

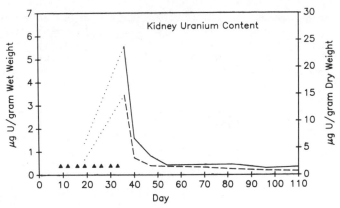

Fig. 1. Kidney uranium content during and after exposure to UO_2F_2. Values shown are mean renal uranium content (n = 2) expressed as ug U/g wet kidney (left) or ug U/g dry kidney (right) for low dose (dashed line) and high doses group (solid link). Solid triangles indicate days on which UO_2F_2 was injected.

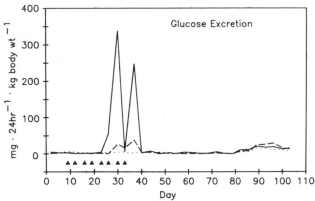

Fig. 2. Urinary excretion of glucose during and after exposure to UO_2F_2. Values shown are means for controls (dotted line), low dose (dashed line) and high dose (solid line) groups. Solid triangles indicate days on which UO_2F_2 was injected.

Table 1. Onset, duration and peak magnitude of functional abnormalities in high dose rats exposed to UO_2F_2.

Urinary Substance	Experiment Day			Peak Magnitude (% of control)
	Onset	Peak	End	
Glucose	30	30	40	7465
Alpha-amino nitrogen	23	37	47	278
Protein	16	30	54	202
Albumin	16	30	44	506
LDH	19	37	44	994
AST	26	30	47	326
NAG	26	30	44	149
GGT	33	37	47	67
AP	37	37	40	72

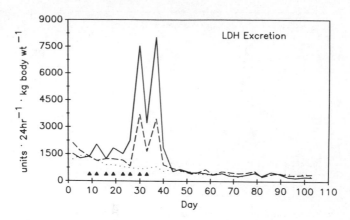

Fig. 3. Urinary excretion of lactate dehydrogenase during and after exposure to UO_2F_2. An enzyme unit is equivalent to one nmole substrate converted per min. See Figure 2 legend for explanation of symbols.

By day 36, three days after the eighth injection of UO_2F_2, injury had progressed to focally severe necrosis and apoptosis of tubular epithelial cells in S3 and, to a lesser extent, in S2 of the low dose rats. Similar but more severe changes were seen in high dose rats with occasional collections of inflammatory cells. Loss of PAS staining in involved segments was now almost complete and was accompanied by a loss of PAS-positive granules. Histological changes were accompanied by increased numbers of mitoses in tubular cells of uranium-treated animals as compared to controls.

Four days later on day 40, 7 days after the eighth injection of UO_2F_2, rats continued to show focally necrotic and apoptotic renal tubular cells in S2 and S3, with small focal inflammatory cell accumulations and focal proliferation of tubular epithelium and regenerative-type low cuboidal cells. Apical brush borders and cytoplasmic granules showed restoration of PAS-positive staining in low dose animals, with only focal failure to stain in the high dose group. At this time, segments of the thick ascending limbs of the loop of Henle exhibited focal necrosis and apoptosis as did rare collecting tubules in the cortex. Mitotic figures were less frequent and no longer increased above controls.

Repair of renal injury had progressed by day 47, 14 days after the eighth injection of UO_2F_2, to the point were only a few dilated segments of pars recta (S2 and S3) and possible increased nuclear size in some tubular epithelial cells were evident. Restoration of PAS-positive staining of brush borders and cytoplasmic granules was complete. Thick ascending limbs of the loop of Henle and collecting tubules were restored. Three weeks after the eighth injection, on day 54, only some possibly enlarged tubular nuclei were seen. Subsequent to day 54, kidneys were essentially normal with only tiny foci of interstitial fibrosis and mononuclear cell infiltrates present in one high dose animal.

DISCUSSION

Uranyl fluoride is the main hydrolysis product of uranium hexafluoride (UF_6) which is used in the industrial production of enriched uranium. Once released into ambient air, UF_6 rapidly hydrolyses to yield UO_2F_2. Thus, UO_2F_2 is the principal form of uranium to which humans are exposed after accidental release of UF_6 gas (1). While human exposure to UO_2F_2 is most likely to occur from inhalation, an injection route was used in the present study. This allowed greater control over absorbed dose for the purpose of exploring relationships between renal uranium levels and severity of nephropathy (4).

A level of renal uranium at 3 ug U/g wet kidney has been proposed as a threshold level for acute renal injury in humans (2,3). In the present study, cellular injury was apparent 3 days after the third injection of UO_2F_2 (day 19), at which time renal uranium burden was 0.7 and 1.4 ug U/g wet tissue in the low and high dose groups, respectively (Figure 1). Injury progressed to relatively severe tubular necrosis (day 36) followed by complete restoration and repair within 35 days after the exposure (day 68). Duration of renal injury in the present study was considerably shorter than that reported elsewhere (4,5) and may reflect the less severe, acute injury produced from the lower exposure level.

Rats in both low and high dose groups showed impaired tubular reabsorption of low-molecular weight solutes, proteinuria and enzymuria which appeared to be related temporally to progression of renal tubular injury. Peak intensity was concurrent with peak severity of tubular necrosis which occurred 3 days after the eighth injection (day 36). Furthermore, changes in renal function were, without exception, greatest in the high dose group, which is also consistent with more severe tubular necrosis in these animals. Considerable variability in the onset of functional changes, peak magnitude and duration of the responses to renal injury is apparent from data presented in Table 1. Tubular injury, as assessed histologically, preceded and persisted beyond the period of certain functional abnormalities.

The results of this study have practical implications for occupational safety and health in the uranium industry. The possibility that the injury threshold in humans is below the proposed 3 ug U/g kidney action level must be seriously considered. This may require development of biological monitoring programs for detecting uranium exposures below 3 ug U/g. Furthermore, use of urinary biochemical endpoints alone has serious limitations for detecting early and late stages of injury from exposures of this magnitude. Timing of evaluation, relative to exposure, is critical if injury is to be detected at all. Finally, an issue that is yet to be addressed is long-term effects of exposures to even low levels of uranium fluoride compounds. Continual release of uranium from bone long after the acute injury phase is over may render individuals more susceptible to injury from later exposures to uranium compounds or other nephrotoxicants.

Values shown are as follows: first day excretion of each substance changed significantly from control, $p < 0.05$ (Onset); day the maximum or minimum value for each parameter was observed (Peak); day each parameter returned to baseline (End) and magnitude of peak response expressed as a percentage of control.

REFERENCES

1. U.S. Nuclear Regulatory Commission, "Assessment of the Public Health Impact from the Accidental Release of UF6 at the Sequoya Fuels Corporation Facility of Gore, Oklahoma, USNRC Report NUREG-1189, Vol. 1, 1986.

2. U.S. Uranium Registry, "Biokinetics and Analysis of Uranium in Man," USUR-05 HEHF-47, 1984.

3. W.L. Spoor and J.N. Hursh, "Protection Criteria," In: Uranium,

Plutonium and Transplutonic Elements, H.C. Hodge, J.N. Stannard and J.B. Hursh, Eds. (Springer-Verlag, New York, 1973), pp. 241-269.

4. P. E. Morrow, L.J. Leach, F.A. Smith, R.M. Gelein, J.B. Scott, H.D. Beiter, F.J. Amato, J.J. Picano, C.L. Yuile and C.T. Consler, "Metabolic fate and evaluation of injury in rats and dogs following exposure to the hydrolysis products of uranium hexafluroide," NUREG/CR-2268, 1981.

5. D.P. Haley, R.E. Bulger and D.C. Dobyan, "The long-term effects of uranyl nitrate on the structure and function of the rat kidney," Virchows. Arch. (Cell Pathol.) 41, 181-192 (1982).

6. R.K. Zalups and G.L. Diamond, "Mercuric chloride-induced nephrotoxicity in the rat: Effect of unilateral nephrectomy and compensatory renal growth," Virchows. Arch. (B. Cell Pathol.), in press.

LOW MOLECULAR WEIGHT PROTEINS IN THE KIDNEY OF COPPER-LOADED RATS

Winston Evering, Susan Haywood and Jim Trafford

Department of Veterinary Pathology, University of Liverpool, P.O. Box 147, Liverpool L69 3BX, England

INTRODUCTION

A high proportion of renal Cu has been identified (Bremner et al., 1977) bound to the LMWP metallothionein in Cu-loaded rats, and to a lesser extent, in Cu-poisoned sheep. Moreover, Cu-MT administered parenterally to rats was found to be excreted efficiently and preferentially by the kidneys, and during dietary supplementation urinary metallothionein (MT) concentrations increased substantially in Cu-loaded rats (Bremner et al. 1978; 1986).

Studies on rats fed a high Cu diet have shown that the metal is apparently excreted from the renal PCT and that temporary degenerative changes are followed by recovery and tolerance to Cu (Haywood 1980; 1985). This apparently protective function of the kidney towards Cu-overload may be associated with either induced renal MT, or a transfer of Cu-MT from the liver to the kidneys (Bremner and Young, 1977). The aim of this work was to attempt to clarify the role of LMWP's in the rat kidney during high Cu-influx and the development of tolerance.

MATERIALS AND METHODS

Male Wistar rats, of uniform age and weight, were fed a high Cu diet: (1g Cu/Kg) for 16 weeks. The rats were killed sequentially and sections of kidney here taken for acid-digestion and histology. Pooled samples were obtained and prepared for chromatography (Mehra and Bremner 1984). Kidney 2 portions for acid-digestion were oven dried at 70°C for 4 days and digested in a mixture (2:1) of nitric and perchloric acid (Haywood, Trafford and Loughran 1985). All digested tissues were subsequently analysed for Cu and Zn by atomic absorption (AA) spectrophotometry.

The pooled kidney samples were homogenised in 2.5 vol 10mM Tris/HCl of pH 7.4 and centrifuged at 35,000xg for 4 hr. The pellets were suspended in 3.5 vol of 1% (v/v) 2-mercaptoethanol in distilled water, freeze-thawed three times and left overnight at 4°C. These samples were then centrifuged for a similar period and their supernatants retained.

The extracts of the soluble and particulate fractions were then chromatographed on sephadex G-75 gel with 10mM Tris/HCl eluant at pH 8.0, and the eluted fractions' absorbance was measured at 280 nm. Their Cu and

Zn content was later determined by AA spectrophotometry.

Formalin fixed blocks were routinely processed and paraffin embedded. Sections of 5-7 um thickness were stained with haematoxylin and eosin (H&E), and Cu was demonstrated histochemically using rubeanic acid and rhodanine stains.

RESULTS

Cu-containing granules and droplets (Fig. 1) were first observed histologically at 4 weeks (167 $\pm$ 17 ug Cu/g) in the cytoplasm of the PCT epithelial cells and in the desquamated cells of such tubules. Necrosis of PCT epithelial cells was most evident at 8 weeks.

Kidney Cu concentrations rose to 449 $\pm$ 89 ug Cu/g (Mean $\pm$ SEM) at 8 weeks and remained unchanged to 16 weeks (Fig. 2). Major and minor absorption peaks in the high and low molecular weight range respectively, were detected in the chromatographic separation profiles of the soluble fractions (Fig. 3). Controls showed the major absorption peaks, however the minor peaks presented as shoulders. The pellet extracts also showed a similar profile, but the fractions corresponding to the minor peaks had higher elution volumes (Fig. 4).

Cu-associated proteins in the cytosolic fractions appeared in both high and low molecular weight bands from 3-16 weeks, achieving maximum levels at 8 weeks (Fig. 3). However, there was a disproportionate concentration of low molecular weight cuproteins (60-70%) in marked contrast to absorptivity. Similar profiles appeared in the particulate fractions, although in much lower concentrations (Fig. 4). Control kidneys showed no significant Cu or Zn associated-LMWP's in either soluble or particulate fractions.

Zn levels remained constant throughout, both with regard to overall concentration and in relative proportions between different soluble and particulate fractions.

DISCUSSION

The important role played by the rat kidney in Cu-overload is indicated by the maintenance of high Cu-concentrations from 8-16 weeks, while the livers of these animals showed maximum Cu values at 5 weeks, after which the Cu levels steadily declined to 16 weeks (unpublished data). The identity and significance of the high molecular weight cUproproteins 'is not known, but they account for the lesser portion of Cu-associated proteins in contrast to the liver (unpublished data).

Cu-associated LMWP's appear to consist of a heavier UV absorbing (280nm) fraction, and a major lighter component which does not absorb at 280nm. Although the chromatographic behaviour of these proteins would imply a molecular weight of about twice that reported for MT (6500 daltons), this protein is known to occur as a prolate ellipsoid which behaves abnormally, in the manner described, during gel filtration (Mehra and Bremner, 1984). It is most probable that the major LMWP component is MT or MT-like polypeptides.

The minor absorption peak showing apparent Cu-association may be the LMWP alpha-2u-globulin (19,000 daltons) found in the male rat kidney (Roy and Neuhaus, 1966). Protein droplets have been incriminated in the pathogenesis of some xenobiotic-induced nephropathies in the male rat, however the extent of their function is unknown. The Cu-staining cytoplasmic bodies observed in this study, identifiable with the hyaline

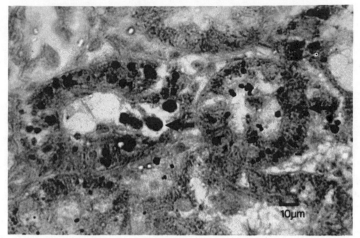

Fig. 1.   Cu-complexes in droplet and granular form are shown in the cytoplasm of the PCT epithelial cells (arrows). Rubeanic acid (Week 8).

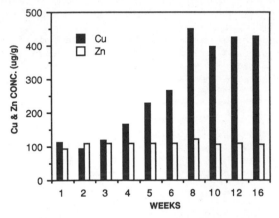

Fig. 2.   Cu concentrations peak at 8 weeks and remain high to 16 weeks. No variation in Zn levels is observed.

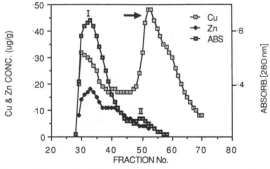

Fig. 3.   Major (I) and minor (II) absorption peaks in the high and low molecular weight range.   Maximum concentration of Cu-associated LMWP's are shown (arrow) from samples after 8 weeks.

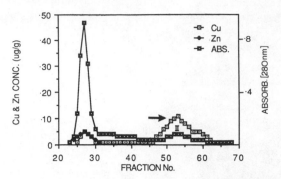

Fig. 4. Minor (II) absorption peak at 8 weeks showing higher elution volume. Cu-associated LMWP's present in low concentrations (arrow).

droplets seen on H&E sections, support the involvement of this protein during Cu-overload.

Constant Zn concentrations associated with increasing Cu content is in marked contrast to gastrointestinal absorption where a mutual antagonism is displayed during wide dietary unbalances of these elements (Cousins, 1985).

Current knowledge concerning alpha-2u-globulin, the role of MT and their respective functions in the detoxification and clearance of Cu during Cu-overload, remains limited. However, it is now reasonable to ascribe an important protective role to LMWP's in the Cu-burdened rat kidney.

ACKNOWLEDGEMENTS

We gratefully acknowledge Dr. I. Bremner of the Rowett Research Institute for his advice and technical assistance. We wish to thank Mrs. M.W. Harling for the histology, Mrs. P. Jenkins for the photography and Mrs. J. Baxter for typing the manuscript.

REFERENCES

I. Bremner, W.G. Hoekstra, N.T. Davies and B.W. Young, Effect of zinc status of rats on the synthesis and degradation of copper-induced metallothionein, Biochem. J. 174:883-892 (1978).

I. Bremner, R.K. Mehra, J.N. Morrison and A.M. Wood, Effects of dietary copper supplementation of rats on the occurrence of metallothionein-I in liver and its secretion into blood, bile and urine, Biochem. J. 235:735-739 (1986).

I. Bremner and B.W. Young, Copper thionein in the kidneys of copper poisoned sheep, Chem.-Biol. Interact. 19:13-23 (1977).

R.J. Cousins, Metabolism of copper and zinc: special reference to metallothionein and ceruloplasmin, Physio. Ren. Am. Physio. Soc. 65:238-309 (1985).

S. Haywood, The effect of excess dietary copper on the liver and kidney of the male rat, J. Comp. Path. 90:213-233 (1980).

S. Haywood, Copper toxicosis and tolerance in the rat I. Changes in copper content of the liver and kidney, J. Path. 145:149-158 (1985).

S. Haywood, J. Trafford and M. Loughran, Copper toxicosis and tolerance in the rat: IV. Renal tubular excretion of copper, Br. J. Exp. Path. 66:699-707 (1985).

R.K. Mehra and I. Bremner, Species differences in the occurrence of copper-metallothionein in the particulate fractions of the liver of copper-loaded animals, Biochem. J. 219:539-546 (1984).

A.K. Roy and O.W. Neuhaus, Identification of rat urinary proteins by zone and immuno-electrophoresis, Proc. Soc. Exp. Biol. Med. 121:894 (1966).

GOLD NEPHROPATHY - EFFECT OF GOLD ON IMMUNE RESPONSE TO RENAL TUBULAR BASEMENT MEMBRANE (TBM) ANTIGEN IN MICE

Shiro Ueda, Yoko Wakashin, Hiromichi Yoshida, Teruo Mori, Yoshio Mori, Ryosaku Azemoto, Makoto Ogawa, Isao Kato, and Masafumi Wakashin

First Department of Internal Medicine, School of Medicine, Chiba University, Chiba, Japan

INTRODUCTION

Renal injuries that follow administration of gold salt in the treatment of rheumatoid arthritis are well recognized (1,2). Changes are seen distributed both in the glomerular and tubular regions studied by light and electron microscopy (1,2). Using guinea pigs, we have reported that injection of gold produces tubulointerstitial nephritis with positive anti-renal tubular basement membrane (TBM) autoantibody and immune complex nephropathy with positive anti-renal tubular epithelial (RTE) autoantibody (3). It is of interest that autoimmune diseases are induced by gold treatment. Measel (4) reported that gold not only had an immunosuppressive effect but also an immunoenhancing effect, depending on dosage. Lando et al. (5) reported that appropriate low doses of cyclophosphamide induce encephalomyelitis in genetically resistant mouse strains, suggesting that low doses cyclophosphamide deletes activity of suppressor T cells. With the assumption that an appropriate dose of gold would have the same effect as cyclophosphamide, we attempted to induce interstitial nephritis (IN) in genetically resistant C57BL/6 (6) mice by pretreatment with gold and immunization with syngeneic TBM antigen in complete Freund's adjuvant. We also studied the effect of gold on immune response to TBM antigen and on development IN in high responder BALB/c mice.

MATERIALS AND METHODS

Animals. Six-week, old inbred mice of two strains, BALB/c and C57BL/6 were purchased from the Shizuoka Laboratory Animal Center (Shizuoka, Japan).

Preparation of Murine TBM Antigen. TBM antigen (Ag) was prepared from normal kidneys from each strain. The purification procedures have already been described (7).

Injection Procedures of TBM Ag and Gold Salt. One hundred mice from each strain were divided into five groups of 20 each. The animals of group 1, 2, and 3 were immunized twice with 50 μg of syngeneic TBM Ag with 0.05 ml of complete Freund's adjuvant (CFA) with a 2-week interval. In groups 2 and 3, in addition to TBM Ag immunization, the animals were injected with 0.01 mg (group 2) or 0.1 mg (group 3) of sodium aurothiomalate (gold) once a week for 4 weeks, starting 1 week before the first TBM Ag immunization.

139

The group 4 animals were given 0.01 mg of gold four times, but were not immunized with TBM Ag. In group 5, the animals were injected with saline and 0.05 ml of CFA without the antigen or gold.

Histological Examination.   Ten animals from each experimental group were sacrificed 8 weeks after the final immunization. Renal tissues were served for routine histological examination by light microscopy. The severity of interstitial changes was graded from 0 to +4 by the degree of mononuclear cell infiltration and tubular damage per cross section of the cortex (0, 0-5%; +1, 5-10%; +2, 10-25%; +3, 25-50%; +4, > 50%).

Direct Immunofluorescent Study of Diseased Kidneys.   Cryostat sections prepared from diseased kidneys were stained with FITC-labelled goat IgG antibody fraction against mouse IgG.

Proliferative Response of Splenic Lymphocytes to TBM Ag.   The spleens were removed from 10 mice of each group 14 days after the final immunization with TBM Ag. Splenic lymphocytes were fractionated on a nylon wool (Fenwal Lab., Morton Grove, IL) column by the method of Julius et al. (8). Using nylon wool non-adherent cells (nonadherent cells), the proliferative response of splenic lymphocytes to TBM Ag in mice immunized with syngeneic TBM Ag was examined. Nonadherent cells ($4x10^5$ viable cells in 200 ml of medium) from mice of each experimental group were cultured in microplate for 5 days with or without 10 pg of syngeneic TBM Ag. One micro-curie of ^{3}H-thymidine was added to each well 16 hr before harvesting with an automated cell harvester with glass fibre fibrosis. Filter disks were removed, placed in scintillation fluid, and the tritium was counted with a Beckman LS-150 liquid scintillation counter. All cultures were carried out in triplicate. Thymidine uptake was expressed as mean cpm and as the stimulation index (SI) as follows: SI = mean cpm with antigen/mean cpm without antigen.

Assessment of In Vivo Effect of Gold on Suppression Activity of Adherent Cells in the Proliferative Response to Non-adherent Cells to TBM Ag.   A preliminary experiment showed T cell fraction in nylon wool adherent cells to have suppressive activity against the proliferative response of non-adherent cells to TBM Ag. Therefore, the suppressive activity from each experimental group was assayed. Nonadherent cells ($4x10^5$ cell in 200 ml of medium) were co-cultured with $1x10^5$ adherent cells under the same conditions as for the monoculture of nonadherent cells. Proliferative responses of the mixed culture were also expressed as stimulation indices, and the suppressive activities of adherent cells were expressed as percentage suppression:

Percentage suppression (PS) =
$$\frac{\text{SI of nonadherent cells culture} - \text{SI of mixed culture}}{\text{SI of nonadherent cells culture}} \times 100$$

Detection and Titration of Anti-TBM Antibody.   Titration of anti-TBM antibody was carried out by enzyme-linked immunosorbent assay (ELISA). Flat-bottom microplates were coated with syngeneic TBM Ag, and 0.2 ml of sample serum diluted 1:1000 with phosphate-buffered 0.15 N NaCl, pH 7.2, containing 0.05% Tween 20 (PBST), was added to each well. After 5 hr of incubation at room temperature, the plates were washed with PBST. Goat anti-mouse gamma-gloholin IgG-peroxidase was diluted 1:1000 with PBST and added to the plates. After overnight incubation, the plates were washed and the amount of peroxidase that bound to the well was determined using 5-aminosalicylic acid as substrate. Reaction was stopped by the addition of 0.05 ml of 1N-NaOH/well after a suitable incubation period at room temperature. The absorbance was measured at 450 nm using a 580 Micro-elisa Auto Reader (Dynatech Inst., Inc., Torrence, CA). A standard curve was obtained using the positive control and its twofold serial dilutions. The titre was calculated by plotting OD on the standard curve. We designated the titre of the positive control to be 200 units (U), and the titres of the samples were accordingly expressed. The specificity of the antisera from the experimental animals was confirmed by indirect immunofluor-escence. The anti-sera was seen to react specifically with TBM of normal kidney (Fig. 1)

RESULTS

Induction of Interstitial Nephritis (IN) in Mice Treated with Gold

Twice immunization with TBM Ag induced typical IN in all BALB/c mice, and mean histological score was +3.5; the main interstitial changes was mononuclear cell infiltration into the interstitium with interstitial fibrosis destruction of TBM and tubules, and periglomerular fibrosis (Fig.1). However, IN was induced in only 10% of C57BL/6 mice. Four weekly injections of 0.01 mg of gold decreased the frequency and the grade of IN in BALB/c mice. The frequency of IN was decreased from 100% to 20% by the gold treatment, and the mean score was lessened from +3.5 to +0.2. The result in treatment with 0.01 mg of gold definitely increased the frequency and the grade of IN in C57BL/6 mice. The frequency increased from 10% to 80%, and the mean score from +0.1 to +2.5 (Table 1). The interstitial changes in C57BL/6 mice were the same as those seen in BALB/c mice immunized with TBM Ag without gold (Fig. 2). Direct immunofluorescent study revealed a linear deposition along TBM of all diseased kidneys in BALB/c and C57BL/6 mice. The effect of gold on the induction of IN in C57BL/6 mice was diminished by an increased dose of gold, namely, 4 injections of gold did not effect significant enhancement of histological damage (Table 1).

Table 1. Effect of gold on induction of IN in mice immunized with TBM Ag.

| | Occurrence of IN (mean histological score) | |
Treated by	BALC/c	C57BL/6
TBM Ag [a] + CPA [b]	10/10 (+3.5)	1/10 (+0.1)
TBM Ag + CFA + Gold [c] (0.04mg)	2/10 (+0.3)	8/10 (+2.5)
TBM Ag + CFA + Gold (0.4 mg)	Not done	2/10 (+0.2)
Gold (0.04 mg)	0/10	0/10
CFA alone	0/10	0/10

a. Each mouse was immunized with 50 ug of syngeneic TBM Ag twice at a two-week interval.

b. Complete Freund's adjuvant (CFA) was injected with TBM Ag or saline.

c. Sodium aurothiomalate (Gold) was injected (0.01 or 0.1 mg/one mouse) once a week 4 times.

Titre of Anti-TBM Antibody in Mice Treated with Gold

Sera were obtained 14 days after the final immunization, and the titre of antibody was assayed by ELISA. Titres of antibody in sera of BALB/c mice were higher than those in C57BL/6 mice when they were immunized with TBM Ag without gold (Table 2). However, when animals were treated with an appropriate dose of gold, the result was in the reverse order. Treatment

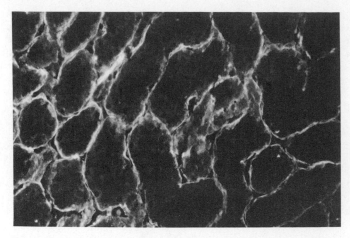

Fig. 1. Immunofluorescent staining of a frozen section of a normal kidney using C57BL/6 anti-C57BL TBM auto-antibody and FITC-labelled anti-mouse IgG. TBM is specifically stained in a linear pattern (indirect staining).

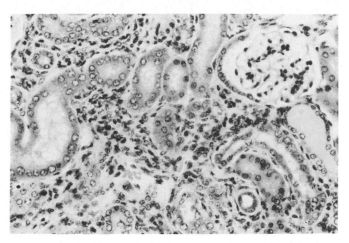

Fig. 2. Photomicrograph of the kidney from a diseased BALB/c mouse treated with TBM Ag without gold, demonstrating typical lesions of interstitial nephritis.

Table 2. Titration of anti-TBM antibody by ELISA

Treated by	Titre of anti-TBM antibody	
	BALC/c	C57BL/6
TBM Ag + CFA	198	105
TBM Ag + CFA + Gold (0.04 mg)	41	226
TBM Ag + CFA + Gold (0.4 mg)	38	87
Gold (0.04 mg)	Not detected	Not detected
CFA alone	Not detected	Not detected

Values are mean units (U) of 10 mice.

142

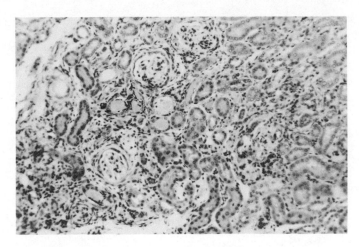

Fig. 3. Photomicrograph of the diseased kidney from a C57BL/6 mouse treated with TBM Ag and gold.

with 0.04 mg of gold increased the titre of sera of C57BL/6 mice from 198 to 226, and decreased that in BALB/c mice from 198 to 41 (Table 2). Anti-TBM antibody was not detected at all in the animals that were injected with gold alone or CFA and saline.

Proliferative Response of Nylon Wool Nonadherent Cells and Suppressive Activity of Adherence Cells In Vitro

The in vitro response of nylon wool nonadherent cells to TBM Ag was examined 14 days after the final immunization. The stimulation index (SI) in BALB/c mice was 8.20 when they were immunized with TBM Ag without gold, and that in C57BL/6 mice was 3.99. The suppressive activity of adherent cells against the proliferative response of nonadherent cells was not strong in BALB/c mice, and that of BALB/c mice was 20% when expressed as percentage suppression (PS). However, the suppressive activity of C57BL/6 mice, low responder to TBM antigen, was very high and PS was about 70% (Table 3). When gold was used, the results of proliferative response were in a reverse order. SI of BALB/c mice was 3.12 when they were immunized with TBM Ag with gold, and that of C57BL mice was 5.14. PS of adherent cells of both strains of mice were decreased by using gold especially in C57BL/6 mice. The PS of adherent cells from C57BL/6 mice was remarkably decreased by treatment with 0.04 mg of gold, to 28% (Table 3).

DISCUSSION

Typical interstitial nephritis (IN) with a strong anti-TBM autoantibody response was consistently induced in genetically resistant C57BL/6 mice by injection of 0.04 mg of gold and TBM Ag. However, the treatment with 0.04 mg of gold alone failed to induce either IN or anti-TBM antibody. The injection of 0.4 mg of gold and TBM Ag could not induce IN and did not have enhancing effect on anti-TBM antibody response in C57BL/6 mice. In contrast, treatment with 0.04 mg of gold had no enhance effect on induction of IN and anti-TBM antibody response in BALB/c mice, but had suppressive effect on them. These results suggest that gold induces pheno-typically different effects in different inbred strains of mouse. When we studied the proliferative response of lymphocytes to TBM antigen by an in vitro culture system, the proliferative response of nylon wool nonadherent cells to TBM Ag was found to be slightly enhanced by in vivo treatment

Table 3. Proliferative response of nylon wool nonadherent cells and suppressive activity of adherent cells in vitro.

PROLIFERATIVE RESPONSE (SI) [a]

Strain/Treated by	Non adherent cell	Non adherent cells + Adherent cells	Percentage [b] Suppression
BALB/c			
1) TBM Ag, CFA	8.20	6.56	20
2) TBM Ag, CFA, Gold (0.04mg)	3.62	3.20	12
3) Gold (0.04mg)	1.42	1.35	5
4) CFA alone	1.01	1.16	-13
C57BL/6			
1) TBM Ag, CFA	3.99	1.17	71
2) TBM Ag, CFA, Gold (0.04mg)	5.14	3.69	28
3) TBM Ag, CFA, Gold (0.4 mg)	2.35	2.20	6
4) Gold (0.04mg)	1.12	1.04	7
5) CFA alone	1.13	1.06	6

a = All samples were obtained 14 days after the final immunization. Proliferative response was expressed as stimulation index (SI). SI = mean cpm with TBM antigen/mean cpm without antigen.

b = Percentage suppression =
$$\frac{\text{(SI of nonadherent cells culture)} - \text{(SI of mixed culture)}}{\text{SI of nonadherent cell culture}} . 100$$

with gold in C57BL/6 mice, and it was suppressed in BALB/c mice. The TBM Agsensitized T cell fraction of nylon wool adherent cells had a suppressive activity on the proliferative response of nonadherent cells to TBM Ag.

This suppressive effect of adherent cells was stronger in resistant C57BL/6 mice and weaker in the susceptible BALB/c mice when gold was not used. The suppression activity of adherent cells was markedly depressed by the treatment with an appropriate dose (0.04 mg) of gold especially in C57BL/6 mice. These results seem to indicate that gold may delete the antigen specific or non-specific suppressor T cells in C57BL/6 mice, and then induce an anti-TBM antibody with high titres and typical IN.

Based on the present study, we able to suggest the existence of helper T cells and suppressor T cells in the immune response to TBM Ag. In high responder BALB/c mice, helper T cells may be superior to the later. On the other hand, in low responder C57BL/6 mice, suppressor T cells may be stronger than helper T cells. Furthermore, gold might depress the activity of all T cells, and the phenotypical effect of gold on immune response to TBM antigen might depend on the dominant T cells population. Therefore, the gold depressed the immune response to TBM antigen in BALB/c mice, in which helper T cells are dominant, and gold enhanced the response in C57BL/6 mice, in which suppressor T cells are dominant.

REFERENCES

1. Lee, J.C., Pushkin, M. and Eyring, E.J. Renal lesions associated with

gold therapy. Light and electron microscopic studies. Arch. Rheum. 8:1-13, 1965.

2. Silverberg, D.S., Kidd, E.G., Shnitka, T.K. and Ulan, R.A. Gold nephropathy. A clinical and pathologic study. Arch. Rheum. 13:812-825, 1970.

3. Ueda, S., Wakashin, M., Wakashin, Y., Yoshida, H., Iesato, K., Mori, T., Akikusa, B. and Okuda, K. Experimental gold nephropathy in guinea pigs: Detection of autoantibodies to renal tubular antigens. Kidney Int. 29: 539-548, 1986.

4. Measel, J.W. Effect of gold on the immune response of mice. Infect. Immunity 11:350-354, 1975.

5. Lando, Z., Teitenbaum, D. and Arnon, R. Induction of experimental allergic encephalomyelitis in genetically resistant strains of mice. Nature 287:551-552, 1980.

6. Rudofsky, U.H., Dilwith, R.L. and Tung, K.S.K. Susceptibility differences in inbred mice to induction of autoimmune renal tubulointerstitial lesions. Lab. Invest. 43:463-470, 1980.

7. Wakashin, Y., Takei, I., Ueda, S., Mori, Y., Iesato, K., Wakashin, M. and Ukuda, K. Autoimmune interstitial disease of the kidney and associated antigen. Purification and characterization of a soluble tubular basement membrane antigen. Clin. Immunol. Immunopathol. 19:360-371, 1981.

8. Julius, M.H., Simpson, E. and Herzenberg, L.A. A rapid method for isolation of functional thymus-derived murine lymphocytes. Eur. J. Immunol. 3:645-649, 1973.

DRUG INDUCED RENAL EFFECTS OF CYCLOSPORINE, AMINOGLYCOSIDE ANTIBIOTICS AND LITHIUM: EXTRAPOLATION OF ANIMAL DATA TO MAN

George A. Porter and William M. Bennett, Department of Medicine, Oregon Health Sciences University Portland, Oregon, USA

INTRODUCTION

Drugs may have either a beneficial or adverse effect on renal function. It is the latter effect we wish to focus on since 10% nephrological consultations involve the possibility of drug-induced renal injury (Porter and Bennett, 1985). Thus information regarding prevalence, clinical presentation, pathophysiological mechanisms of injury and methods of modifying it have become a significant area of research. Most studies are designed to assess the potential risk which a drug possesses for inducing significant nephrotoxicity in a given patient. Since toxicology studies the adverse effects of chemicals on living organisms and assesses the probability of their occurrence, the two expected outcomes of a toxicological analysis are risk assessment and risk prediction. However, clinical toxicology combines the science of toxicology with the art of medicine; thus, the contribution of each is critical in the study of drug-induced nephrotoxicity. Scientifically, both the quantitative and qualitative _in vivo_ and _in vitro_ effect of drugs in the kidney are important contributors to the final assessment. However, the answer most often sought i.e., to predict occurrence in man, must occur in the face of limited scientific data as it involves the extrapolation of one set of exposure conditions to another circumstance involving different species.

Often the first indication that a newly introduced drug is injurious to the kidney comes from isolated case reports or letters to the editor. From such reports, a composite of the nephrotoxic clinical presentation can be formulated. Using the clinical presentation, plus the renal morphology, if known, the drug can be cross referenced to previously studied drug induced renal injury. Once classified, an initial hypothesis as to pathophysiological mechanisms of injury can be constructed along with predictions regarding clinical risk factors. The next step is to establish the relative frequency of adverse renal effects along with the spectrum of clinical presentation. Once a testable hypothesis has been developed regarding the proposed mechanism of renal cell injury, selecting a suitable animal model for experimentation can be accomplished. Animal studies are usually conducted in parallel with prospective clinical investigation and each provides complementary data with the ultimate objective to eliminate or significantly modify the risk of the drug inducing renal injury in patients. Results of animal experimentation will provide the maximum information if all of the following objectives are achieved.

1) That the pattern of drug-induced renal injury in the animal model faithfully reproduces the clinical counterpart being evaluated.

2) That the proposed mechanisms of nephrotoxic injury can be discriminated by the experimental techniques employed.

3) Testing should not be limited to risk factors which are associated with enhanced toxicity, but also of therapeutic manoeuvres which will reduce the toxicity.

The greater the concordance between the measurable features of clinical nephrotoxicity and the animal model being evaluated, the more likely the experimentally derived data regarding prevention and/or modification can be applied to patients. To illustrate this approach to investigating drug-nephrotoxicity, and three examples have been chosen.

AMINOGLYCOSIDE ANTIBIOTICS

Introduction: Aminoglycoside antibiotics are important agents for the treatment of serious gram-negative infections. In addition, they are commonly used in combination with other antibiotics as empirical treatment for immunocompromised patients. Their nephrotoxic potential was recognized soon after their introduction to clinical practice (Appel and Neu, 1978) but because of their clinical efficacy their use continues to be widespread. It is noteworthy that aminoglycoside antibiotics are the most common cause of drug-induced renal failure in hospitalized patients (Porter and Bennett, 1986).

Clinical Presentation Of Aminoglycoside Nephrotoxicity In Man: Non-oliguric renal insufficiency is the most common manifestation of aminoglycoside nephrotoxicity. Less common are a variety of tubular dysfunctional syndromes, i.e., nephrogenic diabetes insipidus, Fanconi syndrome, renal potassium or magnesium wasting; fortunately, oliguric renal failure is quite rare. A drug-induced concentrating defect characterized by polyuria and secondary thirst stimulation precede the detectable risk in blood urea nitrogen and serum creatinine that occur in up to 30% of hospitalized patients treated for more than 5-7 days (Schentag et al, 1982, Smith et al, 1987). Accompanying urinary abnormalities including granular casts and proteinuria, occur with relative frequency but are not of diagnostic assistance (Schentag et al, 1978). Enzymuria is commonly detected between the second and fourth day of administration of aminoglycosides, either to infected patients or human volunteers. In particular, the quantity of beta-2-microglobulin (ß2M) or a variety of proximal tubular brush border enzymes, i.e., N-acetyl-beta-D-glucosaminidase (NAG), alanine aminopeptidase (AAP), etc, increase significantly. Whether such enzymuria represents evidence of nephrotoxicity or simply an epiphenomena paralleling proximal tubular uptake of aminoglycosides remains an unresolved controversy (Gibey et al, 1981).

Reports of renal pathology associated with aminoglycoside nephrotoxicity have been less numerous than those regarding changes in renal function. However, in patients with severe oliguric renal failure of the oliguric form, patchy proximal tubular necrosis has been reported (Bennett et al, 1977). In addition, for patients who satisfy the clinical diagnosis of aminoglycoside nephrotoxicity, autophagocytosis has been observed in proximal tubular cells by electron microscopy. These changes are characterized by prominent cytosegrosomes which contain whorled-material, referred to as myeloid bodies. Similar findings occur in the proximal tubule of patients ingesting a variety of non-nephrotoxic lyophilic drugs, i.e., quinidine. Because of the latter observations, myeloid bodies are not pathognomonic of aminoglycoside-induced nephrotoxic acute renal failure unless there is associated tubular cell necrosis.

A variety of risk factors which predispose to the development of amino-glycoside nephrotoxicity have been identified and are summarized on Table 1. For some factors, i.e., age greater than 60, pre-existing renal disease, liver disease, female sex, little can be done; however, such things as volume depletion, hypotension, concomitant nephrotoxic drugs, acidosis, and hypokalaemia will respond to simultaneous corrective treatment and should reduce risk. Infants and small children tolerate large doses of aminoglycoside drugs without adverse renal effects, while patients with fibrocystic lung disease require large doses to maintain therapeutic serum levels.

TABLE 1.   CLINICAL RISK FACTORS FOR AMINOGLYCOSIDE NEPHROTOXICITY

PATIENT DEPENDENT

1. Dehydration - Volume depletion.
2. Electrolyte abnormalities, K^+, PO_4, Ca^{++}
3. Age
4. Concurrent nephrotoxins
5. Prior aminoglycoside treatment
6. Pre-existing renal disease
7. Liver disease
8. Severe obesity
9. Systemic acidosis
10. Female sex

DRUG DEPENDENT

1. Pharmacokinetics - Tissue uptake
2. Duration of treatment
3. Dosage frequency

Using a pharmacokinetic model with computer assistance, Schentag, et al, (1982) analysed 201 patients given aminoglycoside antibiotics and concluded that those who subsequently developed clinical aminoglycoside nephrotoxicity had significantly greater renal tissue accumulation of either gentamicin or tobramycin during the first 24 hr of dosing despite receiving comparable amounts. Recently, Trollfor (1982) conducted a retro-spective study in which he identified six patients with aminoglycoside nephrotoxicity that reversed despite continued administration of the anti-biotic.

Animal Models of Aminoglycoside Nephrotoxicity: Using a standardized dosing protocol in the Fischer 344 male rat, we and others (Kaloyanides and Pastoviza-Munos, 1980, Houghton et al, 1978, Luft et al, 1975) have been able to induce a predictable and progressive form of aminoglycoside nephrotoxicity which bears a striking resemblance to the clinical description in man (Table 2).

A progressive decline in urinary osmolality occurs after only three days of administration. Abnormal excretion of sodium, potassium, and magnesium develop coincidentally with proximal tubular enzymuria followed in short order by a progressive decline in glomerular filtration rate (GFR) and the appearance of both protein and glucose in the urine (Kluwe and Hook, 1978, Cojocel and Hook, 1983). The changes in tubular reabsorption coincide with measurable changes in organic ion transport (Houghton et al, 1978). This dose dependent, non-oliguric acute renal failure develops over a 7-14 day

TABLE 2.   FEATURES OF GENTAMICIN NEPHROTOXICITY IN MAN AND THE RAT

MAN   RAT

1.   Renal   failure   is   non-   1. Polyuria   and a decreased
oliguric.   Uosm precede fall in GRF.

2.   Renal cortical concentra-   2.   Renal cortical tissue has
tions of gentamicin   exceed   20 times more gentamicin than
serum and medullary levels 5-   serum and 4 times   more than
to 10-fold.   renal medulla.

3.   Proximal tubular necrosis   3.   Ultrastructural   changes
is the predominant lesion. EM   occur early and independent of
shows "myeloid bodies" in most   development   of   proximal
patients irrespective of cli-   tubular necrosis.
nical toxicity.

4.   Recovery of glomerular   4. Glomerular filtration rate
filtration rate is usual with-   improves and proximal   tubular
out dialysis.   regeneration   occurs despite
                                             continued gentamicin adminis-
                                             tration.

period followed by recovery to near normal renal function despite
continued administration of the drug the sole evidence of abnormal renal
function being a persistent urinary concentrating defect (Elliott et al,
1982).   Changes in both the amount and distribution of renal blood flow
(RBF) measured during aminoglycoside nephrotoxicity are characteristic of
non-oliguric acute renal failure (Appel et al, 1981). A host of urinary
enzymes have been measured and those of proximal tubule brush border
origin, i.e., NAG, AAP, are consistently increased following aminoglycoside antibiotics. Patchy proximal tubular necrosis occurs (Houghton
et al, 1976), while cytosegrosomes, including prominent myeloid bodies,
are evident after two days of low-dose gentamicin treatment (Heinert et
al, 1982) but light microscopic abnormalities require a 10-fold increase
in dose. Typically, focal patchy proximal tubular necrosis is maximum at
10 days of treatment with evidence of tubular regeneration coexisting. In
animals given subnecrotic doses of gentamicin, increased cellular turnover
can be demonstrated by in vivo DNA labelling with ^{3}H-thymidine (Laurent et
al, 1983).

Mechanism of Cellular Injury Due to Aminoglycoside Antibiotics: The
pathological expression of severe aminoglycoside toxicity is proximal
tubular cell necrosis. From experimental studies, certain biochemical and
ultrastructural changes leading to cell death have been defined (Tulkens,
1986, Weinberg, 1986). Aminoglycosides reach the proximal tubule via
glomerular filtration. Electrostatic binding occurs at the proximal
tubular brush border and a concentration dependent pinocytotic uptake
ensues with the resulting inclusion vesicles fusing with the lysosomes to
create the intracytosolic cytosegrosomes (DeBroe et al, 1984). The acidic
milieu of the lysosome promote the full expression of the cationic form of
aminoglycoside which enhances the binding of aminoglycosides to the
negatively charged phospholipid bilayers. This binding is associated with
the inhibition of the lysosomal phospholipase A1 and A2 activity (Tulkens,
1986). The latter probably accounts for the formation of myeloid bodies
the osmophylic lamellar material composed of undigested phospholipids. At
this point, several speculations can be entertained to account for
eventual cell death, a process characterized by calcium overload of both
cytosol and mitochondria which uncouples the respiratory chain thus inter-
rupting cell energetics (Weinberg, 1986).   The aminoglycoside-induced

arrest of lysosomal processing and recycling of phospholipids may critically impair membrane renewal thus causing a loss of cell membrane permeability and the cascade of events that leads to cell death (Thurau et al, 1985). Conversely, continued aminoglycoside uptake from the proximal tubule may exceed lysosomal processing capacity and "leak" into the cytosol (Giuliano et al, 1986) where it's cationic characteristic would cause enzyme interruption through competitive inhibition of calcium mediated intracellular processes. Irrespective of which speculative mechanism of cellular injury eventually emerges, aminoglycoside nephrotoxicity shares with ischaemic renal injury the common denominator of irreversible membrane damage progressing to acute renal failure.

Methods of Modification of Acute Aminoglycoside Nephrotoxicity: Since animal models resemble the clinical state of aminoglycoside nephrotoxicity, a natural extension of the experimental studies has been to evaluate techniques for modifying or eliminating the risk of nephrotoxicity (Table 1). The adverse effect of volume depletion was confirmed in both dogs (Adelman et al, 1979) and rats (Bennett et al, 1976). Systemic acidosis is associated with a more severe renal failure (Chen et al, 1976). Although female animals resist aminoglycoside nephrotoxicity (Parker et al, 1980), the contribution of female hormones remains in dispute (Whelton and Solez, 1984). Older animals have increased susceptibility while younger animals demonstrate resistance (McMartin and Wugel, 1982). Animals who receive the same daily dose as multiple injections rather than a single injection have more profound renal injury (Elliott et al, 1982). Potassium depletion enhances the intensity of acute renal failure due to aminoglycoside (Cron et al, 1982), while supplementing dietary calcium is protective (Bennett et al, 1982), as is pretreatment with calcium channel antagonists (Eliahou et al, 1984). Phosphate depletion provides significant protection against experimental renal failure (Eknoyan et al, 1984). Expanding on the observation that both the rapidity and total tissue accumulation of aminoglycoside are important determinates of both clinical and experimental nephrotoxicity (Porter et al, 1983), attempts at selective blockade of aminoglycoside uptake have been undertaken. Polyamines will displace tissue bound aminoglycoside in vitro, but in preliminary experiments prove to be too toxic for in vivo use. Similarly, attempts to substitute less nephrotoxic aminoglycosides in hopes of reducing tubular injury prove to be unsuccessful (Bennett et al, 1986).

An interesting approach to modifying aminoglycoside nephrotoxicity came from Vaamonde et al, (1984), who reported that diabetic animals were resistant to aminoglycoside nephrotoxicity. Disappointingly, Bergeron et al, (1985) were unable to show similar protection when diabetic patients were compared to non-diabetic patients treated with aminoglycoside. Although diuretic-induced volume depletion causes a more severe experimental aminoglycoside-induced renal injury, a similar risk could not be identified for patients given furosemide (Smith and Lietman, 1983). Surprisingly, the pharmacokinetics of gentamicin do not show any age dependence according to the results of Bauer and Bloum (1982). One of the important differences between human aminoglycoside nephrotoxicity and that induced in animals is the cephalosporin- aminoglycoside synergism. While Mannion et al (1981) documented such synergism in humans, attempts by Luft et al, (1976) to achieve it in animals actually produced protection. Recently, English et al (1985) have reported that simultaneous ticarcillin administration will protect against experimental aminoglycoside toxicity. The latter observation may explain the apparent discrepancy between human and animal data. Studies of Sugarman et al (1983) have implicated an additive aminoglycoside nephrotoxicity, in the presence of concomitant cephalosporin treatment compare that combination to one of aminoglycoside plus semi-synthetic penicillin. Thus, the difference they note may have reflected the protection effect of either methicillin or ticarcillin rather than an additive effect of cephalosporin. The role of renal eicosanoids in experimental acute renal failure has received increasing attention. In particular, we have explored dietary fish oil for any protection which it might provide against aminoglycosides nephrotoxicity and found it to be effective but requiring pre-treatment. Finally, we have examined the influence of coexisting infection in aminoglycoside induced renal failure. Rats infected by peritoneal implants were treated with two different dosage regimes, but the same total daily dosage (Woods et al, 1987). The results were similar to our previous dosing observations in uninfected animals (Bennett et al, 1986) in that the multidose schedule gave more profound renal damage than did the once day dose; however, both dosages were equally effective in antibacterial effect.

Summary: Aminoglycoside antibiotics continue to be an important component of the treatment of serious gram-negative sepsis. A variety of risk factors both with regards to the patients treated and the drug itself have been identified and including them in the clinical deliberations can minimize serious toxicity. Animal experimentation continues to yield important information concerning the cellular events which eventuate in tubular cell necrosis. Various techniques for modifying experimental aminoglycoside nephrotoxicity have been identified but must await clinical confirmation.

CYCLOSPORINE

Although cyclosporine has greatly improved the results of clinical solid organ transplantation and shows promise in the therapy of autoimmune disease, nephrotoxicity and hypertension have emerged as major obstacles to the widespread acceptance of this novel immunosuppressive agent.

Clinical Presentations of Cyclosporine Nephrotoxicity: The various clinical presentations of cyclosporine nephrotoxicity are summarized on Table 3. In cadaveric renal transplantation, cyclosporine may cause prolonged oligoanuria. Canafax et al, (1986) have shown that the percentage of patients who require dialysis is not greater in patients who receive cyclosporine as compared to azathioprine, but that those whose initial graft function is delayed have a much more prolonged period of oligoanuria. Transplant biopsies performed during the period of oligoanuria are either normal or in some cases reveal diffuse interstitial fibrosis. The latter finding has been associated with prolonged periods of non-function where the cadaver organ has been retrieved from a non-beating heart donor (Hall et al, 1987). Despite the presence of diffuse interstitial fibrosis, sufficient graft function is usually observed to allow excellent 1 and 2 year allograft survival. The long-term fate of these grafts is less clear. The Canadian Multicentre Study (1985) has identified other risk factors for oligoanuria including pulsatile machine perfusion, prolonged organ storage and most importantly high initial doses of cyclosporine. Reduction of initial cyclosporine dose to 5-8 mg/kg has greatly obviated this type of nephrotoxicity. Some centres prefer to begin cyclosporine only after urine flow is well established. Monitoring of cyclosporine blood levels during the period of oligoanuria is crucial to minimization of this problem, although after 3 weeks of non- function empirical dose reduction is indicated even if blood concentrations are in the "therapeutic" range.

Acute episodes of renal dysfunction occur frequently during cyclosporine immunosuppression (Bennett and Pulliam, 1983). They are usually asymptomatic and are discovered during routine monitoring of renal function. In general, blood pressure is elevated but, in renal transplantation this is not reliable for distinguishing cyclosporine-induced renal dysfunction from allograft rejection. The patient is most often nonoliguric and fractional excretion of sodium is low. Nuclear medicine techniques may show decreased allograft perfusion, however, perfusion deficits are also characteristic of acute renal allograft rejection. Blood levels are statistically higher in patients with cyclosporine-induced renal dysfunction. However, for the individual patient this is of limited value, since many patients who show clinical improvement with dose reduction have low pre-existing blood concentrations (Kahan et al, 1982). Most transplant physicians actively try to exclude rejection and relegate the diagnosis of cyclosporine nephrotoxicity to one of exclusion. Since rejection and cyclosporine nephrotoxicity can coexist, Table 4 shows the features of proven cyclosporine nephrotoxicity compared to those of acute rejection.

TABLE 3.   CLINICAL PRESENTATIONS OF CYCLOSPORINE NEPHROTOXICITY

Prolonged oligoanuria

Episodes of acute renal dysfunction
Chronic depression of glomerular filtration rate
Reversible
Progressive
Hypertension - de novo or aggravating pre-existing
Vasculopathy

Unfortunately, the clinical signs of rejection are subtle or absent in most cases and invasive techniques such as allograft biopsy or empirical manipulation of cyclosporine dosage are required. Low fractional excretion of sodium, absence of enzymuria and impaired potassium excretion suggest renal vasoconstriction as a prominent pathophysiological mechanism in cyclosporine induced acute renal dysfunction. Prompt improvement of function with dose reduction also favours a haemodynamic explanation for this syndrome. The long term consequences of episodes of renal dysfunction are unclear but some workers have suggested that more chronic interstitial changes in renal allografts are related both to cumulative dose and the number of acute episodes of dysfunction (Klintmalm et al, 1985).

Non-transplant patients treated with cyclosporine also have more subtle changes in renal function. In patients with autoimmune disease, for example, creatinine clearance regularly falls gradually. When the drug is withdrawn, renal function returns to baseline even after 1 year of treatment (Von Graffenreid and Harrison, 1985). Some, but not all, of these patients develop de novo hypertension and most have rises in mean arterial pressure even though values remain less than 140/90 (Palestine et al, 1986). Most of these patients have no other reason for the decline in renal function and maintain stable but elevated serum creatinine values during the entire treatment period. When the drug is withdrawn for financial reasons, as in the series of Curtis et al, (1986), there is a prompt increase in effective renal plasma flow. Reduction of dose and combination therapy with other immunosuppressive drugs may minimize the decline in creatinine clearance. The lack of sensitivity of the serum creatinine and creatinine clearance in discerning progressive tubulo-interstitial renal disease make it difficult to dismiss this almost inevitable result of cyclosporine therapy as harmless and "reversible" until long-term follow up is available (Shemesh et al, 1985).

Myers et al (1984) have reported progressive renal insufficiency requiring end stage renal disease management in cardiac allograft recipients treated with cyclosporine. Since these patients have excellent function of their allografts and had no other causes for renal disease, cyclosporine is almost certainly implicated. Although many of these patients had large initial doses by today's standards (14-18 mg/kg), it is disturbing that disease progression has been noted despite dose reduction and strict maintenance of "therapeutic" blood levels. When biopsies have been performed, chronic tubulointerstitial fibrosis and glomerulosclerosis have been observed. In some patients treated for autoimmune uveitis by Palestine et al (1986), these chronic histopathological findings have also been observed. The number of cases evolving within the group of patients thought to have stable, but reversible renal dysfunction as described above, is unknown. The observation has been made that most cases of chronic nephrotoxicity are reported in individuals with full innervation to both kidneys (Porter and Bennett, 1986).

TABLE 4. COMPARISON OF ACUTE REJECTION AND CYCLOSPORINE-ASSOCIATED RENAL ALLOGRAFT DYSFUNCTION

SIGNS OR SYMPTOMS	CSA	REJECTION
Fever, graft tenderness	Absent	Present in 25%
Oliguria	Absent	Present in 50%
Graft swelling (clinical ultrasound, NMR, Fine needle manometry)	Absent	Present in 50%
Hypertension	75%	50%
Blood CSA concentration	Normal or High	Normal
Renal perfusion by isotope scan	Decreased in 75%	Decreased in virtually all
Hyperkalemic metabolic acidosis with hyperchloremia	15%	5%
Fractional excretion of sodium	Low	Low in days 0-1 then increased
Biopsy fine needle aspirates	Subtle features Rejection absence	Diagnostic (usually)

Elevation of blood pressure, either de novo or from previously hyper-tensive levels, is frequently seen in cyclosporine treated patients (Bennett and Norman, 1986). Although renal function is usually also decreased, this is not uniformly true. When measured, plasma renin activity is low and the renin-angiotensin axis is relatively unresponsive to stimulatory manoeuvres such as upright posture and diuretics (Bantle et al, 1985). Cyclosporine dose reduction may be indicated for severe hyper-tension even in the absence of renal dysfunction since Textor et al, (1986) described an accelerated hypertension syndrome in previously normo-tensive bone marrow recipients complicated by neurological symptoms including seizures.

Rarely, patients may present a fulminant syndrome of rapid decline in renal function, severe hypertension, microangiopathic haemolytic anaemia and thrombocytopenia (Shulman et al, 1981). This clinical picture has been associated with the presence of arteriolar changes on renal biopsy. Arcuate and afferent arterioles show mucoid thickening and proliferation

(Mihatsch et al, 1983) of smooth muscle cells leading to obliterative arteriolopathy. The clinical picture resembles the haemolytic uraemic syndrome and usually results in the permanent loss of kidney function. Thrombocytopenia is regularly present and thrombosis of the afferent arteriole has been reported by Shuchman et al (1981). Recurrence of haemolytic uraemic syndrome as well as its de novo occurrence are reported (Bennett and Norman, 1986). The latter may result from a drug effect to enhance clotting in susceptible hosts such as bone marrow transplant recipients. This fortunately uncommon syndrome is not clearly dose related.

Experimental Models of Cyclosporine Nephrotoxicity: Administration of cyclosporine orally or parenterally to various experimental animal species in doses similar to those received by man (on a weight basis) produces little in the way of acute or chronic renal dysfunction. However, when rodents are given 25-50 mg/kg orally or 10-15 mg/kg parenterally for periods of 1 day to 2 weeks, Whiting et al (1982) induced a dose dependent reversible renal dysfunction. Analogous to the clinical situation, decreases in RBF and GFR predominate over evidence of direct tubular injury (English et al, 1987). In the same study, sensitive tubular function parameters such as the fractional excretion of sodium, in vitro renal cortical slice transport of organic ions remain normal despite marked depression of GFR. Histopathological examination of the kidney reveals proximal tubular cell vacuolar changes but little evidence for tubular cell necrosis. In fact, according to Whiting et al, (1982), increases in urinary enzyme excretion reported by some investigators may be artifactual because results were expressed as units per mg creatinine. In rats whose kidneys are made ischaemic by various periods of renal artery clamping, cyclosporine produces more profound renal dysfunction for any given cyclosporine dose.

The ischaemic model seems analogous to the clinical cadaveric transplant situation and holds promise for elucidation of factors which are critical in producing the oligoanuric form of clinical cyclosporine nephrotoxicity. Although the spontaneously hypertensive rat is allegedly quite sensitive to renal dysfunction produced by cyclosporine, there are limited data on the hypertensive properties of cyclosporine in other animal species, nor do common experimental animal develop chronic tubulointerstital fibrosis even with prolonged periods of cyclosporine administration. Lesions of renal arterioles are not commonly observed in experimental animals exposed to acute or chronic cyclosporine administration.

Mechanisms of Cyclosporine Induced Renal Dysfunction: Although it is quite clear from experimental animal models that cyclosporine can produce a dose dependent decrease in RBF due to renal afferent arteriolar vasoconstrict- ion, the factor(s) mediating this phenomenon are unclear. Increases in sympathetic nerve traffic have been observed in cyclosporine treated animals. Denervation, pharmacological alpha-adrenergic blockade and calcium entry blockers can improve renal haemodynamics (Finn, 1987). Converting enzyme inhibitors produce inconsistent effects making a primary role for angiotensin unlikely (Murray et al, 1985). Furthermore, chronic administration of cyclosporine produces suppression not stimulation of the renin and cyclosporine treatment produce increases in vasoconstrictor eicosanoids (Gibbons et al, 1987, Kawaguchi et al, 1985). The use of selective thromboxane synthase inhibitors or dietary fish oil rich in eicosapentanoic acid produce modification of cyclosporine induced renal dysfunction associated with improvement in renal vasodilator/constrictor prostaglandin ratios (Perico et al, 1986, Elzinga et al, 1987). The renal source of increased thromboxane is unclear. The data of Perico et al, (1986) suggest a glomerular source, since RBF changes in their experiments were independent of decreases in GFR. Rogers et al, (1987) have suggested that infiltrating macrophages could be a possible source. Activated macrophages could stimulate various growth factors, fibroblasts and lymphokines providing a theoretical link between acute vasoconstrictive effects of cyclosporine and the more chronic interstitial changes observed in patients. Humes et al, (1987) have demonstrated cyclosporine induced increases in interstitial DNA synthesis and increased mononuclear cell infiltrates in cyclosporine treated rats. The relationship, if any, between renal vasoconstrictive changes and an interstitial cell proliferative response is unclear.

Cyclosporine can produce direct vasoconstrictive responses in isolated vascular smooth muscle (Xue et al, 1987). Whitworth et al, (1987) have demonstrated an increase in mean arterial pressure in conscious sheep without associated renal haemodynamic changes or major increases in cardiac output. Textor et al, (1986) reported a similar phenomenon in bone marrow transplant recipients. Thus, it is possible that cyclosporine by its intracellular interaction with calcium binding proteins could produce hypertension by direct action on resistance vessels to influence intracellular calcium. Obviously, more research is needed in this area.

Caution must be exercised in extrapolating _in vitro_ effects of cyclosporine to _in vivo_ situations. Cyclosporine is extremely hydrophobic and may be activated to metabolites in various target tissues. Phenobarbital and other inducers of hepatic P-450 metabolism reduce experimental cyclosporine nephrotoxicity (Schwass et al, 1986). However, specific activation to toxic metabolites in the kidney has not been excluded. Buss and Bennett (1987) have recently shown inhibition of protein synthesis in renal microsomes with _in vivo_, but not _in vitro_ cyclosporine treatment. This type of action in tubular cells could prevent a normal cellular response to ischaemic insults produced by organ preservation or rejection.

Summary: At present, specific strategies to reduce cyclosporine nephrotoxicity must await a better understanding of basic mechanisms (Bennett, 1985). Details of the renal handling of cyclosporine, possible generation by the kidney of toxic metabolites and the mediators of vasoconstriction are incompletely elucidated. The appealing unifying hypothesis that cyclosporine could activate macrophages which in turn begin a cascade of vasoconstrictive and interstitial events awaits confirmation. Thus, minimization of drug dose consistent with maintaining adequate immunosuppression will remain the clinically prudent approach. Serial blood cyclosporine levels remain useful to provide guidelines for interindividual and intraindividual differences in pharmacokinetics of this valuable immunosuppressive agent.

LITHIUM

The first report of lithium chloride nephrotoxicity comes from an accidental poisoning (Cleveland 1913). However, when Cade (1949) demonstrated successful treatment of manic depressive illness with lithium bicarbonate, the rapid acceptance of this clinically effective treatment brought with it increased risk of nephrotoxicity (Radomski et al, 1950). During the initial decade of lithium therapy it was considered to be a benign drug because of the paucity of adverse reactions that were reported (Lippman, 1982). When nephrotoxicity was recognized, it seemed restricted to individuals who had experience recurring episodes of acute lithium intoxication (Schou et al, 1968). This attitude changed dramatically when Hestbeck and co-workers (1977) reported biopsy proven chronic interstitial nephritis in 14 lithium treated patients who had neither prior acute lithium intoxication nor in whom polyuria was a prominent symptom. This was the first clear implication that continuous lithium therapy might be linked with chronic irreversible renal failure.

The most prominent symptom in patients given therapeutic doses of lithium carbonate are polyuria and secondary polydypsia (Ramsey and Cox 1982). From 12 to 50 percent of patients report polyuria, which is most obvious during the initiation of treatment (Ayd, 1978). Due to the ADH-resistance of the polyuria, it has been characterized as resembling nephrogenic diabetes insipidus. In addition, with continuous treatment, there is a progressive time-dependent fall in maximum urinary concentrating ability (Bendz et al, 1983a).

In a recent literature survey, Bendz (1983b) reported that between 30% and 96% of all patients given lithium will show a submaximal rise in urinary osmolality, i.e. 800 mOsm/kg, to a test dose of either parenteral arginine vasopressin (AVP) or nasal DDAVP. A consistent finding of all studies evaluating lithium-treated patients has the been significant inverse correlation between duration of lithium treatment in years and impaired maximum urinary concentrating capacity following AVP challenge. However, a finding which has confounded the specificity of this being a lithium effect is the observation that patients with affective disorders who have never received lithium treatment also have impaired maximal concentrating capacity (Ellis et al, 1971, Hullin et al, 1979). Since neuroleptic agents, an alternative to lithium in affective disorders, which have been shown to cause impairment of maximum concentrating capacity, the issue remains unsolved (Waller et al, 1984)

The clinical studies summarized by Bendz (1983b) tried to provide answers to several questions concerning long-term lithium therapy and its affect on renal function. For example:-

1) Is acute lithium intoxication a mandatory precondition for chronic lithium nephropathy to develop?

2) Do other neuroleptic drugs contribute to the chronic lithium nephropathy?

3) Is there a correlation between the renal lesion noted from biopsy and dose of lithium, total amount of lithium ingested, or peak blood level?

4) Does age, concomitant drugs, and/or co-existing renal disease contribute to chronic lithium nephropathy?

Neither Hullin and co-workers (1979), nor Donker et al, (1979) reported any significant difference in GFR between lithium patients and control patients with affective disorders. However, in the latter study "control" patients had the unusually low value of GFR, when compared to published norms. Ellis et al, (1971) had previously reported that affective patients receiving neither lithium nor neuroleptic agents have a relative polyuria when compared to normal controls. Grof et al, (1982) in a prospective study failed to detect any change in creatinine clearance following the initiation of lithium therapy but did note that "nonresponders" had larger 24-hr urine volumes and more impressive impairments of maximum concentrating capacity. Evaluating 278 patients on lithium therapy for more than 2 years, Wallin et al, (1982) found that 1 in 2 two patients did not concentrate their urine > 600 mOsm/kg following AVP challenge and this defect correlated directly with the duration of lithium therapy but was independent of associated neuroleptic drugs.

While 17% of their patients had a reduction in GFR which paralleled the fall in maximum concentrating capacity they failed to detect any significant increase in B2M Coopen and co-workers (1980) measured urinary ß2M and NAG creatinine clearance and maximum concentrating capacity, in

101 patients with either affective disorders or age/sex matched controls and found no significant difference for either enzymuria or GFR. Conversely, Tyrer et al, (1983) reported a deterioration of GFR with long-term lithium therapy. While Waller et al, (1984) likewise were unable to demonstrate a correlation between accumulated lithium dose and predictable change in GFR they did note a 10% incidence of abnormal urinary enzyme excretion of either NAG and B2M and confirmed the inverse correlation between maximum urinary concentrating capacity and the duration of lithium treatment. An additional observation was that in 40% of their patients microalbuminuria was present but independent of the duration of lithium treatment. In 7 of the studies summarized by Bendz, (1983b), GFR was measured by 51Cr-EDTA, a technique which is more reliable and sensitive than endogenous creatinine. Collectively, approximately 10% of patients on long-term lithium treatment had GFR's below age-matched published standards. Subsequently, Waller (1984) reported a significant negative correlation between EDTA measured GFR and time on lithium treatment for a population of 179 patients. Thus, although a majority of the study population had an abnormal response to DDAVP challenge, Bendzs' (1983b) summary could find no correlation between renal functional changes and sex, diagnosis, time on treatment, serum lithium levels, the type of lithium preparation used or combined lithium-neuroleptic treatment. A quasi-longitudinal study of GFR in lithium-treated patients was reported by Johnson and co-workers (1984). These authors found no consistent changes in GFR in a group of lithium-treated patients (mean 4.5 yr) who were re-tested 2 years later. However, detection of an interactive effect of time on treatment and GFR may require much longer observations. Lokkegaard et al, (1985), in a cross-sectional study of renal functions in 153 patients treated in excess of 5 years, recorded a modest, but significant, reduction in GFR as a function of time on treatment. The regression line bisected the lower confidence limits for GFR's in reference subjects after 17 yr of lithium treatment. Finally, a prospective study of ^{51}Cr-EDTA measured GFR in 13 consecutive patients who had never received lithium was reported by Jensen and Rickers (1984). Seven of 8 patients tested after one year of treatment had lower GFRs while 3 of the remaining 5 patients had decreases in GFR measured after 2 years of treatment.

In addition to effects on GFR, other investigators have concluded that distal nephron injury occurs. Hansen and co-workers (1981) evaluated enzymuria in patients with documented lithium-induced concentrating defects, and biopsy proven chronic tubulointerstitial disease. Since only one patient had a significant increase in urinary B2M they concluded that the lithium-induced injury probably occurred at a distal tubular site. Expanding on the question of a distal tubular lesion, Batlle et al, (1985) reported a mild distal tubular acidification defect in lithium-treated patients. Since amiloride reversed the acidification defect, a distal site was proposed for the lithium induced concentrating defect. Adding to this is the observed by Penney et al (1981) that the AVP content in the morning urine of lithium treated patients was increased as compared to controls. Gold et al, (1983) evaluated the effect of lithium on central vasopressin release and concluded that rather than having a partial central diabetes insipidus, their subjects had increased vasopressin secretion due to enhanced osmoreceptor sensitivity. The failure of the increased availability of endogenous AVP to activate distal tubular water reabsorption was due to the increased distal tubular urine flow plus the lithium-induced reduction in renal sensitivity to AVP.

A critical study in defining the extent of lithium nephropathy was the histopathological results reported by Hestbech and co-workers (1977) which documented chronic histological changes including diffuse and focal interstitial fibrosis, degenerative and atrophic tubular epithelium and increased frequency of sclerotic glomeruli. Walker et al, (1982) compared lithium treated patients with patients with affective disorders before starting lithium. Using a quantitative technique for assessing the extent of interstitial fibrosis in renal biopsy tissue the interstitial volume for lithium-treated patients was significantly greater than from age-matched healthy kidney donors, but did not differ significantly from specimens obtained from the pre-lithium affective disorder group. The ^{51}Cr-EDTA measure GFR was lower in lithium treated patients than in the pre-lithium affective disorder patients of comparable age, while protein-uria was greater. Changes in GFR did display the expected inverse correlation with age but did not correlate with duration of lithium treatment. However, the reduction in urinary osmolality and maximum concentrating capacity did have a significant inverse correlation with time on lithium. An additional finding was the defect in ammonium chloride induced urinary acidification loading which was present in lithium patients, absent in pre-lithium patients and correlated inversely with time on drug. A new pathological contribution from this study was definition of the "acute, specific lesion of lithium" which consisted of cytoplasmic vacuoles and PAS-positive staining filaments found in the distal tubular and collecting duct cells of patients receiving lithium. Such changes were absent in 5 patients who had stopped chronic lithium ingestion within 3 months of biopsy. More recently by Jorgensen et al, (1984) who compared renal histology from chronic lithium treated patients with age-matched patients having either acute oliguria or slight proteinuria. ^{51}Cr-EDTA GFR were measured and interstitial fibrosis was quantitated. Nine percent of lithium treated patients had GFR's below age adjusted normal subjects. Reduced maximum concentrating capacity correlated inversely with duration of lithium treatment but reduced GFR did not. However, unlike Walker et al, (1982), these authors found no difference in the percent volume of fibrotic tissue in lithium-treated patients as compared to controls. They did note that the percent of sclerotic glomeruli in lithium patients was twice that of control patients. They made no comment as to any "acute specific lesion of lithium." Based upon these two studies, significant interstitial fibrosis probably occurs in less than 10% of any lithium-treated population. The cause of the chronic interstitial nephritis in long-term lithium treatment remains to be explained.

Factors which have been shown to correlate with the lithium-induced concentrating defect include serum-lithium levels, the dosage frequency, and the formulation of the tablet. For example, Plenge et al, (1982) evaluated changes in both renal function and histology by comparing a single total daily dose of lithium versus the same dose given on either a BID or TID regime. Both functional and structural changes were more intense in the patients receiving the divided dose. A study by Schou et al, (1982) evaluated the same endpoint and obtained similar results.

In summary, chronic lithium therapy is associated with a decrease in AVP stimulated maximum urinary osmolality while inducing a polyuria which has the functional characteristics of a nephrogenic diabetes insipidus. The concentrating defect is reversible with lithium withdrawn in most patients but recovery may be prolonged. The polyuria is not life threatening; however, it may predict a future decline in GFR which occurs in approximately 10% of any population treated long-term. The cause of the chronic interstitial nephritis in patients with affective disorders is unclear. Lithium nephrotoxicity maybe more related to the frequency of dose rather than the total daily dose and has prompted current recommendations of once daily dosing of a patient to maintain blood lithium levels at the lower therapeutic levels, i.e., 0.4-0.7 mEq/L. As with other clinical circumstances in which nephrotoxins are administered, it is critical to avoid salt depletion which can disturb the equilibrium of serum lithium and induce acute intoxication. Because of the known discrepancy between serum creatinine and GFR in the elderly, adjustment of lithium intake by monitoring serum lithium level is an effective means of minimizing chronic toxicity in this age population.

<u>Animal Experimentations</u>: Lithium ingestion can cause major alterations in both acid base and electrolyte composition of the urine (Thompson and Schou, 1968, Steele et al, 1976). Myers and associates (1980) have demonstrated a striking parallel between the urinary electrolyte composition following acute lithium loading and that following acute sodium loading, with the exception of the effects on acid secretion which are lithium specific. It is postulated that the similarity between sodium and lithium loading probably represents a volume induced depression of proximal tubular reabsorption. While some authors have suggested that lithium induced kaliuresis is linked to the vasopressin resistant renal concentrating defect, (August et al, 1970) recent micropuncture experiments do not support this contention (Hecht et al, 1978). The proposed mechanism for lithium-induced distal tubular acidosis has been examined by Arruda et al, (1980) using the isolated turtle bladder. These authors were able to exclude a direct lithium inhibition of the hydrogen ion pump under appropriate experimental conditions. Their results indicate that the lithium-induced reduction in hydrogen ion secretion was an indirect effect involving the inhibition of active sodium transport, which resulted in a less favourable electrical diffusion gradient for the outward flow of intercellular hydrogen ion. This may explain why Batlles et al, (1985) were able to correct the concentrating defect of lithium using concomitant amiloride.

The most intense experimental efforts regarding the renal effect of lithium have explored the mechanism of the concentrating defect which characterizes chronic lithium ingestion in man. The principal animal used in such experiments has been the rat. Lithium, given either inter-peritoneally (Martinez-Maldonado et al, 1972) or by diet (Forrest et al, 1974) will induce a vasopressin resistant polyuria after only 7 days. Using the amphibian urinary bladder Harris and Jenner (1972) reported that lithium inhibited AVP mediated water flow when applied from the blood surface while, Singer et al, (1972) found that lithium effectively inhibited AVP-mediated water flow only when applied to the urine surface, and Bentley and Wasserman (1972) were unable to demonstrate any lithium inhibition of AVP-mediated osmotic water flow. While the interaction between lithium and antidiuretic hormone induced water flow has been inconsistent, inhibition of active sodium transport in isolated membrane preparations by lithium has been more consistent.

After receiving lithium in their drinking water for one month, Christensen et al, (1985) microdissected various vasopressin sensitive regions of the rat nephron. For comparison similar tissue was obtained from Brattleboro rats. Tissue cAMP accumulation in response to AVP was significantly reduced in lithium-treated rats in contrast to Brattleboro rats, as was the activity of adenylate cyclase isolated from medullary collecting tubule. In addition, the cortico-papillary urea gradient was markedly diminished in lithium treated rats. Thus, in the rat, lithium reduced the c-AMP response to AVP plus diminished the osmotic gradient between collecting duct and medullary region. This mimics the clinical syndrome of nephrogenic diabetes insipidus. Additional studies concerning the mechanism of lithium-induced urinary concentrating defect in the rat have been provided by the micropuncture studies of Hecht et al, (1978) and Carney et al, (1980). Based upon the tubular fluid to plasma inulin ratio from both proximal and distal tubular puncture sites, Hecht et al, (1978) found a significant depression of fluid reabsorption from proximal convoluted tubules, but not from the pars rectus or loop of Henle in rats with lithium-induced polyuria. These observations are inconsistent with the contention that lithium-induced polyuria is restricted to the distal tubule. Following up on these observations, Carney et al, (1980) actually measured an increase in the percent of water reabsorbed from the distal tubule and collecting duct in rats with lithium induced polyuria and concluded that the physiological response to endogenous AVP in the distal and collecting ducts was intact. Furthermore, they speculated that the failure of exogenous antidiuretic hormone to have an effect on urine osmolality reflects a new state of tubular fluid equilibrium induced by lithium since there was evidence that AVP was exerting its physiological action. Finally, they confirmed the observation of Hecht et al, (1978) of a depressed proximal tubular fluid reabsorption and, in addition, found impairment of the loop of Henle reabsorption. Interference with loop of Henle reabsorption is consistent with reports that lithium interferes with thick ascending limb chloride transport (Martinez-Maldonado and Opava-Stetzer, 1977) and with the reduction of the medullary solute gradient (Jenner and MacNell, 1975). Thus, one can conclude that once lithium-induced polyuria stabilizes, a new steady state for nephron hydrodynamics develops which is characterized by an increased delivery of a sodium chloride-rich fluid into the thick ascending limb of Henle which now has a restricted chloride transport and a reduced medullary solute gradient which prevents the maximum expression of endogenous AVP action on the urinary concentrating capacity. In addition, prolonged lithium treatment causes impairment of adenylate cyclase. Since the collecting duct is under maximum anti-diuretic hormone simulation, no additional affect can be registered with the administration of exogenous antidiuretic hormone.

The main pathological features associated with lithium induced toxicity in the rat have been summarized by Radomski, et al, (1950). These changes are localized to the collecting duct of the distal tubules and consist of cellular and nuclear polymorphism, nuclear hyperchromatism, focal tubular luminal dilatation with occasional tubular cell atrophy (Evans and Ollerich, 1972). Despite long-term lithium administration to the rats with or without neuroleptic agents, no evidence of pure interstitial fibrosis has been verified (Christensen et al, 1981, 1982). Jacobson et al, (1982) were able to detect early changes in structural protein of the renal tubular cells. By performing ^{3}H-Thymidine autoradiographic studies, they substantiated increased DNA synthesis in the collecting duct of lithium-treated rats which antedated the detection of cellular proliferation by conventional light microscopy. The changes were maximal at the junction of the outer and inner medullary regions with little spread into adjacent structures. Recently, Kling et al, (1982) have reported on sequential changes in distal tubular and collecting ducts of rats given lithium for 18 weeks. The late pathological effects are dominated by the proliferation of collecting duct cells with no interstitial inflammation or fibrosis identified. These authors concluded that the proliferating cells of the collecting duct may be more susceptible to an otherwise trivial insult and it is the latter which leads to the occasional chronic tubulo-interstitial nephropathy reported in men. Finally, the histological changes seem to be reversible once lithium is withdrawn, although the more severe the lesion the longer time interval required for such reversal (Christensen et al, 1982).

One can summarize the animal data as showing a consistent but reversible polyuria in rats at serum lithium concentrations well within the therapeutic range. Although this polyuria was originally classified as a functional nephrogenic diabetes insipidus, micropuncture studies suggested that, in addition, this is a proximal defect with functional consequences which impair the concentrating mechanism. This is separate from the lithium-induced effect on the AVP mediated change in collecting duct permeability. The dose dependent structural changes in animals are limited to the distal tubular and collecting duct region with prolonged treatment causing a significant proliferation of collecting duct cells.

Summary: A precise definition of "chronic lithium nephropathy" cannot be rendered at present. The confusion introduced by the finding of chronic interstitial nephritis as being a component of affective disorders further clouds the diagnosis. While it was previously thought that frequent episodes of acute lithium intoxication were a requirement for chronic lithium nephropathy, more recent studies indicate that such is not the case. The possibility also remains that other neuroleptic agents may contribute. Of interest is the unique distal tubular vacuoles which has been shown by Walker and co-workers (1982).

REFERENCES

Adelman, R.D., Spangler, W.L., Beasom, F., Ishizake, G., and Conzelman, G.M., 1979, Furosemide enhancement of experimental gentamicin nephrotoxicity: comparison of functional and morphological changes with activities of urinary enzymes, J. Infect. Dis., 140:342.

Angrest, B.M., Gershon, S., Levitan, S.J., and Blumberg, A.G., 1970, Lithium-induced diabetes insipidus-like syndrome, Compr. Psychiat., 11:141.

Appel, G.B., and Neu, H.C., 1978, Gentamicin in 1978, Am. Intern. Med., 89:528.

Appel, G.B., Siegel, N.J., Appel, A.S., and Hayslett, J.P., 1981 Studies on the mechanism of non-oliguric experimental acute renal failure, Yale J. Biol. Med., 54:273.

Arruda, J.A., Dytko, G., Mola, R., and Kurtzman, N.A., 1980, On the mechanism of lithium-induced renal tubular acidosis: studies in the turtle bladder, Kidney Int., 17:196.

Ayd, F.J., 1978, Lithium-induced kidney damage: an update, Internat. Drug Thera. Newsletter, 13:17.

Bantle, J.P., Nath, K.A., Sutherland, D.E., Najarian, J.S., Ferris, T.F., 1985, Effects of cyclosporin on the renin angiotensin aldosterone system and potassium excretion in renal transplant patients, Arch. Int. Med., 145:505.

Batlle, D.C., von Riotte, A., Gaviria, M., and Grupp, M., 1985, Amelioration of polyuria by amiloride in patients receiving long-term lithium therapy, N. Eng. J. Med., 312:408.

Bauer, L.A. and Bloum, B.A., 1982, Gentamicin pharmacokinetics: Effect of aging in patients with normal renal function, J. Am. Geriatr. Soc., 30:309.

Bendz, H., 1983, Kidney functions in lithium-treated patients: a literature survey, Acta Psychiat. Scand., 68:303.

Bendz, H., Andersch, S., and Aurell, M., 1983, Kidney function in an unselected lithium population, A cross-sectional study, Acta Psychiat. Scand., 68;325.

Bennett, W.M., 1985, Basic mechanisms and pathophysiology of cyclosporine nephrotoxicity, Transpl. Proc., 17:297.

Bennett, W.M. and Norman, D.J., 1986, Action and toxicity of cyclosporine, Ann. Rev. Med., 37:215.

Bennett, W.M., Pulliam, J.P., 1983, Cyclosporine nephrotoxicity, Ann. Intern. Med., 99:851.

Bennett, W.M., Wood, C.A., Houghton, D.C., and Gilbert, D.N., 1986, Modification of experimental aminoglycoside nephrotoxicity, Am. J. Kidney Dis., 8:292.

Bennett, W.M., Gilbert, D.N., Houghton, D., and Porter, G.A., Gentamicin nephrotoxicity in man: morphologic and pharmacological features, West. J. Med., 126:65.

Bennett, W.M., Hartnett, M.N., Gilbert, D.N., Houghton, D.C. and Porter, G.A., 1979, Effect of sodium intake on gentamicin nephrotoxicity in the rat, Proc. Soc. Biol. Med., 151:736.

Bennett, W.M., Elliott, W.C., Houghton, D.C., Gilbert, D.N., DeFehr, J. and McCarron, D.A., 1982, Reduction of experimental gentamicin nephrotoxicity in the rat by dietary calcium loading, Antimirob. Agent Chemother., 22:508.

Bentley, P.J. and Wasserman, A., 1972, The effects of lithium in the permeability of an epithelial membrane, the toad urinary bladder, Biochim. Biophys. Acta, 266:285.

Bergeron, M.G., Lessard, C., Ronald, A., Stiver, G., Van Rooyer, C.E., and Chadwick, P., 1983, Three to eight weeks of therapy with netilmicin: toxicity in normal and diabetic patients, J. Antimicrob. Chemothera., 12:245.

Buss, W., Bennett, W.M., 1987, Cyclosporine in vivo produces a dose dependent inhibition of protein synthesis, Fed. Proc., 46:555.

Cade, J.F.J., 1949, Lithium salts in the treatment of psychotic excitement, Med. J. Aust., 36:349.

Canadian Multicenter Transplant Study Group., 1983, A randomized clinical trial of cyclosporine in cadaveric renal transplantation, New Eng. J. Med., 309:809.

Canafax, D.M., Torres, A., Fryd, D.S., Heil, J.E., Strand, M.H., Ascher, N.L., Payne, W.D., Sutherland, D., Simmons, R., Najarian, J.S., 1986, The effects of delayed function on recipients of cadaver renal allografts, Transplantation, 41:177.

Carney, S.L., Wong, L.M., and Dirks, J.H., 1980, Effects of lithium treatment on rat tubule function, Nephron, 25:293.

Chen, P.J.S., Miller, G.J., Long, J.F. and Waity, J.A., 1979, Renal uptake and nephrotoxicity of aminoglycosides during urinary alkalinization in the rat, Clin. Exp. Pharmacol. Physiol., 6:317

Christensen, S., Hansen, B.B., and Faarup, P., 1982, Functional and structural changes in the rat kidney by long-term lithium treatment, Renal Physiol., 5:95.

Christensen, S., Kristensen, A.R., and Faarup, P., 1981, Effects of lithium and neuroleptics and combinations of the two on renal function and structure in rats, Acta Pharmacol. Toxicol., 49:161.

Christensen, S., Kusano, E., Yusufi, A.N.K., Murayama, N. and Dousaa, T.

P., 1985, Pathogenesis of nephrogenic diabetes insipidus due to chronic abnormalities of lithium in rats. J. Clin. Invest., 75:1869.

Cleaveland, S.A., 1913, A case of poisoning by lithium, JAMA, 60, 722.

Cojocel, C., and Hook, J.B., 1983, Effects of acute exposure to gentamicin on renal handling of proteins, Toxicology, 28:347.

Coopen, A., Bishop, M.E., Bailey, J.E., Cattell, W., and Price, R.G., 1980, Renal function in lithium and non-lithium treated patients with affective disorders, Acta Psychiat. Scand., 62:343.

Cronin, R.E., Nix, K.L., Ferguson, E.R., Southern, P.M., and Henrick, W.L., 1982, Renal on composition and Na-K-ATPase activity in gentamicin nephrotoxicity, Am. J. Physiol., 242:F477.

Curtis, J.J., Luke, R.G., Jones, P., Dubovsky, E.V., Whelchel, J.D., Diethelm, A.G., 1986, Cyclosporine in therapeutic doses increases renal allograft resistance, Lancet, 2:477.

DeBroe, M.E.,1984, Paulus, G.J., Verpooten, G.A., Roels, F., Buyssens, N., Wedeen, R., Van Hooj, F. and Tulkens, P.M., Early effects of gentamicin, tobramycin and amikacin on the human kidney. Kidney Int., 25:643.

Donker, A.J.M., Prince, E., Meijer, S., Sluiter, W.J., Van Berkestin, J.W.B.M., Dois, L.C.W., 1979, A renal function study in 30 patients on long-term lithium therapy, Clin. Nephrol., 12:254.

Eknoyan, G., Gentry, L., and Bulger, R., 1984, Attenuation of gentamicin induced acute renal failure by phosphate depletion, Kidney Int. 25:229.

Eliahou, H., Iaina, A. and Serban, I., 1984, Verapamils' beneficial effect and cycle nucleotides in gentamicin-induced acute renal failure, Nephron., 4:323A.

Elliott, W.C., Houghton, D.C., Gilbert, D.N., DeFehr, J., and Bennett, W.M., 1982 Gentamicin nephrotoxicity. I Degree and permanence of acquired insensitivity, J. Lab. Clin. Med., 100:501.

Ellis, G.G., 1971, Coppen, A., and Glen, A.I.M., Urine concentration in depressive illness, J. Neurol. Neurosurg. Psychiat., 34:30.

Elzinga, L., Kelley, V., Houghton, D.C., Bennett, W.M., 1987, Fish oil modifies experimental cyclosporine nephrotoxicity and decreases renal prostaglandins, Transplantation, 43:271.

English, J., Evan, A., Houghton, D.C., Bennett, W.M., 1987, Cyclosporine induced acute renal dysfunction in the rat: evidence for arteriolar vaso-constriction with preservation of tubular function, Transplantation (in press).

English, J., Gilbert, D.N., Kohlhepp, S.J., Kohner, P.W., Mayor, G., Houghton, D.C. and Bennett, W.M., 1985, Alternatives of experimental tobramycin nephrotoxicity with ticarcillin, Antimicrob. Agent Chemothera., 27:897.

Evans, A.P. and Ollerich, D.A., 1972, The effect of lithium carbonate on the structure of the rat kidney, Am. J. Anat., 134:97.

Finn, W.F., 1987, Renal vascular effects of cyclosporine, Transpl. Immunol. Letter, 3:4.

Forrest, J.N., Jr., Cohen, A.D., Torretti, J., Himmelhock, J.M., and Epstein, F.H., 1974, On the mechanism of lithium-induced diabetes insipidus in man and the rat, J. Clin. Invest., 53:1115.

Gibbons, C.P., Wiley, K.N., Lindsey, N.J., Fox, M., Beck, S., Slater, D.N., Preston, F.E., Brown, C.B., Raftery, A.T., Cortical and vascular prostaglandin synthesis during renal allograft rejection in the rat, Transplantation, 43:472.

Gibey, R., Dupond, J.L., Alber, D., Leconte d'Fleus, R., and Henry, J.C., 1981, Predictive value of urinary N-acetyl-beta-D-glucosaminidase (NAG), Alanine-aminopeptidase (AAP) and beta-2-microglobulin (B2M) in evaluating nephrotoxicity of Gentamicin, Clin. Chem. Acta, 116:27.

Giuliano, R.A., Verpooten, G.A., Verbist, L., Wedeen R.P., DeBroe, M.E., 1986, In vivo uptake kinetics of aminoglycosides in the kidney cortex of the rat. J. Pharmacol. Explt. Therap., 236:470.

Gold, B.W., Robertson, G.L., Post, R.M., Kaye, W., Ballenger, J., Rubinow, D., and Goodwin, F.K., 1983, The effects of lithium on osmoregulation of arginine vasopressin sections J. Clin. Endocrin. Metabolism, 56:295.

Grof, P., Hux, M., Pressler, B., and O'Sullivan, K., Kidney Function and response to lithium treatment, Prog. Neuropsychopharmacol. Biol. Psychiat., 6:491.

Hall, B.M., Tiller, D.J., Duggin, G.G., Horvath, J.S., Farnsworth, A., May, J., Johnson, J.R., Shiel, A.G., 1985, Post-transplant acute renal failure in cadaver renal recipients treated with cyclosporine. Kidney Int., 28:178.

Hansen, H.E., Mogensen, C.E., Sorensen, J.L., Norgaard, K., Heilskov, J., and Anderesen, A., 1981. Albumin and beta-2-microglobulin excretion in patients on long-term lithium treatment, Nephron, 29:229.

Harris, C.A. and Jenner, F.A., 1972, Some aspects of the inhibition of the action of antidiuretic hormone by lithium ion in rat kidney and bladder of toad Bufo Marinos, Br. J. Pharmacol., 44:223.

Hecht, B., Kashgarian, M., Forrest, J.N. Jr., and Hayslett, J.P., 1978, Micropuncture study on the effect of lithium on proximal and distal tubule function in the rat kidney, Pfleugers Arch., 377:69.

Heinert, G., Wyrobrik, J., Scherberick, J., Mondorf, W. and Weber, M., 1982, Quantitative histophotometry analyzing significant inductive and alternative features of aminoglycoside application upon kidney tubule proteins, Urol. Int., 37:221.

Hestbech, J., Hansen, H.E., Amdisen, A., and Olsen, S., 1977, Chronic renal lesions following long-term treatment with lithium, Kidney Int., 12:205.

Houghton, D.C., Hartnett, M.N., Campbell-Boswell, M., Porter, G.A., and Bennett, W.M., 1976, A light and electron microscopic analysis of gentamicin nephrotoxicity in the rat, Am. J. Pathol., 82:589.

Houghton, D.C., Plamp, C.E., DeFehr, J.M., Bennett, W.M., Porter, G.A., and Gilbert, D.N., 1978, Gentamicin and tobramycin nephrotoxicity: a morphologic and functioned comparison in the rat, Am. J. Pathol., 93:137.

Hullin, R.P., Culey, V.P., Birch, N.J., 1979, Renal function after long-term treatment with lithium, Br. Med. J., 1:1457.

Humes, H.D., 1987, Renal tubulointerstitial effects of cyclosporine, Transpl. Immunol. Letter, 3:6.

Jacobsen, N.O., Olesen, O.V., Thomsen, K., Ottosen, P.D., and Olsen, S., 1982, Early changes in renal distal convoluted tubules and collecting ducts of lithium-treated rats: light microscopy, enzyme histodensity and ^{3}H-thymidine autoradiography, Lab. Invest., 46:298.

Jenner, F.A. and MacNell, S., 1975, The effect of lithium ions on the antidiuretic action of vasopressin in the rat, Br. J. Pharmacol., 55:527.

Jensen, S.B. and Rickers, H., 1984, Glomerular filtration rate during lithium therapy, A longitudinal study, Acta Psychiat. Scand., 70:235.

Johnson, G.F.S., Hunt, G.E., Duggin, G.G., Harrath, J.S. and Tiller, D.J., 1984, Renal functions and lithium treatment: Initial and follow-up tests in manic depressive illness. J. Affect. Disord. 6:249.

Jorgensen, F., Larsen, S., Spanager, B., Clausen, E., Tango, M., Brinch, E., and Brun, C., 1984, Kidney function and quantitative histological changes in patients on long-term lithium therapy, Acta Psychiat. Scand., 70:455.

Kahan, B.D., Van Buren, C.T., Lin, S.N., Ono, Y., Agostino, G., Lagrue, S.J., Boileau, M., Payne, W.D., Kerman, R.H., 1982, Immunopharmacological monitoring of cyclosporin A treated recipients of cadaveric kidney allografts, Transplantation, 34:36.

Kaloyanides, G.G., Pastoriza-Munoz, E., 1980, Aminoglycoside nephro-toxicity, Kidney Int., 18:571.

Kawaguchi, A., Goldman, M.H., Shapiro, R., Foegh, M.L., Ramwell, P.W., Lower, R.R., 1985, Increase in urinary thromboxane B2 in rats caused by cyclosporine, Transplantation, 40:214.

Kling, M.A., Fox., J.G., Johnston, S.M., Tolkoff-Rubin, N.E., Rubin, R.H., and Colvin, R.B., 1984, Effects of long-term lithium administration on renal structure and function in rats. A destructive tubular lesion, Lab. Invest., 50:526.

Klintmalm, G., Bohman, S.O., Sundelin, B., Wilczek, H., 1985, Interstitial fibrosis in renal allografts after 12 to 46 months of cyclosporin treatment: beneficial effect of low doses in the early post-transplantation period, Lancet, 2:950.

Kluwe, W.M., and Hook, J.B., 1978, Analysis of gentamicin uptake by the rat renal cortical tissue, Toxicol. Appl. Pharmacol., 45:531.

Laurent, G., Maldagne, P., Carlier, M.B., and Tulkens, P.E., 1983, Increased renal DNA synthesis in vivo after administration of low doses of gentamicin in the rat, Antimicro. Agent Chemothera., 24:586.

Lippmann, KS., 1982, Is lithium bad for the kidneys?, Clin. Psychiat., 43:220.

Lokkegaard, H., Andersen, N.F., Henrisken, E., Bartels, P.D., Brahm, M., Baastrup, P.C., Joorgensen, H.E., Larsen, M., Munck, O., Rosmusseu, K.,

1985, Renal function in 153 manic-depressive patients treated with lithium for more than 5 years. Acta Psychiat. Scand. 71:347.

Luft, F.C., Patal, V., Yom, M.N., Patel, B. and Kleit, S.A., 1978, Experimental aminoglycoside nephrotoxicity. J. Lab. Clin. Med., 86:213.

Luft, F.C., Patel, V., Yom, M.N., Patel, N., and Kliet, S.A., Nephrotoxicity of cephalosporin-gentamicin combinations in rats, Antimicrob. Agent Chemother., 4:831.

Mannion, J.C., Block, R., and Popovich, N.G., 1981, Cephalosporin-aminoglycoside synergistic nephrotoxicity: fact of fiction? Drug Intell. Clin. Pharm., 15:248.

Martinez-Maldonado, M. and Opava-Stetzer, S., 1977, Distal nephron function in the rat during lithium chloride infusion, Kidney Int., 12:17.

Martinez-Maldonado, M., Stavroulaki-Tsapara, A., Tsaparas, N., Suki, W., and Eknoyan, G., 1972, Renal effects of lithium administration in rats: alterations in water and electrolyte metabolism and the response to vasopressin and cyclic adenosine monophosphate during prolonged administration, J. Lab. Clin. Med., 51:1081.

McMartin, D.N., and Engel, S.G., 1982, Effect of aging on gentamicin nephrotoxicity and pharmacokinetics in the rat, Res. Commun. Clin. Pathol. Pharm., 38:193.

Mihatsch, M.J., Thiel, G., Spichtin, H.P., 1983, Morphological findings in kidney transplants after treatment with cyclosporine, Transpl. Proc., 15:2821.

Murray, B.M., Paller, M.S., Ferris, T.F., 1985, Effect of cyclosporine administration on renal haemodynamics in conscious rats, Kidney Int., 28:767.

Myers, B.D., Ross, J., Newton, L., Luetscher, J., Perlroth, M., 1984, Cyclosporine associated chronic nephropathy, New Eng. J. Med., 311:699.

Myers, R.B., Morgan, T.O., Carney, S.L., and Ray. C., 1980, Effects of lithium on the kidney, Kidney Int., 18:601.

Palestine, A.G., Austin, H.A., Balow, J.E., Antonovych, T.T., Sabnis, S.G., Preuss, H.G., Nussenblatt, R.B., 1986, Renal histopathological alterations in patients treated with cyclosporine for uveitis, New Eng. J. Med., 314:129.

Parker, R.A., Bennett, W.M., Plamp, C.E., Houghton, C., Gilbert, D.N. and Porter, G.A.., 1980, Resistance of female rats to gentamicin nephrotoxicity, Proc. 11th Int. Cong. Chemother. Antibiot., 1:601.

Penney, M.D., Hullin, R.P., Srinivasan, D.P., and Morgan, D.B., 1981, The relationship between plasma lithium and renal responsiveness to arginine vasopressin in man, Clin. Sci., 61;793.

Perico, N., Benigni, A., Zoja, C., Delaini, F., Remuzzi, G., 1985, Functional significance of exaggerated renal thromboxane A2 synthesis induced by cyclosporin A., Am. J. Physiol., 257:F581.

Plenge, P., 1982, Mellerup, E.T., Bolurg, T.G., Burn, C., Hetmar, O., Ladefoged, J., Larsen, S., and Rafaelsen, O.J., Lithium treatment: does the kidney prefer one daily dose instead of two?, Acta Psychiat. Scand., 66:121.

Porter, G.A., and Bennett, W.M., 1985, The effect of drugs on the kidney In: "Harrison's Principles of Internal Medicine, Update VI: The New Treatment Modalities," R.G. Petersorf, R.D. Adams, E. Braunwald, K.I. Isselbacher, J.B. Martin, and J.D. Wilson, ed., McGraw-Hill Inc., New York.

Porter, G.A. and Bennett, W.M., 1986, Chronic cyclosporine associated nephropathy, Transpl. Proc., 18:204.

Porter, G.A., and Bennett, W.M., 1986, Nephrotoxin-induced acute renal failure, In: Acute Renal Failure, Chap 6., B.M. Brenner, and J.F. Stein, ed., Churchill-Livingstone, New York, London.

Porter, G.A., Bennett, W.M., and Gilbert, D.N., 1983, Unraveling amino-glycoside nephrotoxicity using animal models, J. Clin. Pharmacol., 23:445.

Radomski, J.L., Fuyat, H.N., Nelson, A.A., and Smith, P.K., 1950, The toxic effects, excretion and distribution of lithium chloride, J. Pharmacol. Exp. Thera., 100:429.

Ramsey, T.A. and Cox, M., 1982, Lithium and the kidney: A review. Am. J. Psychiat., 4:139.

Rogers, T.S., Elzinga, L., Bennett, W.M., Kelley, V.E., 1987, Selective enhancement of thromboxane in macrophages and kidneys in cyclosporine A induced nephrotoxicity: Dietary protection by fish oil. Transplantation (in press).

Schentag, J.J., Cerra, F.B., and Plaet, 1982, M.E. Clinical and pharmacokinetic characteristics of aminoglycoside nephrotoxicity in 201 critically ill patients, Antimicro. Agent. Chemother., 21:721.

Schentag, J.J., Suften, T.A., and Plaut, 1978, M.E. Early detection of aminoglycoside nephrotoxicity with beta-2-microglobulin, J. Med., 9:201.

Schou, M., Amdisen, A., Thomsen, K., Vestergaard, P., Hetmar, O., Mellerup, E.T., Plenge, P., and Rafaelsen, O.J., 1982, Lithium treatment regimen and renal water handling: the significance of dosage pattern and tablet type examined through comparison of the results of two clinics with different treatment regimens, Psychopharmacol., 77:387.

Schou, M., Amdisen, A., and Trap-Jensen, J., 1986, Lithium poisoning, Am. J. Psychiat., 124:520.

Schwass, D., Sasaki, A., Houghton, D.C., Benner, K., Bennett, W.M., 1986, Effect of phenobarbital and cimetidine on experimental cyclosporine nephrotoxicity, Clin. Nephrol., 25:S126.

Shemesh, O., Golbetz, H., Kriss, J.P., Myers, B.D., 1985, Limitations of creatinine as a filtration marker in glomerulopathic patients, Kidney Int., 28:830.

Shulman, H., Striker, G., Deeg, H.J., Kennedy, M., Storb, B., Thomas, E.D., 1981, Nephrotoxicity of cyclosporin A after allogeneic marrow transplantation: glomerular thromboses and tubular injury, New Eng. J. Med., 305:1392.

Singer, I., Rotenberg, D., and Puschett, J.B., 1972, Lithium-induced nephrogenic diabetes insipidus: In vivo and in vitro studies, J. Clin. Invest., 51:1081.

Smith, C.R. and Lietman, P.S., 1983, Effect of furosemide on aminoglycoside induced nephrotoxicity and auditory toxicity in humans, Antimicrob. Agents. Chemother., 213:133.

Smith, C.R., Lipsky, J.J., Lasker, O.L., and Lietman, P.S., 1980, Double-blind comparison of the nephrotoxicity and auditory toxicity of gentamicin and tobramycin, New Eng. J. Med, 302:1106

Steele, T.H., Dudgeon, K.L., and Larmore, C.K., 1979, Pharmacological characterization of lithium reabsorption in the rat, J. Pharmacol. Exp. Ther., 196:188.

Sugarman, A., Brown, R.S., Silvia, P., and Rosen, S., 1983, Features of gentamicin nephrotoxicity and effect of concurrent cephalothin in rats, Nephron, 34:239.

Textor, S.C., Fornan, S.J., Borer, W., Carlson, J., 1986, Sequential blood pressure hormonal and renal changes during bone marrow transplant recipients with normal renal function, Clin. Res., 34:44A.

Thompson, K. and Schou, M., 1968, Renal lithium excretion in man, Am. J. Physiol., 215:823.

Thurau, K., Mason, J., and Gstraunthaler, G., 1985, Experimental acute renal failure, In: "The Kidney", Physiology and Pathophyisology, Chap. 81., pg. 1885. D.W. Seldew and G. Giebisch, ed., Raven Press, New York,

Trollfars, B., 1983. Gentamicin-associated changes in renal function are reversible during continuous treatment, J. Antimicrob. Chemother., 12:285.

Tulkens, P.M., 1986, Experimental studies on nephrotoxicity of aminoglycosides at low doses: mechanisms and perspectives, Am. J. Med., 80:105

Tyrer, S.P., Schacht, R.G., McCarthy, M.J., Menard, K.N., Leong S., and Shopsin, B., 1983, The effect of lithium on renal haemodynamic function, Psychol. Med., 13:61.

Vaamonde, C.A., Bier, R.T., Grovea, W., Alpert, H, Kelley, J. and Pardo, V., 1984, Effect of duration of diabetes on the protection observed in the diabetic rat against gentamicin - induced acute renal failure, Miner. Electrol. Metab., 10:209.

Von Graffenreid, B., Harrison, W.B., 1985, Renal function in autoimmune diseases treated with cyclosporine, Transp. Proc., 17:215.

Walker, R.G., Bennett, W.M., Davies, B.M., and Kincaid-Smith, P., 1982, Structural and functional effects of long-term lithium therapy, Kidney Int., 11:S13.

Waller, D.G., Edwards, J.G., Naik, R., and Polak, A., 1984, Renal function during lithium treatment, Q. J. Med., 53:369.

Waller, D.G. and George, C.F., 1984, Lithium and the kidney, Adv. Drug React. Ac. Pois. Rev., 3:65.

Wallin, L., Alling, C., and Aurell, M., 1982, Impairment of renal function in patients on long-term lithium treatment, Clin. Nephrol., 18:23.

Weinberg, J.M.,1986, The role of cell calcium overload in nephrotoxic renal tubular cell injury, Am. J. Kidney Dis., 8:284.

Whelton, A and Solez, K., 1984, Sex and gentamicin-damaged kidneys, <u>In</u>: "Acute Renal Failure: Correlation Between Morphology and Function," pg. 221, A. Welton, and K. Solez, ed., Marcel Dekker, New York

Whiting, P.H., Thomson, A.W., Blair, J.T., Simpson, J.G., 1982, Experimental cyclosporin A nephrotoxicity, <u>Br. J. Exp. Pathol</u>., 63:88.

Whitworth, J.A., Mills, E.H., Coghlan, J.P., Denton, D.A., McDougall, J.G., Nelson, M.A., Spence, C.D., Tresham, J.J., Scoggins, B.A., 1987, The haemodynamic effects of cyclosporine in sheep, <u>J. Exper. Pharm. Physiol</u>. (in press).

Wood, C.A., Kohlhepp, S.J., Bennett, W.M., Porter, G.A., Houghton, D.C., Kohner, P.W., Brummet, R., Gilbert, D.N., 1987, The influence of tobramycin dosage regimen on nephrotoxicity, ototoxicity and antibacterial efficacy in a rat model of subcutaneous abscess, (submitted for publication).

Xue, H., Bukowski, R., McCarron, D.A., Bennett, W.M., 1987, Cyclosporin A induces contraction in isolated rat aorta, <u>Transplantation</u>, (in press).

LITHIUM-INDUCED DISTAL NEPHRON DILATATION IN YOUNG RABBITS WITH ASSOCIATED ENCEPHALITAZOAN CUNICULI RELATED INTERSTITIAL FIBROSIS

C.J. Roe, R.G. Walker, and P.K. Kincaid-Smith

Department of Nephrology, The Royal Melbourne Hospital, Grattan Street, Parkville 3050, Australia

INTRODUCTION

Controversy exists over whether interstitial fibrosis occurs as a consequence of chronically administered lithium. Our group in a previous study (1) using adult NZW rabbits demonstrated the presence of both interstitial nephritis and distal tubular dilatation (microcyst formation) following 12 months lithium chloride administration. The present study was conducted in order to confirm these results and in particular to try to further explore the rabbit as an animal model of renal cystic disease. In this study however, young rabbits were used to examine any potentiating effect of lithium on the developing kidney.

METHODS

Twenty-four just weaned (6 week old) NZW rabbits were divided into two groups. Eighteen animals were treated with lithium (Li) (50-175 mmol LiCl/kg food) to maintain a blood lithium level between 0.50-1.00 mmol/l. Six control (C) animals were given identical food to which LiCl had not been added. Animals were weighed weekly. Every 2 weeks serum lithium estimations were determined on a spectrophotometer for atomic absorption from 1 ml of blood extracted from ear veins. The amount of LiCl in the food was adjusted according to the serum lithium level. Each month 10 ml of blood was extracted for estimation of urea, creatinine, Ca, PO_4, K, Na HCO_3, Cl, albumin, protein and aspartate (AST) and alanine transaminase (ALT). These were determined on an auto analyser. At 6 months an additional 10 ml of blood was tested for antibodies to Encophalitzaoan cuniculi using indirect immunofluorescence. Also at 6 months all animals underwent closed renal biopsy, following premedication with 300 ug atropine sulphate and 0.02 mg acepromazine and anaesthesia using Saffan (alphaxalone 45 mg and alphadolone acetate 15 mg/ml) given as a 1 ml bolus and 0.3 ml incremental doses as required to maintain the animal pain free. Under stile conditions the kidney was palpated and immobilized by an assistant and a percutaneous procedure was employed using a true-cut biopsy needle. The whole procedure was always completed in less than 5 minutes. The 6 month renal biopsy tissue was fixed in mercuric formalin, and processed as previously described (2) and stained with haematoxylin and eosin, Masson's trichrome or periodic acid Schiff. Under light microscopy evidence of chronic interstitial nephropathy (glomerular sclerosis, tubular atrophy, cast formation and interstitial fibrosis) was semi-quantitated using a 0 to 3+ grading system (0 = absent, 1+ = mild, 2+ = moderate, 3+ = severe). In addition distal tubule luminal area was quantitated using a Hewlett Packard Digitizer (9874A) attached to a preprogrammed calculator (9825A) from the median of 25 distal tubule profiles as previously described (1) (range 9-26).

The animals were sacrificed at 12 months, the kidneys removed, photographed and weighed before being processed for histological analysis.

Statistical analysis was performed using the students t-test for unpaired data or the Wilcoxon rank-sum test. The research obtained approval from both the Royal Melbourne Hospital Board of Medical Research and Hospital Animal Ethics Committee.

RESULTS

The results of the current study are for 18 animals which have completed the first 6 months of the protocol.

Animals. One control animal died as a result of a handling accident 7 weeks after commencement. Mean$\pm$SD serum lithium (Figure 1) ranged from 0.43$\pm$0.15 mmol/l to 1.06$\pm$0.27 mmol/l in the lithium treated group. There were no observed episodes of acute lithium intoxication in any animal. The serum lithium level was not detectable in all control animals throughout the study.

Weight gain is demonstrated in Figure 2. Between 12 and 19 weeks the lithium treated group gained weight less rapidly than the control group, but both groups had similar weights at 6 months. This was not associated with inadequate nutrition as albumin and total serum proteins remained normal (see Biochemistry).

Biochemistry. A mild acidosis (serum HCO_3 < 18 mmol/l) was observed in 4 Li animals during the period of observation. However, there were no differences between the lithium treated and control groups in the change (Δ), over the 6 month period, in any of the parameters shown in Table 1. Liver function tests were also transiently abnormal as described below.

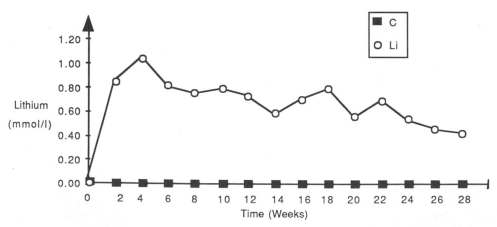

Figure 1.   Serum lithium levels over 28 weeks

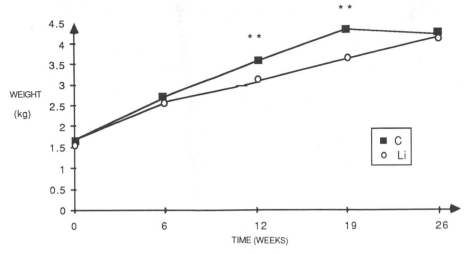

Figure 2. Weight changes over 27 weeks.

Histology. Quantitative. In general the glomeruli, tubules, interstitium and blood vessels were normal or showed only minor abnormalities for both groups. Semi-quantitative scores for pathological changes in cortex and medulla determined from sum of scores (0-3+) from 2 independent observers. Figure 3. Marked perivascular fibrosis in a lithium treated animal. However, interstitial fibrosis was present in nearly all animals and in 10/12 lithium treated and in 2/5 control animals that was distributed mainly in the perivascular areas (Figure 3).

Semi-quantitative and Quantitative. A summary of the quantitative and semi-quantitative histological findings is shown in Table 2. Only mean (±s.d.) internal luminal areas of the distal nephron was significantly greater in the lithium treated compared to control animals.

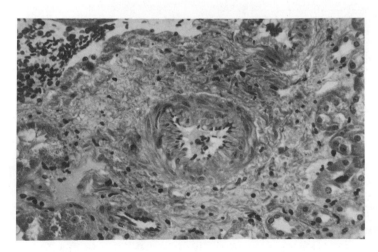

Figure 3. Marked perivascular fibrosis in a lithium trested animal

Table 1.   Biochemistry data from lithium treated animals

	CONTROL	Li	P
Δ urea (mmol/l)	2.9	1.1	NS
Δ creatinine (mmol/l)	0.0	0.0	NS
Δ Ca (mmol/l)	0.0	0.0	NS
Δ PO4 (mmol/l)	-0.7	-0.7	NS
Δ HCO3- (mmol/l)	-4.6	-3.3	NS
Δ Cl (mmol/l)	7.0	4.3	NS
Δ K (mmol/l)	0.1	-4.8	NS
Δ Na (mmol/l)	0.4	-1.0	NS
Δ Alb (gm/l)	3.4	5.3	NS
Δ Protein (gm/l)	-2.0	5.8	NS

Table 2.   Qualitative and semi-quantitative histological changes

	CONTROL			LITHIUM			p
*CORTEX	Median	Range	n	Median	Range	n	
Casts	1.0	0 - 1	5	1.0	0 - 2	10	NS
Tubule Atrophy	0.0	0 - 2	5	0.0	0 - 4	10	NS
Interstitial Fibrosis	1.0	0 - 3	5	2.5	0 - 6	10	NS
Glomerular Sclerosis	0.0	0 - 1	5	0.0	0 - 5	10	NS
**MEDULLA							
Casts	0.5	0 - 1	4	0.0	0 - 1	9	NS
Tubule Atrophy	0.0	0 - 1	4	0.0	0 - 1	9	NS
Interstitial Fibrosis	2.0	1 - 3	4	2.0	0 - 5	9	NS

*2 Li biopsies insufficient cortex
** 3 Li & 1 C biopsies insufficient medulla

MEAN DISTAL TUBULE LUMINAL AREAS
Square Units Mean ± s.d.

		n
CONTROL	1.5 ± 0.8	5
LITHIUM	3.4 ± 0.6	10
	p < 0.001	

Evidence of E. Cuniculi Infection.   When the animals were tested at   6 months all control and 10 of 12 lithium treated rabbits were antibody positive for E. cuniculi infection. Additionally, ALT was abnormal in all rabbits and AST was abnormal in 4/6 control and 9/12 lithium treated animals.

DISCUSSION

Although the 6 month renal biopsy histology was mostly normal in both groups, there were two important abnormalities. First, there was a significant increase in internal luminal area of the distal tubule in Li rabbits.   This may reflect tubule dilatation occurring secondary to a lithium-induced diuresis or may be a distinct lithium effect.   There were however no frank cystic changes (i.e. tubules greater than x10 normal size).   Further clarification of these observations may be apparent following evaluation at 12 months of lithium administration.

The second abnormality was the presence of interstitial fibrosis most marked in a perivascular location (Figure 3).   This lesion occurred in both groups of animals so cannot be attributed to lithium administration alone.   A similar lesion has been described in animals infected with the intra-cellular parasite Encephalitzoan cuniculi (3).   This organism in addition to causing chronic interstitial nephritis also causes acute ecephalitis, acute pneumonitis and acute hepatitis. No animal experienced clinical evidence of encephalitis, 2 Li animals had mild respiratory infections which resolved spontaneously. All the animals had reversible abnormalities of liver function tests and all but 2 Li animals were antibody positive at 6 months to E. cuniculi. Accordingly, it would appear that all these animals have become infected with this organism. This organism may therefore be an important aetiologic agent in the development of the observed interstitial fibrosis.

CONCLUSION

Six months lithium administration with serum lithium levels in the ranges similar to the therapeutic range in man was well tolerated in young rabbits. Distal nephron tubule dilatation had occurred without the development of frank cystic change. An interstitial fibrosis had occurred which may largely be due to infection with E. cuniculi. We would suggest that the presence of this common organism in rabbits should be taken into account when using NZW rabbits as a model of lithium nephrotoxicity.

REFERENCES

1. R.G. Walker, M. Escott, I. Birchall, J.P. Dowling, P. Kincaid-Smith, Chronic progressive renal lesions induced by lithium, Kidney Intern. 29:865-881 (1986).

2. T.H. Mathew, D.C. Mathews, J.B. Hobbs, P. Kincaid-Smith, Glomerular lesions after renal transplantation, Am. J. Med. 59:177-190 (1975).

3. J.C. Cox, H.A. Gallichio, An evaluation of indirect immunofluorescence in the serological diagnosis of Nosema cuniculi infection, Res. Vet. Sci. 22:50-52 (1977).

URINARY PHOSPHOLIPIDS PATTERNS AFTER TREATMENT WITH AMINOGLYCOSIDE ANTIBIOTICS AND CIS-PLATINUM

S. Ibrahim, Z. Kallay, F. Clerckx-Braun, J. Donnez, Ph. Jacqmin, and P.M. Tulkens

Lab. de Chimie Physiologique and International Institute of Cellular and Molecular Pathology, Unite de Pharmacocinetique et Lab. de Biopharmacie Clinique, Service de Gynecologie-Obstetrique; Universite Catholique de Louvain and Cliniques Universitaires St Luc, Bruxelles, Belgium

INTRODUCTION

Oto- and nephro-toxicity are the two main limiting factors in the clinical use of aminoglycoside antibiotics. The earliest renal alteration induced by aminoglycosides is the development of a phospholipidosis in proximal tubular cells related to the inhibition of the activities of lysosomal phospholipases and sphingomyelinase (see Tulkens, 1986 for review). Josepovitz et al. (1986) reported that large doses of aminoglycosides, the use of which is associated with the rapid onset of widespread tubular necrosis and kidney dysfunction, induce a marked urinary excretion of phospholipids in rats. We have observed that this excretion already occurs in animals treated at low, clinically relevant doses (Ibrahim & Tulkens, 1986), suggesting that it was not solely due to tubular necrosis and shedding of phospholipid-overloaded cell casts in the lumen. We have therefore examined the phospholipid excretion in humans treated with normal doses of an aminoglycoside, in the absence of significant alteration of the renal function. In parallels we have examined the phospholipid excretion in rats treated with another nephrotoxin acting on proximal tubular cells but which does not cause phospholipidosis, namely cis-platinum.

MATERIALS AND METHODS

Animals. Female Sprague-Dawley rats (200-250 mg) were injected with either gentamicin (supplied as the gentamicin complex GEOMYCIN used in human clinical practice in Belgium; Essex Belgium s.a., subsidiary of the Schering Corporation, N.J.) at 10 mg/(kg.day) for 10 days, or with cis-platinum (supplied as an sample for non-clinical investigations by Bristol Laboratories, Syracuse, N.Y.) at 2 mg/(kg.day) for 4 days. The daily doses were administered in one injection per day (qD). Controls received 0.9% NaCl on the same schedule. 24h urines were collected by placing animals individually in metabolic cages.

Patients. Nine young women suffering from pelvic inflammatory disease (who had not received an aminoglycoside before being referred to our hospital) were enrolled in the present study. Spot urine was obtained at day 0 (prior therapy) and 24h urines were collected at days 1, 4 and 7 during therapy. The antibacterial treatment consisted of netilmicin

(NETROMYCIN, Essex Belgium s.a., subsidiary of the Schering Corporation, N.J.) at an initial dose of 6.6 mg/(kg.day) given either in 1 injection (QID) or 3 injections (TID) per day, ampicillin (4 g/day, BID) and tinidazole (0.8 g/day, QID). For the patients treated on a TID schedule with netilmicin, dosage was readjusted if necessary to maintain the serum peak concentration (extrapolated at t=o) between 5 and 7 mg/l.

Assay of phospholipids. The whole 24h rat urine sample (7-15 ml) of each animal, or a 100 ml aliquot of each human urine sample was centrifuged at 25,000 rpm for 1h and the pellet suspended in 0.5-1.0 ml of water. Total lipid phosphorus was extracted and measured as described by Laurent et al. (1982). Individual phospholipids were separated by unidimensional thin-layer chromatography on silical gel 60 (Merck AG, Darmastadt, W.-Germany). For the separation of phosphatidylethanolamine (PE) and sphingomyelin (SM), elution was performed with choroform:methanol:ammonia:water (24:16:2:1, v/v). Phosphatidylinositol (PI), phosphatidylserine (PS), and phosphatidylcholine (PC) were separated by two successive developments in chloroform:methanol:acetic acid:water (65:50:1:4, v/v). The position of each phospholipid on the plates was established by comparison with reference standards chromatographed on the same plates and visualized by iodine vapour. The zones of the plates corresponding to the phospholipids to be measured were scrapped off and the samples mineralized with 60% perchloric acid at 210°C for 90 min.

Other analyses. At the end of the treatment, the animals were killed and the renal cortex collected, fixed and treated for histopathological examination using standard procedures.

RESULTS

Table I shows the excretion of phospholipids in rats. After 4 days of of treatment with gentamicin, or 2 days with cis-platinum, the excretion of all measured phospholipids was increased approximately 2- to 3-fold compared to baseline values 4-fold for phosphatidylethanolamine). When the treatment was continued for gentamicin, phospholipiduria became more pronounced for all phospholipids, reaching a 6- to 8-fold increase, except for sphingomyelin. Earlier studies have demonstrated that a 10 days treatment with gentamicin at 10 mg/(kg.day) induces a conspicuous lysosomal phospholipidosis (Laurent et al., 1982), but no widespread cortical necrosis (Kosek et al., 1974), even though a 5- to 6-fold increase in DNA cortex synthesis can be evidenced (Laurent et al., 1983), partly corresponding to a tubular repair process following focal tubular necrosis (Toubeau et al., 1986). In comparison to gentamicin-treated animals, rats receiving cis-platinum for 4 days showed considerably less phospholipid excretion. Yet, histopathological examination revealed that this treatment with cis-platinum induced widespread necrosis of proximal tubules, as previously described by Maids & Harrington (1978).

Table II shows the urinary excretion of phospholipids in women treated with netilmicin. Whereas all phospholipids measured were increased, their pattern was different from that observed in gentamicin-treated rats, with a highly predominant excretion of phosphatidylinositol. As in rats, however, sphingomyelin excretion was the least enhanced. During treatment, no patient experienced increase in serum creatinine over 0.1 mg %, and creatinine clearance was not significantly decreased (data not shown). Only minor dosing readjustment was needed to maintain patients assigned to the TID schedule within acceptable peak and through serum concentrations (5-7 mg/l and less than 1 mg/l, respectively). Patients treated on a qD schedule showed peak levels comprised between 16 and 24 mg/l. In all cases, the serum half-life of the aminoglycoside remained comprised between 1.5 and 2h.

Table I. Urinary excretion of phospholipids in gentamicin- or cis-platinum-treated rats

amount of phospholipid excreted per day
(% of day 0)*

Drug	Duration of treatment	PI [a]	PS	PC	PE	SM
G [b]	4 d.	280+32	166+19	231+20	381+47	210+29
	10 d.	864+53	783+90	745+45	603+30	338+18
C [c]	2 d.	219+30	210+45	234+23	228+49	277+65
	4 d.	327+70	240+113	357+116	284+50	301+58

* All values are significantly different from day 0 (p < 5%; n = 5)
a PI, phosphatidylinositol; PS, phosphatidylserine; PC, phosphatidyl-choline;
b PE, phosphatidylethanolamine; SM, sphingomyelin gentamicin:10 mg/(kg.day)
c cis-platinum: 2 mg/(kg.day)

Table II. Urinary excretion of phospholipids in netilmicin-treated women

Phospholipid excreted per g creatinine and
per day (in % of values at day 1)*

Duration of treatment	PI [a]	PS	PC	PE	SM
4 days	250+150	140+60	113+63	125+63	116+53
7 days	688+410	263+142	358+187	246+121	239+113

* the phospholipid:creatinine ratio at day 0 (prior therapy; spot urine) was not significantly different from that at day 1; all values shown at day 7 are significantly different from those at day 1 (p < 5%; n = 9).

a same abbreviations as in Table I.

DISCUSSION

The results of our study show that aminoglycoside treatment causes a highly significant increase in the urinary excretion of phospholipids at low, clinically relevant doses in both rats and humans. Compared to the report of Josepovitz et al. (1986), our use of low doses allows us to rule out massive cortical necrosis as the cause of aminoglycoside-induced phospholipiduria. Further, we also show that necrosis per se, as induced by cis-platinum, causes only a modest phospholipiduria, compared to that seen with gentamicin-treatment. Actually, the pattern of urinary phospholipids in gentamicin-treated animals is largely similar to that of the excess of phospholipids found in cortex during treatment with this aminoglycoside (Ibrahim et al., 1985). In humans, no significant alteration of the kidney function was observed, suggesting that the treatment used had not caused widespread histological damage. Netilmicin is known to cause marked lysosomal phospholipidosis in humans (De Broe et al., 1983). Altogether, these findings suggest that phospholipiduria induced in animals and patients mostly results from exocytosis or regurgitation of the lysosomal contents from proximal tubular cells, although focal necrosis may also partly contribute to it. Further studies are necessary to establish whether the differences in urinary phospholipids patterns seen between humans and rats relates to a species difference, or to the use of netilmicin vs gentamicin.

Several urinary constituents have been used to monitor aminoglyco-side-induced tubular alterations, such as beta-2-microglobulin, N-acetyl-beta-hexosaminidase, casts etc. Significant increase of their urinary content, however, has been observed in many other situations of renal intoxication or disturbance, including renal and/or urinary tract infection. Phospholipiduria may be a more specific index of aminoglycoside-induced alteration of tubular cells. Its usefulness for detecting patients at risk of intoxication will need, however, to be critically assessed.

ACKNOWLEDGEMENTS

We thank Dr S. Abid and Prof. P. Maldague for help in performing the histopathological examinations. This work was supported in part by the Belgian FRSM (grant no. 3.4516.79) and FNRS (grant no. 1.583.86) and by Essex Belgium, s.a., Brussels, Belgium. S.I. is the recipient of a doctoral fellowship of the Kufa College of Medicine, Al-Mustansiriayah University, Baghdad, Iraq Z.K, was ICF fellow; and P.M.T. is Maitre de Recherches of the Belgian FNRS.

REFERENCES

De Broe, M.E., G.J. Paulus, G.A. Verpooten, R.A. Giuliano, F. Roels & P.M. Tulkens. 1983. Early toxicity of aminoglycosides in human kidney: a prospective, comparative study of amikacin, gentamicin, netilmicin and tobramycin. In: Proceedings of the 13th International Congress of Chemotherapy, Vienna vol.86. K.H. Spitzy & K. Karrer, edit. 86/11-24.

Ibrahim, S., M.B. Carlier, G. Laurent & P.M. Tulkens. 1985. Quantitative analysis of the phospholipid composition of rat kidney cortex after treatment with gentamicin, dibekacin, netilmicin and tobramycin at low doses (10 mg/kg). In: 25th Intersc. Conf. Antimicrob. Agents & Chemother., Minneapolis, Minn. Abstract no. 708.

Ibrahim, S. & P.M. Tulkens. 1986. Increased urinary excretion and change of patterns of phospholipids in gentamicin-treated rats. In: 26th Intersc. Conf. Antimicrob. Agents & Chemother, New Orleans, La.

Josepovitz, C, R. Levine, T. Farrugella & G. Kaloyanides. 1986. Comparative effects of aminoglycosides on renal cortical and urinary phospholipids in the rat. Proc. Soc. Exp. Biol. Med. 182:1-5.

Kosek, J.D., R.I. Mazze & M.J. Cousins. 1974. Nephrotoxicity of gentamicin. Lab. Invest. 30:48-57.

Laurent, G., M.B. Carlier, B. Rollman, E. Van Hoof & P. Tulkens. 1982. Mechanism of aminoglycoside-induced lysosomal phospholipidosis: in vitro and in vivo studies with gentamicin and amikacin. Biochem. Pharmacol. 31:3861-3870.

Laurent, G., P. Maldague, M.B. Carlier & P. Tulkens. 1983. Increased renal DNA synthesis in vivo after administration of low doses of gentamicin to rats. Antimicrob. Agents Chemother. 24:586-593.

Madias, N.E. & J. Harrington. 1978. Platinum nephrotoxicity. Am. J. Med. 65:307-314.

Toubeau, G., G. Laurent, M.B. Carlier, S. Abid, P. Maldague, J. Heuson-Stiennon & P.M. Tulkens. 1986. Tissue repair in rat kidney cortex during short treatment with aminoglycosides at low doses: a comparative biochemical and morphometric study. <u>Lab. Invest</u>. 54:385-393.

Tulkens, P.M. 1986. Experimental studies on nephrotoxicity of aminoglycosides at low doses: mechanisms and perspectives. <u>Am. J. Med</u>. 80:105-114.

COMPARATIVE UPTAKE AND LYSOSOMAL PHOSPHOLIPIDOSIS INDUCED BY GENTAMICIN COMPONENTS C1, C1a, AND C2

Z. Kallay*, M.B. Carlier, B. Rollmann, P. Maldague and P.M. Tulkens

Lab. de Chimie Physiologique and International Institute of Cellular and Molecular Pathology; Lab. d'Analyse des Medicamentsf Laboratoire de Cytologie et Pathologie Experimentales Universite Catholique de Louvain, Bruxelles, Belgium. * Present address: Institute of Experimental Pharmacology, Slovak Academy of Sciences, Bratislava, Czechoslovakia

INTRODUCTION

Aminoglycosides are nephrotoxic and this adverse effect has triggered many efforts towards the design and/or the screening of less toxic derivatives (see Price, 1986 for a recent review). Yet, the first broad-spectrum and still widely used aminoglycoside, gentamicin, is not a pure substance and is actually commercialized as a mixture of three main components, C1, C1a and C2, which differ by the methylation of the N6 and C6 atoms in the 2',6' diaminosugar moiety. Surprisingly enough, little information is available concerning the relative nephrotoxicities of these components. Whereas some reports suggest that gentamicin C1 induces less nephrotoxicity than gentamicin complex in humans (see e.g., Mossegaard et al., 1975), others failed to substantiate such difference (e.g., Forrey et al., 1978). Kohlepp et al. (1984) showed in a comparative study in rats that gentamicin C2 and gentamicin C1a are more nephrotoxic than gentamicin C1 at an equivalent, high dosage (40 mg/kg). The uptake of gentamicin complex by rat kidney cortex, however, is saturable, with an apparent Km in a 10-20 mg/l serum concentration range (Gauliano et al., 1986). No definitive information is yet available concerning the individual components of gentamicin because of analytical difficulties (see in DISCUSSION section below), but it may be surmised that uptake, and therefore toxicities at high doses may not be predictive of the behaviour of gentamicin components at lower, more clinically-relevant doses. In this connection, we investigated the renal uptake of gentamicin C1, C1a and C2 in rats treated at doses of 4 and 10 mg/kg. Since these low doses do not induce marked histological or functional toxicities in rat kidney cortex, we also examined the early lysosomal alterations induced by the gentamicin components, which we previously demonstrated to be a useful and predictive index of aminoglycoside nephrotoxicity (see Tulkens, 1986, for review).

MATERIALS AND METHODS

Male CD/COBS rats (Charles River, France; 175-200g) were used throughout. Gentamicin C1, C1a and C2 components were supplied as sulphate salts by Pierrel SpA, Milano, Italy. Their identity and purity (over 95%) was checked by high-pressure liquid chromatography in comparison with pure samples of the same components kindly prepared by H.G, Vanderhaeghe and P.J. Claes (Laboratorium voor Farmaceutische Scheikunde, Katolieke Universiteit te Leuven, Louvain, Belgium). Each of these components were administered intraperitoneally for 4 and 10 days, at doses of 4, 10 and 20 mg/kg to separate groups of 5 animals each. The daily dose was divided in two injections given at 8 am and 8 pm, respectively. Control animals &k96H received a corresponding volume (0.5 ml) of saline. Animals were killed by decapitation 12 h after the last injection, and the kidney cortex obtained by sharp dissection. Tissue samples for biochemical analyses were immediately frozen and kept at -20°C until homogenised (1:50) in distilled water. Samples for morphological studies were fixed in 2% glutaraldehyde, postfixed with osmium tetroxide, dehydrated and embedded in Epon.

For determination of gentamicin component concentration, we used an adaptation of the method of Anhait (1977). Homogenates were added with dibekacin as internal standard. After deproteinization by addition of trichloroacetic acid (6% w/v; final concentration) and centrifugation, samples were applied to Dowex 50 W-X8 microcolumns (bed volume 0.6 ml). After washing out with 10 ml of 0.1 M-sodium acetate in 0.1 M-sodium sulphate, aminoglycosides were eluted with 0.5 ml of 0.1 N NaOH in 0.1 M-Na_2SO_4 received in 0.025 ml of a mixture of 2 M p-toluene sulphonic acid – 2 M received in 0.025 ml of acid. 0.03 ml of sample was analysed by HPLC using two Nucleosil columns 100-5-C_{18} used in serial arrangement. Elution was performed at a rate of 1 ml/min with a 40% to 80% gradient of a solution containing 0.02 M-sodium p-toluene sulphonate – 0.1 M-sodium sulphate, 0.02 M-sodium acetate and 0.04 M-acetic acid, and the same solution plus 5% acetonitrile. Post-column derivatization was performed with o-phthalaldehyde and detection was made by fluorescence.

Sphingomyelinase and total lipid phosphorus were determined as described by Laurent et al. (1982). Morphological evaluation was performed on plastic sections cut at 0.5 um and stained with toluidine blue. We used a semi-quantitative score (graded from 0 to 3) described in detail by Carlier (1984), which examines (i) the apparent size of the lysosomes; (ii) the intralysosomal accumulation of an heterogeneous, sometimes lamellar and heavily stained material; (iii) the irregularity of the lysosomal contour; (iv) the presence of metachromatic, granular material in the lumen. All scores were summed and expressed by reference to controls.

RESULTS

Table I summarizes the results of both the biochemical and morphological investigations in each treatment group. At day 10, the renal accumulation of gentamicin Cl was significantly and constantly lower than that of the two other components. The difference between Cla and C2 was not significant. At day 4, Cla was more accumulated than either C1 or even C2. The increase in total lipid phosphorus in cortex increased during the time of the treatment and according to the dose used, as described previously for gentamicin complex and other aminoglycosides (Carlier, 1984). Systematically, a lower increase was seen in animals receiving gentamicin C1, compared to the two other components, except at day 4 and at a the dose of 4 mg/kg when, however, the increases observed for all groups are at the limit of the significance. In overall, groups receiving Cla or C2 did not show significant differences in their phospholipid accumulation. Sphoingomyelinase activity decreased in all groups (except, at day 4, for animals treated with the C1 component). In overall, the decrease was more severe for animals receiving the Cla or the C2 components than for those receiving the C1. Lysosomal morphological alterations, as seen in plastic sections, developed according to the dose and the duration of the treatment. Again, lesions were systematically less pronounced in animals treated with the C1 component, compared to those receiving the other components.

Table I. Drug concentration, total lipid phosphorus, sphingomyelinase activity and morphological lysosomal alterations in the kidney cortex of rats treated with gentamicin components.

Component	Dose (mg/kg)	Treatment (days)	Component cortical concentr. (ug/g)	Total Lipid Phosph.	Sphingo-myelinase activity	Lysosomal overload
				------ % of control* -----		
C1	4	4	39±11	106±8	105±6	141
	10	4	167±25	110±7	95±9	170
	20	4	324±97	107±2	89±8	215
	4	10	46±8	103±4	92±5	148
	10	10	215±37	110±7	79±3	335
	20	10	360±20	111±4	72±5	400
C1a	4	4	100±50	108±5	93±11	226
	10	4	240±55	114±5	87±6	296
	20	4	537±96	115±6	76±8	330
	4	10	309±93	107±5	73±4	335
	10	10	318±89	121±5	76±8	500
	20	10	487±120	125±9	63±7	574
C2	4	4	87±7	102±6	89±7	181
	10	4	138±17	116±3	71±8	318
	20	4	298±65	107±5	76±8	307
	4	10	249±22	108±3	84±6	309
	10	10	338±43	122±6	79±7	483
	20	10	401±70	116±3	68±9	474

DISCUSSION

The accurate determination of aminoglycosides concentration in kidney cortex is associated with several difficulties, the major one being the correct monitoring of the respective amounts of extracted and unextracted drug. The bulk of the intracortical aminoglycoside accumulated in vivo is firmly associated with the lysosomes, and it is by no means certain that the same or, a fortiori, another aminoglycoside added in vitro to a homogenate of an untreated animal will bind to and be extracted from cellular constituents as the drug taken up in vivo. Thus, strictly speaking, all methods using external standards are fraught with difficulties, and only determinations using or controlled by means of a radioactive drug should be taken into consideration. Potentially incomplete extraction may be of minor importance when various treatments with the same aminoglycoside are compared (viz., Giuliano et al., 1986). Conversely, studies comparing different aminoglycosides are much more difficult, since extraction may vary from one drug to another, including components of the gentamicin complex. To the condition that we are not fooled by highly discrepant extraction properties, our results would indicate that gentamicin C1a is accumulated more by rat kidney cortex than gentamicin C1, whereas gentamicin C2 shows an intermediate behaviour. Lechatre et al. (1982) also found that the uptake of gentamicin C1 was lower than that of the other components in rabbits. Generally-speaking also, the severity of the lysosomal alterations induced by gentamicin C1 were consistently weaker than those observed for gentamicin C1a. Again, gentamicin C2 had an intermediate behaviour. Since these 3 components of gentamicin show the same inhibitory potency towards lysosomal phospholipases in vitro (Carlier et al, 1983), our data would strongly suggest that that the greater propensity of gentamicin C1a to cause lysosomal phospholipidosis in vivo is related to its probably higher tissue accumulation. Thus, gentamicin C1a content would need to be specially monitored in batches of gentamicin complex from different sources when comparing their nephrotoxic potential, since their composition may largely vary (see White et al., 1983). Conversely, gentamicin C1, and to a lesser extent gentamicin G2, appears safer. In this connection, it is interesting to note that sagamycin, also referred to as gentamicin C2b, in which the N6' aminogroup is methylated as in gentamicin C1 (whereas the N6' of both gentamicins C1a and C2 is a primary amine) is reported to be significantly less toxic than the gentamicin complex (Ohkoshi et al., 1977). The present results are somewhat at variance with those of Kohlepp et al. (1984), who identified gentamicin C2 as the most toxic component in gentamicin complex. This discrepancy may result from the differences in dosage used. Thus, uptake of gentamicin C1a might be more efficient at lower doses (lower apparent K_m ?), whereas more gentamicin C2 would be taken up at larger doses due to a larger maximal transport rate (V_{max}) combined with a higher apparent K_m?

Recommendations concerning gentamicin complex composition should also take the antibacterial potency of each component into consideration. Gentamicin C1 appears slightly less active than gentamicins C1a and C2 in vitro, although it is active against 6'N-acetylating strains which inactivate the two other components (Nagabhushan et al., 1982). Unfortunately, only very limited in vivo data are available concerning the pharmacokinetic and chemotherapeutic properties of the individual gentamicin components. Thus, more extensive work is probably necessary before definitive and comprehensive conclusions can be reached as to the therapeutic indexes of gentamicin components.

ACKNOWLEDGEMENTS

This work was supported in past by the Belgian FRSM (grant no. 3.4516.79) and FNRS (grant no. 1.583.86), and by a grant-in-aid from Pierrel SpA, Milano, Italy. Z.K. was ICP.fellow, and P.M.T. is Maitre de Recherches of the Belgian FNRS.

REFERENCES

Anhalt, J.P. 1977. Assay of gentamicin in serum by high-pressure liquid chromatography. Antimicrob. Agents chemother. 11:651-655.

Carlier, M.B., G. Laurent, P.J. Claes, H.J. Vanderhaeghe & P.M. Tulkens. 1983 Inhibition of lysosomal phospholipases by aminoglycoside antibiotics: comparative studies in vitro. Antimicrob. Agents Chemother 23:440-449.

Carlier, M.B. 1984. La phospholipidose renale induite par les aminoglycosides: etude biochimique et morphologique. Thesis, Universite Catholique de Louvain. 121 pp.

Forrey, A.W., B.T. Meijsen-Ludwick, M.A. O'Neil, B.M. Maxwell, A.D. Blair & R.E. Cutler. 1978. Nephrotoxicity: a comparison in humans of gentamicin and gentamicin C1 administration. Toxicol. Appl. Pharmacol. 44:453-462.

Giuliano, R.A., G.A. Verpooten, L. Verbist, R. Wedeen, M,E. De Broe. 1986 In vivo uptake kinetics of aminoglycosides in the kidney cortex of rats. J. Pharmacol. Exp. Ther. 236:470-475.

Kohlhepp, S.J., M.O. Loveless, P.W. Kohnen, D.C. Houghton, W.M. Bennett &

D.N. Gilbert. 1984. Nephrotoxicity of the constituents of the gentamicin complex. J. Infect. Dis. 149:605-614.

Laurent, G., M.B. Carlier, B. Rollman, F. Van Hoof, P. Tulkens. 1982. Mechanism of aminoglycoside-induced lysosomal phospholipidosis: in vitro and in vivo studies with gentamicin and amikacin. Biochem. Pharmacol. 31:3861-3870.

Lechatre, G., L. Merle, J.P. Valette, J. Tromchet, J.P. Charmes G G. Nicot. 1982. Study of the renal accumulation of gentamicin C1, C1a and C2 components in the rabbit. ICRS Medical Science 10:857-858.

Mosegaard, A.. P.G. Welling & P.O. Madsen. 1975. Gentamicin and gentamicin C1 in the treatment of complicated urinary tract infections: comparative study of efficacy, tolerance and pharmacokinetics. Antimicrob. Agents Chemother. 7:328-332.

Nagabhushan, T.L., G.H. Miller & M.J. Weinstein. 1982. Structure-activity relationships in aminoglycoside-aminocyclitol antibiotics. In: The amino-glycosides: microbiology, clinical use and toxicology. A. Whelton and H.C. Neu, edit., Marcel Dekker, Pub., New York. 3-27.

Ohkoshi, M., K. Nashimo, J. Ishigami & F. Miki. 1977. Summary of basic and clinical studies on KW-1062 conducted in Japan. Chemotherapy (Tokyo) 25:1781-1800.

Price, K.E. 1986. Aminoglycoside research 1975-1985: prospects for development of improved agents. Antimicrob. Agents Chemother. 29:543-548.

Tulkens, P.M. 1986. Experimental studies on nephrotoxicity of aminoglyco-sides at low doses: mechanisms and perspectives. Am. J. Med. 80:105-114.

White, L.O., A. Lovering & D.S. Reeves. 1983. Variations in gentamicin C1, C1A, C2 and C2A content of some preparations of gentamicin sulphate used clinically as determined by high-performance liquid chromatography. Ther. Drug Monit. 5:123-126.

UPTAKE AND SUBCELLULAR DISTRIBUTION OF POLY-L-ASPARTIC ACID, A PROTECTANT AGAINST AMINOGLYCOSIDE-INDUCED NEPHROTOXICITY, IN RAT KIDNEY CORTEX

Zoltan Kallay* and Paul M. Tulkens   Laboratoire de Chimie Physiologique and International Institute of Cellular and Molecular Pathology, Universite Catholique de Louvain, Bruxelles, BELGIUM.   * Present address: Institute of Experimental Pharmacology, Slovak Academy of Sciences, Bratislava, Czechoslovakia

INTRODUCTION

Williams & Hottendorf (1985), and Williams et al. (1986) have observed that the co-administration of poly-L-aspartic acid protects rats against gentamicin- or amikacin-induced nephrotoxicity. Yet, they found that co-administration of polyaspartic acid increased the total amount of amino-glycoside accumulated by kidney cortex, although less drug was recovered in fractions enriched in brush-border and basolateral membranes. We showed that polyaspartic acid significantly protects against gentamicin-induced lysosomal phospholipidosis (Beauchamp et al., 1986), an early renal alteration which we previously demonstrated to be a specific and predictive index of aminoglycoside nephrotoxicity related to the accumulation of the these drugs in lysosomes (see Tulkens et al., 1985, and Tulkens, 1986, for review). Beauchamp et al. (1986), and more recently Gilbert et al. (1987) also confirmed that polyaspartic acid did not decrease, but rather increased the amount of gentamicin stored by kidney cortex. The latter results are in contradiction with the original hypothesis of Williams & Hottendorf (1985) who selected polyaspartic acid as a potential competitor for gentamicin uptake by kidney, based on the observation that it interferes with gentamicin binding to renal membrane vesicles in vitro. In this context, we have investigated and report here on the uptake and subcellular distribution of polyaspartic acid and gentamicin in renal cortex after in vivo infusion of these compounds to rats.

MATERIALS AND METHODS

Poly-L-aspartic acid (Mr 15,000; Sigma Chem. Co., St Louis, Mo.) was labelled by acetylation of its terminal aminogroup with [^{3}H] acetic anhydride (pH 7.9, 15 min at room temperature). After exhaustive dialysis, the specific radioactivity of the final product was 296 kBeq/mg. Female Sprague-Dawley rats (200-240 g) were infused, as described by Giuliano et al. (1984), with labelled polyaspartic acid (250 mg/kg), gentamicin (100 mg/kg) or the combination of polyaspartic acid and gentamicin, over a 12 h period. All compounds were dissolved in 0.9% saline, and the solutions were infused at a flow rate of 1.025 ml/h. Two hours after the end of the infusion, the animals were killed by decapitation, and the kidney cortex was collected along with the other main organs. Tissue samples were homogenised (1:50) in distilled water. For cell fractionation experiments, the kidney cortex was homogenised in ice-cold 0.33 M phosphate-buffered sucrose and the homogenate subjected to differential and isopycnic centrifugation as described by Aubert-Tulkens et al. (1979) and Giurgea-Marion et al. (1986). Enzymes and constituents were assayed according to Proverbio & del Castillo (1981) and Giurgea-Marion et al. (1986). Gel filtration was carried out on Sephadex G50 (Pharmacia AB, Uppsala, Sweden) in 3 mM phosphate buffer.

RESULTS

Organ distribution of poly-L-aspartic acid. Based on total ^{3}H determination, the distribution of polyaspartic acid and/or of its non-volatile metabolites was (in % of the administered dose and per g or ml of organ): kidney cortex, 4.1; kidney medulla, 1.8; spleen, 0.3; heart, 0.3; liver, 0.2; lungs, 0.7; muscle, 0.1, and serum, 0.1. Kidney cortex thus concentrates polyaspartic acid and/or its degradation products. Upon filtration through Sephadex G50 columns, 43% and 61% of the radioactive material found in serum and kidney cortex, respectively, was collected in the same fractions as intact polyaspartic acid, whereas the remaining part was eluted in the fractions containing low molecular weight molecules. Based on these data, we calculated that the kidney cortex contained approx. 1.5 mg of polyaspartic acid per g of wet tissue, i.e. approx. 1.6-fold the amount of gentamicin (0.9 mg/g; Beauchamp et al,, 1986). Thus, the polyaspartic acid:gentamicin mass ratio observed in cortex was of the same order of magnitude as to that used in the infusion solution (2.5:1).

Subcellular distribution of polyaspartic acid and gentamicin. Figure 1 shows the density distribution patterns of ^{3}H, gentamicin, sphinomyalinase (lysosomes), alanylaminopeptidase (brush-border), and Na+/K+ ATPase (basolateral membrane) in sucrose gradients, after isopycnic centrifugation of post-nuclear supernatant prepared from homogenates of kidney cortex of rats infused with the combination of [^{3}H]-polyaspartic acid and gentamicin. Upon gel filtration, most of the radioactive material collected in to low density fractions was of low molecular weight, whereas most of the ^{3}H recovered in the high density fractions (1.17-1.25) eluted as intact polyaspartic acid. When only the latter is considered (thick line in Figure 1), it clearly appears that the distribution patterns of polyaspartic acid largely overlaps that of gentamicin, and that it also overlaps that of the lysosomal enzyme sphingomyelinase. Conversely, all three patterns are clearly distinct from those of alanylaminopeptidase or Na+/K+ ATPase.

DISCUSSION

The behaviour of poly-L-aspartic acid, as revealed by the distribution of both low molecular weight and large molecular weight ^{3}H, is consistent with its uptake, accumulation and partial degradation in the lysosomes of kidney cortex, followed by diffusion of the degradation products (most likely small peptides or single N-[^{3}H]-acetyl-aspartic acid) into the cytosol, as observed for many other peptides and proteins capable of filtering through the glomerular barrier. Gentamicin is also taken up by kidney cortex and accumulates in lysosomes (Just et al., 1977; Silverblatt & Kuehn, 1979; Giurgea-Marion et al., 19863. The present data therefore strongly suggest that polyaspartic acid and gentamicin become concentrated together within the same organelles in kidney cortex, namely the lysosomes. Conversely, our data fail to disclose any preferential association of gentamicin and/or polyaspartic acid to brush border or basolateral membrane two hours after cessation of the infusion.

Since lysosomes only represent a minor proportion of the total cell volume, even after treatment with gentamicin and polyaspartic acid at the

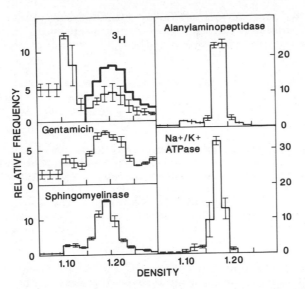

Figure 1. Isopycnic centrifugation of post-nuclear supernatant from kidney cortex of rats infused with gentamicin (100 mg/kg) and [³H]-labelled poly-L-aspartic acid (250 mg/kg) for 12 h. Animals were killed 2 h after the end of the infusion. The figure shows the relative frequency of each constituent, as a function of the density, and the surface of each histogram is therefore consistently equal to 1 (see Giurgea-Marion et al., 1986 for details on methods and calculation procedures). For the ³H distribution, the thin line (----) refers to the total radioactivity distribution, whereas the thick line (===) refers to the distribution of the large molecular weight radioactivity (approx. 50% of the total amount of radio-activity collected). The vertical bars show the SD (n=3).

doses used in this study (see Beauchamp et al., 1986), gentamicin and polyaspartic acid probably become highly concentrated therein and could easily bind to each other. Electrostatic interactions will be favoured by the acid pH (5-5.5) prevailing in lysosomes, since gentamicin will be fully protonated (the pK_a of its amino groups spanning between 5.5 and 9) whereas polyaspartic acid will still remain fully charged. Intralysosomal binding of gentamicin to polyaspartic acid could decrease its capacity to bind to phospholipids and to impair the lysosomal catabolism of phospholipids (see discussion in Laurent et al., 1982 and Carlier et al., 1983), as is indeed demonstrated in vivo. This would in turn result in protection against further toxicity (Tulkens, 1986). Ongoing in vitro and in vivo studies may help to clarify these issues.

ACKNOWLEDGEMENTS

This work was supported in part by the Belgian Fonds de la Recherche Scientifique Medicale (grants no. 3.4516.79 and 3.4551.86). Z.K. was ICP Fellow, and P.M.T. is Maitre de Recherches of the Belgian Fonds National de la Recherche Scientifique.

REFERENCES

Aubert-Tulkens, G., F. Van Hoof & P. Tulkens. 1979. Gentamicin-induced lysosomal phospholipidosis in cultured rat fibroblasts. Lab. Invest. 40:481-493.

Beauchamp, D., G. Laurent, P. Maldague, P.M. Tulkens. 1986. Reduction of gentamicin nephrotoxicity by the concomitant administration of poly-L-aspartic acid and and poly-L-asparagine in rats. Arch. Toxicol. Suppl.9:306-309.

Carlier, M.B., G. Laurent, P.J. Claes, H.J. Vanderhaeghe, P.M. Tulkens. 1983. Inhibition of lysosomal phospholipases by aminoglycoside antibiotics: comparative studies in vitro. Antimicrob. Agents Chemother. 23:440-449.

Giuliano, R.A., G.J. Paulus, R.A. Verpooten, V. Pattyn, D.E. Pollet, P.M. Tulkens & M.E. De Broe. 1984. Recovery of cortical phospholipidosis and necrosis after acute gentamicin loading in rats. Kidney Int. 26:838-847.

Giurgea-Marion, L., S. Toubeau, G. Laurent, J. Heuson-Stiennon & P.M. Tulkens. 1986. Impairment of lysosome-pinocytic vesicle fusion in rat kidney proximal tubules after treatment with gentamicin at low doses. Toxicol. Appl. Pharm. 86:271-285.

Laurent, G., M.B. Carlier, B. Rollman, F. Van Hoof, P. Tulkens. 1982. Mechanism of aminoglycoside-induced lysosomal phospholipidosis: in vitro and in vivo studies with gentamicin and amikacin. Biochem. Pharmacol. 31:3861-3870.

Tulkens, P.M., J.M. Ruysschaert, R. Brasseur, M.B, Carlier, J.P. Claes, G. Laurent & H.J. Vanderhaeghe. 1985. Computer models and structureactivity data for the prediction of aminoglycoside-induced nephrotoxicity. In: Renal Heterogeneity and Target Cell Toxicity. P.H. Bach and E.A. Lock, edit., J. Wiley & Sons, Chichester. 303-313.

Tulkens, P.M. 1986. Experimental studies on nephrotoxicity of aminoglycosides at low doses: mechanisms and perspectives. Am. J. Med. 80:105-114.

Williams, P.D. & G.H. Hottendorf. 1985, Inhibition of renal membrane binding and nephrotoxicity of gentamicin by polyasparagine and poly-aspartic acid in the rat. Res. Comm. Chem. Pathol. Pharmacol. 47:317- 320.

Williams, P.D., G.H. Hottendorf & D.B. Bennett. 1986. Inhibition of renal membrane binding and nephrotoxicity of aminoglycosides. J. Pharmacol. Exp. Ther. 237:919-925.

AMINOGLYCOSIDE ANTIBIOTICS INHIBIT THE PHOSPHATIDYLINOSITOL CASCADE IN RENAL PROXIMAL TUBULAR CELLS: POSSIBLE ROLE IN TOXICITY

George J. Kaloyanides and Leslie S. Ramsammy

Division of Nephrology and Hypertension, Department, Department of Medicine, State University of New York at Stony Brook, Stony Brook, NY 11794 and Veterans Administration Medical Center, Northport, NY 11768

INTRODUCTION

A growing body of evidence supports the conclusion that aminoglycoside antibiotics (AG) interact with phosphoinositides. For example AG have been shown to bind to phosphoinositides in model membranes (1-5) by a mechanism best explained by an electrostatic interaction (3,5). The strong avidity of these drugs for phosphatidylinositol-4,5-bisphosphate (PIP_2) (1,5,6) has led to the hypothesis that PIP_2 serves as the biological receptor for these agents (6-8). AG have been shown to induce a phosphatidylinositol (PI)-enriched phospholipidosis in rat renal cortex (9,10) and in cells grown in culture (11,12), a phenomenon which may be related to the observation that AG have the capacity to inhibit a PI-specific phospholipase C (13-15). Moreover, neomycin has been shown to block the hydrolysis of PIP_2 and the generation of inositol trisphosphate (IP3) in response to agonist stimulation in vitro (16,17) and to depress the synthesis and turnover of $[^{32}P]PIP_2$ in vitro and in vivo (1,18,19). These observations indicate that AG have the potential to perturb the PI cascade, which serves as the transmembrane signal transducing mechanism for a number of agonists (20). Inhibition of the PI cascade by AG might cause profound derangements in the regulation of a number of intracellular processes and thereby contribute to the toxicity of these agents. As a first step in testing this hypothesis we examined the capacity of gentamicin to disrupt the PI cascade in primary cultures of rabbit proximal tubular cells (RPTC) and in the renal cortex of the rat.

METHODS

Primary cultures of RPTC were prepared as described by Taub (21) and grown in plastic culture dishes (60 mm diameter) at $37^{\circ}C$ under an atmosphere of 5% CO_2 and room air in Delbecco's modified Eagle's medium to which was added insulin (5 ug/ml), transferrin (5 ug/ml) and hydrocortisone ($5\times10^{-8}M$). Experiments were performed after the cells attained confluency which usually occurred between 7 and 10 days. To assess the effect of gentamicin on agonist stimulation of IP_3 generation monolayers were incubated in medium containing $[^3H]$myoinositol for 48 hr to label the phosphoinositide pool. Then, the cells were incubated in fresh medium with or without gentamicin ($10^{-3}M$). LiCl ($10^{-3}M$) was added to the cultures 24 hr prior to agonist stimulation. On the morning of the experiment the cells were suspended in a test tube containing 2 ml of fresh medium and preincubated at 37°C for 3 min. After stimulation by agonists (10^{-6}) preincubated at 37°C for 3 min. the addition of perchloric acid (final concentration 5%). Labelled inositol phosphates were separated by sequential elution from a Dowex formate column (22) and assayed in a liquid scintillation counter.

In separate cells grown for 48 hr in medium containing gentamicin $(10^{-3}M)$, we examined the effect of parathyroid hormone (PTH) $(10^{-6}M)$ on the redistribution of protein kinase C from the cytosolic to the membrane fraction prepared by centrifuging sonicated cells at 75,000 xg for 6 min. Protein kinase C was assayed as the difference between ^{32}P phosphorylation of exogenous histone I in the presence and absence of phosphatidylserine and Ca^{++} (23). In other gentamicin-exposed cells we examined the effect of PTH $(10^{-6}M)$ on cAMP generation. Five min after stimulation with PTH the cells were pelleted, resuspended in buffer, sonicated and assayed for cAMP by RIA.

Male Sprague-Dawley rats were injected s.c. with 0.9% NaCl or gentamicin (100 mg/kg b.wt. per day) for 2 days and sacrificed 24 hr later. Fifteen min prior to sacrifice the rats were injected i.p. With 0.9% NaCl or 2 U of PTH. Protein kinase C activity was assayed in the cytosolic and membrane fractions of the renal cortex.

RESULTS

In control cells PTH stimulated a significant increase in IP_3 at 1 and 2 min and a significant increase of IP but only at 2 min whereas no change in IP_2 was detected (Figure 1). The response at 2 min was maximal as no further increase was observed at 5 min. In cells exposed to gentamicin for 48 hr baseline levels of individual inositol phosphates were not different from those of control cells and no significant changes from baseline were detected in response to PTH (Figure 1).

In cells exposed to gentamicin for 48 hr cAMP increased from a baseline level of 64 ± 4.7 to 87 ± 1.7 pmol/mg protein (P < 0.01). This response was not statistically different from that of control cells (69.3 ± 5.1 to 101.3 ± 5.8 pmol/mg protein).

PTH had no effect on total protein kinase C activity of control cells, but it stimulated a significant redistribution of enzyme activity from the cytosolic to the membrane fraction (Table 1). In cells exposed to gentamicin for 48 hr, PTH had no significant effect on total, cytosolic or membrane protein kinase C activity (Table 1).

In control rats PTH had no effect on total protein kinase C activity in renal cortex but it stimulated a significant redistribntion of protein kinase C from the cytosolic to the membrane fraction (Table 2). In rats injected with gentamicin for 2 days PTH failed to alter either total activity or the distribution of protein kinase C activity between the cytosolic and membrane fractions (Table 2).

Angiotensin II (AII), phenylephrine (PE), bradykinin (BK) and arginine vasopressin (AVP) also stimulated generation of IP_3 in FPTC (Table 3). In cells exposed to gentamicin for 24 hr, these agonist failed to augment IP_3 formation (Table 3).

DISCUSSION

The objective of these experiments was to test the hypothesis that AG inhibit the PI cascade in renal proximal tubular cells. In previous studies we demonstrated that RPTC grown in primary culture accumulate

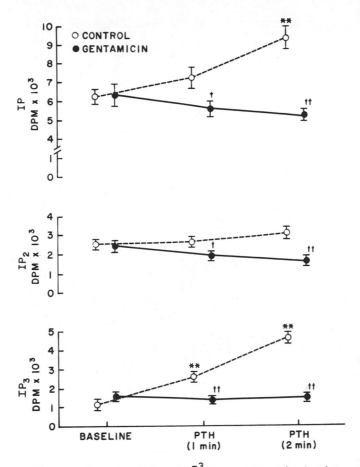

Figure 1. Effect of gentamicin (10^{-3}M) on PTH stimulation of inositol phosphates in primary cultures of RPTC. Data represent mean±S.E. (N=5) in dpm/culture plate. ** significantly different from baseline, P < 0.01 and †† significantly different from control, P < 0.01

Table 1. Effect of PTH on protein kinase C activity in RPTC[a]

	TOTAL		CYTOSOLIC		MEMBRANE	
PTH	−	+	−	+	−	+
Control	171	174	192	150*	126	192**
	±27	±8	±9	±14	±9	±18
Gentamicin	161	148	170	183	154	146
	±21	±22	±8	±12	±26	±22

a. Data represent mean±S.E. (N = 5) expressed a pmol/mg protein.
* significantly different from baseline, P < 0.05.
** Significantly different from baseline, P < 0.01.

Table 2. Effect of PTH on protein kinase C activity in rat renal cortex[a].

| | TOTAL | | CYTOSOLIC | | MEMBRANE | |
| | - | + | - | + | - | + |
PTH						
Control	62	66	105	98*	35	44**
	± 2	± 2	± 3	± 1	± 2	± 1
Gentamicin	64	64	102	105	37	38
	± 3	± 3	± 2	± 2	± 1	± 1

a. Data represent mean$\pm$S.E. (N = 6) expressed as pmol/mg protein.
*   significantly different from baseline, $P < 0.05$.
**   significantly different from baseline, $P < 0.01$.

Table 3. Effect of gentamicin on agonist stimulation of IP3 generation in RPTC[a].

AGONIST	CONTROL	IP_3	GENTAMICIN
NONE	1483 ± 65	NS	1540 ± 92
PTH 10^{-6}M	2503 ± 111	$P < 0.01$	1345 ± 64
AII 10^{-6}M	2959 ± 283	$P < 0.01$	1688 ± 121
PE 10^{-6}M	2660 ± 90	$P < 0.01$	1608 ± 119
BK 10^{-6}M	3814 ± 255	$P < 0.01$	1655 ± 166
AVP 10^{-6}M	3106 ± 309	$P < 0.01$	1410 ± 178

a. Data represent the mean$\pm$S.E. (N = 5) expresssed as dpm/culture plate. PTH, parathyroid hormone: AII, angiotensin II: PE, phenylephrine: BK, bradykinin: AVP, arginine vasopressin.

gentamicin in high concentration and develop a PI-enriched phospho-lipidosis in association with the characteristic lysosomal ultrastructural lesion, the myeloid body (12). Moreover, we showed that the phospholipid-osis was due in large measure to impaired degradation of phospholipid (12). In other experiments we found that by 12 days of exposure to 10^{-3}M gentamicin primary cultures of RPTC manifested unequivocal evidence of cell injury including decreased total protein, decreased incorporation of [^{14}C]leucine into protein, decreased total DNA, decreased incorporation of [^{14}C]thymidine into DNA, and decreased trypan blue exclusion (unpublished observations). These results suggested that primary culture of RPTC would be a suitable model for examining the effects of gentamicin on agonist-stimulation of the PI cascade. Moreover, this cell culture model affords obvious technical advantages over the intact kidney in terms of achieving uniform labelling of the phosphoinositide pool and of measuring the generation of IP_3 over brief time intervals in response to agonist stimulation.

PTH has been shown to activate the PI cascade as well as adenylate cyclase in renal proximal tubular cells (24-26). Therefore we chose in our initial studies to examine whether gentamicin had any inhibitory effect on PTH generation of IP_3 in RPTC grown in primary culture. We demonstrated that 10^{-6}M PTH activated the PI cascade in RPTC as assessed by the increased generation of IP_3 and that it also activated the adenylate cyclase system as evident by the increased generation of cAMP. In RPTC exposed to 10^{-3}M gentamicin for only 24 hr PTH failed to stimulate a rise in IP, whereas the rise in cAMP was not different from that of control cells. We interpret the rise in cAMP as evidence that gentamicin did not prevent PTH from interacting with its plasma membrane receptor and the failure of PTH to stimulate IP_3 generation reflects an effect of gentamicin at a step distal to agonist-receptor binding. The data are consistent with our hypotheses that gentamicin binds to PIP_2 and prevents its hydrolysis by phospholipase C.

Activation of the PI cascade also leads to the generation of diacyl-glycerol which stimulates protein kinase C activity by promoting redistribution of the enzyme from the cytosolic to the membrane fraction (20). We demonstrated that PTH stimulated redistribution of protein kinase C in RPTC grown in culture and that gentamicin completely blocked this response. Thus, we have obtained evidence that gentamicin inhibited both arms of the PI cascade as predicted by our hypothesis that gentamicin inhibits the hydrolysis of PIP_2.

These experiments were performed in a cell culture model using a concentration of gentamicin (10^{-3}M) considerably higher than that used clinically or in in vivo toxicology studies. In order to determine whether these observations obtained in vitro hold relevance for the in vivo situation, we examined the effect of gentamicin on PTH-stimulated redistribution of protein kinase C activity in rat renal cortex. We chose a dose of PTH which has been shown to stimulate a maximal phosphaturic response in the rat (27). We chose a dose of gentamicin (100 mg/kg per day x2) which we have shown causes a reproducible degree of proximal tubular cell injury in the rat if continued for 4 to 6 days (28,29). We observed that PTH did stimulate recruitment of protein kinase C from the cytosolic to the membrane fraction of rat renal cortex but that this effect was completely inhibited in rats injected with two doses of gentamicin. We interpret these data as evidence that gentamicin at a dose known to cause nephrotoxicity in rats in vivo also inhibits the PI cascade.

Finally we demonstrated that inhibition of the PI cascade by gentamicin was not limited to PTH but that all agonists known to activate the PI cascade in renal proximal tubular cells including angiotensin II (30), phenylephrine (30), and bradykinin (31) were also inhibited. Unexpectedly, we found that AVP also stimulated the PI cascade in RPTC and that this effect was blocked by gentamicin. AVP has been shown to activate the PI cascade via the V_1 receptor (32), but this receptor has not been identified in proximal tubular cells. It is unclear whether the V_1 receptor becomes expressed in primary cultures of RPTC or whether the high concentration of AVP (10^{-6}M) used in our experiments stimulated hydrolysis of PIP_2 by a non-specific mechanism.

In summary, we have obtained evidence that gentamicin at doses known to cause toxicity in vitro in primary cultures of RPTC and in vivo in rat renal cortex induced a generalized inhibition of agonist-stimulation of the PI cascade. Particularly noteworthy is the fact that inhibition of the PI cascade in primary cultures of RPTC and in rat renal cortex occurred early in the course of gentamicin exposure before the appearance of typical functional or morphological lesions of injury and necrosis. Thus, perturbation of the PI cascade could be a proximal event in the injury cascade of aminoglycoside toxicity.

The mechanism by which a generalized disruption of the PI cascade contributes to AG toxicity is open to speculation at this time. It is known that IP_3 through its effect on mobilizing intracellular Ca^{++} activates a calmodulin-dependent protein kinase activity which has a broad substrate specificity and participates in the regulation of a number of enzymes (33). Derangements in the regulation of these enzymes may contribute to the toxicity of AG. Activation of protein kinase C by DAG has been shown to interact synergistically with calmodulin-dependent protein kinase (33). Protein kinase C also participates in the response to growth factors (34) by stimulating Na^+/H exchange (35) and by inducing ornithine decarboxylase (36) the first and rate limiting enzyme in the synthesis of polyamines (37). Ornithine decarboxylase and polyamines participate in the regulation of cell growth and regeneration (37). Thus, depression of this key enzyme might compromise the capacity of proximal tubular cells to mount an appropriate and effective response to derangements in the function/structure of subcellular membranes and organelles induced by AG. In view of the critical role of the PI cascade in the regulation of a number of intracellular processes, the potential impact of inhibition of this transmembrane signaling mechanism on the integrity and viability of the cell would appear to be substantial.

ACKNOWLEDGEMENTS

This research was supported by grant AM 27061 from the ADDHO Institute of the National Institutes of Health and by the Research Service of the Veterans Administration.

REFERENCES

1. J. Schacht, N.D. Weiner and S. Lodhi, Interaction of aminocyclitol antibiotics with polyphosphoinositides in mammalian tissues and artificial membranes, In: Cyclitols and Phosphoinositides, W.W. Wells and F. Eisenberg, ed., Academic Press, New York (1978).

2. R. Brasseur, G. Laurent, J.M. Ruysschaert and P. Tulkens, Interactions of aminoglycoside antibiotics with negatively charged lipid layers, Biochem. Pharmacol. 33:629 (1984).

3. L. Chung, G. Kaloyanides, R. McDaniel, A. McLaughlin and S. McLaughlin, Tnteraction of gentamicin and spermine with bilayer membranes containing negatively charged phospholipids, Biochemistry 24:442 (1985).

4. L. Ramsammy and G.J. Kaloyanides, Effect of gentamicin on the transition temperature and permeability to glycerol of phosphatidyl-inositol-containing liposomes, Biochem. Pharmacol. 36:1179 (1987).

5. S. Au, N.D. Weiner and J. Schacht, Aminoglycoside antibiotics preferentially increase the permeability in phosphoinositide-containing membranes: a study with carboxyfluorescein in liposomes. Biochim. Biophys. Acta 902:80 (1987).

6. J. Schacht, Isolation of an aminoglycoside receptor from guinea pig inner ear tissues and kidney, Arch. Otorhinolaryngol. 224:129 (1979).

7. J. Schacht, Molecular mechanisms of drug-induced hearing loss, Hearing Res. 22:297 (1986).

8. M. Sastrasinh, T.C. Rnauss, J.M. Weinberg and H.D.Humes, Identification of the aminoglycoside receptor of renal brush border membrane, J. Pharmacol. Exp. Ther. 222:350 (1982).

9. S. Peldman, M. Wang and G.J. Kaloyanides, Aminoglycosides induce a phospholipidosis in the renal cortex of the rat: An early manifestation of nephrotoxicity, J. Pharmacol. Exp. Ther. 220:514 (1982).

10. C. Josepovitz, T. Farruggella, R. Levins, B. Lane and G.J. Kaloyanides, Effect of netilmicin on the phospholipid composition of

subcellular fractions of rat renal cortex. *J. Pharmacol. Exp. Ther*. 235:810 (1985).

11. D. W. Schwertz, J. I. Greisberg and M.A. Venkatachalam, Gentamicin-induced alterations in pig kidney epithelial (LLC-PK1) cells in culture, *J. Pharmacol. Exp. Ther*. 236:254 (1986).

12. C. Josepovitz, L. Ramsammy, B. Lane and G.J. Kaloyanides, Gentamicin inhibits degradation and stimulates synthesis of phosphatidylinositol in primary culture of rabbit proximal tubular cells. *Kidney Int*. 31:369 (1987).

13. J.J. Lipsky and P.S. Lietman, Aminoglycoside inhibition of a renal phosphatidylinositol phospholipase C, *J. Pharmacol. Exp. Ther*. 220:287 (1982).

14. K.Y. Gostetler and L.B. Hall, Inhibition of kidney lysosomal phospho-lipases A and C by aminoglycoside antibiotics: Possible mechanism of aminoglycoside toxicity. *Proc. Natl. Acad. Sci. USA* 79:1663 (1982).

15. D.W. Schwertz, J.I. Ereisberg and M.A. Ventkatachalam, Effects of aminoglycosides on proximal tubule brush border membrane phosphatidyl-inositol-specific phospholipase-C, *J. Pharmacol. Exp. Ther*. 231:48 (1984).

16. H. Streb, J.P. Heslop, R.F. Irvine, I. Schulz and M.J. Berridge, Relationship between secretagogue-induced Ca^{++} release and inositol poly-phosphate production in permeabilized pancreatic acinar cells. *J. Biol. Chem*. 260:7309 (1985).

17. W. Siess and E.G. Lapetine, Neomycin inhibits inositol phosphate formation in human platelets stimulated by thrombin but not other agonists, *FEBS* 267:53 (1986).

18. P. Marche, S. Komtouzov and A. Girard, Impairment of membrane phospho-inositide metabolism by aminoglycoside antibiotics: streptomycin, amikacin, kanamycin, dibekacin, gentamicin and neomycin, *J. Pharmacol. Exp. Ther*. 227:415 (1983).

19. P. Marche, B. Olier, A. Girard, J.-P. Fillastre and J.-P. Morin, Aminoglycoside-induced alterations of phosphoinositide metabolism 31:59 (1987).

20. M.J. Berridge, Inositol trisphosphate and dicylglycerol: two interact-ing second messengers, *Ann. Review Biochem*. 56:159 (1987).

21. M. Taub, Growth of primary and established kidney cell cultures in serum-free media, *In*: Methods for Serum-Free Culture of Epithelial and Fibroblastic Cells, Alan R. Liss, Inc., New York (1984).

22. C.P. Downes and R.B. Michell, The polyphosphoinositide phosphodiester-ase of erythrocyte membranes, *Biochem. J*. 198:133 (1981).

23. R. Minakuchi, Y. Takai, B. Yu and Y. Nishizuka, Widespread occurrence of calcium-activated, phospholipid dependent protein kinase in mammalian tissues, *J. Biochem*. 89:165 (1981).

24. R.V. Farese, P. Bidot-Lopez, A. Sabir, and J.S. Smith, Parathyroid hormone acutely increases polyphosphoinositides of the rabbit kidney cortex by a cycloheximide-sensitive process. *J. Clin. Invest*. 65:1523 (1980).

25. E.A. Hruska, D. Moskowitz, P. Esbrit, R. Civitelli, S. Westbrook and M. Huskey, Stimulation of inositol trisphosphate and diacylglycerol production in renal tubular cells by parathyroid hormone, J. Clin. Invest. 79:230 (1987).

26. H. Rasmussen, I. Rojima, W. Apfeldorp and P. Barrett, Cellular mechanism of hormone action in the kidney: messenger function of calcium and cyclic AMP, Kidney Int. 29:90 (1986).

27. E. Pastoriza-Munoz, R.E. Colindres, W.E. Lassiter and C. Lechene, Effect of parathyroid hormone on phosphate reabsorption in the rat distal convolntion., Am. J. Physiol. 235:F321 (1978).

28. L. Soberon, R.L. Bowman, E. Pastoriza-Munoz and G.J. Kaloyanides, Comparative nephrotoxicities of gentamicin, netilmicin and tobramysin in the rat, J. Pharmacol. Exp. Ther. 210:324 (1979).

29. L. Ramsammy, G.-Y. Ling, C. Josepovitz, R. Levine and G.J. Kaloyanides, Effect of gentamicin on lipid peroxidation in rat renal cortex, Biochem. Pharmacol. 34:3895 (1985).

30. G. Wirthensohn and W. G. Guder, stimulation of phospholipid turnover by angiotensin II and phenylephrine in proximal convoluted tubules micro-dissected from mouse nephron, Pflugers Arch. 404:94 (1985).

31. J.A. Shayman and A.R. Morrison, Bradykinin-induced changes in phosphatidylinositol turnover in cultured rabbit papillary collecting tubules, J. Clin. Invest. 76:978 (1985).

32. D.A. Troyer, D.W. Schwertz, J.I. Rreisberg and M.A. Venkatachalam, Inositol phospholipid metabolism in the kidney, Ann. Review Physiol. 48:51 (1986).

33. H. Rasmussen, The calcium messenger system. New Engl. J. Med. 314:1164 (1986).

34. Y. Nishizuka, Studies and perspectives of protein kinase C, Science 233:305 (1986).

35. W.H. Moolenar, Effects of growth factors on intracellular pH regulation, Ann. Rev. Physiol. 48:363 (1986).

36. A.M. Jetten, B.R. Ganong, G.R. Vandenbark, I.E. Shirley and R.M. Bell, Role of protein kinase C in diacylglycerol-mediated induction of ornithine decarboxylase and reduction of epidermal growth factor binding. Proc. Natl. Acad. Sci. USA 82:1941 (1985).

37. M.A. Grillo, Metabolism and function of polyamines, Int. J. Biochem. 17:943 (1985).

SILYMARIN AMELIORATES GENTAMICIN NEPHROTOXICITY

M.K. Chan* and W.L. Ng

Department of Medicine* and Department of Pathology, University of Hong Kong, Queen Mary Hospital, Hong Kong

INTRODUCTION

Gentamicin (GM) nephrotoxicity is most evident in the proximal tubules which sustain injury as a result of membrane-related events (1-3). Silymarin (SL), an extract from the plant milk thistle, has been shown to exert membrane protective effects (4). The possibility that silymarin may prevent or ameliorate GM-induced nephrotoxicity is investigated in a rat model.

METHODS

Non-inbred, male Sprague-Dawley rats weighing from 180-260g, were randomly divided into 3 groups of 10 animals, and housed 5 to a cage. Group 1 animals each received a daily intraperitoneal (i.p.) injection of 100 mg/kg of GM sulphate for 28 days or until it was sacrificed. Group 2 animals were given 15 mg/kg of SL daily by mouth for 6 days. Then a daily i.p. injection of GM, 100 mg/kg, was given as in group 1, for up to 28 days. Oral administration of SL continued in the same dosage while the animals received GM. Group 3 animals were given both SL and GM from the start of the experiment, 28th day. All animals were fed Purina chow and given water ad libitum. 24-h urine samples were collected on days 0, 3, 6, 8, 10, 12, 14 from group 1 rats. Because rats in groups 2 and 3 lived to the 28th day, urine was also collected on day 21 and 28 from these animals. In addition, group 2 rats had urine collected on day -6, i.e. before the administration of SL. The urine samples were stored at -40°C until assayed for total protein concentration by colourimetry, for N-acetyl-ß-Glucosaminidase (NAG) activities (6), for ß2-microglobulin concentrations using a kit from Pharmacia, and for creatinine concentrations by the rate of chromogen formation with picric acid. Blood was obtained from the retro-orbital plexuses of the rats on the same days when urine was collected and the serum separated and stored pending assay for creatinine. Necropsies were carried out on sacrificed or dead animals. Tissue blocks were taken from both kidneys for light and electron microscopy and remaining kidney tissue were separated into cortex and medullary tissues, snapped frozen in liquid nitrogen and stored at -70°C pending assay for tissue GM concentrations. The kidney tissue were weighed and homogenised. The suspensions were centrifuged at a speed of 3000 r.p.m. for 20 minutes. The supernatant was collected and the GM concentration measured using a Syva CP 5000. The results were expressed as micrograms of GM per gram of wet kidney tissue. SL was supplied by Madaus & Co. The tablets were pulverised and sonicated in distilled water. The suspension was then filtered to get rid of the film coat of the tablets and finally made up to a concentration of 30 mg/ml. Differences among groups were evaluated with the Mann-Whitney U test. In the same animal before and after treatment differences were determined by the paired-t test or Chi^2. A $p < 0.05$ (two-tailed) was regarded as significant.

RESULTS

Body weight. Group 1 animals became uraemic and listless after GM injections and lost weight from day 6 onwards so that the mean weights on day 12 and day 14 respectively was significantly ($p < 0.0001$) lower than the starting weight. Six animals died and the rest were moribund and sacrificed on day 14. Animals in groups 2 and 3 did not gain weight in the first 2 weeks of GM administration. However, the animals were more active and their mean weights on days 12 and 14 were significantly higher than the corresponding values of group 1 animals. One animal in group 2 died of anaesthesia and another in group 3 died of uraemia within 2 weeks. The rest continued to thrive and gain weight despite the continued GM administration. Thus on or before day 14, 6 of 10 animals given GM alone died while only 2 of 20 animals that had also received SL died. The difference was significant ($p < 0.01$, Chi^2).

Urinary NAG. Baseline 24-h urine NAG excretions were comparable among all 3 groups of rats. Group 1 rats showed a marked increase in NAG excretion which peaked on day 8, the difference from the baseline value being highly significant ($p < 0.0001$). Urinary NAG excretion also increased in groups 2 and 3, but not as markedly as in group 1. In general, the difference in urinary NAG excretion between SL treated rats and rats which received GM alone was statistically significant from day 6 onwards. There was no statistically significant difference in urinary NAG excretion between SL-pretreated and SL-cotreated rats.

Urinary protein excretion. In group 1 rats, urinary protein excretion increased after GM administration in parallel with NAG and reached highly statistically significant difference from baseline values on day 8, 10 and 12. In SL-treated rats, the same phenomenon was observed for urinary protein and NAG excretion.

Urinary ß2-microglobulin. Urinary ß2-microglobulin also increased after GM injection and the difference from baseline values reached statistical significance on days 8, 10 and 12. However, because of wide disperse of data, the p values were not significant. Five rats each in groups 2 and 3 had urinary ß2-microglobulin excretion determined. There was a large scatter of data, so that although values observed after GM injections were higher than pretreatment values, the difference was not statistically significant. No significant difference was observed in urinary ß2-microglobulin excretion between SL-treated rats (either pretreatment or cotreatment) and rats that received GM alone.

Serum creatinine. All 3 groups had comparable serum creatinine concentrations to start with. Group 1 rats became uraemic and their mean serum creatinine concentration reached a peak of 0.23 mmol/l on day 12, which was highly significantly different from baseline values. The increase in serum creatinine concentrations in groups 2 and 3 was not as marked as was in group 1.

Creatinine clearance. The mean baseline creatinine clearance was comparable in all 3 groups, being 0.60 for group 1, 0.52 for group 2 and 0.53 for group 3 rats. Creatinine clearance decreased from day 6 onwards in group 1 rats and the difference from baseline values was highly significant. Creatinine clearances in groups 2 and 3 also decreased after GM administration, but the difference from the baseline was not statistically significant. The difference in creatinine clearance between the SL-treated rats and that of the rats which received only GM was highly significant.

The biochemical data are summarized in Table 1. For clarity, values on day 6 and day 21 and ß2-microglobulin values are omitted.

Table 1. Mean Biochemical Values in Rats given Gentamicin with or without Silymarin

		Days after intraperitoneal gentamicin administration							
		-6	0	3	8	10	12	14	28
Weight	1.	-	219	225	208	193	181^b	169^a	-
(g)	2.	213	219	239	228	223^c	223^c	220^c	292^a
	3.	-	210	209	198	201	195	199^c	293^a
NAG	1.	-	274	735^a	1680^a	1143^a	1165^a	-	-
(mU/24h)	2.	236	240	543^b	$750^{a,c}$	$626^{b,c}$	$562^{b,c}$	375^b	362^b
	3.	-	260	613^a	813^a	$751^{a,c}$	453^c	368	441^b
Protein-	1.	-	8.5	11.5	32.0^a	32.7^a	28.0^a	-	-
uria	2.	6.2	8.6	12.4	$16.3^{b,c}$	$17.3^{b,c}$	$13.1^{b,c}$	9.9	14.4
	3.	-	6.0	7.5	$11.4^{b,c}$	$9.1^{b,c}$	$12.6^{b,c}$	7.9	10.0
Ccr	1.	-	0.60	0.64	0.32^a	0.12^a	0.17^a	-	-
(ml/min/	2.	0.55	0.52	0.51	0.41	0.59^c	0.52^c	0.48	0.88
100g)	3.	-	0.53	0.53	0.49	0.38^c	0.25^b	0.59	0.56
Creatinine	1.	-	0.03	0.035	0.09^a	0.22^a	0.23^a	-	-
(mmol/l)	2.	0.04	0.05	0.046	0.08^b	0.06^c	0.06^c	0.06	0.03
	3.	-	0.04	0.043	0.06	0.06^c	0.08^{bc}	0.04	0.04

a = Difference from baseline, p < 0.005
b = Difference from baseline, p < 0.03
c = Difference from corresponding value in group 1, p < 0.01

Tissue GM concentrations. The GM concentrations in homogenised kidney tissues from all 3 groups of rats are given in Table 2. In a pilot study, 5 rats given GM alone as in group 1 and 5 rats treated as in group 2 were sacrificed on day 6 and the mean tissue GM concentration was, respectively, 477 and 467 ug/g of kidney tissue. The tissue GM concentration in group 1 rats averaged 477 ug/g around day 14. The mean tissue GM concentration on day 28 was 459 ug/g in group 2 and 295 ug/g in group 3 respectively. SL did not interfere with GM assay since in 5 rats sacrificed after 5 days of SL the tissue GM concentration was less than 1 ug/g. The tissue GM concentration on day 28 in group 3 rats was significantly lower than all the other values.

Morphology of the kidney. Sections from kidneys in all 3 groups showed tubular necrosis on light microscopy. On electron microscopy, numerous cytosegregosomes containing myelin-like bodies were seen in sections from group 1 animals. In kidney sections from groups 2 and 3, the myelin-like bodies were not so conspicuous and not as numerous (Fig. 1).

DISCUSSION

Proximal tubular dysfunction is characteristic of GM induced nephro-toxicity and in severe cases the glomerular ultrafiltration coefficient is

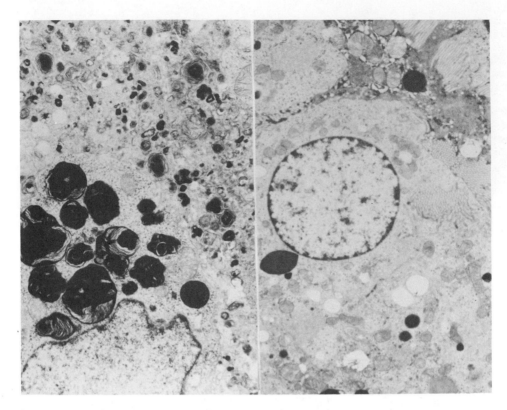

Fig. 1. Typical electron micrographs of proximal renal tubular cells of rats given gentamicin alone (left-hand side) and of those receiving gentamicin and silymarin at the same time (right-hand side). Note the numerous and prominent myelin-like figures which are characteristic of gentamicin nephrotoxicity.

Table 2. Gentamicin Concentrations [a] (ug/g wet tissue) in Renal Cortex of Rats

	Group 1	Group 2	Group 3
Day 6[b]	477±61 (n=5)	467±53 (n=5)	–
Day 14	477±48 (n=9)	–	–
Day 28	–	459±57 (n=9)	295±28 (n=9)[c]

a All values in mean±s.e.m.
b In a pilot study, five rats in each group were sacrificed on day 6.
c Different from value on day 14 in group 1 (p < 0.01) and from corresponding value in group 2 (p < 0.05).

c is not mentioned on original

reduced. All these features were apparent in our study. Urinary NAG and urinary protein excretion increased. ß2-Microglobulin also showed a significant rise. Creatinine clearance decreased and serum creatinine concentrations rose. The rats lost weight and died of uraemia. Pretreatment with SL did not affect renal function and could not prevent GM nephrotoxicity. However, both pretreatment and cotreatment with SL significantly reduced the degree of GM-induced nephrotoxicity functionally and morphologically. Qualitatively the number of myelin-like bodies was reduced and a semiquantitative analysis is in progress. What is most significant is that the SL-treated rats did not lose weight and were able to survive up to at least 28 days despite continued GM administration. Although it has been reported that rats which survive the initial nephrotoxic insult by GM can withstand the continued administration of the drug without succumbing to uraemia, our rats received much higher doses of GM (100 mg/kg/day) and were more frequently bled than the animals in previous studies (8), even though SL was given by mouth, the volume of fluid administered never exceeded 0.2 ml per day. Thus the observed reduced GM nephrotoxicity in SL-treated rats could not be explained by volume expansion.

The mechanism of the protective effects afforded by SL is not clear. The proximal tubules are prone to damage by GM because the cells accumulate the drug by pinocytosis. That SL does not affect the early accumulation of GM in kidney tissues is evident from our demonstration that GM concentrations in renal cortical homogenates on day 6 did not differ significantly between SL treated rats and rats that received GM alone. That SL does not modulate the initial events of GM nephrotoxicity is reflected by the fact that in SL treated rats, urinary NAG and protein excretion did increase after GM injections and that the difference in the mean values of these parameters from those of rats given GM alone reached significance only from day 8 onwards. Thus it is more likely that SL enhances renal tubular regeneration. Tubular regeneration is obvious in GM nephrotoxicity as soon as tubular necrosis occurs. SL has been shown to increase hepatic cellular regeneration after subtotal hepatectomy (9).

Aminoglycosides are important antibiotics for gram-negative sepsis. Clinically evident nephrotoxicity occurs in about 8.7-14% of patients treated with aminoglycosides, although different aminoglycosides have different nephrotoxic potentials (10). Although GM nephrotoxicity can be reduced by loading animals with calcium chloride (11), such pretreatment is of little value in clinical practice. Furthermore, calcium chloride reduces receptor binding of GM and may reduce the anti-microbial activity of drug (12). Thus it is especially significant that we have shown that not only pre-, but also co-treatment, with SL reduces GM nephrotoxicity. SL has been used in various forms of toxic hepatitis (13) without side effects. It apparently possesses a "membrane-stabilizing" effect (4) and can act as a scavenger for oxygen radicalsl (4). The dose of SL commonly used is 5 mg/kg whereas that of GM is 1-3 mg/kg. We have used 3 times the normal dose of SL and over 30 times the dose of GM in our experiments. It is conceivable that GM nephrotoxicity in patients can be reduced by cotreatment with clinically achievable doses of SL. While admitting that the usual dosing principles of aminoglycoside therapy and risk factors of nephrotoxicity should not be ignored, we suggest that a trial of SL is warranted in patients who have multiple risk factors and for whom aminoglycoside therapy cannot be avoided.

ACKNOWLEDGEMENT

The study was supported by grant no. 335/041/0031 (University of Hong Kong) and a grant from the Wing Lung Bank Medical Research Fund. The technical assistance of Joseph Leung and Patrick Yip in the biochemical measurements, of Allan Cheung in measuring tissue gentamicin concentrations and of S.F. Wong in the care of the rats is gratefully acknowledged.

REFERENCES

1. J.C. Kosek, R.I. Mazze, M.J. Cousins, Nephrotoxicity of gentamicin, Lab Invest 30:48-57 (1974).

2. F.O. Luft, V. Patal, M.N. Yum, B. Patel, S.A. Kleit, Experimental aminoglycoside nephrotoxicity, J Lab Clin Med 86:213-220 (1975).

3. J.M. Wellwood, D. Lovell, A.E. Thompson, J.R. Tighe, Renal damage caused by gentamicin: a study of the effects of renal morphology and urinary enzyme excretion, J Path 118:171-182 (1976).

4. G. Ramellini, J. Meldolesi, Stablization of isolated rat liver plasma membranes by treatment in vitro with silymarin, Arzneim-Forsch (Drug Res) 24:544-552 (1977).

5. J.J. Sedmak, S.E. Grossberg, A rapid, sensitive, and versatile assay for protein using Coomassie Brilliant Blue G250, Anal Biochem 79:544-552 (1977).

6. D. Maruhn, Rapid colorimetric assay for ß-galactosidase and N-acetyl-ß-glucosaminidase in human urine, Clin Chim Acta 73:453-561 (1976).

7. C. Bayliss, H.K. Rennke, B.M. Brenner, Mechanism of the defect in glomerulo ultrafiltration associated with gentamicin administration, Kidney Int 12:344-353 (1977).

8. D.N. Gilbert, D.C. Houghton, W.M. Bennett, C.E. Plamp, K. Reger, G.A. Porter, Reversibility of gentamicin nephrotoxicity in rats: recovery during continuous drug administration (40397), Proc Soc Exp Biol Med 160:99-103 (1979).

9. E. Magliulo, P.G. Carosi, L. Minoli, S. Gorini, Studies on the regenerative capacity of the liver in rats subjected to partial hepatectomy and treated with silymarin, Arzneim-Forsch (Drug Res) 23:161-167 (1973).

10. G. Kahlmeter, J.I. Dahlager, Aminoglycoside toxicity - a review of clinical studies published between 1975 and 1982, J Antimicrob Chemother 13 (Suppl A):9-22 (1984).

11. W.M. Bennett, W.C. Elliot, D.C. Houghton, D.N. Gilbert, J. DeFehr, D.A. McCavron, Reduction of experimental gentamicin nephrotoxicity by dietary calcium loading, Antimicrob Agent Chemother 22:508-512 (1982).

12. L.E. Bryan, H.M. Van Den Elzen, Effects of membrane-energy mutations and cations on streptomycin and gentamicin in susceptible and resistant bacteria, Antimicrob Agents Chemother 12:163-177 (1977).

13. B. Tuchweber, W. Trost, M. Salas, R. Sieck, Prevention of Praeseodymium-induced hepatotoxicity by silybin, Toxicol Appl Pharmacol 38:559-570 (1976).

14. A. Bindoli, L. Cavallini, N. Siliprandi, Inhibitory action of silymarin of lipid peroxide formation in rat liver mitochondria and microsomes, Biochem Pharmacol 26:2405-2409 (1977).

POSSIBLE ROLE OF THE RENIN-ANGIOTENSIN SYSTEM IN THE DEVELOPMENT OF
GENTAMICIN NEPHROTOXICITY IN THE RAT

J.P. Morin, N. Thomas, H. Toutain, H. Borghi and J.P. Fillastre

INSERM U-295, Universite de Rouen, B.P. 97-76 800 Saint Etienne
Du Rouvray, France

INTRODUCTION

The possible involvement of the renin angiotensin system in the
development of drug induced renal failure was investigated by inhibiting
the activity of Angiotensin Converting Enzyme (ACE) with Perindopril, a
new specific and potent inhibitor of ACE (1). The anti-hypertensive
activity of Perindopril is similar to that of Ramipril and greater than
that of Enalapril (2). The pattern of gentamicin induced kidney damage is
now well established (3,4) and thus allowed the use this drug to produce a
model of drug induced renal failure with proximal tubule injury. This
study was performed in Wistar rats and consisted of the evaluation of
renal morphological, biochemical and functional parameters.

EXPERIMENTAL PROTOCOL

Perindopril was given orally as a single daily administration of 2 mg/kg
in 1 ml water. Gentamicin was given daily as a single ip injection of 50
mg/kg in 0.4 ml of isotonic saline.

Four groups of animals were designated as follows (Fig. 1). Group A (n =
25): Control: daily administration of 1 ml water (po) from day -15 to day
+15, daily injection of 0.4 ml isotonic saline (ip) from day 0 to day +15.

Group B (n = 37): Gentamicin: daily administration of 1 ml water (po) from
day -15 to day +15, daily injection of Gentamicin (ip) 50 mg/kg from day 0
to day +15.

Group C (n = 25): Perindopril: daily administration of Perindopril (po) 2
mg/kg from day -15 to day +15, daily injection of 0.4 ml isotonic saline
(ip) from day 0 to day +15.

Group D (n = 37): Perindopril + Gentamicin: daily administration of
Perindopril (po) 2 mg/kg from day -15 to day +15, daily injection of
Gentamicin (ip) 50 mg/kg from day 0 to day +15.

Animals from groups A and C were sacrificed at 0 (n = 6), 7 (n = 6), 15 (n
= 6), and 22 days (n = 7); and animals from groups B and D were sacrificed
at 2 (n = 6), 4 (n = 6), 7 (n = 6), 10 (n = 6), 15 (n = 6) and 22 days (n
= 7).

Seven animals from each group were housed individually in diuresis cages from day −2 up to day +22. The urinary excretion of creatinine, sodium, potassium, calcium, cyclic AMP (radiocompetition assay using erythrocyte membranes) and N-acetyl-ß-D-glucosaminidase (NAG) excretions was measured daily throughout the study. The blood levels of creatinine and ACE activity using Hippuryl-Histidyl-Leucine substrate (5) were measured on the day of sacrifice. Biochemical analysis of renal cortex was performed on the day of sacrifice and consisted of assay of alanine aminopeptidase (3), cathepsin B (3), NAG (3), sphingomyelinase (using chromogenic substrate as described in ref 6) and antibiotic concentration (microbiological assay using Bacillus subtilis ATC 6633 as test organism) in homogenates of renal cortex (1:100 w/v) in distilled water.

Fragments of kidney cortices were processed for light and electron microscopy.

RESULTS

All animals in groups A, B, and C survived whereas 5 animals in group D died between day 6 and 10. Creatinine clearance remained unchanged in groups A and C throughout the study, was slightly decreased (by 20%) from day 2 to day 7 in group B and drastically decreased in group D (by 80% at day 7) from day 2 to day 15. All surviving animals had recovered normal creatinine clearances at day +22.

Serum ACE activity (fig 3) was slightly decreased at days 10 and 15 in group B after Gentamicin treatment. In Group C, inhibition of serum ACE activity was established at day 0 (40 to 50% of control levels), was sustained up to day +15 and was reduced upon treatment withdrawal: (80% of control levels at day 22). In group D, inhibition of serum ACE was established at day 0 (46% of control levels) and was further enhanced on day 7 (13% of control levels) and was sustained at day 15. Partial recovery of serum ACE activity was seen upon treatment withdrawal (67% of control levels at day +22).

Urinary parameters: In group B, diuresis (Fig. 2) increased from day 7 to reach a sustained level (100% increase) between day 10 and 15. This returned to control value at day +22. A slight polyuria (30% increase of diuresis) occurred in group C from day 0 to day +15. Diuresis returned to normal values upon treatment withdrawal. In group D, diuresis was increased between day 4 and day 6. At days 7 and 8, two of the seven animals had diuresis < 1 ml/24 hours and died at day 9, two of the 7 animals became polyuric with diuresis between 26 and 56 ml/24 hours and the remaining animals of the group had normal diuresis and became polyuric at day 10. Mean polyuria was sustained at high levels (25 − 45 ml/24 hours) between days +13 and +22 (Fig. 2).

Urinary calcium and cyclic AMP excretion (Fig. 5) remained stable in groups A and C throughout the study. In groups B and D urinary calcium excretion increased from day 2 concomitant with a decrease of urinary excretion of cyclic AMP leading to a large decrease of the urinary cyclic AMP / calcium excretion ratio (Fig. 3). This ratio was affected to a greater extent in group D than in group B.

Urinary excretion of sodium and potassium were not affected in groups A and C, they were slightly decreased in group B between days 2 and 8 and severely decreased between days 4 and 12 in group D. Urinary excretion of NAG (Fig. 4) remained stable in groups A and C, and was increased by 50 to 100% of control values in group B between days 6 and 14. A biphasic pattern is seen in group D: Urinary NAG excretion increased from day 2, reached a first peak value at day 6, decreased to a trough value at day 10, increased to a second peak value at day 16 and declined slowly until day 22.

Renal cortex biochemistry: Renal cortex activity of alanine aminopeptidase (Fig. 6) was not affected in groups A, B and C but was decreased from day 4 to 22 in group D. This activity did not recover upon treatment withdrawal up to day 22.

Renal cortex activity of cathepsin B (Fig. 7) was not affected in groups A and C. This activity was decreased from day 2 to day 22 in group B, with a trough level at day 7 (66% of control value). In group D, cathepsin B activity was decreased from day 2 to day 22, with a trough level at day 7 (36% of control value).

Renal cortex activity of NAG (Fig. 8) was not affected in groups A and C. This activity was slightly decreased in groups B and D, with a trough level at day 7 (about 70% of control value). Similar patterns were seen between groups B and D for this parameter.

Renal cortex activity of sphingomyelinase (Fig. 9) was not affected in groups A and C. This activity was decreased very early in group B with a trough level at day 2 (41 % of control value), recovered control levels at days 7 and 10, was again decreased at day 15 (55% of control value) and recovered control levels upon treatment withdrawal. In group D, the impairment of sphingomyelinase activity was less marked and delayed when compared to group B: a trough was seen at day 4 (52% of control value) after which sphingomyelinase activity was partially restored at days 7 and 10 and again declined at days 15 and 22.

Renal cortex accumulation of Gentamicin (Fig. 10) was more pronounced in group D than in group B at days 2, 4, 7, 15 and 22. Gentamicin concentrations were similar for both groups at day 10.

Pathology: No modification of morphological appearance was observed either by optical or electron microscopy in Group A throughout the study. In group C very mild lesions were seen in the deep cortex consisting essentially in dilatation of intracellular spaces of proximal tubules. These lesions were more clearly shown at the ultrastructural level. No lesion of the ultrastructural morphology of epithelial cells was seen.

In group B, the typical feature of aminoglycoside induced renal injury was seen. Lesions were maximal at days 4 and 7 and consisted of focal necrosis of proximal tubule cells which were scored as moderate lesions. Ultra-structural examination revealed a partial loss of the proximal tubule cell brushborder and an extensive overloading of their lysosomes with myeloid bodies.

In group D, extensive lesions of renal cortex were seen as soon as day 2. At day 4, marked dilatation of intercellular spaces and necrosis of proximal tubule cells were seen by both light and electron microscopy. Maximal lesions were seen at day 7: renal cortex structure was markedly disturbed: tubule cells were necrotic, numerous tubules were obstructed with cell debris and/or colloids, and epithelial intercellular spaces and vasa recta appeared dilated suggestive of extensive osmotic nephrosis. Lysosomal overloading with myeloid bodies appeared to be less marked than in group B at the same time. Despite continuation of the treatment, the morphological appearance was improved at days 10, 15 and 22. At day 22, cortical lesions were still clearly seen.

DISCUSSION

Perindopril treatment at the dose of 2 mg/kg produced a clear pharmacological effect: serum ACE inhibition was stable between day 0 and day 15 in group C. No renal toxicity of Perindopril was seen: no clear effect of the drug on renal function or structure was seen under our experimental conditions in group C. These findings are consistent with previously published data (7), which show that ACE inhibition enhance renal plasma flow without changing glomerular filtration rate, and may also improve the capacity of the kidney to excrete sodium. One should however keep in mind that there are some limits to these beneficial effects: in the case of low perfusion pressure, autoregulation of glomerular filtration rate cannot be maintained and renal failure may occur. Gentamicin administration during the blockade of the renin angiotensin system led to extensive renal injury with two superimposed features:-

i) proximal tubule cell necrosis with lysosomal phospholipidosis which is a well known feature of gentamicin induced nephrotoxicity, and
ii) dilatation of the vascular compartment and of intercellular spaces of tubular epithelial cells which may result from enhanced modification of the renal haemodynamic or ultrafiltration capacity induced by the the blockade of the renin angiotensin system (decrease of K_f or of oncotic pressure in peritubular capillaries) during gentamicin induced renal failure.

Several mechanisms involving prostaglandins, the renin-angiotensin system or the kallikrein-kinin systems have been implicated in the pathogenesis of acute renal failure. Some data are available on aminoglycoside induced renal failure:-

i) Indomethacin, an inhibitor of prostaglandin synthesis caused a further decline of renal function in aminoglycoside treated rats suggesting that prostaglandins may have a protective effect against aminoglycoside-induced nephrotoxicity (8) while they do not seem to play a significant role in the control of renal function in normal rats (9,10)
ii) Higa et al (8) showed that the use of aprotinin, a kallikrein inhibitor, in aminoglycoside treated rats had no additional effect on their renal function.
iii) Schor et al (11) showed that aminoglycosides may stimulate the renin angiotensin system, and
iv) Klotman et al (12) demonstrated that the co-administration of Captopril and gentamicin in potassium depleted Sprague Dawley rats further increased the deleterious effects of Gentamicin. This was not seen in potassium repleted animals.

Luft et al (13) reported a further decrease of creatinine clearance in rats receiving Captopril + Gentamicin as in rats receiving Gentamicin alone. Kimbrough et al (14) showed that activation of the renin-angiotensin system was an essential condition for the control of renal function by angiotensin II which took place in sodium-depleted animals and not in sodium-repleted animals.

The observation that neither inhibition of prostaglandin synthesis nor inhibition of the renin-angiotensin system induce any significant changes of the renal function of the normal rat, but cause a further decline of renal function in aminoglycoside treated animals suggest that the integrity of these systems may play an important role in the limitation of kidney injury during drug induced nephrotoxicity.

210

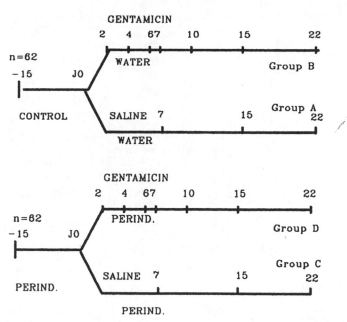

Figure 1. Scheme of treatment protocol where 6 animals were killed at each time point.

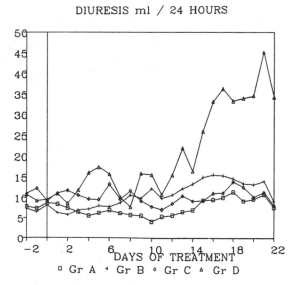

Figure 2. Time course of diuresis where data is represented as mean of 6 animals housed individually for the duration of the study.

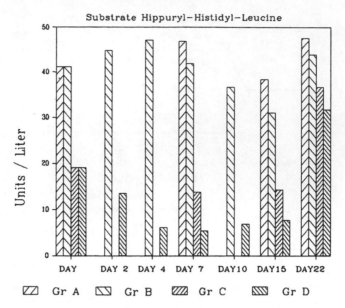

Figure 3. Serum ACE activity of 6 animals at the time of sacrifice

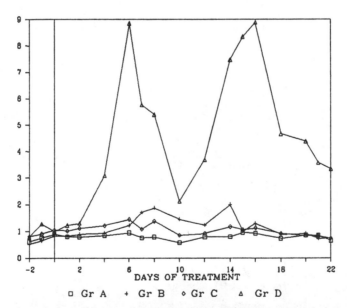

Figure 4. Urinary NAG excretion mU/uMole creatinine

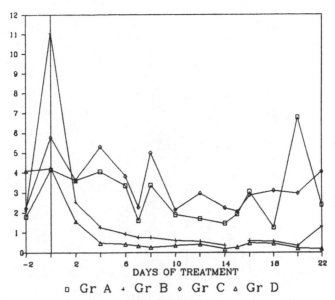

Figure 5. Urinary cAMP/calcium excretion expressed as nMole cAMP/uMole calcium.

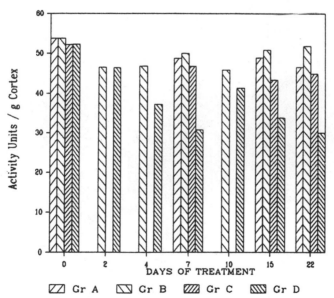

Figure 6. Renal cortex content of alanine aminopeptidase in units of activity per g of cortical tissue. Mean of 6 values.

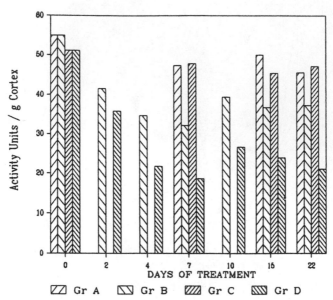

Figure 7. Renal cortex content of cathepsin B units of activity per g of cortical tissue. Mean of 6 values.

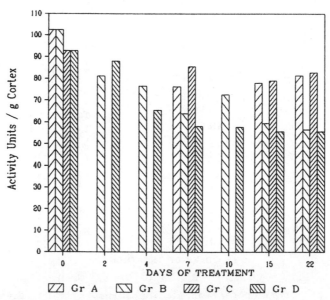

Figure 8. Renal cortex content of NAG in units of activity per g of cortical tissue. Mean of 6 values.

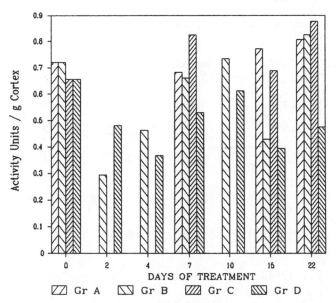

Figure 9. Renal cortex content of sphingomyelinase in units of activity per g of cortical tissue. Mean of 6 values.

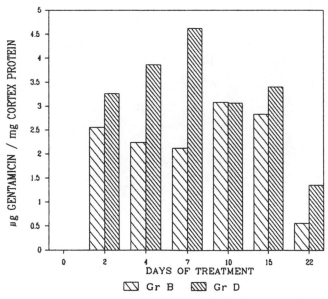

Figure 10. Renal cortex content of gentamicin in ug concentration per mg of cortical tissue. Mean of 6 values.

BIBLIOGRAPHY

1.   LAUBIE M., SCHIAVI P., VINCENT M., SCHMITT H.   J. Cardiovasc. Pharmacol. 1984:8, 1076.

2.   UNGER T., MOURSI M., GANTEN D., HERMAN K., LANG R.E.   J. Cardiovasc. Pharmacol. 1986:8, 276.

3.   MORIN J.P., VIOTTE G., VANDEWALLE A., VAN HOOF F., TULKENS P., FILLASTRE J.P.   Kidney Int. 1980:18, 583.

4.   BENNETT W.M.   Nephron 1983:35, 73.

5.   CUSHMAN D.W., CHEUNG H.S.   Biochem. Pharmacol. 1971:20, 1637

6.   GAL A.E, BRADY R.O., HIBBERT S.R., PENTCHEV P.G.   New Engl. J. Med. 1975:293, 632.

7.   BRUNNER H.R., WAEBER B., NUSSBERGER J.   Kidney Int. 1987:31 (S20), S104.

8.   HIGA E.M.S., SCHOR N., BOIM M.A., ATZEN H., RAMOS O.L.   Braz. J. Med. Biol. Res. 1971:18, 355

9.   TERRAGNO N.A., TERRAGNO D.A., McGIFF J.C.   Circ. Res. 1977: 40, 590.

10.   HAYLOR J., LOTE C.J.   J. Physiol. 1980:298, 371.

11.   SCHOR N., ICHIKAWA I., RENNKE H.G., TROY J.L.   Kidney Int. 1981:19, 288.

12.   KLOTMAN P.E., BOATMAN J.E., VOLPP B.D., BAKER J.D., YARGER W.E. Kidney Int. 1985:28,118.

13.   LUFT F.C., ARONOFF G.R., EVAN A.P., CONNORS B.A., WEINBERGER M.H., KLEIT S.A.   J. Pharmacol. Exp. Ther. 1982:220, 433.

14.   KIMBROUGH H.M., VAUGHAN E.D., CAREY R.M., AYERS K.W., Circ. Res. 1977:40, 174.

EFFECT OF FUROSEMIDE AND VERAPAMIL ON GENTAMICIN NEPHROTOXICITY

H. Nakahama, M. Horio, T. Moriyama, Y. Fukuhara, Y. Orita and T. Kamada

Osaka University Medical School, First Department of Medicine, 1-1-50, Fukushima, Fukushima-ku, Osaka 553, Japan

INTRODUCTION

While furosemide (F), a potent loop diuretic, has been known to potentiate gentamicin (G) nephrotoxicity (1), verapamil (V), a calcium entry blocker, has been postulated to attenuate gentamicin nephrotoxicity (2). We have therefore examined the effect of furosemide or verapamil co-administration with gentamicin on renal gentamicin accumulation.

MATERIALS AND METHODS

Groups of Sprague Dawley rats weighing 200-250 g (n = 6) received either gentamicin alone (40mg/kg/day) [group-G], a combination of gentamicin (40mg/kg/day) and furosemide (5mg/kg/day) [group-GF] or a combination of gentamicin (40mg/kg/day) and verapamil (100 ug/kg/day) [group-GV] subcutaneously in two divided doses. Groups of rats were also given either normal saline [group-C], furosemide alone [group-F], or verapamil alone [group-V] to serve as controls. Animals were fed with standard rat laboratory chow and allowed water ad lib. Rats were sacrificed after 10 experimental days. The kidney cortices were removed for determination of renal gentamicin concentration and renal calcium content. We employed haematoxylin-eosin staining for ordinary light microscopic examination and Von Kossa staining for the detection of calcium deposition in the tissue. Renal gentamicin concentration was determined by substrate labelled fluorescence immunoassay (SLFIA, TDA-gentamicin, Ames Sankyo Inc., Tokyo, Japan), after the renal cortex was homogenised with thirty volumes of Tris-Hepes buffer (pH 7.4) by Virtis-23 homogenizer. Renal calcium content was determined by atomic absorption spectrometry. Renal function was assessed on day-1, day-6 and day-10 by blood urea nitrogen (BUN) and serum creatinine levels.

Values are expressed as mean$\pm$SD. Dunnet's or Scheffe's multiple comparison analyses were used in the statistical evaluation of the data and p values of less than 0.05 were taken to indicate statistically significant differences.

RESULTS

The summary of body weight gain (%), BUN and serum creatinine levels is shown in Table 1.

Group-F and group-GF rats showed a significant growth retardation as compared with group-C (p < 0.05). No significant difference in renal function was found among the groups studied. The renal gentamicin concentration in group-GF (414±85 ug/g wet tissue) was significantly (p < 0.05) higher than that in group-G (172±38 ug/wet tissue) and that in group-GV (193±59 ug/wet tissue). The difference between [group-G] and group-GV was not significant (Fig. 1). No significant difference in renal calcium content was found among the groups studied (Fig. 2).

Although, light microscopically, moderate degeneration and necrosis of proximal tubular cells were found in group-G, GV and GF, little calcium deposits were found on Von Kossa's calcium staining (Fig. 3). No difference in the degrees of proximal tubular damage was found among the groups G, GV and GF.

Table 1. Weight gain, blood urea nitrogen and serum creatinine at sacrifice. n = 6 mean±SD

	C	G	GV	V	GF	F
BW(%)	30±4	22±15	25±8	36±8	5±13*	14±6*
BUN(mg/dl)	20±3	76±57	48±31	19±3	76±69	12±3
s-Cr(mg/dl)	0.6±0.4	1.7±1.3	1.1±0.4	0.9±0.6	1.8±1.5	0.4±0.1

* p < 0.05 compared with group-C
furosemide (F); gentamicin (G); verapamil (V)

DISCUSSION

Most of the studies that have investigated the effect of furosemide on gentamicin nephrotoxicity indicate that furosemide enhances gentamicin nephrotoxicity. The mechanism by which furosemide enhances gentamicin nephrotoxicity remains unclear, however. In the present study, we have

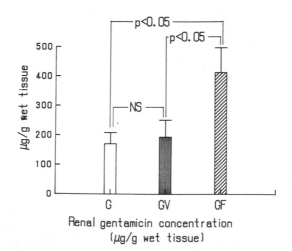

Figure. 1 Concentration of gentamicin in the renal cortex homogenates at sacrifice. n = 6 mean±SD

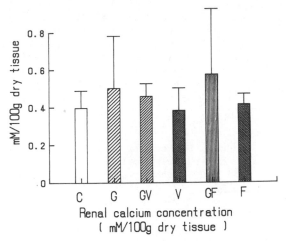

Figure. 2. Renal calcium content at sacrifice, n = 6 mean±SD

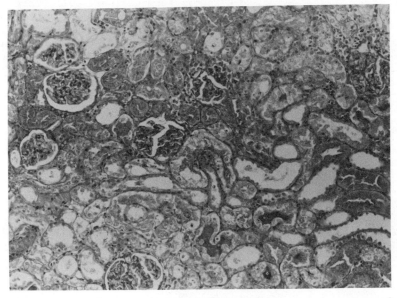

Figure. 3. A light microscopic examination of the renal cortex of a group-GF rat at sacrifice. Moderate degenaration and necrosis of the proximal tubular cells were present.

clearly shown that furosemide facilitates gentamicin accumulation in kidney tissues. This facilitation of gentamicin accumulation may well be a factor for enhanced nephrotoxicity. The reason for no significant impairment of renal function in group-GF despite higher renal gentamicin concentration may be that the observation period of 10 days could have been too short for the renal function impairment to become overt. We have already reported that furosemide facilitates renal gentamicin accumulation and thereby causes renal failure within five days (3). Thus it seems that susceptibility to gentamicin nephrotoxicity varies among experimental animal species.

While verapamil is proposed to be effective as a protective agent in various models of ischaemic acute renal failure (4) and subtotally nephrectomized rats (5) the protective effect of verapamil on aminoglycoside nephrotoxicity has been a controversial subject. In the present study, we could not observe any effect of verapamil on renal gentamicin accumulation or on renal calcium content, which is proposed to be elevated in association with gentamicin nephrotoxicity (6). Thus we could not draw any conclusion on the effect of verapamil.

REFERENCES

1. R.D. Adelman, W.L. Splanger, F. Beasom, G. Ishizaki and G.N. Conzelman. Furosemide enhancement of experimental gentamicin nephrotoxicity; comparison of functional and morphorogical changes with activities of urinary enzyme. J. Infect. Dis. 140:342 (1979)

2. H. Eliahou, A. Iaina, I. Serbon, S. Gaveno and S. Kapuler. Verapamil's beneficial effect and cyclic nucleosides in gentamicin-induced acute renal failure (ARF) in rats (abstract). Proc. IX Int. Cong. Nephrol. 323A (1984)

3. Y. Orita, Y. Fukuhara, H. Nakahama, M. Horio, T. Moriyama and T. Kamada. Enhanced nephrotoxicity of gentamicin by furosemide. In: Diuretics II. Chemistry, Pharmacology and Clinical Applications. J.B. Puschett ed., Elsevier Science Publishing Co. Inc. New York. (1987)

4. T.J. Burke, P.E. Arnold, J.A. Gordon, R.E. Bulger, D.C. Dobyan and R.W. Schrier. Protective effect of intrarenal membrane blockers before or after renal ischemia. J. Clin. Invest. 74:1830 (1984)

5. D.C. Harris, W.S. Harnond, T.J. Burke and R.W. Schrier. Verapamil protects against progression of experimental chronic renal failure. Kidney Int 31:41 (1987)

6. R.E. Cronin, K.L. Nix, E.R. Ferguson, P.M. Southern and W.L. Henrich. Renal cortex ion composition and Na-K ATPase activity in gentamicin nephrotoxicity. Am. J. Physiol. 242:F477 (1982)

RENAL PHOSPHOLIPIDOSIS IN RATS AFTER GENTAMICIN AND PEFLOXACIN COADMINISTRATION AT LOW DOSES

M.-B. Carlier, Z. Kallay* and P.M. Tulkens

Laboratoire de Chimie Physiologique and International Institute of Cellular and Molecular Pathology, Universite Catholique de Louvain, Bruxelles, Belgium . * Present address: Institute of Experimental Pharmacology, Slovak Academy of Sciences, Bratislava, Czechoslovakia

INTRODUCTION

Fluoroquinolones constitute a new class of highly active, wide spectrum antimicrobials (see Wolfson & Hooper, 1985; and Hooper & Wolfson, 1985 for review), among which pefloxacin is one of the first to have reached wide clinical usage. Since up to 60% of the administered dose of pefloxacin is eliminated through the kidney, it appears important to examine its potential nephrotoxicity. Moreover, pefloxacin can be administered in combination with an aminoglycoside in order to broaden the spectrum covered by the antiinfective therapy and/or to decrease the risk of emergence of bacterial resistance to either of these drugs (Pechere et al., 1987). Combination of other antibiotics with an aminoglycoside may increase (viz. vancomycin; Wood et al.,1986; Francq-Dufief et al., 1987), or decrease (viz. fosfomycin or piperacillin; Laurent et al., 1985; Carlier et al., 1987) aminoglycoside toxicity. In this connection, we have examined and report here on the influence of pefloxacin on the development of lysosomal phospholipidosis, an early, sensitive and predictive index of aminoglycoside-induced nephrotoxicity in animals and man (see Tulkens, 1986, for review).

MATERIALS AND METHODS

Female Sprague-Dawley rats (180-200 g) were injected for 4 and 10 days with gentamicin at 4 and 10 mg/(kg.day) alone or in combination with pefloxacin at 50 and 100 mg/(kg.day). Gentamicin was given i.p., whereas pefloxacin was administered s.c. All biochemical analyses of the cortical tissue were performed exactly as described earlier (Laurent et al., 1982). Morphological evaluations were made on plastic sections, using a semi-quantitative approach described by Carlier (1984). In brief, slides were scored (from 0 to 3) for (i) enlargement of lysosomes of proximal tubular cells; (ii) accumulation of heterogeneous, toluidine blue-stained material in lysosomes of proximal tubular cells; (iii) irregularity of lysosomes shape of proximal tubular cells; (iv) occurrence of metachromatic, granular material in the lumen of proximal tubules; and (v) hyperchromicity of lysosomes in distal tubules and collecting ducts. Scores for the 5 types of lesions in all animals in each treatment group were summed, and expressed as percent of controls.

RESULTS

Table I shows the results obtained after 10 days of treatment concerning the analysis of the biochemical and morphological parameters characteristically modified during the development of gentamicin-induced phospholipidosis in animals and man (Laurent et al., 1982; De Broe et al., 1984; Carlier, 1984). The co-administration of pefloxacin moderately enhanced the accumulation of total phospholipids and slightly aggravated the impairment of phospholipase A1 activity. These effects, however, were at the limit of the significance and were not dose-dependent with respect to pefloxacin. Conversely, pefloxacin slightly protected against gentamicin-induced inhibition of sphingomyelinase activity. Morphological examination disclosed a modest, time-dependent protective effect of pefloxacin against the development of lysosomal alterations related to gentamicin treatment.

Table 1. Influence of the co-administration of pefloxacin (50 or 100 mg/kg per day) on the phospholipidosis-induced by gentamicin (10 mg/kg per day). Rats were treated BID during 10 days. All values are im % of controls (rats receiving no gentamicin and no pefloxacin) ± SD when applicable (n = 5)

Parameter	Gentamicin		
	+ Saline	+ Pefloxacin	
		50 mg/kg	100 mg/kg
A. Biochemical analyses			
Total phospholipids	113±1.4	119.6±6.1	115.3±5.0
Sphingomyelinase activity	85.5±3.9	90.7±11.3	94.4±8.8
Phospholipase A1 activity	82.0±12.5	68.8±4.2	71.7±10.8
B. Morphological evaluation*	372	359	300

* summed scores of all animals (15) per treatment group; see Material and Methods for score definition.

DISCUSSION

With the dosage and duration of treatment used, gentamicin induced marked lysosomal alterations, without occurrence of widespread necrosis or functional alterations, as reported earlier by us and other investigators (Kosek et al., 1974; Laurent et al., 1982). This protocol, therefore, allowing to test for both an increase, or a decrease of gentamicin specific toxicity, since the former will precipitate the sequence of events leading from lysosomal phospholipidosis to tubular necrosis (which may then become detectable), whereas the latter will be easily recognized as a protective effect against gentamicin-induced phospholipidosis (see Beauchamp et al., 1986 and Carlier et al., 1987, for two examples of the action of nephroprotectants). On this basis, pefloxacin coadministration did not markedly modify gentamicin toxicity. Because the doses used are clinically-relevant, we suggest that these results are predictive of the situation prevailing in humans. The present approach, however, is limited to the detection of a direct effect of pefloxacin on gentamicin intrinsic toxicity. Other techniques investigating the kidney cortex necrosis / regeneration processes are being applied to test for indirect effects of pefloxacin on tubular or interstitial integrity when co-administered with gentamicin (see Laurent et al., 1987, for discussion), and the results will be presented elsewhere.

ACKNOWLEDGEMENTS

This work was supported in part by the Belgian FRSM (grants no.   3.4516.79
and no.   3.4551.86),   and by Rhone-Poulenc sante,   paris, France. Z.K. was
ICP fellow, and P.M.T. is Maitre de Recherches of the Belgian FNRS.

REFERENCES

Beauchamp, D., G. Laurent, P. Maldague & P.M. Tulkens. 1986. Reduction of
gentamicin nephrotoxicity by the concomitant administration of poly-L-
aspartic acid and and poly-L-asparagine in rats. Arch. Toxicol.
Suppl.9:306-309.

Carlier, M.B. 1984. La phospholipidose renale induite par les aminoglycosides: etude biochimique et morphologique. Thesis, Universite Catholique
de Louvain. 121 pp.

Carlier, M.B., Z. Kallay, B. Rollmann & P.M. Tulkens. 1987. Reduction of
aminoglycoside-induced renal alterations in rats by coadministration of
piperacillin at clinically-relevant doses. In: Proceedings of the 15th
International Congress of Chemotherapy, Istanbul, Turkey. Ecomed. In
press.

Francq-Dufief, M.P., G. Laurent, G. Toubeau, J.A. Heuson-Stiennon & P.M.
Tulkens. 1987. Animal evaluation of the nephrotoxic potential associated
with aminoglycoside x vancomycin combinations at low doses. In: 27th
Intersc. Confer. Antimicrob. Agents Chemother., New York, N.Y. Abstract
no. 23.

Hooper, D.C. & J.S. Wolfson. 1985. The fluoroquinolones: pharmacology
clinical uses, and toxicities in humans. Antimicrob. Agents Chemother.
28:716-721.

Laurent, G., D. Beauchamp, M.B. Carlier, P.M. Tulkens, H. Loibner P.
Stutz. 198S. Use of fosfomycin salt of an aminoglycoside (S87351) to
decrease its toxicity towards rat kidney cortex. In: 26th Congress of the
European Society of Toxicology, Kuopio, Finland. Abstract mo. P22.

Laurent, G., P. Maldague, G. Toubeau, J.AW Heuson-Stiennon & P.M. Tulkens.
1987. Kidney tissue repair after nephrotoxic injury : biochemical and
morphological characterization. CRC Crit. Rev. Anat. Sci. In press.

Pechere, J.C., M. Michea-Hamzehpour, R. Auckenthaler S P. Regamey. 1987.
Ways for limiting emergence of resistance during quinolones therapy of
experimental pseudomonas. In: 27th Intersc. Confer. Antimicrob. Agents
Chemother., New York, N.Y. Abstract no. 448.

Tulkens, P.M. 1986. Experimental studies on nephrotoxicity of aminoglycosides at low doses: mechanisms and perspectives. Am. J. Med. 80:105-114.

Wolfson, J.S. & D.C. Hooper. 1985. The fluoroquinolones: structures,
mechanisms of action and resistance, and spectra of activity in vitro.
Antimicrob. Agents Chemother. 28:581-586.

Wood, C.A., S.J. Kohlhepp, P.W. Kohnen, D.C. Houghton & D.N. Gilbert.
1986. Vancomycin enhancement of experimental tobramycin nephrotoxicity.
Antimicrob. Agents Chemother. 30:20-24.

223

MORPHOLOGICAL AND FUNCTIONAL IMPAIRMENT OF THE DEVELOPING RAT KIDNEY EXPOSED TO GENTAMICIN IN UTERO

Thierri Gilbert*, Martine Lelievre-Pegorier*, Bernadette Nabarra** and Claudie Merlet-Benichou*

*INSERM U13, Hopital Claude Bernard, 75944 Paris CEDEX 19 and ** INSERM U25 and CNRS LA122, Hopital Necker-Enfants Malades, 75015 Paris, France

INTRODUCTION

Aminoglycoside antibiotics used to treat severe bacterial infection during pregnancy can cross the placenta. The effects of in utero exposure to these compounds is receiving increasing attention. It was shown that in the foetal animal, as in the adult, the kidney was the major site of gentamicin accumulation (1). In foetal guinea-pigs whose mothers were given daily 4 mg/kg of gentamicin for the seven days immediately following the period of nephrogenesis, intrarenal gentamicin concentration was found to be about 2 ug/g of tissue. More than two weeks after the treatment to the mother has ceased, the antibiotic released from all maternal and foetal tissues continued to accumulate in the developing kidney, especially as the renal blood flow and glomerular filtration rate increased with age (2). In pups born of gentamicin-treated mothers, impairments of the growth and the function of the proximal tubules were observed, but the damage was transitory (2).

In other experiments, pregnant rats were injected daily with 75 mg/kg of gentamicin for the second half of gestation, which corresponds in this species to the period of early nephrogenesis (3,4). In most of the newborn animals, intrarenal gentamicin concentration was about 2 ug/g of tissue and the number of nephrons was reduced by about 25% (4). In the present study we report morphological and functional patterns of renal maturation in developing rats exposed to gentamicin in utero and exhibiting a reduction in the number of nephrons.

MATERIAL AND METHODS

Pregnant Sprague-Dawley rats of known mating dates received one daily intramuscular injection of 75 mg/kg gentamicin in saline, for 12 days from the 10th day of gestation to its term. Another group of pregnant females received an equivalent volume of saline during the same period of gestation. All animals have free access to a standard laboratory chow and tap water. The females were allowed to deliver spontaneously.

In newborn pups taken within 4 hours of birth, the kidneys were prepared for electron microscopic observation. They were fixed by intra-cardiac perfusion with 6% glutaraldehyde in 0.1M sodium cacodylate buffer, pH 7.4 according to Larsson (5). After washing, small pieces of the kidney were cut and post-fixed in 1% osmium tetroxide in 0.1M cacodylate buffer, dehydrated and embedded in epoxy resin. Ultrathin sections were stained either with uranyl acetate and lead citrate or with silver according to Movat (6) and were examined with a Philips EM 200 at 60 Kv.

Clearance experiments were performed in 14-day-old pups which had a normal, or slightly lower than normal, birth weight. As previously shown in these pups, the number of nephrons was reduced by about 25%. Other pups in which the reduction could reach 50% were often severely growth retarded. Either they died or their mother killed them. Pups were anaesthetized intraperitoneally with 10 mg/100g with Inactin (Promonta, West Germany). After tracheotomy, an external jugular vein, a femoral artery, and the ureters were catheterized. The animals were infused with isotonic saline (1.3% of body weight). They were then given a priming dose of 10 uCi of $[^3H]$ inulin per 100g (specific activity, 150 uCi/mg; New England Nuclear Corp., Boston, Mass.) and 10 uCi of $[^{14}C]$ urea (specific activity, 50 mCi/mmol; Departement des radioelements, CEN Saclay), immediately followed by an appropriate sustaining dose of both these labelled molecules in saline, administered at a rate of 10 Ìl/min per 100g throughout the experiment. Urine was collected 60 min after the priming dose and for 3 periods of 45 min each. Arterial blood samples were taken during each period. Blood samples were immediately centrifuged, and the plasma was stored for analysis. After the addition of saline, the erythrocytes were injected into the animals. In the plasma and urine samples, the concentrations of $[^3H]$ inulin and $[^{14}C]$ urea were determined by using a liquid scintillation counter (LKB Instruments) in Instagel solution (Packard).

The phosphate concentration was measured by the method of Chen (7), and osmotic pressure was determined by cryometry by the method of Razsay and Brown (8). At the end of the experiments, both kidneys were removed and weighed. In the left kidney, the number of nephrons was determined by the method of Damadian (9). In the right kidney, the glomeruli and proximal tubular segments were microdissected after maceration of renal tissue by the method of de Rouffignac (10). Glomerular volume and proximal tubular length were then measured as already described (11).

RESULTS AND DISCUSSION

In the kidney of newborn rats exposed to gentamicin in utero, focal tubular lesions of the mature nephrons, lying in the deep cortex were observed (4). Prominent myeloid bodies in the lysosomes of the proximal tubular cells, dedifferentiation of their apical microvilli and cellular debris in the tubular lumen were observed. These lesions resembled those usually observed in the mature young or adult rat kidney after gentamicin administration (12-15). The subcapsular nephrogenic zone of the kidney was of normal histological appearance, but observation by electron microscopy reported here, revealed ultrastructural alterations of cells of the metanephric blastema and of nephron anlagen. They affected the mitochondria (Fig. 1), the Golgi apparatus and the endoplasmic reticulum, where numerous deposits of myelin like material was found, suggesting that phospholipidosis has occurred as it does in the lysosomes of mature cells exposed to gentamicin (16). Nuclear lesions were also observed, which involved the nuclear envelope and/or the nuclear content (Fig. 2). It is worthwhile to note that such alterations of cellular organelles, including the nuclei, were found in otherwise normal cells of the metanephric blastema and nephron anlagen of the subcapsular cortical zone, where no characteristic features of gentamicin nephrotoxicity was observed.

In the adult kidney cells exposed to gentamicin, neither nuclear anomalies nor the presence of myelin like material in cytoplasmic organelles other

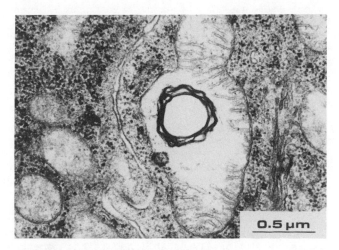

Fig. 1. Subcellular lesion in renal tissue of a newborn rat issued from gentamicin-treated mother. The mitochondria exhibits dense myelin-like material. The other parts of the mitochondria are well defined. (x50000, bar represents 0.5 μm).

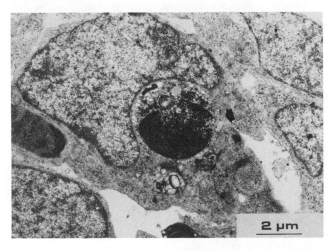

Fig. 2. Nuclear lesion in the subcapsular zone of the kidney of a newborn rat exposed to gentamicin in utero. A normal nucleus and a degenerated mass of chromatin (arrow) are present in a same metanephric blastema cell. (x9000, bar represents 2 μm).

than lysosome has been observed. In cells of the undifferentiated and differentiating renal tissues, endocytosis apparatus is either absent or still poorly functioning (17,18). The fact that no lysosomal sequestration of the drug could occur in these tissues, might have deprived the other cellular organelles or membranes of its possible protective role (19). Alternatively, subcellular lesions observed in the nephrogenic subcapsular tissues might be specific for these tissues, independently of the absence of functioning vacuolar apparatus.

Although the present study did not address the mechanism of reduction in nephron mass in animals exposed to gentamicin in utero, histological observation of the kidneys clearly showed that no widespread necrosis was present which might indicate that nephrons or nephron anlagen have formed and subsequently degenerated. As already pointed out (4,20) the reduction in the number of nephrons at birth was probably due to early reduction either of the rate of dichotomous divisions of the ampullae or the rate of nephron formation in the blastema, or both. In this respect, it is worthy to note that, while no structural or ultrastructural lesion of the collecting ducts, including their terminal ampullae, was observed at birth, numerous and varying ultrastructural alterations had occurred in the blastema cells. The question therefore arises whether similar alterations affecting the blastema in earlier stages of development might have altered its response to the induction signal.

It was previously shown that, in the postnatal rat kidney (4), similar to the developing guinea-pig kidney exposed to gentamicin in utero (2) an elevated antibiotic concentration was maintained for more than 2 weeks after the last injection to the mother. In the rat, nephrogenesis continues for about a week after birth and in 14-day-old animals issued from gentamicin-treated mothers the final number of nephrons was found to be reduced. It is not definitely established at the moment whether the postnatal part of nephrogenesis was, as the foetal part, also impaired or whether the reduction in the final number of nephrons resulted from the reduction in the rate of early nephrogenesis. However, recent data obtained in young animals injected with gentamicin from birth to 14 days, clearly indicate that high intrarenal concentration of the antibiotic failed to modify the rate of nephrogenesis during the postnatal period (4). In addition, as would be expected from a reduction in the rate of nephrogenesis (which would be due to a reduction in the rate of the early dichotomous divisions of the ampullae) the percentage of reduction in the final number of nephrons was about the same as the percentage of reduction in the number of nephrons at birth.

The present study shows that, despite their reduced number of nephrons, 14-day-old rats from mothers treated with aminoglycosides exhibited a normal kidney weight (Table 1). Compensatory growth of the glomeruli and proximal tubules have occurred for both the juxtamedullary and the superficial nephrons (Fig. 3). In pups of the gentamicin group, neither the mean glomerular filtration rate nor the renal handling of water, urea and phosphate, and the capacity to concentrate urine was not significantly different from control pups (Table 1). In animals exposed to gentamicin in utero, cellular injuries, such as focal loss of brush border microvilli, cellular debris partially filling the lumen, and marked increase in the number and size of vacuoles, were still present two weeks after birth in the proximal tubules of the juxtamedullary nephrons and the proximal tubules of the superficial nephrons which have formed after birth (4).

Our data clearly show that neither the drug present in cells nor the injury it causes them in rats exposed to gentamicin in utero, prevents the morphological or functional adaptation of the nephrons to their small number. Thus in 14-day-old animals functional compensation was likely to be fully achieved.

Long-term follow-up of the kidney morphology and function of rats exposed to gentamicin in utero was undertaken in our laboratory. Preliminary data show that while glomerular filtration rate expressed per g of kidney or body weight remained constant from 3 to 12 months in the control animals, it significantly decreased in the gentamicin group. In the 6-month-old animals of both groups, proteinuria was similar (20 ± 4 mg/d, n = 4 versus 19 ± 3 mg/d, n = 4), but at 12 months, it was nearly 4-fold higher in rats exposed to gentamicin in utero than in control (38 ± 10 mg/d, n = 5 versus 142 ± 27 mg/d, n = 5). Evidence of accelerated focal and segmental

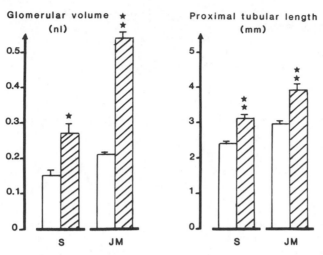

Fig. 3.   Glomerular volume and proximal tubular length for superficial
(S)   and   juxtamedullary (JM) nephrons in 14-day-old rats born of saline
(open bars) or gentamicin (hatched bars) treated mothers.   84 and 108
nephrons   were   microdissected and measured in 7 control and gentamicin
animals, respectively.   *** p < 0.01 and p < 0.001 compared to the values
in controls.

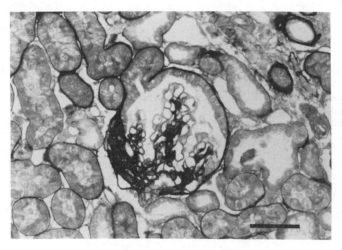

Fig. 4.   Glomerulus of a 12-month-old rat exposed in utero to gentamicin.
Segmental   glomerular   sclerosis is evident.   Note the thickening of the
Bowman's capsule.   1um-paraffin section stained with   Jone's   reticulin
(x400, bar represents 50 um).

glomerular sclerosis was observed in animals of the gentamicin group (Fig.
4).   Proximal tubular cells exhibited various alterations.   Studies are
in progress to determine whether the delay or progressive decrease in
renal   function   would   have been the same in kidneys having a reduced
nephron mass, but not previously exposed to gentamicin.

TABLE 1. Overall kidney function in 14-day-old rats born of saline or gentamicin-treated mothers.

Body wt g	Kidney wt mg	Glom No.	UFR (ul/min)	U/P In	GFR (ul/min)	FE% H_2O	Urea	PO_4	Uosm
Control (n = 7)									
31.0	183	34316	0.87	84	45.9	1.36	31.9	31.1	705
±1.6	±9	±1504	±0.20	±10	±3.6	±0.19	±2.9	±2.9	±64
Gentamicin (n = 9)									
30.0	185	25220[a]	0.69	70	41.5	1.90	30.2	36.9	587[b]
±0.8	±6	±2182	±0.15	±11	±5.1	±0.35	±6.4	±7.0	±34

Glom. No., Number of glomeruli per kidney; UFR, urinary flow rate; U/P In, urine-to-plasma concentration ratio for inulin; GFR, glomerular filtration rate; FE%, fractional excretion of water, urea and phosphates expressed as percent of their filtered load; Uosm, urine osmolarity. Values are means with their standard error. [a] $p < 0.01$ compared to the values in control animals. [b] mean of 3 values.

SUMMARY

In rats born of gentamicin treated mothers, the number of nephrons present at birth, as well as the final number of nephrons were reduced. At birth, the subcapsular nephrogenic zone exhibited focal alteration of cytoplasmic organelle membranes, as well as nuclear lesions, in cells of the nephron anlagen and of the undifferentiated blastema which were otherwise of normal appearance. In both the newborn and the 14-day-old animals, the proximal tubular cells of the mature nephrons exhibited extensive damage resembling that described in tubular cells of adult rats exposed to gentamicin. As soon as 14 days, morphological and functional adaptation of the nephrons to their small number was evident. But, as in other model of reduction in nephron mass, glomerular sclerosis develops prematurely in older animals issued from gentamicin-treated mothers.

REFERENCES

1. M. Lelievre-Pegorier, R. Sakly, A. Meulemans and C. Merlet-Benichou, Kinetics of gentamicin in plasma of non-pregnant, pregnant, and foetal guinea-pigs and itS distribution in foetal tissues, Antimicrob. Agents Chemother. 28:565 (1985).

2. M. Lelievre-Pegorier, T. Gilbert, R. Sakly, A. Meulemans, and C. Merlet-Benichou, Effects of foetal exposure to gentamicin on the kidneys of young guinea-pigs, Antimicrob. Agents Chemother. 31:88 (1987).

3. J.P. Mallie, H. Gerard and A. Gerard, Gentamicin administration to pregnant rats. Effect on renal development in utero, Dev. Pharmacol. Ther. 7:89 (1984).

4. T. Gilbert, M. Lelievre-Pegorier, R. Malienou and C. Merlet-Benichou, Effects of prenatal and postnatal exposure to gentamicin on renal differentiation in the rat, Toxicol. 43:301 (1987).

5. L. Larsson, Effects of different fixatives on the ultrastructure of the developing proximal tubule in the rat kidney, J. Ultrastruct. Res. 51:140 (1975).

6.   H. Movat, Silver impregnation methods for electron microscopy, _Am. J. Clin. Pathol_. 35:328 (1961).

7.   P.S. Chen, T.Y. Toribara and H. Warner, Microdetermination of phosphorus, _Anal. Chem_. 28: 1756 (1964).

8.   J.A. Ramsay and R.H.J. Brown, Simplified apparatus and procedures for freezing-point determination upon small volumes of fluid, _J. Sci. Instrum_. 32:372 (1955).

9.   R.V. Damadian, E. Shawayri and N.S. Bricker, On the existence of non-urine-forming nephrons in the diseased kidney of the dog, _J. Lab. Clin. Med_. 65:26 (1965).

10.   C. De Rouffignac, S. Deiss and J.P. Bonvalet, Determination du taux individuel de filtration glomerulaire des nephrons accessibles et inaccessibles h la microponction, _Pflugers Arch_. 315:273 (1970).

11.   C. Merlet-Benichou, M. Pegorier, M. Muffat-Joly and C. Augeron, Functional and morphologic patterns of renal maturation in the developing guinea-pig, _Am. J. Physiol_. 241:F618 (1981).

12.   J.C. Kosek, R.I. Mazze and M.J. Cousins, Nephrotoxicity of gentamicin, _Lab. Invest_. 30:48 (1974).

13.   F.C. Luft, V. Patel, M.N. Yum, B. Patel and S.A. Kleit, Experimental aminoglycoside nephrotoxicity, _J. Lab. Clin. Med_. 86:213 (1975).

14.   D.C. Houghton, M. Hartnett, M. Campbell-Boswell, G. Porter and W. Bennett, A light and electron microscopic analysis of gentamicin nephrotoxicity in rats, _Am. J. Pathol_. 82:589 (1976).

15.   R.H. Cowan, A.F. Jukkola and B.S. Arant, Pathophysiologic evidence of gentamicin nephrotoxicity in neonatal puppies, _Pediatr. Res_. 14:1204 (1980).

16.   G. Aubert-Tulkens, F. Van Hoof and P.M. Tulkens, Gentamicin induced lysosomal phospholipidosis in cultured rat fibroblasts, _Lab. Invest_. 40:481 (1979).

17.   L. Larsson and A.B. Maunsbach, Differentiation of the vacuolar apparatus in cells of the developing proximal tubule in the rat kidney, _J. Ultrastruct. Res_. 53:254 (1975).

18.   J. Schaeverbeke and M. Cheignon, Differentiation of glomerular filter and tubular reabsorption apparatus during foetal development of the rat kidney, _J. Embryol. Exp. Morph_. 58:157 (1980).

19.   P.D. Williams, P. D. Holohan and C.R. Ross, Gentamicin nephro-toxicity. I. Acute biochemical correlates in rats, _Am. J. Pathol_. 61:234 (1981).

20.   T. Gilbert, B. Nabarra and C. Merlet-Benichou, Light and electron microscopic analysis of the kidney in newborn rats exposed to gentamicin in utero, _Am. J. Pathol_. in press (1987).

MORPHOLOGICAL AND FUNCTIONAL EFFECTS IN RAT NEONATES OF AMINOGLYCOSIDES GIVEN TO THE MOTHER DURING GESTATION

J.P. Mallie (1), H. Smaoui (2), Cl. Billerey (3), M. Cheignon (2) and J. Schaeverbke (2)

(1) Lab. de Nephrologie, Universite Nancy 1B.P. 184 F-54505 Vandoeuvre Cedex; (2) Lab. de Biologie Cellulaire, Universite Paris 7, Tour 23-33 2 Place Jussieu, F-75251 Paris Cedex 05 and (3) Lab. d'Anatomie Patholo-gique 2 Place Saint Jacques F-25030 Besancon Cedex, France

INTRODUCTION

Aminoglycosides are widely used to treat gram-negative infections, which occur frequently in pregnant women and require the use of these antibiotics. The nephrotoxicity of aminoglycosides is an important consideration in the clinical use of these drugs, that has led to numerous studies (Price, 1986). However, little attention has been paid to a possible nephrotoxic effect of these antibiotics on the foetus, although they are able to cross the placental barrier.

We have reported previously that gentamicin administration to pregnant rats is followed by a slowing down of the glomeruli differentiation with pathological evidence for an in-utero induced nephrotoxicity (Mallie et al 1984, 1985). Tubular lesions and modifications of the nephrogenesis have been recently published (Mallie et al 1986, Gilbert et al 1987).

This study was undertaken to verify the nephrotoxic effects on function, to assess the effects of other aminoglycosides and to establish if glomerular differentiation could be altered very early. Only 33% of definite nephrons are mature at birth in rats, thus every stage of maturation can be seen in a neonate kidney.

Using techniques allowing the measurement of renal function in neonates (Kavlock and Gray 1982) we investigated the effects of netilmicin or amikacin given to pregnant rats. The early nephrogenesis was also studied at a glomerular level, using specific techniques in neonates born to mothers who were given gentamicin (Cheignon et al 1987).

PROTOCOL

This study was conducted using mated female Wistar rats. Day 1 of pregnancy was the day that sperm was found in vaginal smear. Drugs were administered on day 7 to 11 (organogenesis) and 14 to 18 (beginning of nephrogenesis). Commercial preparations of antibiotics were used: netilmicin (Netromicine, Laboratoires UNICET) 60 mg/kg/d, amikacin (Amiklin, Laboratoires BRISTOL) 180 mg/kg/d, and gentamicin (Gentalline, Laboratoires UNICET) 75 mg/kg/d. A similar volume of saline (7%) was given to control pregnant females.

<u>Netilmicin, amikacin and control groups</u>. Studies on this groups were done in order to measure the functional effects of these drugs and then the morphological aspects of the developing kidney.

The day after birth (day 1 of life) neonates were subjected to a basal clearance evaluation following techniques described by Kavlock and Gray (1982, 1983). Diuresis was stated per hr/g body weight and creatinine clearance was calculated using the standard formula. At the conclusion of the experiment, the kidneys were removed, one prepared for electron microscopy and the other for light microscopy (semi-thin sections).

<u>Gentamicin groups</u>. Examinations were concentrated on the aspects of the glomerular basal membrane (GBM) at different ages of differentiation. Studies were performed in 1-day old neonates from either treated or control mothers. Kidneys were investigated using electron microscopy. A cationic probe: polyethyleneimine (PEI) was injected i.v. to some neonates at least 20 minutes before sacrifice. PEI characterizes the heparan sulphate proteoglycans (anionic sites) of the glomerular membrane (Bakala 1987).

Anionic ferritin (A.F., molecular weight 480,000 and pI: 4.1-4.6) was injected i.v. to some other neonates. This marker does not cross the lamina densa of the glomerular membrane of fully differentiated glomeruli in controls.

RESULTS

<u>Effects of netilmicin and amikacin</u>. Controls and netilmicin-treated mothers gave birth after a normal duration of gestation while 3 out of 10 amikacin-treated mothers had a gestation shortened by 1 day and gave birth to premature pups.

As compared to controls: Body weight (Fig. 1) was slightly increased in netilmicin and amikacin-term neonates ($p < 0.05$ respectively). Diuresis was increased ($p < 0.01$) in all amikacin pups. However if we exclude the premature pups no increase was noted. Plasma creatinine was increased in netilmicin neonates ($p < 0.001$). Creatinine clearance (Fig. 2) was decreased after both aminoglycosides ($p < 0.001$ respectively); nevertheless if we exclude the premature pups it was normal in the amikacin term neonates.

Pathology showed slight alterations of proximal tubules after either netilmicin or amikacin: cytoplasmic vacuoles, conspicuous PAS positive inclusions, lysosomal hypertrophy and focal atrophy of brush borders. Myeloid bodies were found loose in the cytoplasm, in mitochondria, brush borders and in lysosomes. After netilmicin focal lumen dilations and numerous myeloid bodies were seen (Fig. 3) while amikacin led to larger vacuoles (Fig. 4).

<u>Gentamicin-induced alterations</u>. The pattern of glomerular different-iation appeared unchanged in kidneys of neonates born to gentamicin-treated mothers. However alterations were noted in their glomeruli whatever the stage of differentiation: The fibrillar material of the GBM and the anionic sites (shown by PEI as the cationic probe) were more abundant in prenatally exposed animals than in controls (Fig. 5). In the deepest glomeruli, ie. fully differentiated, the same features were observed.

The development of permselectivity was found to be altered. In the normal maturing glomeruli AF does cross the GBM; it is then stopped by the lamina densa when the latter is developed. For similar stages of

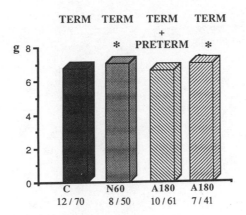

Figure 1. Body weight of rat neonates on day 1 of life after mothers have
been given aminoglycosides during the gestation.

Control: C, netilmicin: N, amikacin: A. In the amikacin group neonates
were born after a normal duration of gestation (term) or after a shorter
gestation (preterm).   The lower line indicates the number of litters and
the number of pups studied in each group. * p < 0.05

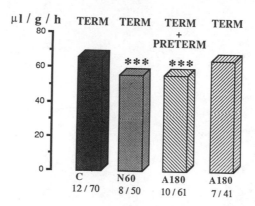

Figure 2. Creatinine clearance in rat neonates on day 1 of life. See Fig.
1 for groups. *** p < 0.001

differentiation, the passage of AF was greater after gentamicin than in
controls and its passage was not stopped in fully differentiated
glomeruli.

Typical changes after gentamicin such as dense deposits and myeloid bodies
in the lysosomes as previously described by others in adults (Houghton et
al 1976, Solez et al 1983) were observed in the proximal tubules. We also
noticed a decrease in endocytosis vesicles at the apical part of the
cells.   In both structures, glomeruli and tubules, myelin figures were
often observed, mainly in the Golgi apparatus of which sacculae were more
numerous and dilated.

DISCUSSION

Morphological alterations of the kidneys of neonates were noted when
pregnant rats were given aminoglycosides (Mallie et al 1984, 1985, 1986,

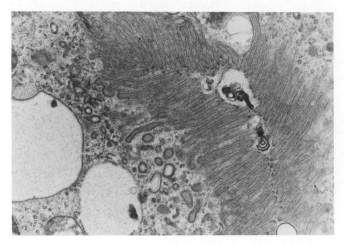

Figure 3.   Kidney of rat neonate in-utero exposed to netilmicin.   Proximal tubule cells and lumen: numerous myelin figures in lysosomes, brush border and lumen.

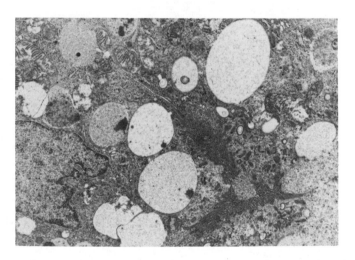

Figure 4.   Kidney of rat neonate in-utero exposed to amikacin.   Proximal tubule cells and lumen: numerous and large cytoplasmic vacuoles.

1987, Gilbert et al 1987).   Tubular lesions resemble closely those reported in adults (Houghton et al 1976,   Solez et al 1983) or in neonates receiving antibiotics directly (Provoost et al 1985).   Teratological studies   do not usually consider this aspect of   in-utero-acquired nephrotoxicity (Bamonte et al 1979,   Weinberg et al 1981) characterized by both morphological and functional aspects.

The body weight of pups after netilmicin and in term neonates after amikacin is increased as compared to the controls.   This is different from the decrease always noted after gentamicin.   A different impairment of the development of the concentration gradient depending on the   aminoglycoside used could be responsible of different water metabolisms in pups.

After netilmicin the creatinine clearance is decreased while it is not after amikacin,   althought only in term neonates; the plasma creatinine is

236

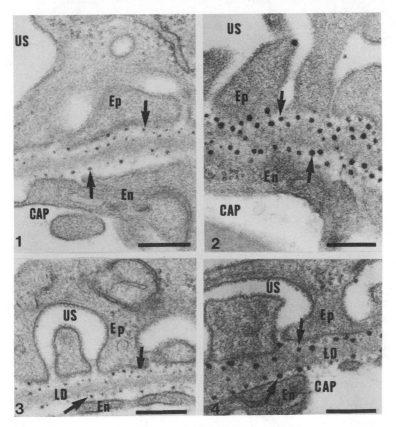

Figure 5. Maturing (5-1, 5-2) and mature (5-3, 5-4) glomeruli of neonates born to control and gentamicin-treated females. Pups were injected intravenously by polyethyleneimine. In both cases, basement membrane material and anionic sites appear more abundant in prenatally exposed animals (on the right) than in control (on the left).

CAP: capillary lumen, En: endothelial cell, Ep: epithelial celi, LD: lamina densa, US: urinary space. Magnification: Bar = 0.5um

increased after netilmicin. These results suggest a greater toxicity of netilmicin than amikacin.

The shorter gestation after amikacin in some cases needs further investigation. We reported elsewhere (Mallie et al 1987) that the blood biology of pregnant females is not significantly modified after amino-glycosides when using this protocol.

Netilmicin and amikacin lead to morphological features close to those reported after gentamicin (Mallie et al 1986); nevertheless the slight differences in pathology noted after these antibiotics must be reconciled with differences observed using functional tests. These results illustrate the fact that a prediction of clinical features based on routine pathology findings is not easy.

The alterations of the maturing glomeruli are difficult to explain. The developing GBM is modified as compared to the control (Cheignon et al 1987, Bakala et al 1987). A hypersecretion of GBM constituents could be possible since the Golgi apparatus seems hyperdeveloped; but a local hyperhydration cannot be excluded. The impaired permselectivity seems to be directly related to the morphological alterations of the GBM development.

Thus this aminoglycoside-induced nephrotoxicity in pups after antibiotics have been given to the mother is characterized by tubular and glomerular alterations, but the relative extent of damage shown to the glomeruli is greater in this model than that found in post maturational investigations which are commonly conducted.

In view of a possible development of the use of aminoglycosides (Price, 1986) an improvement in the quality of these agents could be hoped for from a better knowledge of their effects.

ACKNOWLEDGEMENTS

This work was supported in part by the Institut National de la Sante et de la Recherche Medicale (INSERM Grant 865010) and by Universite of Paris 7.

REFERENCES

Bakala H., Cornet S., Cheignon M., Djaziri R. and Schaeverbeke J., 1987, Basement Membrane Proteoglycans and Anionic Sites in the Fetal Rat Kidney during Late Gestation. J. Morphol. (to be published).

Bamonte F., Al biero L. and Ongini E., 1979, Reproductive and Teratological Studies with a New Aminoglycosides: Netilmicin (Sch-20569). Acta Pharmacol. Toxicol., 45: 145-151.

Cheignon M., Bakala H., Cornet S., Djaziri R. and Schaeverbeke J., 1987, Localization of Basement Membranes Glycoproteins in the Rat Kidney during Fetal Development. Biol. Cell., 60:(to be published).

Gilbert Th., Leiievre-Pegorier M., Malienou R., Meulemans A. and Merlet-Benichou Cl., 1987, Effects of Prenatal and Post-natal Exposure to Gentamicin on Renal Differentiation in the Rat. Toxicology, 43:301-313.

Houghton D.C., Hartnett M., Campbell-Boswell M., Porter G. and Bennett W.M., 1976, A light and Electron Microscopic Analysis of Gentamicin Nephrotoxicity in Rats. Am. J. Pathol., 82:589-612.

Kavlock R.J. and Gray J.A., 1982, Evaluation of Renal Function in Neonatal Rats. Biol. Neonate, 41:279-288.

Kavlock R.J. and Gray J.A., 1983, Morphometric, Biochemical and Physiopathological Assessment of Perinatally Induced Renal Dysfunction. J. Toxicol. Envir. Health, 11:1-3.

Mallie, J.P., Gerard H. and Gerard A., 1984, Gentamicin Administration to Pregnant Rats: Effect on Fetal Renal Development in utero. Dev. Pharmacol. Ther., 7:89-92.

Mallie, J.P., Gerard H. and Gerard A., 1985, Developing kidney and in-utero exposure to gentamicin, in: "Renal Heterogeneity and Target Cell Toxicity, P.H. Bach and E.A. Lock eds., John Wiley & Sons, Chichester, pp 365-368.

Mallie, J.P., Gerard H. and Gerard A., 1986, In-utero Gentamicin-lnduced Nephrotoxicity in Rats. Fediatr. Pharmacol., 5:229-239.

238

Mallie, J.P., Coulon G., Billerey Cl. and Faucourt A., 1987, In-utero Induced Aminoglycosides Nephrotoxicity in Rat Neonates. Kidney International (accepted).

Price K.E., 1986, Aminoglycosides Research 1975-1985. Prospects for Development of lmproved Agents. Antimicrob. Ag. Chemother., 29:543-548.

Provoost A.P., Adejuyigbe O. and Wolff E.D., 1985, Nephrotoxicity of Aminoglycosides in Young and Adult Rats. Pediatr. Res., 19:1191-1196.

Solez K., Racusen L.C. and Olsen S., 1983, The Pathology of Drug Nephrotoxicity. J. Clin. Pharmacol., 23:484-490.

Stolte H. and Alt J.M., 1982, The choice of animals for nephrotoxic investigations, In: "Nephrotoxicity, Assessment and Pathogenesis", P.H. Bach et al., eds., John Wiley & Sons, Chichester, pp 102-112.

Weinberg E.H., Fleld W.E., Gray W.D., Klein M.F., Robbins G.R. and Schwartz E., 1981, Preclinical Toxicologic Studies of Netilmicin. Arzneim Forsch. Drug Res., 31:816-822.

GENTAMICIN-STIMULATED INCREASE IN PARA-AMINOHIPPURATE UPTAKE IN RENAL CORTICAL SLICES AND ISOLATED PROXIMAL TUBULAR CELLS

E.M. Gordon, S.M. McDougall, P.H. Whiting and G.M. Hawksworth

Clinical Pharmacology Unit and Department of Chemical Pathology, University of Aberdeen, Foresterhill, Aberdeen AB9 2ZD, UK

INTRODUCTION

A deleterious effect on renal tubular transport is an important criteria for establishing the nephrotoxic potential of a drug or chemical. In this context the transport of the organic ions p-aminohippurate (PAH) and tetraethylammonium (TEA) into renal cortical slices has been extensively studied (Hirsch, 1976). For example, Kluwe and Hook (1978) have suggested that renal cortical slice transport of organic anions is a sensitive indicator of gentamicin-induced nephrotoxicity.

The use of isolated proximal tubular (PT) cells in suspension for toxicity studies as described by Gordon et al (1987) requires that the cells retain uptake and efflux mechanisms both at the brush border and basolateral membranes. Although the cells may lose their polarity in suspension (Ojakian and Herzlinger, 1984), more importantly they have been shown both morphologically and functionally to retain an intact brush border. This paper describes a study which compares the rate of organic acid uptake in isolated PT cells with the well accepted renal cortical slice preparation. Isolated PT cells would overcome many of the disadvantages involved in the use of cortical slices. The cells would remain in contact with substrates and toxins in the incubation medium unlike those in the cortical slices, with which it has been shown that the lumen collapse within a short period of time (Chahwala and Harpur, 1966). This study also examined the effect of 10 day gentamicin treatment on PAH uptake in isolated PT cells and in renal cortical slices. It is well established that the early transient rise in PAH uptake seen after gentamicin treatment acts as a sensitive index of nephrotoxicity (Kaloyanides and Pastoriza-Munoz, 1980). The aim of the study was to determine whether this could also be demonstrated with PT cells, which provide a more defined system for the study of compounds exhibiting toxicity specific for the PT.

METHODS

Adult male Sprague Dawley rats (initial mean weight 320g) were used throughout. They were housed in temperature controlled conditions and allowed free access to food and water. Groups (n = 5) of animals received either gentamicin sulphate (50 mg/kg body weight) or saline (0.9% w/v) daily by a single intraperitoneal injection (0.3ml) for up to 14 days. Renal function, determined by measurement of creatinine clearance rates, and urinary N-acetyl-ß-D-glucosaminidase (NAG) activity, a sensitive indication of renal parenchymal damage, was measured pretreatment (day 0) and on days 4, 7, 10 and 14 (Whiting and Simpson, 1983). Creatinine clearance rates and NAG enzymuria are expressed as ml/h/kg body weight and IU/mmol urinary creatinine respectively.

Cortical slices were prepared with a Vibroslice (Campden Instruments, London) to give 6-8 slices of cortical tissue per kidney (200ìm thick, 15-20 mg/slice). PT cells were isolated by collagenase incubation (30 min, $37^{\circ}C$) followed by Percoll density gradient centrifugation (20,000g, 30 min) as described previously by Gordon et al (1987). Cell yield was $8\pm3\times10^6$ cells/kidney and viability was > 90% as assessed by Trypan blue exclusion. Incubations were carried out at $37^{\circ}C$ in an atmosphere of $95\%O_2/5\%CO_2$ with 60 mg sliced tissue/5ml buffer or 10^6 cells/ml buffer. The incubation with medium used was Krebs Ringer bicarbonate buffer, pH 7.4 containing 11 mM glucose. Inclusion of sodium acetate (10 mM) at pH 7.4 resulted in maximal PAH uptake when compared to either the absence of acetate or at a pH of 8.2 (Gerencer et al, 1977) and therefore was included during the incubations. Incubation were carried out for 20 or 30 min for cells and slices respectively with ^{14}C-PAH (10-500 uM). Cells and slices were recovered after the incubation period by either filtration (0.1 um mesh) for the cells and by blotting for the slices; before solubilisation for scintillation counting. Protein determinations were carried out using the method of Lowry et al (1951). Gentamicin treatment was without significant effect on the protein content of either cells or slices (results not shown). Consequently, the values for net uptake rate of PAH in cells and slices were comparable in terms of the amount of protein present. The results were therefore expressed as nmol PAH/g tissue/30 min for slices and as nmol PAH/10^6 cells/20 min.

RESULTS

The effect of gentamicin on creatinine clearance rates and NAG enzymuria is shown in Table 1. NAG enzymuria was significantly elevated by day 4, and this increase was maintained over the experimental course. However, reduced creatinine clearance rates were only observed on day 10 with a slight, but insignificant, improvement being noted on day 14. Consequently animals treated with gentamicin for either 4 or 10 days, and demonstrating evidence of renal cell damage but with either normal or reduced kidney function, were used for studies of renal cortical slice or cell PAH uptake.

Table 1. The effect of gentamicin on creatinine clearance and NAG enzymuria

Days Treatment	Creatinine Clearance		NAG Enzymuria	
	Sal	Gen	Sal	Gen
Pretreatment	448±46	1385±124	70±8	72±9
4	509±48	445±59	86±9	183±53**
10	348±110	189±84*	86±14	365±211*

Results are expressed as the mean±SD and there were 5 determinations per group. Saline (Sal) and gentamicin (Gen) treated groups were compared at each time point using Student's 't' test; *, p < 0.05; **, p < 0.01. Results for days 7 and 14 are not shown.

The net rate of uptake of PAH into cortical slices from gentamicin treated animals was significantly raised at all concentrations tested, when compared with saline treated animals (Fig. 1), only on day 10 (3.2±0.3

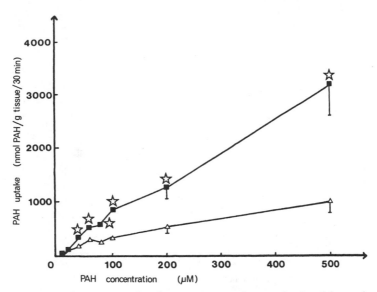

Figure 1. Rate of PAH uptake into rat renal cortical slices in untreated
(△) rats and following gentamicin treatment for 10 days (■). Results
are shown as mean + SEM and were compared with untreated values using
Student's 't' test, (☆ , p < 0.01).

compared to 0.98±0.09 umol/g tissue/30 min at a PAH concentration of 500
uM; mean±SEM). By day 14, PAH uptake had, however, returned to values
similar to those shown by saline treated control animals (results not
shown).

The PT cell preparation, achieved following collagenase incubation and
Percoll density centrifugation, demonstrated a > 90% purity and viability.
Electron microscopy also revealed that these cells had retained the
integrity of both their brush border and basolateral membranes throughout
this preparation. The initial viability of PT cells obtained following
gentamicin pretreatment was also not significantly changed from those
cells prepared from control animals, neither did the viability of the
cells from either control or gentamicin treated animals significantly
decrease over the incubation period. Maximal PAH uptake into isolated PT
cells was observed following a 20 min incubation in Krebs Ringer
bicarbonate buffer containing 10 mM sodium acetate and 11 mM glucose. The
net rate of PAH uptake into cells prepared from gentamicin treated animals
(Fig. 2) was significantly elevated when compared with control values,
only on day 10 and at PAH concentrations of 200 and 500 uM (40.0±12.9
compared with 6.5 ± 1.0 nmol/10^6 cells/20 min; mean±SEM).

DISCUSSION

In the past renal tissue slices have been widely used in a variety of
physiological, biochemical and toxicological studies to both demonstrate
and investigate the effects of many environmental chemicals and drugs on
the kidney (Elliot et al, 1981). In this context renal slices, obtained
from both cortex and medulla, have been used to assess the effects of
potential toxicants on both the transport function, using several
prototype ions including PAH and TEA (Hirsch, 1976), and metabolic
activity, for example gluconeogenesis and ammonia production, of the
kidney. However, many nephrotoxic agents display site specificity and may
only cause damage to either the proximal or distal segments of the

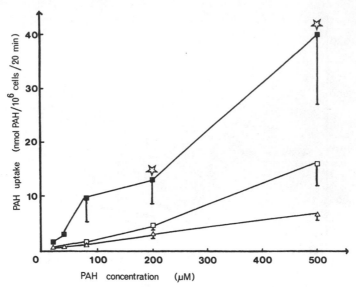

Figure 2. Rate of PAH uptake into the proximal tubular cells in untreated (△) rats and following gentamicin pretreatment (50 mg/kg/day) for 4 days (□) and 10 days (■). Results are shown as mean±SEM, and were compared with untreated values using Student's 't' test, (☆, p < 0.01).

nephron. Examples of the former include aminoglycoside antibiotics (Kaloyanides and Pastoriza-Munoz, 1980) and cephaloridine (Kuo and Hook, 1982), while papillary necrosis is associated with the administration of paracetamol (Mohandas et al, 1984). Pure preparations of renal tubular cells and/or fragments may therefore be a more appropriate means of studying this site specific toxicity to the kidney.

We have previously described the preparation and characterization of homogenous proximal tubular cell suspensions (Gordon et al, 1987, and this volume) and proposed their use in toxicity studies. Many toxic agents affect tubular transport mechanisms both in vivo and in vitro, indeed, Kluwe and Hook (1978) have suggested that increased PAH uptake into renal slices is one of the most sensitive indications of gentamicin-induced nephrotoxicity, an agent acting specifically on the proximal convoluted tubule (Kosek et al, 1974).

In the present study gentamicin-induced renal dysfunction was most severe between days 7 and 10 as evidenced by elevated NAG enzymuria, present on day 4 and reaching a peak by day 10 and a reduced creatinine clearance rate present from day 10 onwards. The presence of elevated NAG enzymuria, a sensitive indication of renal cell damage, before reduced kidney function was observed has also been demonstrated by other workers (Wellwood et al, 1976; Whiting and Simpson, 1983). The uptake of PAH into cortical slices reached a maximum on day 10, at all PAH concentrations tested which coincided with the highest urinary NAG activities. Furthermore, as saturation of the transport mechanism was not achieved in the present study it was not possible to derive Km values. However, Lapkin et al (1977) have suggested a value of 0.25-0.20 mM for the slice uptake of PAH.

The viability of proximal tubular cells prepared from either gentamicin-treated or control animals as assessed by Trypan blue exclusion, was similar and maintained at > 90% over the experimental course. Compared to cells prepared from control animals, those from gentamicin-treated animals also demonstrated increased PAH uptake only on day 10; at rates similar to those observed for slices, expressed on the basis of protein content. PAH efflux from renal slices, shown by Bennett et al, (1980) to be reduced following gentamicin treatment, was not however measured in the present study.

The similar PAH uptake profiles observed in both cell and slice preparations from normal and gentamicin-treated animals is consistent with the maintenance of functionally intact luminal and basolateral membranes. This provides partial validation for the proposal that the cell preparations are appropriate for toxicity studies. These preparations have already been used in other studies (see Gordon et al, this volume) which demonstrate the presence of 3-methylcholanthrene inducible forms of cytochrome P450-dependent mono-oxygenase activity and maintenance of intracellular reduced glutathione levels at > 50% for 2 hr at 37°C.

The results presented above confirm that proximal tubular cell preparations, prepared by Percoll density centrifugation following a limited collagenase digestion, retain their structural, functional and metabolic integrity, which makes them an appropriate system for studies designed to elucidate the underlying mechanisms of drug-induced nephrotoxicity.

REFERENCES

Bennett, W.M., Plamp, C.E., Parker, R.A., Gilbert, D.N., Houghton, D.C. and Porter, G.A., 1980, Alterations in organic ion transport, induced by gentamicin nephrotoxicity in the rat, J. Lab. Clin. Med., 95:32.

Chahwala, S.B. and Harpur, E.S., 1986, Rat renal tubules - Gentamicin nephrotoxicity, J. Pharm. Meth., 15:21.

Elliot,W.C., Parker, R.A., Houghton, D.C., Gilbert, D.N. and Bennett, W.M.T 1981, Comparative nephrotoxicity of dibekacin and gentamicin in rats, Res. Commun. Chem. Pathol. Pharmacol., 33:419.

Gerencer, G.A., Chaisetseree, C. and Hong, S.K., 1977, Acetate influence upon transport kinetics of p-aminohippurate at 37°C in rabbit kidney slices, Proc. Soc. Exp. Biol. Med., 154:397.

Gordon, E.M., Whiting, P.H., Simpson, J.G. and Hawksworth, G.M.; 1987, Isolation and characterisation of rat renal proximal tubular cells, Biochem. Soc. Trans., 15:457.

Gordon, E.M. Whiting, P.H., Simpson, J.G. and Hawksworth, G.M., 1987, Isolated rat renal proximal tubular cells: a model to investigate drug-induced nephrotoxicity, this volume.

Hirsch: G.H., 1976, Differential effects of nephrotoxic agents on renal transport and metabolism by use of in vitro techniques, Environ. Health Perspect., 15:89.

Kaloyanides, G.J. and Qastoriza-Munoz, E., 1980, Aminoglycoside nephro-toxicity, Kid. Int., 18:571.

Kluwe, W.M. and Hook, J.B., 1978, Analysis of gentamicin uptake by rat renal cortical slices, Toxic. Appl. Pharm., 45:531.

Kosek, J.C., Mazze, R.I. and Cousins, M.J., 1974, Nephrotoxicity of gentamicin, Lab. Invest., 30:48.

Kuo, C. and Hook, J.B., 1982, Depletion of renal glutathione content and nephrotoxicity of cephaloridine in rabbits, rats and mice, <u>Toxic. Appl. Pharm.</u>, 63:292.

Lapkin, R. T Bowman, R. and Kaloyanides, G.J., 1977, Effect of gentamicin on p-aminohippurate metabolism and transport in rat kidney slices, <u>J. Pharmacol. Exp. Ther.</u>, 201:233.

Lowry, O.H., Rosebourgh, N.J.; Farr, A.L. and Randall, R.J., 1951, Protein measurement with the Folin phenol reagent, <u>J. Biol. Chem.</u>, 193:265.

Mohandas, J., Marshal, J.J., Duggin, G.G., Hoevarth, J.S. and Tiller, D.J., 1984, Differential distribution of glutathione and glutathione-related enzymes in rabbit kidney: Possible implications in analgesic nephropathy, <u>Biochem. Pharm.</u>, 33:1801.

Ojakian, G.K. and Herzlinger, D.A., 1984, Analysis of epithelial cell surface polarity with monoclonal antibodies, <u>Fed. Proc.</u>, 43:2208.

Mellwood, J.M., Lovell, D., Thompson, A.E. and Tighe, J.R., 1976, Renal damage caused by gentamicin: a study of the effects on renal morphology and urinary enzyme excretion, <u>J. Pathol.</u> 118:171.

Whiting, P.H. and Simpson, J.G., 1983, The enhancement of cyclosporin A-induced nephrotoxicity by gentamicin, <u>Biochem. Pharm.</u>, 32:2025.

246

INVESTIGATION OF GENTAMICIN NEPHROTOXICITY USING RENAL BRUSH BORDER

MEMBRANE VESICLES

C. Godson and M.P. Ryan

Department of Pharmacology, University College Dublin, Belfield, Dublin 4,
Ireland

INTRODUCTION

A number of in vitro model systems are available to investigate
nephrotoxicity. As many nephrotoxic agents initially interact with cell
membrane components, the use of membrane vesicles may be particularly
appropriate to studying initial interactions and mechanisms of
nephrotoxicity at the cell membrane level. In renal tubules, transcellular
transport consists of at least three components: transport across the
apical (luminal, brush border) membrane, transport across the cytosol,
transport across the serosal (contraluminal, peritubular, baso-lateral)
membrane. In studies with whole tissue or isolated cells, it is not
possible to resolve these components of transport. However, isolation of
vesicles formed by the brush border and the basolateral membrane have made
it possible to study and define transport processes located in either
brush border or basolateral membranes. In this paper we report on
aminoglycoside interaction with brush border membrane vesicles prepared
from rat renal cortex.

The aminoglycosides (AG) are widely used in the treatment of gram negative
infections. Nephrotoxicity is a dose-limiting feature of gentamicin (G)
therapy. We have previously reported on gentamicin-induced nephrotoxicity
in cystic fibrosis patients (Godson et al., 1986). The renal pathogenesis
of the AG can be attributed to their selective accumulation within renal
proximal tubular cells. Reabsorption via the brush border membrane is
thought to constitute the dominant route of tubular accumulation (Williams
et al., 1986). Because the initial event in the renal tubular reabsorption
of AG involves binding to the brush border membrane the use of brush
border membrane vesicles (BBMV) may provide a particularly useful model
for studying in vitro the mechanisms of gentamicin-induced nephrotoxicity.
As renal leakage of calcium is a feature of gentamicin nephrotoxicity, the
effects of gentamicin on calcium transport in brush border membrane
vesicles was a special focus of this work.

METHODS

The brush border and the basolateral membranes differ in many respects
including morphology, enzyme content, protein-, lipid- and carbohydrate-
composition, hormone receptors and transport properties.

These differences are exploited in isolation and characterization procedures. The kidney is a very heterogeneous tissue and careful anatomical separation of tissue zones before membrane isolation can reduce the heterogeneity. In this study, kidneys were removed from male Wistar rats and cortex dissected out and homogenised using a polytron-type homogenizer. Homogenization was carried out at $4^{\circ}C$ in a mannitol and EGTA medium. Addition of mannitol and EGTA to the incubation medium can help in reducing membrane damage. Brush border isolation methods are mainly based on differential precipitation of other subcellular organelles with calcium or magnesium. The addition of calcium or magnesium does not lead to precipitation of brush border membranes due to the high negative surface charge densities. (Booth and Kenny, 1974; Biber et al., 1981). The method employed in this study was essentially that of Biber et al. (1981). The flow chart for the isolation procedure is shown in Figure 1. Purity of the BBMV was assessed by marker enzyme assays. The relative specific activities of gamma-glutamyl transpeptidase (GGT) and alkaline phosphatase were used as indices of BBMV purification. Contamination of the membrane preparations was checked as follows:- Na-K-ATPase-basolateral membranes; succinate dehydrogenase - mitochondria; aryl sulphatase and ß-N-acetyl-glucosaminidase - lysosomes. Morphology of BBMV was examined by electron microscopy. The BBMV preparation was fixed in glutaraldehyde and post-fixed in OsO_4. Ultra-thin sections were stained with lead citrate and uranyl acetate.

The effects of gentamicin on calcium binding and transport by the vesicles were investigated as follows:

1. Time course of Ca uptake by BBMV: BBMV (200 mg membrane protein) were preincubated with gentamicin (12.5-200 ug ml) at $25^{\circ}C$ for 10 min. 0.1 mM $^{45}CaCl_2$ was added to the membrane suspension and Ca uptake into the vesicles stopped after 2, 5, 10, 20, and 40 min by addition of 2 ml ice-cold incubation mixture and rapid filtration through polyethyleneimine (PEI) coated glass-fibre (GF/F) filters (Bruns et al., 1983).

2. Initial rate of Ca uptake by the BBMV: BBMV were preincubated at various concentrations of gentamicin (12.5-200 ug ml) at $25^{\circ}C$. CaCl was added to the membrane suspension at final concentrations 0.25-3 mM $CaCl_2$. Uptake of Ca was stopped after 20 secs by rapid filtration through GF/F filters. K_m and V_{max} were determined using ROSFIT computer programme (Greco et al., 1982).

3. Ca efflux by BBMV: BBMV were preloaded with ^{45}Ca (0.1 mM) for 60 min at $4^{\circ}C$. Efflux was initiated by a 10-fold dilution of the membrane suspension with incubation buffer. Gentamicin (12.5- 200 ug/ml) was added at this point. Efflux was stopped by rapid filtration at various time points.

4. Ca binding by BBMV: BBMV were preincubated with gentamicin (12.5-200 ug/ml) at $25^{\circ}C$. Various concentrations of $^{45}CaCl_2$ (5-2.5 mM) with and without 400-fold excess CaCl were added. After 60 min at $25^{\circ}C$ binding was stopped by rapid filtration. The amount of unbound calcium contained within the intravesicular space was determined after estimating the intravesicular volume by the Na-dependent D-glucose uptake (Aronson & Sacktor, 1975). Binding of ^{45}Ca to BBMV was calculated by substracting the ^{45}Ca unbound within the vesicular space from Ca uptake. The calcium binding data was analysed using EBDA and ligand computer programme.

RESULTS

BBMV purification: The marker enzyme results are shown in Table 1. The marker enzymes for BBMV, gamma-glutamyl transpeptidase and alkaline phosphatase were enriched from crude homogenate 12.7 ± 0.4 and 8.7 ± 0.2 fold

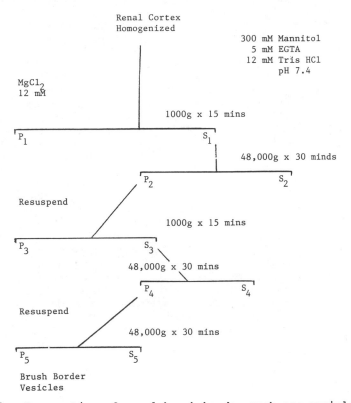

Renal Cortex
Homogenized

300 mM Mannitol
5 mM EGTA
12 mM Tris HCl
pH 7.4

MgCl$_2$
12 mM

1000g x 15 mins

P$_1$ S$_1$

48,000g x 30 minds

P$_2$ S$_2$

Resuspend

1000g x 15 mins

P$_3$ S$_3$

48,000g x 30 mins

P$_4$ S$_4$

Resuspend

48,000g x 30 mins

P$_5$ S$_5$

Brush Border
Vesicles

Fig. 1. Preparation of renal brush border membrane vesiclses

respectively. Contamination with basolateral membranes was low as indexed by the relative specific activity of 0.64 ± 0.07 for Na-K-ATPase. Contamination with mitochondria and lysosomes was minimal as indexed by relative specific activities of succinate dehydrogenase (0.5 ± 0.02) and ß-N-acetylglucosaminidase (0.11 ± 0.1). Electron microscopy revealed a high yield of sealed vesicles orientated right-side out. The results for the time course of ^{45}Ca uptake are shown in Table 2. In the control situation, ^{45}Ca uptake increased up to the 20 min time period. Gentamicin (200 ug/ml) caused a significant decrease in ^{45}Ca uptake at all time periods studied.

Table 1. Purification factors for markers enzymes in brush border vesicles compared to homogenate

Gamma-glutamyltranspeptidase	12.7 ± 0.4
Alkaline phosphatase	8.7 ± 0.2
Na-K-ATPase	0.64 ± 0.07
Succinate dehydrogenase	0.50 ± 0.01
Aryl sulphatase	0.39 ± 0.07
ß-N-Acetylglucosaminidase	0.11 ± 0.01

Results are expressed as enzyme specific activities in brush border vesicles divided by enzyme specific activities in the homogenate. Results shown are mean$\pm$s.e.m.

Table 2.   Effect of gentamicin on time course of ^{45}Ca uptake in brush border membrane vesicles.

Time (mins)	Control	Gentamicin (200 ug/ml)
2	1.8±0.1	1.1±0.1*
5	2.6±0.3	1.5±0.1*
10	3.7±0.3	2.0±0.1*
20	5.5±0.5	2.7±0.3*
40	5.5±0.5	3.0±0.4*

Results are expressed are nmol Ca/mg protein and are shown as mean±s.e.m. * indicates significant difference ($p < 0.05$) from control values.

The effects of gentamicin on the initial rate of Ca uptake are shown in Table 3.   Gentamicin in the concentration range 25-200 ug/ml reduced the initial rate of calcium uptake by the BBMV in a dose-dependent manner. The K_m of ^{45}Ca uptake was not affected by gentamicin. The results for ^{45}Ca efflux from BBMV are shown in Table 4. Most of the efflux occurred in the first five min. Gentamicin (200 ug/ml) did not significantly alter the ^{45}Ca efflux. The results for binding of ^{45}Ca to brushborder vesicles are shown in Table 5. Computer-derived best fits of the Scatchard analysis of Ca binding revealed two binding sites. Gentamicin (200 ug/ml) reduced specific binding of ^{45}Ca to BBMV. Gentamicin reduced the number of both low and high affinity sites without significantly altering K_D values.

Table 3.   The effects of gentamicin on initial rate of ^{45}Ca uptake into rat renal brush border membrane vesicles.

Gentamicin (ug/ml)	V_{max} (nmol mg/20 sec)	K_m
0	9.32±1.09	1.06±0.22
12.5	10.91±1.33	1.73±0.6
25	8.41±1.38	1.58±0.28
50	4.48±0.57*	1.30±0.18
100	3.28±0.33*	1.09±0.18
200	2.58±0.50*	0.69±0.05

Results shown are mean±s.e.m.   * indicates significant difference from control values.

Table 4.   Time course of ^{45}Ca efflux from brush border membrane vesicles.

Time (mins)	Control	Centamicin (200 ug/ml)
0	3.0±0.4	2.7±0.2
2	2.2±0.1	2.2±0.2
5	1.9±0.2	1.8±0.3
20	1.8±0.1	1.9±0.1

Results are expressed as nmol Ca/mg protein remaining in the vesicles at the times indicated.   Results are given as mean±s.e.m.

Table 5. Scatchard analysis of ^{45}Ca specific binding to brush border membrane vesicles.

		Control	Gentamicin (200 ug/ml)
K_{D1}	$(10^{-5}M)$	1.98	1.66
K_{D2}	$(10^{-5}M)$	3.22	3.09
B_1		1.73	0.78
B_2		11.29	7.03
% specifically bound		83.1	69.0

DISCUSSION

The isolation procedure used in this study provided a high yield of sealed, right-side-out orientated membrane vesicles. The marker enzyme assays indicated good purity of brush border membrane vesicles with little contamination by basolateral vesicles. Contamination with mitochondria and lysosomes was also very low. The investigations showed that gentamicin interfered with calcium transport in brush border membrane vesicles. Gentamicin (200 ug/ml) reduced ^{45}Ca brush border 40 min period. Reductions in ^{45}Ca uptake were also seen at lower concentrations of gentamicin. The effect appeared dose-dependent in the concentration range (12.5-200 ug/ml). Kinetic analysis of the initial rate of ^{45}Ca uptake revealed a reduction in V_{max} by gentamicin, but no significant alteration in K_m. These findings suggest that the inhibition by gentamicin of calcium uptake is of a non-competitive nature. This suggestion was further strengthened by the binding studies. These findings indicated two binding sites for calcium on the brush border membranes. Gentamicin (200 ug/ml) decreased specific binding of calcium to the brush border membrane. It reduced the number of both low and high affinity sites without affecting K_D values. Gentamicin did not inhibit the efflux of calcium from pre-loaded vesicles. Brush border membrane vesicles have also been used by other investigators to study gentamicin nephrotoxicity. Sastrasinh et al. (1982) identified that the binding site of aminoglycosides in rat renal brush border membranes was phospholipid in nature. Williams et al. (1986) demonstrated very good correlations between in vitro binding of aminoglycosides to brush border membrane vesicles and in vivo nephrotoxicity of the aminoglycosides. They demonstrated that inhibition of membrane binding of aminoglycosides by polyamino acids such as polyaspartate was also reflected by reduced nephrotoxicity. These findings suggest that binding of aminoglycosides to brush border membranes may be crucial events in initiating nephrotoxicity. Our findings with calcium binding and transport may facilitate elucidation of the mechanism(s) of aminoglycoside-induced nephrotoxicity.

ACKNOWLEDGEMENTS

This work was supported by the Cystic Fibrosis Association of Ireland

REFERENCES

Aronson, P.S., and Sacktor, B., 1975, The Na gradient transport of D glucose in renal brush border membranes. J. Biol. Chem., 250:6032-6039.

Biber, J., Stieger, B., Haase, W., and Murer, H., 1981, A high yield preparation from rat kidney brush border membranes. Different behaviour of lysosomal markers. Biochem. Biophys. Acta., 647:169-176.

Booth, A.G., and Kenn, A.J., 1974, A rapid method for the preparation of microvilli from rabbit kidney. <u>Biochem. J.</u>, 142:575-581.

Bruns, R.F., Lawson-Wendling, K. and Pugsley, T.A., 1983, A rapid filtration assay for soluble receptors using polyethylenimine coated filters. <u>Anal. Biochem.</u>, 132:74-81.

Godson, C., Ryan, M.P., Brady, H. and FitzGerald, M.X., 1986, Investigation of gentamicin nephrotoxicity in cystic fibrosis patients. <u>Irish J. Med. Sci</u>., 155:133.

Greco, W.R., Priori, R.L., Sharma, M., and Korythynik, W., 1982, An enzyme kinetics non-linear regression curve fitting package for micro-computers. <u>Comput. Biomed. Res</u>., 15:39-45.

Sastrasinh, M., Knauss, T. C., Weinberg, J.M. and Humes, H.D., 1982, Identification of the aminoglycoside binding site in rat renal brush border membranes. <u>J. Pharmacol. Exp. Therap</u>., 222:350-358.

Williams, P.D. Hottendorf, G.H. and Bennett, D.B., 1986, Inhibition of renal membrane binding and nephrotoxicity of aminoglycosides. <u>J. Pharmacol. Expt. Therap</u>. 237:919-925.

TIME DEPENDENT NEPHROTOXICITY OF AMIKACIN

C. Dorian, Ph. Catroux, J.C. Cal and J. Cambar

Groupe d'Etude de Physiologie et Physiopathologie Renales, Faculte de Pharmacie, Place de la Victoire, Bordeaux, France

INTRODUCTION

The present study considers a chronobiological approach in optimizing the clinical use of a drug know to induce nephrotoxicity, amikacin. Nephrotoxicity is probably the most frequent untoward effect encountered in patients treated with aminoglycoside antibiotics. Kidney dysfunction induced by these drugs primarily results from acute tubular necrosis. The risk of morbidity may be further aggravated by the widespread use of aminoglycosides such as advanced age, hypovolaemia, renal disease, previous treatment with aminoglycosides or concomitant administration of other nephrotoxic substances. Other factors may interfere such as dose, duration of drug treatment, frequency and time of administration (Fillastre, 1986). The aim of this study is to determine the importance of the latter.

MATERIALS AND METHODS

Male Wistar rats (180-200g), were housed in collective cages by groups of five animals for a minimum of one week, then in individual metabolism cages, 8 days before the test. Environmental conditions were carefully controlled throughout the experiment (October): relative humidity (50-55%), temperature ($25\pm1^{\circ}C$), food and water "ad libitum", synchronized by artificial light (12L/12D). At 4 difference fixed times during a 24 hr period (08:00 - 14:00 - 20:00 or 02:00), a total of 40 animals received an ip injection of amikacin (1.2g/kg). Urines were collected at 6-hr intervals during 2 consecutive days before (control period) and 3 after amikacin administration. Different urinary parameters were used to assess the nephrotoxicity severity induced by this drug: the urinary excretion of water, sodium, potassium, proteins, and enzymes i.e. gamma-glutamyl-transferase (GGT) and alkaline phosphatase (ALP), two brush border enzymes, and N-acetyl-beta-D-glucosaminidase (NAG) a lysosomal one. The difference between the enzymuria after and before the intoxication (delta

IU/6hr) is presented as a result. A classical statistical analysis was performed on the data.

RESULTS

The injection of 1.2g/kg of amikacin at each of the 4 time points produced an acute tubular injury. Indeed, urinary GGT, ALP and NAG excretion increased significantly which suggested the loss of brush border membranes and tubular necrosis. However, this increase in enzymuria varied greatly as a function of the time point at which the drug was given. Statistically significant variations were found between increase rates when amikacin was given at 14:00 and at 3 other time for each of the three enzymes. Forty-eight hr after amikacin administration the enzymuria began to decrease and reached normal values within the four days of the amikacin injection. Urinary excretion of GGT exhibited a peak 6 to 12 hr after intoxication, in rats dosed at any of the four circadian times. In contrast, for the lysosomal enzyme, the increase occurred as early as the first 6 hr after amikacin. Enzymuria increase was particularly important when amikacin was administered at 14:00 (4.5-fold for GGT, 10-fold for NAG – Fig. 1)

DISCUSSION

The results of this study evidence that the renal response to amikacin is circadian stage dependent. Such findings are consistent with those on heavy metals (Levi, 1982, Cal et al., 1984) and on other aminoglycosides (Pariat, 1984). The first step of any chronotoxicological study consists of acute investigations. Circadian variations in the toxicity of amino-glycosides did not, however, appear only to be due nephrotoxicity (Dorian et al., 1985). The cause of death was probably neuromuscular blockade inducing respiratory paralysis (Fiekers, 1983). In subacute studies, however, it is possible to evaluate specific indices of renal injury, including enzymuria. Morphologically, kidney dysfunction induced by aminoglycosides appears to be associated with the necrosis of proximal tubules. This is consistent with the fact that this section of the nephron is the primary site of drug accumulation. The transfer of the aminoglycosides through the luminal membranes of the proximal tubule seems to be the most important way of their entering the cell. After binding on brush border, aminoglycosides are taken up in pinocytotic vesicles and transferred to lysosomes (Cojocel and Hook, 1985). The aminoglycosides binding to anionic sites on brush border membranes involve the elimination of specific enzymes such as GGT and ALP. The increased urinary excretion of GGT and ALP may reflect accelerated turnover of brush border membrane. The transfer and accumulation in lysosomes of the aminoglycosides explain the increase lysosomal enzymuria. This one may be derived from exocytosis of phagolysosomes with release of lysosomal enzymes into the tubular lumen (during the first 6 hr after a high dose) or from frank proximal tubular cell necrosis (from 6 to 12 hr after dosing). Amikacin, as other amino-glycosides, induces a decrease in urine concentrating ability (proceeding GFR impairment) detected in animals by polyuria. The assessment of urinary electrolytes (Na and K) show a fall in sodium excretion. A dys-function of Na-K pump could interfere to explain the excretion variations, but the mechanism is still unclear. Proteinuria, according to several authors, in the case of aminoglycosides is accompanied by both glomerular and tubular damages. Our results corroborate these facts. All these parameters varied as a function of the time of drug injection, but the most important and early sign for detection of nephrotoxicity is the high levels of enzymes in urine.

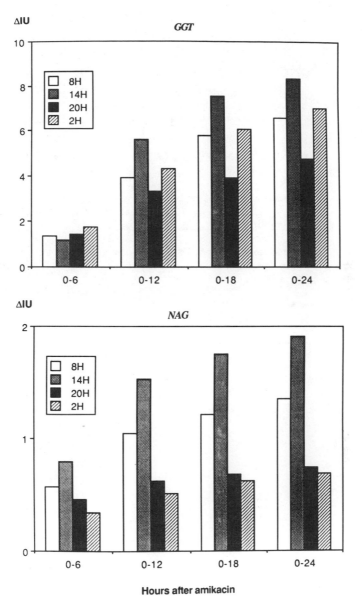

Fig. 1   Accumulated urinary activity of GGT and NAG as a function of the time of amikacin injection.

REFERENCES

Cal, J.C., Desmouliere, A., Cambar, J., 1984, Etude comparative des variations circadiennes de la mortalite induite par le chlorure mercurique et le sulfate de cadmium chez la souris, <u>Ann. Pharm. Franc</u>., 42:487.

Cojocel, C., Hook, J.B., 1985, Aminoglycoside nephrotoxicity, <u>Phar. Sci.</u>, 4:174.

Dorian, C., Cal, J.C., Cambar, J., 1985, Etude de la chronotoxicite de l'amikacine, <u>Pathol. Biol</u>., 33:377.

Fiekers, J.F., 1983, Effects of the aminoglycosides antibiotics, streptomycin and neomycin on neuromuscular transmission. I Presynaptic considerations, II Postsynaptic considerations, <u>J. Pharmacol Exp Ther</u>., 225:487.

Fillastre, J.P., 1986, La nephrotoxicite des aminoglycosides, <u>La Lettre de l'Infectiologue</u>, 1, 5:143.

Levi, F., 1982, Chronopharmacologie de trois agents doues d'activite anticancereuse chez le rat et la souris. Chronoefficacite et chronotolerance., <u>These Doc. Sci. Nat., Paris VI</u>.

Pariat, C., 1986, Etude experimentale de la chronosusceptibilite renale de trois aminoglycosides (gentamicine, dibekacine, et netilmincine)., <u>These Doc. Sci. Pharm., Poitiers</u>.

EFFECT OF LATAMOXEF [MOXALACTAM] ON TOBRAMYCIN BINDING TO KIDNEY BRUSH BORDER MEMBRANES IN RATS.

Ryoji Kojima, Mikio Ito and Yoshio Suzuki

Department of Pharmacology, Faculty of Pharmacy, Meijo University, Nagoya 468, Japan

INTRODUCTION

Latamoxef (LMOX) [moxalactam] has previously been shown to protect rat kidneys from tobramycin (TOB)-induced nephrotoxicity [1,2], and the mechanism for the protection may be involved in the suppression of intrarenal TOB accumulation by combination with LMOX. Therefore, to clarify the mechanism by which LMOX suppresses the intrarenal TOB accumulation in vivo, we have hypothesised that positively charged TOB may be able to interact with negatively charged LMOX by ionic binding in vivo and the interaction may inhibit the binding of TOB to acidic phospholipids forming brush border membranes (BBMs). The inhibition of TOB binding to BBMs may contribute to the decrease in the intrarenal TOB accumulation. Recently, we have demonstrated that TOB directly interacts with LMOX in vitro, [3] and the interaction is associated with the suppression of intrarenal TOB accumulation by combination with LMOX in vivo.

In the present study we have investigated the effect of LMOX on TOB binding to BBMs isolated from the rat renal cortex to confirm our hypothesis.

MATERIALS AND METHODS

Preparation of BBMs. BBMs were isolated from rat kidney cortex by the methods of Evers [4] and Inui [5]. Briefly, the renal cortex of male Sprague-Dawley rats weighing about 230 g was separated and homogenised in 2 mM HEPES/Tris containing 10 mM mannitol (pH 7.1) using Waring blender. After homogenization, 10 mM $CaCl_2$ was added to the homogenate. The homogenate was centrifuged at 500 x g for 12 min. and the resultant supernatant was recentrifuged to obtain BBMs fraction. Isolated BBMs were suspended in 20 mM HEPES/Tris (pH 7.4) containing 100 mM mannitol.

Measurement of enzyme activities. Alkaline phosphatase (ALP) and gamma-glutamyl transpeptidase (gamma-GTP), marker enzymes of BBMs, were measured by the methods of Bessey [6] and Tamaoki [7], respectively. The activity of Na^+-K^+ ATPase locating in basolateral membranes was assayed by slightly modifying the methods described by Jacobson [8] and Lo [9]. N-acetyl-beta-D-glucosaminidase (NAG), a lysosomal enzyme, and succinate dehydrogenase, a mitochondrial enzyme, were measured by the methods of Hasebe [10] and Green [11], respectively. Lactate dehydrogenase (LDH) activity was determined using a LDH LInia-Neo 3a kit (Shinotest, Japan) to assess the degree of contamination of cytosolic fractions. The membrane proteins were measured by using a BIO-RAD protein assay.

Electron microscopy of isolated BBMs. Isolated BBMs were stained with 2.5% ammonium molybdate by the method of Brenner and Horne (12) for negative staining and observed under LEM-2000 electron microscope.

Binding assay. The binding of TOB to BBMs was assayed according to the method of Ishikawa (13). In brief, 200 ul of membrane suspension was incubated at $4^{\circ}C$ for 10 min with TOB (0.4 mM, 200 ul) in 2 mM HEPES/Tris (pH 7.4). The amount of TOB bound to BBMs was measured by a substrate-labelled fluorescent immunoassay.

RESULTS

Purity of isolated BBMs. Table 1 summarizes the specific activities of enzymes in the homogenate and BBMs fraction. As shown in Table 1, the relative specific activities of ALP, gamma-GTP and $Na^{+}-K^{+}$ were 11.5, 14.5 and 0.60, respectively. NAG, SDH and LDH in BBMs fraction were minimal. This result indicates that BBMs are highly purified with less contamination of basolateral membranes and other subcellular fractions.

Table 1. Purity of brush border membranes

Marker enzyme	Specific activity		Relative
	Homogenate	BBM fraction	Specific activity
γ-glutamyl transpeptidase	μmol/hr/mg protein		
	3.67 ± 0.16	53.62 ± 3.43	14.6
Alkaline phosphatase	μmol/hr/mg protein		
	0.04 ± 0.002	0.46 ± 0.03	11.5
$Na^{+}-K^{+}$ATPase	μmol/hr/mg protein		
	0.42 ± 0.07	0.25 ± 0.04	0.60
N-acetyl-β-D-glucosaminidase	μmol/hr/mg protein		
	11.59 ± 0.37	2.21 ± 0.12	0.19
Succinate dehydrogenase	μmol/hr/mg protein		
	1.26 ± 0.02	0.04 ± 0.02	0.03
Lactate dehydrogenase	U/hr/mg protein		
	250 ± 30	40 ± 5	0.02

Data are expressed as means±S.E. for five separate experiments.

Electron microscopy of BBMs. Fig. 1 shows the electron micrograph of BBMs isolated from rat renal cortex. It was evident that isolated BBMs formed vesicles.

Effect of LMOX on TOB binding to BBMs. No obvious changes in TOB binding to BBMs were observed when the aliquots of TOB (0.4 mM) and LMOX (0.4, 0.8 and 2 mM) were simultaneously added to a BBMs fraction. However, the addition of LMOX (4, 10, 20 and 30 mM) to the fraction suppressed the TOB binding to BBMs by 13 to 16% (Fig. 2).

Effect of preformed complex of TOB and LMOX on TOB binding to BBMs. The addition of each reaction mixture of TOB (0.4 mM) and LMOX (4 and 10 mM), which was preincubated for 3 hr at $37^{\circ}C$ for the purpose of interaction, significantly suppressed the TOB binding to BBMs by 24-50%. There was a greater suppression of the TOB binding to BBMs as compared with the result in Fig. 2 (Fig. 3).

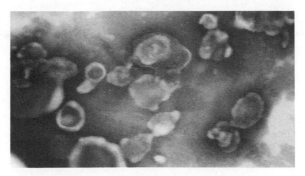

Fig. 1. Electron micrograph of isolated BBMs. BBMs were stained with 2.5 % ammonium molybdate (magnification; X 72,000).

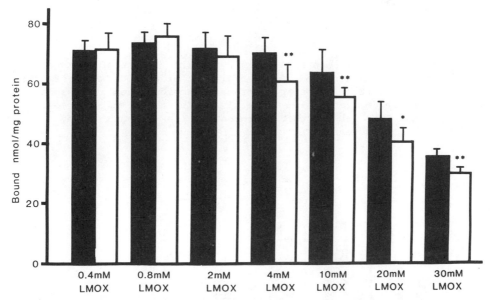

Fig. 2. Effect of LMOX on TOB binding to BBMs. ■: TOB (0.4 mM) and NACl, □: TOB (0.4 mM) and LMOX. *: P<0.05, **: P<0.01 compared to TOB (0.4 mM) and NaCl.

Binding of [^{14}C]LMOX to BBMs. Table 2 shows the binding of [^{14}C]LMOX to BBMs. Membranes vesicles (20 ul, 193 ug of protein) suspended in 2 mM HEPES/Tris (pH 7.4) were incubated at 4 and 37°C for 10, 30 and 60 min. with substrate mixture (20 ul) comprising 2 mM HEPES/Tris (pH 7.4) and 50 uM [^{14}C]LMOX. As shown in Table 2, LMOX bound to BBMs temperature- and time-dependent.

Effect of pretreatment with LMOX on TOB binding to BBMs. There were no significant differences in TOB binding between the two cases, namely pretreatment with LMOX and simultaneous treatment with LMOX (Fig. 4).

Table 2. Binding of $[^{14}C]$LMOX to BBMs

| | incubation time (min) | | |
	10	30	60
		nmol/mg protein	
4°C	13.60 ± 7.87	38.96 ± 9.27	42.22 ± 11.02
37°C	38.62 ± 11.42	67.51 ± 8.04	82.41 ± 20.76

Data are expressed as means ± S.E. for three separate experiments.

DISCUSSION

In the present study, we have investigated the effect of LMOX on TOB binding to BBMs. The method of Ca precipitation provided BBMs fraction with less contamination of other membranes fractions such as basolateral membranes as demonstrated in Table 1. In addition, the electron micrograph of BBMs showed that BBMs used in the present study formed vesicles but not fragments (Fig. 1).

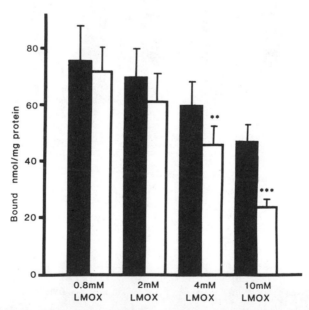

Fig. 3. Effect of preformed complex of TOB and LMOX on TOB binding to BBMs. ■: TOB (0.4 mM) and LMOX, □: reaction mixture of TOB (0.4 mM) and LMOX. **: P < 0.01, ***: P < 0.001 compared to TOB (0.4 mM) and LMOX.

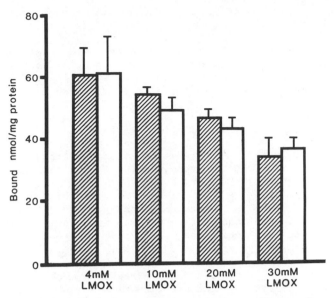

Fig. 4. Effect of pretreatment with LMOX on TOB binding to BBMs. ☐ : pretreatment with LMOX, ⊘ : simultaneous treatment with LMOX.

The addition of LMOX (4, 10, 20 and 30 mM) to the BBMs fraction suppressed the TOB binding to BBMs by about 15% (Fig. 2), indicating that LMOX inhibits the TOB binding to BBMs. In order to determine the mechanism by which LMOX inhibits the TOB binding to BBMS, we examined the effect of preformed complex of TOB and LMOX on TOB binding to BBMs. Before the binding studies, TOB and LMOX were preincubated for 3 hr at 37°C for the purpose of interaction. The addition of reaction mixture significantly suppressed the TOB binding to BBMs by 24-50% (Fig. 3). This result suggested that the interaction of TOB with LMOX was associated with the suppression of TOB binding to BBMs. However, the possibility existed that LMOX might bind to BBMs and inhibit the TOB binding to the receptor, acidic phospholipids including phosphatidylinositol, on the membranes. Therefore, using ^{14}C-labelled LMOX, we analysed the binding of LMOX to BBMs by the rapid filtration technique. As shown in Table 2, LMOX bound to BBMs with temperature- and time-dependent manner. Thus, if the binding to LMOX to BBMs inhibits the TOB binding to receptor on BBMs, pretreatment with LMOX to BBMs would have suppressed the TOB binding to the membranes more than when TOB and LMOX were simultaneously added to BBMs fraction. However, as shown in Fig. 4, there were no significant differences in the TOB binding to BBMs between the two cases. This indicated that LMOX bound to BBMs is not associated with the suppression of the TOB binding to BBMs by LMOX although LMOX binds to the membranes.

In conclusion, these results indicate that the interaction of TOB with LMOX is associated with the suppression of TOB binding to BBMs isolated from the rat renal cortex. This suggests that the decrease in the intra-renal TOB accumulation by combination with LMOX in vivo results from the inhibition of TOB binding to BBMs by the interaction between TOB and LMOX.

REFERENCES

1. R. Kojima, M. Ito, and Y. Suzuki, Studies on the nephrotoxicity of aminoglycoside antibiotics and protection from these effects (3).

Protective effect of latamoxef against tobramycin nephrotoxicity and its protective mechanism, Japan. J. Pharmacol. 42:397 (1986).

2. R. Kojima, M. Ito, and Y. Suzuki, Studies on the nephrotoxicity of aminoglycoside antibiotics and protection from these effects (4). Effect of tobramycin alone and in combination with latamoxef on the stability of rat kidney lysosomal membranes, Japan. J. Pharmacol. 43:73 (1987).

3. R. Kojima and Y. Suzuki, Interaction of tobramycin with latamoxef in vitro, Japan. J. Pharmacol. 39:Suppl. 316 (1985).

4. C. Evers, W. Haase, H. Murer, and R. Kinne, Properties of brush border vesicles isolated from rat kidney cortex by calcium precipitation, Membrane Biochem. 1:203 (1978).

5. K. Inui, T. Okano, M. Takano, S. Kitazawa, and R. Hori, A simple method for the isolation of basolateral plasma membrane vesicles from rat kidney cortex. Enzyme activities and some properties of glucose transport, Biochim. Biophys. Acta 47:150 (1981).

6. O.A. Bessey, O.H. Lowry, and M.J. Brock, A method for the rapid determination of alkaline phosphatase with five cubic millimetres of serum, J. Biol. Chem. 146:321 (1946).

7. H. Tamaoki, S. Minato, S. Takei, and K. Fujisawa, A clinical method for the determination of serum gamma-glutamyl transpeptidase, Clin. Chim. Acta 65:21, (1975).

8. M.P. Jacobson, H.J. Rodriguez, W.C. Hogan, and S. Klahr, Mechanism of activation of renal Na^+-K^+ ATPase in the rat: effect of reduction of renal mass, Am. J. Physiol. 239:F281 (1980).

9. C.S. Lo, T.R. August, U.A. Liberman, and I.S. Edelman, Dependence of renal Na^+-K^+-adenosine triphosphatase activity on thyroid status, J. Biol. Chem. 251:7826 (1976).

10. K. Hasebe, Biochemical studies on synovial fluid, Fukushima J. Med. Sci. 15:35, (1968).

11. D.E. Green, S. Mii, and P.M. Kohout, Studies on the terminal electron transport system. I. succinic dehydrogenase, J. Biol. Chem. 217:551 (1955).

12. S. Brenner and R.W. Horne, A negative staining method for high resolution electron microscopy of viruses, Biochim. Biophys. Acta 34:103, (1959).

13. Y. Ishikawa, K. Inui, and R. Hori, Gentamicin binding to brush border and basolateral membranes isolated from rat kidney cortex, J. Pharmacobio-Dyn. 8:931, (1985).

AMPHOTERICIN-B NEPHROTOXICITY IS DECREASED BY INTRAVENOUS FLUCYTOSINE IN THE RAT

H.Th. Heidemann, K.-H. Brune, L. Gjessing, and E.E. Ohnhaus

I. Medizinische Klinik, Christian-Albrechts-Universitat, D-2300 Kiel 1, Federal Republic of Germany

INTRODUCTION

Amphotericin-B is the most useful drug of the treatment of systemic mycotic infections. The clinical use however is limited because of the side effect to cause nephrotoxicity. The mechanisms by which amphotericin-B induced renal impairment are not yet known. Since the acute vascular effects of amphotericin-B on the kidney can be ameliorated by sodium chloride loading, furosemide and aminophylline, it has been suggested that amphotericin-B activates the tubular glomerular feed-back (Gerkens and Branch, 1980; Heidemann et al., 1983). The antifungal efficacy of the treatment can be increased by a combination of amphotericin-B plus flucytosine (Bennett et al., 1979). Intravenous flucytosine is dissolved in saline. It was therefore the aim of this study to investigate the effect of flucytosine on amphotericin-B nephrotoxicity.

METHODS

Thirty six male Sprague Dawley rats (230-270 g) were sodium depleted (Furosemide 10 mg/kg ip., low sodium rat chow). The animals had drinking water _ad libitum_. 3 days before the start of the experiment each rat received a jugular (silastic) and an intraperitoneal cannula (silicon rubber) under Nembutal[R] anaesthesia (60 mg/kg ip.) Catheters were extended to the neck.

The rats were divided into 5 groups and received the following treatments for 7 days:

I.   Amphotericin-B + glucose 5%
II.   Amphotericin-B + flucytosine (solved in NaCl 0.9%)
III.   Amphotericin-B + NaCl 0.9%
IV.   Amphotericin-B + flucytosine (solved in glucose 5%)
V.   Vehicle $_{(ampho)}$ + glucose 5%

Dosage: Amphotericin-B 5 mg/kg/day ip.; flucytosine 150 mg/kg/12 hr iv (solution 10 mg/ml); NaCl 0.9%, 15 ml/kg/12 hr iv; glucose 5%, 15 ml/kg/12 hr iv.

Before and at the end of the experiment 24-hr urine was collected and a blood sample was taken in the middle of the collecting period to measure creatinine and calculate creatinine clearance. At the end of the experiment the following parameters were measured: Serum: Haematocrit, sodium, potassium, creatinine and BUN. Urine: Volume, sodium, potassium and creatinine.

RESULTS

Amphotericin-B caused a marked reduction in kidney function. After 7 days of treatment the serum creatinine and serum blood urea nitrogen concentrations were significantly elevated in comparison to the vehicle treated rats (Table 1). The treatment had no effect on serum sodium concentrations, however, the serum potassium concentration and the haematocrit were significantly elevated (Table 1).

Table 1. The effect of amphotericin-B(A) plus flucytosine(F) or NaCl on serum sodium, potassium, haematocrit, creatinine and BUN (X ± SEM). (* p = 0.05 in comparison to vehicle, # p = 0.05 in comparison to amphotericin-B + glucose).

	S_{Na}	S_K	HKT	S_{Cr}	S_{BUN}
	mmol/l	mmol/l	%	mg/dl	mg/dl
A + GLU	146 ± 4	8.9 ± 0.9*	45.9 ± 1.2*	1.01 ± 0.19	110 ± 27*
A + F(NaCl)	148 ± 4	5.8 ± 0.9	41.7 ± 1.2	0.42 ± 0.05	49 ± 4*'#
A + NaCl	151 ± 3	5.4 ± 0.4	40.4 ± 0.9	0.54 ± 0.07*	57 ± 9*'#
A + F(GLU)	140 ± 4	5.8 ± 0.3	41.6 ± 0.7	0.44 ± 0.02	65 ±11*'#
VEH	148 ± 2	5.5 ± 0.5	41.4 ± 1.2	0.40 ± 0.03	18 ± 1

The urine volume was unchanged in comparison to the vehicle treated rats (Table 2). The total sodium excretion into the urine was elevated as well as the fractional sodium excretion, whereas the total potassium excretion was decreased (Table 2). The creatinine clearance was markedly reduced in comparison to its own baseline values as well as in comparison to the vehicle treated controls (Fig. 1).

The treatment of amphotericin-B with either flucytosine solved in saline or normal saline, or flucytosine solved in glucose (Fig. 1, Tables 1 and 2). Electrolyte disturbances could not be observed and the haematocrit values were not different from controls (Table 1). The serum creatinine concentrations were within the normal range and the BUN concentrations were significantly lower than in the animals treated with amphotericin-B plus glucose (Table 1). The total sodium excretion into the urine was elevated in comparison to the vehicle group, whereas the potassium excretion was decreased (Table 2). The fractional sodium excretions of these three groups were significantly lower in comparison to the amphotericin-B plus glucose group, they were however elevated in comparison to the controls. The urine volumes were significantly elevated in comparison to the vehicle group (Table 2).

Flucytosine as well as sodium chloride inhibited the drop in creatinine clearance due to chronic amphotericin-B administration (Fig. 1).

264

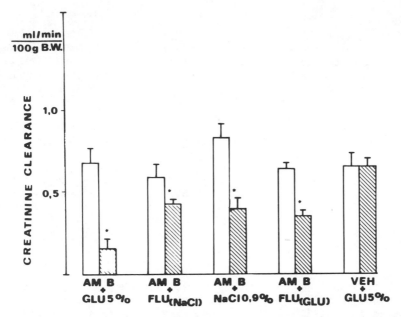

Fig. 1. The effect of glucose 5%, or flucytosine solved in NaCl 0.9%, or NaCl 0.9%, or flucytosine solved in glucose 5% on amphotericin-B induced renal impairment. Creatinine clearances were measured before and after the various treatments.

* = p 0.05 in comparison to vehicle, * = p 0.05 in comparison to amphotericin-B + glucose 5%, X ± SEM.

Comparing pre- and post-treatment values the relative change of creatinine clearance was the least in the animals co-administered flucytosine solved in saline (23.7 ± 7.5%) and significantly higher in the animals receiving amphotericin-B plus sodium chloride 0.9% and amphotericin-B plus flucytosine solved in glucose (48.6 ± 11.4 and 44.4 ± 6.7% respectively).

Table 2. The effect of amphotericin-B (A) plus flucytosine (F) or NaCl on urine volume, sodium and potassium excretion, and fractional sodium excretion (X ± SEM).

	U_{Vol}	$U_{\cdot Na}$ x Vol	U_K x Vol	FE_{Na}
	ml	mmol	mmol	%
A + GLU	16.6 ± 3.3	0.39 ± 0.09*	0.68 ± 0.16	0.86 ± 0.31*
A + F (NaCl)	41 ± 0.11*	0.52 ± 0.11*	0.72 ± 0.08*	0.22 ± 0.04*'#
A + NaCl	31.4 ± 4.3*	0.41 ± 0.07*	0.87 ± 0.24	0.19 ± 0.02*'#
A + F (GLU)	35.1 ± 4.7*	0.27 ± 0.05*	0.93 ± 0.21*	0.19 ± 0.04*'#
VEH	17.8 ± 4.8	0.005 ± 0.002*	1.90 ± 0.17	0.002 ± 0.0004

* p = 0.05 in comparison to vehicle, # p = 0.05 in comparison to amphotericin-B + glucose

DISCUSSION

The most serious side effect of amphotericin-B treatment is nephrotoxicity. The mechanism by which amphotericin-B induces renal impairment
is not known yet. It has been shown previously that salt loading helps to
reverse nephrotoxicity which has already developed (Heidemann et al.,
1983). We now present results which suggest that the frequency of that
adverse effect can be substantially reduced by concomitant intravenous
flucytosine treatment. In addition we can show that this beneficial
effect is due to the flucytosine itself as well as the sodium chloride
serving as its vehicle.

Amphotericin-B causes a decrease in creatinine clearance and an increase
in fractional sodium excretion indicating glomerular as well as tubular
dysfunction. Both these effects can be minimized by co-treatment with
flucytosine or normal saline. The relative changes of creatinine
clearances moreover indicate an additive protective effect of the
flucytosine and saline.

The various treatments have no effect on the serum sodium concentrations.
The serum potassium concentrations, however, were markedly elevated in the
animals treated with amphotericin-B plus glucose 5%. This is in agreement
with Cheng et al. (1982) who also found elevated potassium concentrations
after high amphotericin-B doses. Other investigators have found normal or
low potassium levels (Gorge and Andreole, 1971). In our experiment all
animals treated with amphotericin-B had low potassium excretions,
suggesting that this low output contributes to the high concentrations in
the serum.

The animals treated with amphotericin-B plus glucose 5% had a slight,
however, significantly elevated haematocrit, which can be explained by
volume contraction. No data is available whether or to what extent this
might contribute to the renal impairment.

The chronic effects of amphotericin-B on renal function can be prevented
or reversed in humans by the simple manoeuvre of chronic salt loading
(Branch et al., 1987; Heidemann et al., 1983). The acute vascular effects
of amphotericin-B on kidney function can be ameliorated by sodium chloride
and furosemide in the dog (Gerkens and Branch, 1980) and by aminophylline
in the dog and rat (Gerkens et al., 1983; Heidemann et al., 1983). Since
these three interventions are also known to inhibit tubulo-glomerular
feed-back, thus contributing to its nephrotoxicity. The beneficial effect
of chronic sodium chloride loading on amphotericin-B nephrotoxicity in the
rat is therefore in agreement with the above mentioned hypothesis.

The finding that flucytosine decreases amphotericin-B nephrotoxicity is
new. The mechanism by which this drug is protective is not known yet.
Enhanced excretion of amphotericin-B due to flucytosine is highly unlikely
since only 1-3% is excreted through the kidneys. The most likely
explanation is an intravenous interaction of the two drugs. Most of the
flucytosine is excreted by the kidneys and amphotericin-B acutely
decreases renal blood low and GFR, therefore a haemodynamic interaction
might be possible and has to be investigated.

The observation that intravenous flucytosine decreases amphotericin-B
nephrotoxicity has important clinical relevance, independent of the
mechanism. The combination of these two drugs should be the systemic
antifungal treatment of choice since it is more effective (Bennett et al.,
1979) and is less nephrotoxic.

REFERENCES

Bennett, J.E., Dismukes, W.E. and Duma, P.J., 1979. A comparison of amphotericin-B alone and combined with flucytosine in the treatment of cryptococcal meningitis, N. Engl. J. Med., 301:126.

Branch, R.A., Jackson, E.K., Jacqz, E., Stein, R., Ray, W.A., Onhaus, E.E., Meusers, P. and Heidemann, H., 1987. Amphotericin-B nephrotoxicity in humans decreased by sodium supplements with co-administration of ticarcillin or intravenous saline, Klin. Wochenschr., 65:500.

Cheng, J.-T., Witty, R.T., Robinson, R.R. and Yarger, W.E., 1982. Amphotericin-B nephrotoxicity: Increased renal resistance and tubular permeability, Kidney international, 22:626.

Gerkens, J.F. and Branch, R.A., 1980. The influence of sodium status and furosemide on canine acute amphotericin-B nephrotoxicity, J. Pharmacol. Exp. Ther., 214:306.

Gerkens, J.F., Heidemann, H. Th., Jackson, E.K. and Branch, R.A., 1983. Effect of aminophylline on amphotericin-B nephrotoxicity in the dog, J. Pharmacol. Exp. Ther., 224:609.

Gorge, T.H. and Andriole, V.T., 1971. An experimental model of amphotericin-B nephrotoxicity with renal tubular acidosis, J. Lab. Clin. Med., 78: 713.

Heidemann, H. Th., Gerkens, J.F., Jackson, E.K. and Branch, R.A., 1983. Effect of aminophylline on renal vasoconstriction produced by amphotericin-B in the rat, Nanyn Schmiedeberg's Arch. Pharmacol., 324:148.

Heidemann, H. Th., Gerkens, J.F., Spickard, W.A., Jackson, E.K. and Branch, R.A., 1983a. Amphotericin-B nephrotoxicity in humans decreased by salt depletion, Am. J. Med., 75:476.

APPARENT AMOXAPINE NEPHROTOXICITY: DEPENDENCE ON RHABDOMYOLYSIS AND

ACIDOSIS

Larry T. Welch

School of Pharmacy, Ferris State College, Big Rapids, MI 49307

INTRODUCTION

The tricyclic antidepressant, amoxapine, has been released for distribution in the USA and in Europe. Acute renal failure has sometimes followed (Pumariega et al, 1982) attempts at suicide using this drug, but the incidence has been unpredictable and ranged from 10-15%, which suggests that other factors in addition to high doses of amoxapine and seizures may be involved. The available data in the literature shows that severe acidosis was frequently associated with amoxapine overdose. Goldberg and Spector (1982) described a patient whose blood pH dropped to 6.78 within 2 hr of ingesting nearly 60 mg/kg of amoxapine. Similarly, Rogol et al (1984) reported a blood pH of 6.83 in an infant considered to be overdosed with amoxapine. Shepard (1983) reported a profound acidosis in a 15 month child that had accidentally ingested 25 mg/kg of the drug and developed a blood pH of 6.91. In light of the frequent occurrence of acidosis following overdosage with amoxapine, the possibility exists that it may serve as a major contributing factor in the development of amoxapine-associated renal impairment. We therefore determined the effect of acidosis on the ability of high dosage amoxapine and seizures to produce apparent renal impairment in the rat. Because of the central role of muscle injury in atraumatic rhabdomyolytic acute renal failure in vivo, we also examined the potential of amoxapine to directly produce muscle injury in vitro.

METHODS

All experiments were undertaken on fasting, male Sprague-Dawley rats weighing 125-175 g. In some experiments, the effects of acidosis on serum creatinine levels in animals receiving amoxapine and a shock were examined. Amoxapine was given as a large but subseizure-producing dose (200 mg/kg po) concurrently with ammonium chloride (300 mg/kg ip) or isotonic saline in control groups. This was followed at 1 hr by electro-shock-induced seizures (60 mAmp low voltage AC current for 200 mSec via standard earclips from a Model 2-C Electroshock Apparatus - Hans Technical Associates). Twenty four hours later, renal function was indirectly estimated by measurement of the levels of creatinine in plasma from control and treatment groups. Plasma levels of creatinine were determined by use of a diagnostic kit from Sigma Chemical Company (No. 555) as was creatine phosphokinase (No. 47). The potential cytolytic

effects of amoxapine on muscle, heart, brain and kidney in vitro were
examined by kinetic measurement of the marker enzymes creatine phosphokinase and/or lactic dehydrogenase (Sigma kit No. 226).

With in vitro experiments, the tissues were placed in cold $2^{o}C$ isotonic
saline and thin slices of brain and heart were made with the aid of a
Stadie-Riggs hand microtome. Slices of tissue or pieces of hemidiaphragm
were placed in an oxygenated Krebs-Ringer phosphate solution which
contained amoxapine at a concentration of 3 mM. The tissues were
incubated for 60 min at $37^{o}C$. Aliquots of the incubation media were
analysed for the level of activity of one or both of the marker enzymes.
In one set of experiments, the time course of the myolytic effects of
electroshock alone was examined in vivo. Rats were shocked as described
above, and sacrificed at various times up to 24 hours. Samples of blood
were drawn at the time of sacrifice to determine the activity of creatine
phosphokinase.

RESULTS

Figure 1 shows the results of coupling acidosis with a seizure and a high
(but sub-seizure-producing - SSP) dose of amoxapine on the development of
renal impairment in the rat. The data indicate that when acidosis is
present, the administration of amoxapine at an SSP dose in conjunction
with an induced seizure, results in a significant ($p < 0.05$) increase in
the concentration of creatinine in plasma at 24 hr. The effect of giving
a high dose of amoxapine as well as an induced seizure, but without
acidosis, was associated with a plasma concentration of creatinine which
was no different than that of control animals ($p > 0.05$). Because
seizure-associated myolysis could conceivably be construed as a source of
the elevated level of plasma creatinine in the experiments depicted in
Figure 1, we examined the effect of a shock-induced seizure on the
temporal concentrations of creatine phosphokinase in plasma for 24 hr
after the seizure. Figure 2, indicates that the level of CPK rises
significantly ($p < 0.05$) to a maximum within 15 min of the time of seizure
and returns essentially to normal by 8 hours. At eight, 16 and 24 hr
after the seizure, the values for CPK concentration in plasma were not
significantly different ($p > 0.05$) from that of the control group. Using
release of CPK as an index of myolysis in vivo, we tested the effect(s) of
acidosis on the development of rhabdomyolysis in response to amoxapine and
electroshock. The results are shown in Figure 3. Acidosis produced a
statistically significant diminution ($p < 0.05$) of the release of creatine
phosphokinase. However, the plasma levels of creatine phosphokinase were
still 2-3 times greater ($p < 0.05$) than those in subjects of the control
group. To examine the possibility that amoxapine might have some direct
cytolytic effect on muscle tissue, independent of seizures, we assessed
the consequences of incubating pieces of rat diaphragm in oxygenated Krebs
phosphate buffer solution at pH 7.4. As may be noted in the left hand
panel of Figure 4, amoxapine caused a dramatic and significant ($p < 0.05$)
rise in the release of creatine phosphokinase. To ascertain that the
effect was not peculiar to either the drug or the kinase, we tested the
drug under similar conditions, but measured the release of another
cytolytic marker enzyme, lactic dehydrogenase. The right panel of Figure
4, demonstrates a large and significant ($p < 0.05$) release of lactic
dehydrogenase, similar to that seen with creatine phosphokinase. To find
out whether the effect of amoxapine on the release of creatine
phosphokinase from muscle was unique to that tissue, the drug was also
examined for cytolytic activity using isolated, surviving slices of brain
and heart. The release of creatine phosphokinase during incubation in
vitro, as shown in Figure 5, was not significantly ($p > 0.05$) different
from that in control, incubations with addition of isotonic saline.
These data indicate that the direct cytolytic effects of amoxapine are

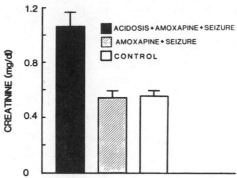

Figure 1. Effect of acidosis on plasma creatinine at 24 hr in rats exposed to amoxapine and seizure. Bars = mean ± SE, n = 6

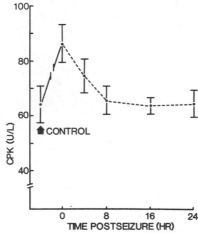

Figure 2. Effect of seizures on the release of creatine phosphokinase (CPK) in the rat with time. Points = mean ± SE, n = 6

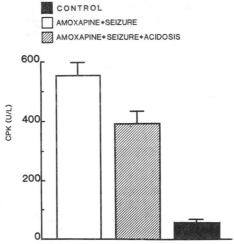

Figure 3. Effect of acidosis on the release of creatine phosphokinase (CPK) in rats exposed to seizure and amoxapine. Bars = mean ± SE, n = 6

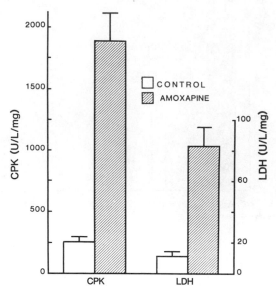

Figure 4. Effect of amoxapine in vitro on release of creatine phosphokinase (CPK) and lactic dehydrogenase (LDH) from muscle. Bars = mean + SE, n = 6

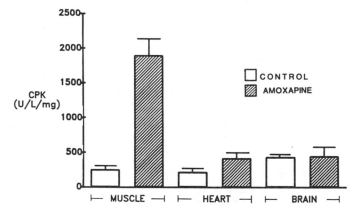

Figure 5. Effect of amoxapine on release of creatine phosphokinase (CPK) from various tissues in vitro. Bars = mean + SE, n = 6

limited to skeletal muscle among the tissues tested.

DISCUSSION

Amoxapine, has received special attention in the last several years due to its reported propensity to produce siezures and in some overdose patients, acute renal failure (abreo et al, 1982: Thompson and Dempsey, 1983: Jennings et al, 1983; Pumariega et al. 1983; Chu et al, 1985; Frendin and Swainson, 1985). In evaluating a series of approximately 100 amoxapine-overdosed patients, Jennings et al (1983) reported that renal failure developed in only 10-15%. Because renal failure does not occur uniformly following amoxapine overdose, we wondered what factor(s) controlled its expression. Data from the reports of renal failure above and those of Goldberg and Spector (1982); Shepard (1983); and Rogol et al (1984) suggest that amoxapine's major high dose effects include seizures, rhabdomyolysis, myoglobinuria and acidosis. However, the factors which are required to precipitate deterioration of renal function in association with amoxapine overdose are unclear. Two significant questions about amoxapine-associated renal impairment are:-

1) can amoxapine directly injure muscle tissue and
2) is acidosis essential in the development of amoxapine-associated acute renal failure.

This study suggests that no renal impairment occurs secondary to high doses of amoxapine associated with seizures unless acidosis is present. These data require further confirmation of the effects of acidosis using a more direct method of assessment of glomerular filtration rate. Nevertheless, there is good reason to believe that acidosis may exert its apparent deleterious effects through its influence on the formation of ferrihaemate from myoglobin (Honda, 1983). While myoglobin is relatively non-nephrotoxic, it may become highly toxic when dehydration, acidemia, or both coexist (Perri and Gorini 1952; Lalich, 1952; Garcia et al, 1981). These reports indicate that aciduria is a prerequisite for myoglobin nephrotoxicity and, that dehydration and a concentrated urine potentiate the nephrotoxic effect of myoglobin in the presence of an acid urine. At a urine pH of 5.6 or less, myoglobin produces ferrihaemate (Bunn and Jandl, 1966). With exertion-related muscle injury and myoglobinuria, ferrihaemate may precipitate from concentrated, acidic urine and thus impair renal function (Knochel, 1981). Blachar et al, (1981) showed that intravenous administration of muscle extracts decreases systemic blood pressure and glomerular filtration rate. Garcia et al (1981) showed that intravenous infusion of myoglobin in rats produces an early, consistent fall in glomerular filtration rate under a variety of conditions. These workers also noted that intratubular cast formation was increased by a low urinary pH, an observation consistent with the possibility that ferrihaemate may be a mediator of myoglobinuric acute renal failure. Anderson et al (1942) demonstrated that ferrihaemate given intravenously can produce a variety of changes including dilatation, haemorrhage, and microthrombi in small vessels, and cellular infiltration, proliferation, and fibrin deposition in glomeruli. Since the addition of acidosis to high dosage amoxapine plus a seizure, produced evidence of renal impairment (Figure 1), as well as evidence of rhabdomyolysis (Figure 2), the deterioration of renal function might have resulted from the release of myoglobin and the subsequent formation ferrihaemate.

The present work also shows that acidosis produced a small but significant reduction in the degree of rhabdomyolysis in response to a seizure caused by a high dose of amoxapine. If the rhabdomyolysis that results from a seizure plus a high dose of amoxapine, occurs secondary to the seizure per se, acidosis may reduce the sensitivity of the central nervous system to a given level of electroshock. An alternate possibility would be a reduced level of development of rhabdomyolysis in the presence of acidosis, assuming that a direct injury to muscle is caused by amoxapine. To whatever extent the rhabdomyolysis demonstrated in figure 3 is due to a direct myolytic effect of amoxapine, the mitigating effect of acidosis could be due to a diminished amount of the nonionic species of amoxapine diffusing into muscle. Amoxapine with a pKa of 7.7 (personal communication, Dr. Morrison, Lederle Laboratories) would certainly be amenable to pH-induced shifts in the amounts of the nonionic species present when the pH of blood changes for example from 7.4 to 6.8 however, it should be appreciated that the degree of myolysis which occurs even in the presence of acidosis may still be sufficient to account for the release of sufficient amounts of myoglobin that could in turn lead to ferrihaemate formation in quantities adequate to explain the nephrotoxic effects brain tissue with in vitro testing. These data are consistent with the possibility that amoxapine's effects on renal impairment may be mediated in part by direct drug-induced injury to muscle as well as that which occurs secondary to seizure activity.

In summary, in vivo studies with the antidepressant, amoxapine, have shown that amoxapine at a high dose combined with a shock-induced seizure is insufficient to produce renal impairment in the rat. When acidosis was superimposed on the above conditions, an elevation of serum creatinine was observed. In vitro studies with amoxapine showed that the drug had significant cyolytic effects on isolated rat diaphragm, but only modest effects on heart and brain tissue. It is suggested that the nephrotoxic effects of amoxapine when observed, may be mediated by direct and indirect release of myoglobin which in the presence of acidosis can lead to renal impairment.

ACKNOWLEDGEMENTS

To Sandra L. Schultz for technical assistance and support, in part, by NIH grant 1 R15 AM36713-01.

REFERENCES

Abreo, A., Shelp, W.D., Kosseff, A., L Thomas, S.; Amoxapine-associated rhabdomyolysis and acute renal failure: case report, J Clin Psy 14:213 (1982).

Anderson, W. A. D., Morrison, D.B., Williams, E.F.; Pathologic changes following injections of ferrihemate (hematin) in dogs. Arch Pathol 33:589-602 (1942).

Blachar, Y., Fong, J.S., De Chadarevian, J.P., Drummnd, K.N.; Muscle extract infusion in rabbits: A new experimental model of the crush syndrome. Circ Res 49:114-24 (1981).

Bunn, H.F., Jandl, J.H.; Exchange of heme among hemoglobin molecules. Proc Natl Acad Sci USA 56:974-8 (1966).

Chu, C., Wadle, C.V., Ruedrich, S.L.; Amoxapine-associated acute renal failure. So Med J, 78:761 (1985).

Frendin, T.J., Swainson, C.P.; Acute renal failure secondary to non-traumatic rhabdomyolysis following amoxapine overdose. New Zeal Med J 98:690-1 (1985).

Garcia, G., Snider, T., Feldman, C., Clyne, D.; Nephrotoxicity of myoglobin in the rat: Relative importance of urine pH and prior dehydration, Kidney Int (Abstract) 19:200 (1981).

Goldberg, M.J., Spector, R.; Amoxapine overdose: Report of two patients with severe neurologic damage. Ann Int Med 96:463-4 (1982).

Honda, N.; Acute renal failure and rhabdomyolysis. Kidney Int 23:888-98 (1983).

Jennings, A., Levey, A., Harrington, J.; Amoxapine-associated acute renal failure. Arch Int Med 143:1525-27 (1983).

Knochel, J.P.; Rhabdomyolysis and myoglobinuria, In: "The Kidney in Systemic Disease" (2nd ed.) Suki, W.N., Eknoyan, G., eds., John Wiley & Sons, New York:

Lalich, J.J.; The influence of in vitro hemoglobin modification on hemoglobin-uric nephrosis in rabbits. J Lab Clin Med 40:102-10 (1952).

Perri, G.C., Gorini, P.: Uremia in the rabbit after injection of crystalline myoglobin. Br J Exp Pathol 33:440-44 (1952).

Pumariega, A.J., Muller, B., Rivers-Bulkeley, N.; Acute renal failure secondary to amoxapine overdose. JAMA 248:3141:42 (1982).

Rogol, A.D., Schoumacher, R., Spyker, D.A.; Generalized convulsions as the presenting sign of amoxapine intoxication. Clin Ped 23:235-37 (1984).

Shepard, F.M.; Amoxapine intoxication in an infant: Seizures arrested with diazepam. So Med J 76:543-44 (1983);

Thompson, M., Dempsey, W.; Hyperuricemia, renal failure, and elevated creatine phosphokinase after amoxapine overdose. Clin Pharm 2:579-81 (1983).

MECHANISMS OF CYCLOSPORIN A NEPHROTOXICITY - RAT TO MAN

Hans Dieperink, Henrik Starklint, Ejvind Kemp and Paul Peter Leyssac

Laboratory of Nephropathology, Odense University Hospital, DK 5000 Odense C, Denmark

INTRODUCTION

Cyclosporin A (CyA) is a cyclical undecapeptide of fungal origin (1-4), and has been used as an immunosuppressive agent in clinical medicine since 1978 (5,6), where it has been of prime importance in the improvement of organ transplantation results. CyA's future role in the treatment of autoimmune disease is now subject to intensive studies. However, the nephrotoxicity of the drug is a major obstacle to its successful use.

FIRST SUSPICION OF NEPHROTOXICITY

The possibility that CyA might decrease renal function was first suggested from clinical studies by Calne (5) and Powles (6). Information concerning CyA-nephrotoxicity in preclinical experiments had not been available: "An unexpected side effect of CyA encountered in clinical practice was nephro-toxicity" (7), which was not noticed in the preclinical animal studies (8,9). Workers at Sandoz (10) did however subsequently report predictive nephrotoxicity such as vacuolation, necrosis and regeneration of proximal tubule cells in rats given high doses of CyA. According to a more compre-hensive toxicology reports (11), rats given CyA had slightly increased serum urea and creatinine in addition to structural proximal tubular damage. These preclinical toxicology data were submitted to the Danish Health Autority in 1981 (12). However, the suggestion that CyA was nephro-toxic was initially not widely accepted because the clinical studies were without appropriate control groups, and nephrotoxicity in laboratory animals was seen only after huge doses. The first irrefutable evidence was the demonstration of decreased inulin clearance in rats given low or moderate doses of CyA (13,14).

Since then, the mechanism of CyA nephrotoxicity has been intensively investigated and it may now be one of the best described toxic nephro-pathies. This survey will extract the information available concerning the causal relationship between CyA administration and renal damage.

THE EFFECT OF CYA ON RENAL FUNCTION

Several observations favours a theory according to which a haemo-dynamic response is of the first importance: immediately following intravenous CyA-infusion, renal vascular resistance increased (15,16), renal blood and

plasma flow decreased (17), GFR declined and proximal fractional reabsorption (PFR) increased (17). The decrease in renal perfusion and filtration
was avoided when the animal was pre-treated with phenoxybenzamine (15).
After 14 days on CyA, rat GFR and end proximal delivery, as measured by
lithium clearance (CLi), was decreased, while PFR increased (14,17-22).
The increase in PFR (14,17) could not be explained by tubular obstruction
because CyA had decreased proximal intratubular pressure (17), and was
therefore concluded to be secondary to a reduced ultrafiltration. It was
speculated (14) whether reduced net ultrafiltration pressure or/and
decreased glomerular surface and permeability (K_f) was the prime reason.

Interestingly enough, CyA has the same effect on the renal function of
humans and rats. Patients given CyA in the treatment of extrarenal disease
(23) had reduced GFR and CLi, while PFR was increased. Also indicative of
a glomerular or haemodynamic impairment, short-term (2 weeks) CyA nephrotoxicity was reduced by a vasoactive drug, nifedipine (20). Renal
denervation (15) and prazosin (24) ameliorated the decrease in GFR and
renal blood flow. Increased renal vascular resistance of kidneys transplanted to patients immunosuppressed with CyA was recently demonstrated.
Thus, indirect evidence has favoured a primary vascular effect. Furthermore, scanning electron microscopy showed CyA-induced constriction of the
afferent glomerular arteriole (25), and CyA induces contraction in other
vascular beds (26).

Thus, the best preliminary thesis may be that a predominant afferent
arteriolo-constriction reduces the effective ultrafiltration pressure.
According to recent data from the Schor (published in this proceedings),
'chronic' CyA treatment reduced intraglomerular capillary pressure due to
an predominant increase in afferent arteriolar pressure. Also efferent
resistance was increased, but as it is known that CyA has a direct vasoconstrictory effect on extrarenal vessels too, this was no surprise. Myers
(27) showed a trend toward restricted transglomerular transport of neutral
various-sized dextrans in CyA-treated heart-transplanted patients, pleaded
for the case of an effect on K_f. However, in these human experiments there
was no statistical significant difference, and crucial parameters of
nephron function (such as glomerular transmembrane hydraulic pressure
difference) were unknown factors assumed to be constants. Schurek (28)
studied the recovery of kidney function in single kidneys after unilateral
nephrectomy, and found that the effective hydraulic permeability of the
glomerular membrane (nl/s mmHg mm^2) increased by almost 40% whether CyA
was given or not, while a small increase of the glomerular capillary
surface was suppressed under CyA. However, very little is know of the
mechanisms by which glomerular surface is increased following reduction of
the total renal mass. It is possible that kidneys with a lower blood flow
due to vasoconstriction will not adapt the glomerular capillary surface as
much as kidneys with normal haemodynamics.

The nephrotoxicity of CyA may partly be due to or involve changes in the
nervous system. Siegl (29) observed tremor, dysesthesia, tachycardia,
hyperglycemia, elevated blood pressure, increased plasma renin activity,
and sodium and potassium retention in spontaneous hypertensive rats given
CyA. They introduced the theory that CyA stimulated the sympathetic
nervous system, and thereby initiated increased activity of renin, angiotensin and aldosterone. Murray (15,24) confirmed the importance of the
sympathetic nervous system, as renal denervation of rats prior to CyA
ameliorated the increased renal vascular resistance and decreased blood
flow observed concomitantly in the innervated contralateral They found
also that the alpha-adrenergic antagonists phenoxybenzamine and prazosin
were able to ameliorate renal blood flow and GFR. Dieperink et al (17)
were unable to confirm this effect of phenoxybenzamine, but these results
were obtained in a slightly different model and did not refute the con-

clusions of Murray. Moss (30) has confirmed the finding that denervated kidneys are protected from the decrease in GFR observed in innervated kidneys after CyA-infusion. They measured the effect of acute intravenous infusion of CyA on efferent genitofemoral and efferent and afferent renal nerve activity, in anesthetized rats. CyA increased efferent nerve activity in both nerves studied, suggesting a generalized sympathetic activation. Afferent activity was increased from denervated kidneys. Thus, the increase in general afferent nerve activity was caused in part by a direct CyA effect. Furthermore, salt excretion from innervated kidneys was decreased by CyA infusion, while in contrast denervated kidneys excreted more. The authors interpreted this finding as a compensatory mechanism that maintained sodium balance during salt retention by the innervated kidney. The main finding of this study, increased sympathetic nerve activity linked to decreased GFR and decreased absolute and fractional salt excretion of innervated kidneys, was consistent with observations of increased PFR. Increased nerve activity, without changes in renal blood flow or GFR, increased proximal tubular reabsorption and decreased sodium clearance (31).

The transplanted kidney is denervated, which, according to these data, to some extent should protect from the nephrotoxic effects of CyA. However, according to clinical data transplanted kidneys are rather liable to the nephrotoxicity. This discrepancy may be due to an increased sensitivity of the denervated organ to non-nervous stimulation (30).

CHANGES IN RENAL STRUCTURE.

The changes in renal function may be linked to the later development of renal structural damage. Direct observations on the kidney surface of rats given CyA for short periods of time showed that they look very much like what is seen during acute partial suprarenal aortic constriction (17,32): nephron heterogeneity with focal groups of partially or totally collapsed proximal convolutions, proximal tubular transit time on average being markedly increased, and in a minority of the proximal tubules complete cessation of fluid flow is apparent. After several weeks of CyA treatment, focal retracted areas, as scattered pinpricks, can be seen with the naked eye on the kidney surface (33). Histologically these pinpricks corresponded to triangular areas of subcapsular fibrosis with the bases formed by the renal capsule. In relation to the subcapsular fibrosis some collapsed, basophilic tubules were seen with degenerating tubular epithelium and thickening of the basement membrane. In some cases, the fibrosis was more widespread and extended towards the medullary area as 'striped' interstitial fibrosis.

Humans also develop focal interstitial fibrosis. Palestine (34) obtained biopsy specimens from 17 patients who had been treated for autoimmune uveitis with CyA, and for comparison analyzed biopsies from patients with idiopathic haematuria, selected to match the CyA-treated patients in terms of sex and age. The CyA-patients had all striped interstitial fibrosis, usually associated with tubular atrophy. Fifteen patients had, in addition, thickened arterioles, with interstitial swelling or hyaline change. There was a inverse linear relation between GFR at the time of biopsy and the severity of the lesions. Klintmalm (35) studied the effect of prolonged CyA treatment on renal transplant morphology. A total of 38 biopsies were performed on 28 patients at 1,2,3 or 4 years after transplantation, at a time of stable renal function. Only 2 out of a total of 8 biopsies taken at the time of transplantation showed slight interstitial fibrosis, while 27 of the 28 patients had interstitial fibrosis (focal or diffuse) after 1 to 4 years on CyA. Atrophic changes of the tubules were always found in areas with interstitial fibrosis. Dose-dependent progression of renal interstitial fibrosis was indicated by increased severity of fibrosis in patients who had received more than 1800 mg/kg of CyA during the first 6 months after transplantation. Bergstrand (36) reviewed 90 kidney transplant biopsies, 55 of which were from patients immunosuppressed with CyA. This material was presumably identical to the one presented by Mihatsch (37). The selection of the biopsies was biased, firstly because they were choosen by the participants for inclusion in the material. A number of specified parameters were used for the evaluation. In each case, the pathologist also included a judgement of therapy group. Thirty-six out of a total of 55 CyA-biopsies were correctly diagnosed, while 23 out ot a total of 35 biopsies from azathioprine-immunosuppressed patients were correctly diagnosed. A chi-square test implemented on the above mentioned data shows that the evaluation based on the pre-fixed criteria had allowed the authors to reject the null-hypothesis that there was no difference whether or not CyA had been given (chi-square = 7.14, P < 0.01, not included in the report). The retrospective comparison of relative frequencies of the pre-specified parameters showed convincingly that none of them were specific to CyA-treated patients. However, if claiming that for the individual parameter there should be a 10% frequency difference between the groups in order to declare the parameter as "typical" to either CyA- or azathioprine-immunosuppressed patients, striped interstitial fibrosis was typical to CyA (29.7 vs. 17.7%, P < 0.007), while interstitial blood extravasation (21.2 vs 4.5 %, P < 0.003) and diffuse interstitial cell infiltrate (49.2 vs. 35.2 %, P < 0.02) were typical to azathioprine. It was claimed that the interstitial fibrosis was especially diagnosed in patients given CyA in excess of 100 days. However, it may seem peculiar that less than 30% of the patients given CyA developed the 'typical' CyA-lesion, but it should be noted that in the animal studies it was found that the CyA-induced changes were to be found especially in the subcapsular cortex, which is usually not represented in biopsy specimens.

COMPARATIVE PHYSIOLOGY AND MORPHOLOGY

Considering the initial confusion with regard to the nephrotoxic effect of CyA, it may seem surprising that the results from the recent studies cited above suggest that the renal functional and histopathological changes can be explained by one hypothesis, as concluded below. Evidently, other mechanisms may be involved too. CyA has a direct vasoconstrictory effect, and increases the vascular sensitivity to other stimulation. This results in a (mainly) preglomerular vasoconstriction, and net ultrafiltration pressure decreases. Proximal fractional reabsorption increases, and tubular flow rates and end proximal delivery decreases. Due to nephron heterogeneity there is varying tubular hypoperfusion, and focal tubular collapse. These collapsed tubules degenerates, as does the tubular basal membrane, while peritubular interstitial fibrosis develops. In more severe cases, with adjoining changes in groups of nephrons, the fibrosis proceeds to focal subcapsular or 'striped' interstitial fibrosis. While the vaso-constriction is reversible after drug withdrawal, the interstitial fibrosis persists. However, in the available studies with restricted observation periods, even in more severe cases only a low percentage of the nephrons are lost. Therefore, one of the main problems to be solved in the future is whether continued CyA administration may ultimately result in renal failure.

REFERENCES

1. J.F. Borel, C. Feurer, H.U. Gubler and H. Stahelin, Biological effects of cyclosporin A: A new antilymphocytic agent, _Agents Actions_, 6:468 (1976).

2. H. Dreyfuss, E. Harri, H. Hofmann, H. Kobel, W. Pache, and H.

Tscherter, Cyclosporin A and C, <u>Eur J Appl Microbiol</u>, 3:125 (1976).

3. T.J. Petcher, H.P. Weber, and A. Ruegger, Crystal and molecular structure of an iodo-derivate of the cyclic undecapeptide cyclosporin A, <u>Helv chim Acta</u>, 59: 1480 (1976).

4. K. Hillier, Cyclosporin A, <u>Drugs Future</u>, 4:567 (1979).

5. R.Y. Calne, D.J.G. White, S. Thiru, D.B. Evans, P. McMaster, D.C. Dunn, G.N. Craddock, B.D. Pentlow, and K. Rolles, Cyclosporin A in patients receiving renal allografts from cadaver donors, <u>Lancet</u>, 2:1323 (1978).

6. R.L. Powles, A.J. Barrett, H. Clink, H. E. M. Kay, J. Sloane, and T.J. McElwain, Cyclosporin A for the treatment of graft-versus-host disease in man, <u>Lancet</u>, 2:1327 (1978).

7. R.Y. Calne, Cyclosporin, <u>Nephron</u>, 26:57 (1980).

8. A.J. Kostakis, D.J.G. White, and R.Y. Calne, Toxic effects in the use of cyclosporin A in alcoholic solution as an immunosuppressant of rat heart allografts, <u>IRCS surgery transplantation</u>, 5:243 (1977).

9. R.Y. Calne, D.J.G. White, K. Rolles, D.P. Smith and B.M. Herbertson, Prolonged survival of pig orthotopic heart grafts treated with cyclosporin A: <u>Lancet</u>, 1:1183 (1978).

10. B. Ryffel, Experimental toxicological studies wiyh cyclosporin A, <u>In:</u> "Cyclosporin A", D.J.G. White, ed., Elsevier, Amsterdam (1982).

11. B. Ryffel, P. Donatsch, M. Madorin, B.E. Matter, G. Ruttiman, H. Schon, R. Stoll, and J. Wilson, Toxicological evaluation of cyclosporin A, <u>Arch Toxicol</u>, 53:107 (1983).

12. B. Ryffel, OL 27-400 summary of toxicity data, Sandoz Ltd, Basle, Switzerland (1981).

13. A.S. Tonnesen, R.W. Hamner, and E.J. Weinmann, Cyclosporine and sodium and potassium excretion in the rat, <u>Transplant Proc</u>, 15, suppl.1:2730 (1983).

14. H. Dieperink, H. Starklint, P.P. Leyssac, Nephrotoxicity of cyclosporin A - an animal model. A study of the nephrotoxic effect of cyclosporin on overall renal and tubular function in conscious rats, <u>Transplant Proc</u>, 15, suppl.1:2736 (1973).

15. B.M. Murray, M.S. Paller, and T.F. Ferris, Effect of cyclosporine administration on renal hemodynamics in conscious rats, <u>Kidney Int</u>, 28:767 (1985).

16. B.A. Sullivan, L.J. Hak, and W. F. Finn, Cyclosporine nephrotoxicity: studies in laboratory animals, <u>Transplant Proc</u>, 14, suppl.1:145 (1985).

17. H.H. Dieperink, P.P. Leyssac, H. Starklint, E. Kemp, Nephrotoxicity of cyclosporin A. A lithium-clearance and micropuncture study in rats, <u>Eur J Clin Invest</u>, 16:69 (1986).

18. H. Dieperink, P.P. Leyssac, E. Kemp, D. Steinbruchel, H. Starklint, Glomerulotubular function in cyclosporine A treated rats, <u>Clin Nephrol</u>, 25, suppl.1:S70 (1986).

19. H. Dieperink, E. Kemp, P.P. Leyssac, H. Starklint, M. Wanscher, J.

Nielsen, K.A. Jorgensen, V. Faber, and H. Flachs. Ketoconazole and cyclo-sporine A: combined effects on rat renal function and on serum and tissue cyclosporine A concentration, Clin Nephrol, 25, suppl.1:S137 (1986).

20. H. Dieperink, P.P. Leyssac, H. Starklint, K.A. Jorgensen, and E. Kemp, Antagonist capacities of nifedipine, captopril, phenoxybenzamine, prostacyclin and indomethacin on cyclosporin A induced impairment of rat renal function, Eur J Clin Invest, 16:540 (1986).

21. H. Dieperink, P.P. Leyssac, H. Starklint, and E. Kemp, Glomerulo-tubular function in cyclosporin A treated rats. A lithium clearance, occlusion time/transit time and micropuncture study, Proc Eur Dial Trans Assoc, 21:853 (1985).

22. H.H. Dieperink, P.P. Leyssac, H. Starklint, E. Kemp, Effects of cyclo-sporin A, gentamicin and furosemide on rat renal function. A lithium clearance study, Clin Exp Pharm Toxicol, in the press.

23. H. Dieperink, P.P. Leyssac, E. Kemp, H. Starklint, N. E. Frandsen, N. Tvede, J. Moller, P. Buchler Frederiksen, N. Rossing, The nephrotoxicity of cyclosporin A in humans. Effects on glomerular filtration and tubular reabsorption rates, Eur J Clin Invest, in the press.

24. B.M. Murray, and M.S. Paller, Beneficial effects of renal denervation and prazosin on GFR and renal blood flow after cyclosporine in rats, Clin Nephrol: 25, suppl.1:S37 (1986).

25. J. English, A. Evan, D. Houghton, and W.M. Bennett, Experimental cyclosporine (CSA) nephrotoxicity: evidence for renal vasoconstriction with preservation of tubular function, Clin Res, 34:594A (1986).

26. H. Xue, R.D. Bukoski, D.A. McCarron, and W. Bennett, Cyclosporine induces contraction in isolated vascular smooth muscle, Fed Proc, 45:669 (1986).

27. B.D. Myers, J. Ross, L. Newton, J. Luetscher, and M. Perlroth, Cyclo-sporine-associated chronic nephropathy, N Engl J Med, 311:699 (1984).

28. H.J. Schurek, K.H. Neumann, W.P. Jesinghaus, B. Aeikens, and K. Wonigeit, Influence of cyclosporine A on adaptive hypertrophy after unilateral nephrectomy in the rat, Clin Nephrol, 25, suppl.1:S144 (1986).

29. H. Siegl, B. Ryffel, R. Petric, P. Shoemaker, A. Muller, P. Donatsch, and M. Mihatsch, Cyclosporine, the renin-angiotensin-aldosterone system, and renal adverse reactions, Transplant Proc, 15, suppl.1:2719 (1983).

30. N.G. Moss, S.L. Powell, and R.J. Falk, Intravenous cyclosporine activates afferent and efferent renal nerves and causes sodium retention in innervated kidneys in rats, Proc Natl Acad Sci, 82:8822 (1985).

31. U. Abildgaard, N.-H. Holstein-Rathlou, and P.P. Leyssac, Effect of renal nerve activity on tubular sodium and water reabsorption in dog kidneys as determined by the lithium clearance method, Acta Physiol Scand, 126:251 (1986).

32. K.H. Gnutzmann, K. Hering, and H.-U. Gutsche, Effect of cyclosporine on the diluting capacity of the rat kidney, Clin Nephrol, 25, suppl.1:S51 (1986).

33. H. Dieperink, E. Kemp, and H. Starklint, Cyclosporin A in high dosages induces renal interstitial fibrosis in the rat, *Transplant Proc*, in the press.

34. A.G. Palestine, H.A. Austin, J.E. Balon, T.T. Antonovych, S.G. Sabnis, H.G. Preuss, and R.B. Nussenblatt, Renal histopathologic changes in patients treated with cyclosporine for uveitis, *N Engl J Med*, 314:1986.

35. G. Klintmalm, Interstitial fibrosis in renal allografts after 12 to 46 months of cyclosporin treatment beneficial effects of lower doses early after transplantation, *In:* "Cyclosporin A nephrotoxicity in human transplant patients", G. Klintmalm, Huddinge, Sweden, Repro print AB, Stockholm (1984).

36. A. Bergstrand, S.O. Bohman, A. Farnsworth, J.M. Gokel, P.H. Krause, W. Lang, M.J. Mihatsch, B. Oppedal, S. Sell, R. K. Sibley, S. Thiru, R. Verani, A. C. Wallace, H.U. Zollinger, B. Ryffel, G. Thiel, and K. Wonigeit, Renal histopathology in kidney transplant recipients immuno-suppressed with cyclosporin A: results of an international workshop, *Clin Nephrol*, 24:107 (1985).

37. M.J. Mihatsch, A brief review of histopathology in kidney transplant recipients immunosuppressed with cyclosporin A: *Scand J Urol Nephrol*, 92, suppl:95 (1985).

THE EFFECTS OF CYCLOSPORIN A ON THE URINE EXCRETION OF SPECIFIC PROTEINS IN HUMANS

Anne Dawnay, Michael Lucey, Carolyn Thornley, Robert Beetham, Bill Cattell and Roger Williams

Departments of Chemical Pathology and Nephrology, St Bartholomew's Centre for Research, St Bartholomew's Hospital, London EC1A 7BE and The Liver Unit, King's College Hospital, London SE5 8RX, UK

INTRODUCTION

Cyclosporin A (CyA) is widely used as an immunosuppressant following organ transplantation and in the treatment of various autoimmune disorders. A major disadvantage is its nephrotoxicity which is probably of multi-factorial origin, involving acute, reversible haemodynamic changes and irreversible tubulointerstitial injury and focal glomerulosclerosis (Cohen et al, 1984; Klintmalm et al, 1984; Myers et al, 1984; Palestine et al, 1986). There is no satisfactory animal model for CyA nephrotoxicity and its assessment in CyA treated renal transplant recipients is complicated by the coexistence of other renal disorders. For these reasons, we have chosen to study a group of patients being treated with long-term CyA for an autoimmune disorder, primary biliary cirrhosis (PBC).

The monitoring of serum creatinine alone cannot detect subclinical dysfunction and early tubulointerstitial disease, whereas low level albuminuria and tests of renal tubular proteinuria are more sensitive. Therefore we have investigated the effect of CyA on different parts of the nephron using appropriate marker molecules to demonstrate malfunction viz. glomerular (albumin), proximal tubular (ß-2-microglobulin, retinol binding protein, N-acetyl-ß-D-glucosaminidase) and distal tubular (Tamm-Horsfall glycoprotein).

PATIENTS

Ten patients with PBC (1 male, 9 female; mean age 56 years, range 40-68) were treated with 3-4 mg/kg/day CyA for between 19 and 31 months (median 26). All had a normal serum creatinine before treatment. The dose was reduced by 50 or 100 mg/day if serum creatinine rose to greater than 0.17 mmol/L; if trough whole blood CyA levels exceeded 800 ug/L; or if hypertension developed. Results were compared with 18 PBC controls (2 male, 16 female; mean age 51 years, range 39-70). The serum bilirubin was not significantly different ($p > 0.10$) between the CyA (median 25 umol/L, range 12-130) and control (median 39 umol/L, range 5-168) groups. The median trough CyA level was 325 ug/L (range 194-663). One patient on CyA and one control had hypertension at the time of study. The study was approved by the Ethical Committee of King's College Hospital and informed consent obtained from all participants.

METHODS

A blood sample and concurrent random urine were obtained from each patient. Serum and urine were analysed for creatinine, Tamm-Horsfall glycoprotein (THG) as described else where (Dawnay et al, 1980; Dawnay et al, 1982), retinol binding protein (RBP) using the method of (Beetham et al, 1985), ß-2-microglobulin (ß2m) using an unpublished radioimmunoassay method and urine for N-acetyl-ß-D-glucosaminidase (NAG, EC 3.2.1.30) by the technique of (Tucker et al, 1975) and albumin (Silver et al, 1986a). Unless abnormal, urine ß2m results were discarded if the pH was less than 6 (2 CyA, 2 control) based on the degradation of the molecule (Bernard et al, 1982). Reference ranges for these analytes were derived from data on 86 normal subjects (40 male, 46 female; mean age 40 years, range 17-65) with normal serum creatinine, urea and liver function tests. To take account of variations in urine flow rate, urine ß2m, RBP and albumin were expressed as a ratio to urine creatinine (upper limit of reference range 30 and 13 ug/mmol creatinine and 2.8 mg/mmol creatinine respectively). The excretion rates of urine NAG and THG, both of which are synthesised by the kidney, were expressed per mL of creatinine clearance (CCr) to account for variations both in the amount of functioning renal tissue and in urine flow rate (reference ranges $\leq$ 0.8 U/mL Ccr and 0.15-0.50 g/mL Ccr respectively). Other reference ranges: serum creatinine 0.05-0.12 mmol/L; serum THG 90-320 ug/L; serum RBP 29-66 mg/L; serum ß2m 1.0-2.6 mg/L. Trough levels of whole blood CyA were measured by radioimmunoassay using the Sandoz cyclosporin RIA-kit. Non-parametric statistics; the Spearman rank correlation coefficient and the Mann-Whitney U-test for the significance of the difference between groups (Siegel, 1956).

RESULTS

Serum creatinine was significantly higher ($0.02 < P < 0.05$) in the CyA group (median 0.10 mmol/L, range 0.06-0.18) compared with controls (0.07, 0.05-0.12). The patients on CyA had an elevated serum creatinine, one remaining at 0.16 mmol/L in spite of dose reduction and the other being 0.18 mmol/L on the test day.

Serum levels of THG were within the reference range in all patients except one, but were significantly lower ($p < 0.002$) in the CyA treated group (median 111 ug/L, range 37-173) compared with controls (212, 132-304) are shown in Fig. 1. The urine excretion rate of THG (THG/Ccr) was also significantly lower ($0.02 < P < 0.05$) in the CyA group (median 0.33 ug/mL Ccr, range 0.16-0.81) compared with controls (0.49, 0.21-0.88), see Fig. 1. In one CyA treated patient with an elevated serum creatinine and in seven controls, the excretion rate was higher than the reference range. In neither group was there any correlation ($p > 0.1$) between serum creatinine and either serum or urine THG.

The urine excretion rate of NAG (NAG/Ccr) was not significantly different ($p > 0.10$) between the two groups and was elevated in all patients (median 2.5 U/mL Ccr, range 0.9-39).

Quantitative measurement of urine albumin excretion yielded no significant difference between the two groups ($p > 0.10$). One control and one CyA treated patient (the latter having hypertension in spite of reduction in the dose of CyA) had low level albuminuria (14.6 and 4.6 mg/mmol creatinine respectively) not detectable by dipstick. A further, hypertensive patient in the control group had a grossly elevated excretion of 80 mg/mmol creatinine.

There was no significant difference ($p > 0.05$) between the two groups in either the serum levels of ß2m and RBP or in their urine excretion (Table

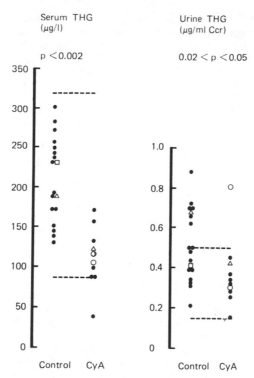

Fig. 1. A comparison of levels of serum and urine THG in control patients with PBC and in CyA treated patients. The dotted lines indicate the limits of the reference ranges. One patient (□) had gross albuminuria, two had low level albuminuria (△) and two had an elevated serum creatinine (○).

1) although the latter tended to be higher in the CyA treated patients with an elevated serum creatinine. These low molecular weight urine proteins and serum ß2m were often elevated while the serum RBP was most commonly reduced. There was no correlation (p > 0.05) between serum and urine levels of either protein in either group.

DISCUSSION

Our results demonstrate considerable abnormalities in markers of both the proximal and distal tubules in patients with PBC. Although tubular abnormalities in the handling of hydrogen ions (McFarlane et al, 1979) and uric acid (Izumi et al, 1983) are recognized in PBC, those described here have not been documented previously. These results will be discussed in more detail elsewhere but serve to demonstrate how necessary it is to use an appropriate control group.

The only significant effects of treatment with CyA were to increase the serum creatinine, a common occurrence found by others (Cohen at al, 1984), and to decrease serum and urine THG, a glycoprotein confined to the thick ascending limb of the loop of Henle and the distal convoluted tubule (Sikri et al, 1981). No significant change was found in urine protein markers of glomerular and proximal tubular segments. In rat models of acute CyA nephrotoxicity, increased excretion of NAG was found (Whiting et

Table 1. A comparison of the urine excretion and serum concentration of ß2m and RBP in control and CyA treated patients. Results are shown as median (range). There was no significant difference between the two groups (all p > 0.05).

	Control	CyA
Urine ß2m (ug/mmol creatinine)	14.6 (6.7-64)	29 (6.8-670)
Urine RBP (ug/mmol creatinine)	10.8 (3,3-63)	22 (7.5-825)
Serum ß2m (mg/L)	3.9 (2.4-6.3)	3.3 (2.0-6.6)
Serum RBP (mg/L)	34 (10.5-55)	51 (16.5-74)

al, 1986). However, such experimental models do not always produce renal dysfunction that is similar to that seen clinically (Bennett and Pulliam, 1983; Thiel, 1986), especially after chronic use of CyA. The elevated levels of serum ß2m in our study are in agreement with previous reports on PBC (Beorchia et al, 1981; Nyberg et al, 1985) and probably originate from increased production by activated T lymphocytes. Immunosuppression with steroids (Beorchia et al, 1981) and D-penicillamine (Nyberg et al, 1985) were found to decrease serum ß2m levels. A similar effect might have been expected with CyA but was not observed when compared with the control group. However, any such decrease may have been masked by the impaired glomerular function in those on CyA which would tend to elevate serum ß2m. The generally low levels of serum RBP in all patients most likely reflects decreased liver synthesis and/or release. This may be due to the liver disease per se or secondary to protein or vitamin A deficiencies (Rask et al, 1980). The lack of correlation between the serum and urine levels of these low molecular weight proteins suggests that their increased urine excretion was not simply due to the increased filtered load exceeding tubular absorptive capacity.

The changes in THG could have several explanations. In a previous study of patients with chronic renal disease (Thornley et al, 1985), a significant reduction in the number of functioning nephrons was shown to decrease serum THG while having a variable effect on the amount excreted into the urine per mL Ccr. However, in the present study, glomerular function was only mildly impaired by CyA and the lack of correlation between serum creatinine and either serum or urine THG suggests that independent mechanisms maybe operating. Also, in a study of renal transplant recipients, the serum THG was lower in those treated with CyA than in those on prednisolone and azathioprine (Avis et al, 1985), although both groups had comparable levels of serum creatinine. In that study, as here, the two groups were more easily separated on the basis of their serum THG levels than on serum creatinine. CyA has been reported to cause significantly greater tubular atrophy in a renal transplant recipients than steroids and azathioprine (Thiru et al, 1983) and, in patients with glomerulonephritis, excretion of urine THG per functioning nephron is significantly lower in those with tubular atrophy than in those with well preserved tubules on biopsy (Thornley et al, 1985). Impaired function of the thick ascending limb of the loop of Henle has been reported in some (Gnutzmann et al, 1986), but not all (Muller-Suur and

Davis, 1986) studies in rats following treatment with CyA and the reduction in serum and urine THG in our patients could be a biochemical manifestation of this. The effects on THG may therefore reflect either a toxic effect of CyA on the kidney tubules or tubular atrophy which may be secondary to arteriolar toxicity (Thiel, 1986).

A pharmacological effect of CyA on THG cannot be ruled out as, apart from the amount of functioning renal tissue, the factors which affect THG synthesis and secretion remain to be elucidated. It has recently been reported that the protein portion of the immunosuppressive glycoprotein uromodulin is identical to THG (Hession et al, 1987) and that this protein binds both recombinant interleukin 1 and tumour necrosis factor and may thereby regulate their activities. The effect of CyA on THG may therefore be specifically linked with its immunosuppressive actions. These principally involve inhibition of T cell proliferation by blocking the production of lymphokines, especially interleukin 2. A secondary consequence of these effects may be reduced interleukin 1 production by macrophages (Wenger, 1986). Whether lymphokines can in any way affect the synthesis and release of THG is unknown but warrants further investigation and would help elucidate the mechanism by which CyA affects THG.

REFERENCES

Avis, P. J. G., Williams, J. D., Salaman, J. R., Asscher, A. W., and Newcombe, R., 1985, Tamm-Horsfall protein concentration in cyclosporin treated renal transplant recipients, Lancet, 1:154.

Beetham, R., Dawnay, A., Landon, J., and Cattell, W., 1985, A radio-immunoassay for retinol binding protein in serum and urine, Clin. Chem., 31:1364.

Bennett, W., and Pulliam, J., 1983, Cyclosporine nephrotoxicity, Ann. Intern. Med., 99:851.

Beorchia, S., Vincent, C., Revillard, J., and Trepo, C., 1981, Elevation of serum beta-2-microglobulin in liver diseases, Clin. Chim. Acta, 109:245.

Bernard, AF Moreau, D., and Lauwerys, R., 1982, Comparison of retinol binding protein and beta-2-microglobulin determination in urine for the early detection of tubular proteinuria, Clin. Chim. Acta, 126:1.

Cohen, D., Loertscher, R., Rubin, M., Tilney, N., Carpenter, C., and Strom, T., 1984, Cyclosporine: a new immunosuppressive agent for organ transplantation, Ann. Intern. Med., 101:667.

Dawnay, A ., McLean, C ., and Cattell, W ., 1980, The development of a radioimmunoassay for Tamm-Horsfall glycoprotein in serum, Biochem. J., 185:679.

Dawnay, A., Thornley, C., and Cattell, W., 1982, An improved radio-immunoassay for urinary Tamm-Horsfall glycoprotein, Biochem. J., 206:461.

Gnutzmann, K., Hering, K., and Gutsche, H-U., 1986, Effect of cyclosporine on the diluting capacity of the rat kidney, Clin. Nephrol., 25(S1):S51.

Hession, C., Decker, J., Sherblom, A., Kumar, S., Yue, C., Mattaliano, R., Tizard, R., Kawashima, E., Schmeissner, U., Heletky, S., Chow, E., Burne, C., ShaW, A., and Muchmore, A,, 1987, Uromodulin (Tamm-Horsfall glyco-protein): A renal ligand for lymphokines, Science, 237:1479.

Izumi, N., Hasumura, Y., and Takeuchi, J., 1983, Hypouricaemia and hyper-uricosuria as expressions of renal tubular damage in primary biliary cirrhosis, Hepatology, 3:719.

Klintmalm, G., Bohman, S., Sundelin, B., and Wilczek, H., 1984, Interstitial fibrosis in renal allografts after 12 to 46 months of cyclosporin treatment, Lancet, 2:950.

McFarlane, I., Tsantoulas, D., Cochrane, A., Eddleston, A., and Williams, R., 1979, Renal tubular acidosis and Tamm-Horsfall glycoprotein, In: "Immune Reactions in Liver Disease", A. Addleston, ed., Pitman, London.

Muller-Suur, R., and Davis, S., 1986, Effect of cyclosporine A on renal electrolyte transport, Clin. Nephrol., 25(S1):S57.

Myers, B., Ross, J., Newton, L., Luetscher, J., and Perlroth, M., 1984, Cyclosporine associated chronic nephropathy, New Engl. J. Med., 311:699.

Nyberg, A., Loof, L., and Hallgren, R., 1985, Serum beta-2-microglobulin levels in primary biliary cirrhosis, Hepatology, 5:282.

Palestine, A., Austin, H., Balow, J., Antonovych, T., Sabnis, S., Preuss, H., and Nussenblatt, R., 1986, Renal histopathologic alterations in patients treated with cyclosporine for uveitis, New Engl. J. Med., 314:1293.

Rask, L., Anundi, H., and Bohme, J., 1980, The retinol binding protein, Scand. J. Clin. Lab. Invest., 40(S154):45.

Siegel, S., 1956, "Non-parametric Statistics for the Behavioural Sciences", McGraw-Hill Kogakusha, Tokyo.

Sikri, K., Foster, C., MacHugh, N., and Marshall, R., 1981, Localisation of Tamm-Horsfall glycoprotein in the human kidney using immunofluorescence and immunoelectronmicroscopical techniques, J. Anat., 132:597.

Silver, A., Dawnay, A., Landon, J., and Cattell, W., 1986, Immunoassays for low concentrations of albumin in urine, Clin. Chem., 32:1303.

Thiel, G., 1986, Experimental cyclosporine A nephrotoxicity: a summary of the International Workshop, Clin. Nephrol., 25(S1):S205.

Thiru, S., Maher, E., Hamilton, D., Evans, D., and Calne, R., 1983, Tubular changes in renal transplant recipients on cyclosporine, Transplant. Proc., 15(S1):2846.

Thornley, C., Dawnay, A., and Cattell, W., 1985, Human Tamm-Horsfall glycoprotein: urinary and plasma levels in normal subjects and patients with renal disease determined by a fully validated radioimmunoassay, Clin. Sci., 68:529.

Tucker, S., Boyd, P., Thompson, A., and Price, R., 1975, Automated assay of N-acetyl-beta-glucosaminidase in normal and pathological human urine, Clin. Chim. Acta, 62:333.

Wenger, R., 1986, Cyclosporine, In: "Progress in Clincal Biochemistry and Medicine", W. Berger, ed., Springer-Verlag, Berlin.

Whiting, P., Thomson, A., and Simpson, J., 1986, Cyclosporine and renal enzyme excretion, Clin. Nephrol., 25(S1):S100.

RENAL TUBULAR FUNCTION IN EXPERIMENTAL AND CLINICAL CYCLOSPORIN (CsA)

NEPHROTOXICITY

P.H. Whiting, D.J. Propper, J.G. Simpson, J. McKay, M.C. Jones and G.R.D. Catto

Departments of Chemical Pathology, Pathology and Medicine, University of Aberdeen, Foresterhill, Aberdeen AB9 2ZD, UK

INTRODUCTION

The use of cyclosporin A (CsA) in both organ transplantation and in the treatment of autoimmune disease may ultimately be limited by the drug's nephrotoxic properties (Klintmalm et al, 1981). Indeed a major clinical problem has been the differentiation of rejection from CsA-induced nephro-toxicity, following renal transplantation. This nephrotoxicity is characterised by impaired renal function and histologically, predominantly by tubular changes (Blair et al, 1982; Thiru et al, 1983). Although the pathogenesis of CsA-induced nephrotoxicity is still unclear, alterations in glomerulotubular function have been demonstrated (Battle et al, 1986; Gnutzman et al, 1986; Dieperink et al, 1986a,b).

The intrarenal control mechanisms regulating glomerular filtration rate (GFR) are triggered by alterations in the constitution of the distal tubular fluid, which depend to a large extent on the functional integrity of the proximal regions of the nephron. Lithium clearance studies may provide a definitive assessment of electrolytes and water handling by the renal tubules as this cation undergoes tubular reabsorption only in the proximal regions of the nephron in amounts equal to that of Na and H_2O (Thomsen, 1984).

This study therefore examines the relationship between lithium clearance rate and the development of CsA-nephrotoxicity in rats given a known toxic dose of the drug. Lithium clearance studies were also conducted in renal allograft recipients treated with CsA.

METHODS

Animal Studies. Groups of male Sprague-Dawley rats (n = 6, initial mean weight 300g) received either CsA (50 mg/kg body weight) or its vehicle (10% ethanol in olive oil) daily by gavage (0.3ml) for 14 days. Although animals were allowed free access to both food and drinking water the latter contained 5 mmolar LiCl from day 1 onwards. Urine free of faecal contamination was obtained from rats kept in individual metabolic cages overnight (16hr). Blood samples, obtained from the tail tip under light ether anaesthesia, on days 0 (pretreatment), 4, 7, 10 and 14, were allowed to clot at $37^{\circ}C$ for 1 hr before serum was expressed by centrifugation. Urine flow rate (ml/h/kg body weight; UFR), glycosuria, NAG (N-acetyl-ß-D-glucosaminidase) enzymuria and trough serum CsA levels (16hr post dose) were measured at the above time points.

Patient Studies. Three groups of patients were studied and their characteristics, renal function and treatment are given in Table 1.

Table 1. Details of the patient groups studied

	GROUP 1	GROUP 2	GROUP 3
Treatment	Normal volunteers	Azathioprine	Cyclosporin A
Sex	11M 9F	6M 4F	8M 2F
Mean age (years)	33 (22-50)	50 (26-65)	49 (15-78)
Mean time since transplant (months)	-	57 (16-114)	10 (3-15)
Mean serum creatinine (umol/l)	84 (67-113)	136 (93-235)	168 (76-400)
Mean prednisolone dose (mg/24 hours)	-	14 (10-20)	16 (5-20)

Range of values given in parentheses.

Measurements and Calculations. Lithium clearance rates were measured as described by Thomsen (1984) using a lithium carbonate dose of 750mg, and creatinine and glucose concentrations and NAG, as described previously (Duncan et al, 1986). Lithium concentrations were measured by flame emission using an IL 943 Flame Photometer (Instrumentation Laboratories Ltd., Marrington, UK). Serum CsA levels were measured by RIA using kits provided by Sandoz Ltd.

Creatinine clearance (CCr) was used as a measure of GFR and lithium clearance (CLi) as an estimate of the delivery of iso-osmotic fluid from the end of the proximal tubule to the loop of Henle. Consequently CCr-CLi reflects the absolute reabsorption of iso-osmotic fluid in the proximal tubule and 1-CLi/CCr (as %) the proximal fractional reabsorption.

The Mann-Whitney U Test and the Student's 't' test were used where appropriate and Pearson Product-Moment tests were used to detect correlations. Regression coefficients were calculated by linear regression analysis and the lines (obtained were compared using Snedecor's F-test. P values of < 0.05 were considered significant.

RESULTS

Animal Studies. The nephrotoxicity associated with CsA administration was characterised by a progressive fall in Ccr, significant from day 4 onwards (Fig. 1), which resulted in a 50% reduction in clearance rates, compared to vehicle treated animals, by day 14. Significant NAG enzymuria was also noted from day 4 onwards and an increased UFR was present on days 10 and 14. Significant glycosuria was noted in 3/6, 3/6 and 5/6 animals on days 7, 10 and 14 respectively (Table 2). Vehicle treatment had no effect on the latter 3 parameters (results not shown). Compared to treatment with vehicle alone, CsA produced significant reductions in CLi at all time points, with a corresponding increase in proximal fractional reabsorption. However, the absolute iso-osmotic proximal tubular reabsorption (CCr-CLi)

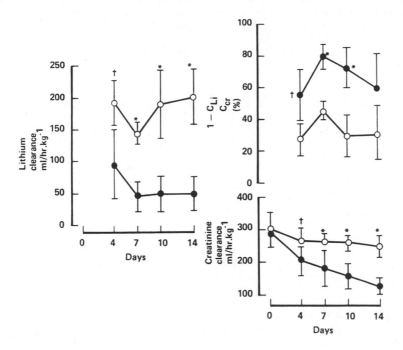

Fig. 1. The effect of CsA on proximal tubule fractional reabsorption (1-CLi/CCr), creatinine and lithium clearance rates. Results are expressed as Mean±1SD with 6 estimations per group. Vehicle (○) and CsA-treated (●) groups were compared; †, $p < 0.05$; **, $p < 0.01$.

was not significantly affected by CsA treatment. Trough serum CsA concentrations on days 4, 7, 10 and 14 were similar at 3.96±1.42, 4.24±0.96, 5.16±1.48 and 4.71±0.86 ug/ml (Mean±1SD) respectively.

Table 2. The effect of CsA on renal function

| | Days Treatment | | | | |
	0	4	7	10	14
UFR	3.32	3.65	3.47	7.03[a]	7.98[a]
	±1.23	±1.95	±3.41	±3.59	±3.72
Glycosuria	0.71	0.81	6.56	13.56	23.28
	±0.10	±0.26	±5.31	±12.70	±21.52
NAG	60	211	221	210	322
	±9	±59	±74	±63	±80
CCr-CLi	NP	109	137	108	72
		±33	±55	±27	±36

Results are expressed as the mean±SD with 6 estimations per group, UFR and clearance rates are expressed as ml/h/kg, while glycosuria and NAG are expressed as mmoles or IU per mmol urinary creatinine respectively. Results compared to Day 0 values; a, $p < 0.05$; b; $p < 0.01$; NP, not performed.

<u>Patient Studies</u>.   Mean CCr was significantly higher in normal volunteers
than in either of the two transplant groups (Table 3).   There was however
no significant difference in CCr between the patients treated with either
azathioprine (Group 2) or CsA (Group 3).   Mean CLi was similar in groups 1
and 2 and significantly higher than in group 3.   Proximal tubular
fractional reabsorption rates were similar in groups 1 and 3 but
significantly lower in group 2.

Table 3.   Renal function in the Patient Groups

Group	CCr	CLi	1-CLi/CCr
Group 1	169	41.0	75.7
(Normal Volunteers)	±16	±6.0	±3.0
Group 2	97	37.0	62.5
(Azathioprine treated)	±28	±13.6	±5.2
Group 3	72	18.0	73.4
(Cyclosporin A-treated)	±30	±10.1	±8.1

p values

1 vs 2	< 0.002	NS	< 0.002
1 vs 3	< 0.002	< 0.002	NS
2 vs 3	NS	< 0.02	< 0.05

The results are expressed as the mean±SD and clearance values are
expressed as ml/min/100kg.   Statistical analysis using the Mann Whitney
U test.   NS: not significant. For further details see text.

A correlation between CLi and CCr for groups 1, 2 and 3 was established
with r values of 0.709 (p < 0.01), 0.926 (p < 0.001) and 0.709 (p < 0.01)
respectively. The linear regression equations were calculated as y = -
0.74+0.25x, y = -3.04+0.41x and y = 3.09+0.19x for groups 1, 2 and 3
respectively. The regression line obtained for group 3 was significantly
different from those obtained for the other two groups (p < 0.05 for
both).   There was however no significant difference between these latter
two groups.

DISCUSSION

The results of the animal study have demonstrated that proximal tubular
dysfunction, as assessed by measurements of lithium clearance rate, occurs
early in the development of CsA-induced nephrotoxicity and is accompanied
by significant reductions in creatinine clearance.   The observation that
urinary NAG activity, an enzyme found predominantly in the proximal
tubule, and glycosuria were increased also supports this view.   Lithium
clearance rate is a measure of the delivery of isoosmotic fluid from the
end of the proximal renal tubule to the loop of Henle (Thomsen, 1984) and
this technique has already provided information regarding tubular function
in CsA-treated animals (Dieperink et al, 1983; 1986a and b). These workers
demonstrated that CsA treatment at doses up to 50 mg/kg caused a reduction
in lithium and inulin clearance rates, and also absolute iso-osmotic
proximal tubular reabsorption with an increased proximal fractional
reabsorption, following treatment for 13 days.   They concluded that CsA
caused a decreased ultrafiltration pressure followed by an inadequate
adaptive reduction in absolute proximal tubular reabsorption.

The results of the present study partially confirm those of Dieperink and
his colleagues. Quantitatively similar alterations in lithium clearance
rate and proximal fractional reabsorption were observed, but absolute iso-

osmotic reabsorption in the proximal tubule remained unchanged and UFR was significantly increased following CsA administration. The reasons for these differences are not clear but may be related to the use of conscious catheterized rats, which had undergone a period of phenobarbital anaesthesia and inulin infusion, by Dieperink and his colleagues, or to a synergistic effect of lithium on CsA-induced tubular dysfunction following its continuous availability in the drinking water in the present study. Furthermore, serum lithium levels did not approach 0.6 mmol/l, the concentration at which both polyuria and tubular functional disturbances were noted by Carney et al (1980), until after day 10 and the renal dysfunction and histological changes observed following CsA has similar to that noted in other recent studies from our laboratory (McAuley et al, 1987a and b).

In contrast to the conclusions of Dieperink and his colleagues, the results presented here are more consistent with the production of a tubulotoxic effect which alters the tubulo-glomerular feedback mechanisms. Each of these processes would heighten the other. An effect on tubular cell "tight junctions" however, cannot be excluded. There is other evidence that CsA exerts a direct effect on the renal tubules. Abnormal diluting ability and H^+ ion handling (Battle et al, 1986; Gnutzman et al, 1986) have been demonstrated and the distal tubular modification of urinary water and electrolyte composition may be important in the development of CsA-induced renal dysfunction (Gerkens et al, 1984; McAuley et al, 1987a and b).

This conclusion is also supported by the results from patients. CsA treated renal allograft recipients demonstrated both reduced lithium clearance rates and also the presence of a different relationship between lithium and creatinine clearance rates compared to either normal volunteers or azathioprine treated patients, which were similar. This infers that CsA treatment produces an altered ionic environment in the proximal tubule which would precipitate an altered tubulo-glomerular feedback response via the distal tubule. It is this alteration in proximal tubular function which may be an appropriate means of detecting and/or confirming the presence of CsA-induced nephrotoxicity.

REFERENCES

Battle, D.C., Gutterman, C.T Tarka, J. and Prasad, R., 1986, Effect of short-term cyclosporine A administration on urinary acidification, Clin. Nephrol., 25 (Suppl. 1):S69.

Blair, J.T.; Thomson, A.W., Whiting, P.H., Davidson, R.J.L., and Simpson, J.G., 1982, Toxicity of the immune suppressant cyclosporine A in the rat, J. Path., 135:163.

Carney, S.L., Wong, N.M.L., and Dirks, J.H., 1980, Effect of lithium treatment on rat renal tubule function, Nephron, 25:293.

Dieperink, H., Kemp, E., Leyssac, P.P. and Starlint, H., 1986a, Cyclosporine A: effectiveness and toxicity in a rat model, Clin. Nephrol., 2S (Suppl. 1):S46.

Dieperink, H., Leyssac, P.P., Kemp, E., Steinbruckl, D. and Starklint, H., 1986b: Glomerulotubular function in cyclosporine A treated rats, Clin. Nephrol., 25 (Suppl. 1):S70.

Dieperink, H., Starklint, H. and Leyssac, P.P., 1983, Nephrotoxicity of cyclosporin - an animal model: study of the nephrotoxic effect of cyclosporine on overall renal and tubular function in conscious rats, Transplant. Proc., 15 (Suppl.1):2736.

Duncan, J. I., Thomson, A.M., Simpson, J.G. and Whiting, P.H.; 1986, Comparative toxicological study of cyclosporine and Nva^2-cyclosporine in Sprague-Dawley rats, Transplantation, 42:395.

Gerkens, J.F., Bhagwandeen, S.B., Dosen, P.J. and Smith, A.J., 1984, The effect of salt intake on cyclosporine-induced impairment of renal function in rats, Transplantation, 38:412.

Gnutzman, K.H., Hering, K. and Gutsche, H.-U., 1986, Effect of short term cyclosporine on the diluting capacity of rat kidney, Clin. Nephrol., 25 (Suppl. 1):S51.

Klintman, G.B.M., Iwatsuki, S. and Starzl, T.E., 1981, Nephrotoxicity of cyclosporine in liver and kidney transplant recipients, Lancet, 1:470.

McAuley, F.T., Simpson, J.G., Thomson A.W. and Whiting, P.H., 1987a, Cyclosporin A-induced nephrotoxicity in the rat: relationship to increased plasma renin activity, Agents Actions, 21:209.

McAuley, F.T., Whiting, P.H., Thomson, A.M. and Simpson, J.G., 1987b; The influence of enalapril or spironolactone on experimental cyclosporin nephrotoxicity, Biochem. Pharmac., 36:699.

Thiru, S., Maher, E.R., Hamilton, D.V., Evans, D.B. and Calne, R.Y., 1983, Tubular changes in renal transplant recipients on cyclosporine, Transplant. Proc., 15 (Suppl. 1):2846.

Thomsen, K., 1984, Lithium clearance: a new method for determining proximal and distal tubular reabsorption of sodium and water, Nephron, 37:217.

296

THE EFFECT OF BILIARY CANNULATION OR LIGATION ON CYCLOSPORIN A (CsA) NEPHROTOXICITY IN THE RAT

S.D. Heys, J.I. Duncan, and P.H. Whiting

Department of Chemical Pathology, University of Aberdeen, Foresterhill, Aberdeen AB9 2ZD7 UK

INTRODUCTION

Although Cyclosporin A (CsA) has become widely accepted as the agent of choice for the control of organ allograft rejection, its attendant nephrotoxicity may still limit its clinical use (Flechner et al, 1983). This property of CsA has, to date, restricted its evaluation as an immunotherapeutic agent in areas of clinical medicine other than transplanation (eg autoimmune disorders). This nephrotoxicity is characterised in both animals and man by a reduction in glomerular filtration rate and by structural damage to the renal proximal tubules (Mihatsch et al, 1985; Blair et al, 1982; Thomson et al, 1984). The pathogenesis of CsA-induced nephrotoxicity, however remains unclear as does the identity of the toxic species, be it parent molecule and/or a metabolite(s).

The major route of CsA metabolism is via the hepatic cytochrome P-450 dependent monooxygenase system (Maurer, 1985; Augustine and Zemaitis, 1986; Moochhala and Renton, 1986) which results in the production of monohydroxy, di-hydroxy and N-demethylated derivatives with preservation of the cyclic oligopeptide structure (Maurer et al, 1984). In addition, metabolite 18 results from an intramolecular cyclisation of metabolite 17 which is hydroxylated at amino acid 1. Furthermore, the major route of excretion of CsA is the bile with > 99% of the total 'CsA content' being made up of metabolites (Maurer et al, 1984), and enterohepatic recycling of CsA and its metabolites is also suspected (Kahan et al, 1983).

Previous studies from our laboratory have indicated that the metabolites of CsA are non-nephrotoxic (Cunningham et al, 1985) and Ryffel and his colleagues (1986) failed to demonstrate any nephrotoxicity when metabolite 17, a major human metabolite, was administered to rats over a period of 14 days.

The aim of this investigation then was to study the development of CsA-nephrotoxicity in animals with either an excess or absence of hepatic-derived CsA metabolites, achieved following either biliary ligation or cannulation respectively.

METHODS

Animals. Adult male Sprague-Dawley rats (initial mean weight 250g), bred in the University Animal Department, were used throughout. The rats, housed under conditions of constant temperature (22°C) with a 12hr lighting cycle were fed Oxoid pasteurised breeding diet and water ad libitum.

Cyclosporin A (CsA). CsA (75mg/kg body weight) or its vehicle (10% ethanol in olive oil) was administered daily to the conscious animal by a single intraperitoneal injection (0.3ml).

Biliary Ligation and Cannulation. The rats were premedicated with 200 units of atropine, given subcutaneously, and anaesthesia induced with 1ml of chloral hydrate (0.5% w/v) administered by intraperitoneal injection. Anaesthesia was maintained by a combination of intraperitoneal chloral hydrate and inhaled diethyl ether as required. The abdomen was opened by a midline incision and the abdominal walls and liver retracted to expose the common bile duct, portal vein and hepatic artery which were lying in the free edge of the lesser omentum running from the porta hepatis to the duodenum. The common bile duct was carefully dissected away from the portal vein and hepatic artery and ligated distally with a 7/0 silk suture (Ethicon Ltd.). This allowed the proximal bile duct to become distended with bile prior to opening the anterior wall with microsurgical scissors. The cannula was then inserted into the bile duct and sutured to its anterior wall again with a 7/0 silk suture. It was then positioned along the posterior abdominal wall before being brought out through the antero-lateral abdominal musculature and then tunnelled subcutaneously to emerge on the dorsum of the rat in the midline. The cannula was carefully positioned so that bile flow was directed away from both the eyes and ears of the animals, the area of skin around the exit site being sprayed with Op-site wound dressing to minimize bile-induced skin irritation. The above technique was also used for biliary ligation except the bile duct was simply ligated and divided between two 7/0 silk sutures without inserting the cannula. The abdominal wound was then closed in one layer (muscle and skin) with a continuous 3/0 vicryl suture, (Ethicon Ltd.).

Protocol. Groups of animals underwent either laparotomy, biliary ligation or biliary cannulation and 24hr later received CsA or its vehicle daily for 4 days; in addition all animals received bile salts (0.25% w/v) in the drinking water. At the end of the study period animals were bled, under ether anaesthesia, by cardiac puncture, following an overnight stay (16hr) in individual metabolic cages. During this period biliary contamination of the urine was avoided by lengthening the cannula and collecting the bile in a seperate container.

Serum indicies reflecting both renal and hepatic function, were measure using a SMAC analyser (Technicon Ltd., Basingstoke, UK) and urine creatinine concentration, creatinine clearance rates and N-acety-ß-D-glucosaminidase (NAG) activity was estimated as described previously (Blair et al, 1982). Whole blood, trough, CsA levels were measured by HPLC using the method described by Annesley et al, (1886).

Statistics. The significance of the differences between group means was determined using the Student's 't' test. A value of $p < 0.05$ was accepted as being statistically significant.

RESULTS

A similar degree of renal dysfunction and NAG enzymuria was noted in those groups of animals that had undergone either laparotomy or biliary ligation and treated with CsA (Table 1). However, animals having undergone biliary cannulation demonstrated reduced renal function and increased NAG enzymuria following CsA treatment compared to the other two groups.

Animals with a biliary cannula which became blocked or ceased to function demonstrated similar biochemical changes to the ligation group.

Table 1. The Effect of Surgical Manipulation on CsA-induced Nephrotoxicity

Group	Urea mmol/l	Creatinine umol/l	Creatinine clearance ml/hr/kg body weight	NAG enzymuria IU/mmol
Laparotomy				
Veh	5.4	40	441	92
(5)	±0.4	±3	±57	±33
CsA	9.3 b	60 b	219 b	215 a
(8)	±2.4	±9	±44	±115
Biliary Ligation				
Veh	5.5	51	274	117
(5)	±0.5	±12	±69	±10
CsA	10.5	57	216	199 b
(5)	±2.9	±3	±34	±39
Biliary Cannulation				
Veh	5.5	43	381	91
(4)1	±0.6	±2	±21	±12
CsA	16.5 *b	152 *b	64 *b	326 *b
(4)	±3.2	±45	±11	±87
Unsuccessful Cannulation				
CsA	9.8	57	231	142
(3)	±1.9	±1	±18	±24

Results are expressed as the mean±SD and the number of animals is given in parentheses.
CsA- and vehicle-treated (Veh) groups compared; a, $p < 0.05$; b, $p < 0.01$.
CsA groups compared; *, $p < 0.01$.

Serum estimates of liver function are shown in Table 2. While total protein levels were reduced following CsA treatment in only the laparotomy group, albumin concentrations were only lowered in the biliary ligation group. The latter group also demonstrated a considerable hyperbilirubin-aemia which was increased by CsA treatment, and higher serum levels of aspartate transaminase. Serum gamma-glutamyl transferase activity was only present in the biliary ligation group. The other two groups demonstrated only a mild hyperbilirubinaemia following CsA treatment. Once again those animals with blocked or non-functional biliary cannulae demonstrated similar biochemistry to the ligation group.

Trough whole blood parent compound CsA concentrations were similar at 4.20±1.19, 5.47±0.91 or 4.71±1.05 mg/l (Mean±SD) in the laparotomy, ligation and cannulation groups respectively.

Table 2. The Effect of Surgical Manipulation on CsA-induced Hepatotoxicity

Group	Total Protein g/l	Albumin g/l	Bili umol/l	AST IU/l	AP IU/l	GGT IU/l
Laparotomy						
Veh (5)	58 ±1	34 ±2	2 ±1	138 ±21	268 ±13	ND
CsA (5)	52 b ±3	33 ±1	10 c ±3	133 ±64	236 ±60	ND
Biliary Ligation						
Veh (5)	56 ±1	29 ±3	204 ±38	552 ±282	483 ±173	70 ±15
CsA (5)	55 ±1	29 * 42	284 b* ±23	937 a* ±391	304 ±46	46 a ±19
Biliary Cannulation						
Veh (5)	58 ±2	34 ±1	2 ±0	122 ±10	287 ±47	ND
CsA (4)	57 ±1	33 ±1	5 a ±2	139 ±42	139 ±31	ND
Unsuccessful Cannulation						
CsA (3)	54 ±2	30 ±2	314 ±39	301 ±87	308 ±55	21 ±7

The results are expressed as the mean±SD and the number of animals is given in parentheses. CsA- and vehicle (Veh)-treated groups compared; a, $p < 0.05$; b, $p < 0.01$; c, $p < 0.001$. CsA-treated groups compared; * $p < 0.01$; ** $p < 0.001$. ND, none determined; Bili; bilirubin; AST, aspartate transaminase; AP; alkaline phosphatase; GGT, gamma-glutamyltransferase.

DISCUSSION

The results of this study demonstrate that biliary cannulation, which would allow the removal of the CsA metabolites in the bile from the body and so prevent any enterohepatic circulation, produced a more severe drug-induced nephrotoxicity than that observed in animals treated with CsA and which had undergone either laparotomy or biliary ligation. For example, the endogenous creatinine clearance rates and NAG enzymuria observed in the cannulation group following CsA treatment were approximately 4-fold decreased or 2-fold increased respectively, compared to observed values in the other two experimental groups.

Biliary ligation would be expected to increase circulating CsA metabolites in the circulation by effectively blocking their major excretory route. Consequently, if any of these metabolites possessed nephrotoxic properties then renal function would have been comparatively worse in the CsA-treated biliary ligated animals compared to the other two drug-treated groups. This was not the case. However, biliary ligation would produce hyper-bilirubinaemia and ultimately hepatocellular damage.

Predictably CsA, a known hepatotoxin, caused an exacerbation of this toxicity as evidenced from the serum concentrations of albumin and bilirubin and the activities of AST and GGT.

Although the HPLC analysis of whole blood samples revealed similar parent CsA concentrations in all treated groups, metabolite levels appeared to be greatly increased in ligated animals, with low levels being observed in the other two groups. However, quantitation and identification of these metabolites was not possible due to the non-availability of pure standards.

One other possible explanation for the exacerbation of CsA-nephrotoxicity following biliary cannulation would the the effect of volume depletion. Approximately 12-15ml of bile were produced daily with a potential loss of both body water and electrolytes. However, the animals in the cannulation groups received 5ml of normal saline twice daily over the experimental period. The mean fractional excretion of sodium in these animals prior to surgery was 0.97% and it fell to 0.69 and 0.77 in the CsA- and vehicle-treated animals, respectively by day 4. The effects of volume depletion can not therefore be totally excluded in these animals.

Biliary cannulation then, by removing non-toxic metabolites, will deplete species that may compete with the parent CsA molecule at the site or sites of toxicity. These may include binding to receptors on cell membranes, organelles or intracellular macromolecules (Hess and Colombani, 1986) enzymes, including for example Phospholipase A2 (Niwa et al, 1986), or the macula densa with the well documented effects on the Renin Angiotensin Aldosterone System (McAuley et al, 1987a and b). However, the results of this study confirm previous results from both this and other laboratories (Cunningham et al, 1984 and 1985; Ryffel et al 1986) that the parent CsA molecule is the nephrotoxic species although the renal or extrahepatic generation of a toxic metabolite(s) cannot be excluded.

REFERENCES

Annesley, I., Matz, K.I Balogh, L. and Clayton, G.D., 1986, Liquid chromatographic analysis for cyclosporine with use of a microcolumn and small sample volume, Clin. Chem., 32:1407.

Augustine, J.A. and Zemaitis, M.A., 1986, The effects of cyclosporine A (CsA) on hepatic microsomal drug metabolism in the rat, Drug Metab. Dispos. 14:73.

Blair, J.T., Thomson, A.W., Whiting, P.H., Davidson, R.J.L. and Simpson, J.G., 1982, Toxicity of the immune suppressant cyclosporine A in the rat, J. Path., 135:163.

Cunningham, C., Burke, M.D., Wheatley, D.N., Thomson, A.W., Simpson, J.G. and Whiting, P.H., 1985, Amelioration of cyclosporine-induced nephro-toxicity in rats by induction of hepatic drug metabolism, Biochem. Pharmac., 34:573.

Cunningham, C., Gavin, M.P., Whiting, P.H., Burke, M.D., McIntyre, F., Thomson, A.W. and Simpson, J.G.: 1984, Serum cyclosporin levels, hepatic drug metabolism and renal tubulotoxicity, Biochem. Pharmac., 33:2857.

Flechner, S.M., Buren, C.V., Kerman, R.H. and Kahan, B.D., 1983, The nephrotoxicity of cyclosporine in renal transplant recipients, Transplant. Proc., 15:2689.

Hess, A.D. and Colombani, P.M., 1986, Mechanism of action of cyclosporine: Role of calmodulin, cyclophilin, and other cyclosporine-binding proteins, Transplant. Proc., 18:219.

Kahan, B.D., Reid, M. and Newburger, J., 1983, Pharmacokinetics of cyclo-sporine in human renal transplantation, Transplant. Proc., 15:446.

Niwa, Y., Kang, T., Taniguchi, S., Miyachi, Y., and Sakane, T., 1986, Effect of cyclosporin A on the membrane associated events in human leukocytes with special reference to the similarity with dexamethasone, Biochem. Pharmac., 35:947.

Maurer, G. T 1985: Metabolism of cyclosporine, Transplant. Proc., 17 (Suppl. 1):19.

Maurer, G., Loosli, H.R., Schreier, E., and Keller, B., 1984, Disposition of cyclosporin in several animal species and man, Drug Metab. Dispos., 12:120.

McAuley, F.T., Simpson, J.G., Thomson, A.W. and Whiting, P.H., 1987a, Cyclosporin A-induced nephrotoxicity in the rat: Relationship to increased plasma renin activity, Agents Actions, 21:209.

McAuley, F.T., Whiting, P.H., Thomson, A.M. and Simpson, J.G., 1987b, The influence.of enalapril or spironolactone on experimental cyclosporin nephrotoxicity, Biochem. Pharmac., 36:699.

Mihatsch, M.J., Thiel, G., Basler, V., Ryffel, B.: Landmann, J., von Overbeck, J., and Zollinger, H.U., 1985, Morphological patterns in cyclo-sporine-treated renal transplant patients, Transplant. Proc., 17 (Suppl. 1):101.

Moochhala, S.M. and Renton, K.M., 1986: Inhibition of hepatic microsomal drug metabolism by the immunosuppressive agent cyclosporin A, Biochem. Pharmac., 35:1499.

Ryffel, B., Hiestand, P., Foxwell, B., Donatsch, P., Boelsterli, H.J., Maurer, G. and Mihatsch, M.J., 1986, Nephrotoxic and immunosuppressive potentials of cyclosporine metabolites in rats, Transplant. Proc., 18 (Suppl. 5):41.

Thomson, A.M., Whiting, P.H. and Simpson, J.G., 1984, Cyclosporine: immunology, toxicity and pharmacology in experimental animals, Agents Actions, 15:306.

Whiting, P.H., Burke, M.D. and Thomson, A.W., 1986, Drug interactions with Cyclosporine: Implications from animal studies, Transplant. Proc., 18 (Suppl. 5):56.

CYCLOSPORINE A-INDUCED LIPID PEROXIDATION IN RAT RENAL MICROSOMES AND EFFECT ON GLUCOSE UPTAKE BY RENAL BRUSH BORDER MEMBRANE VESICLES

G. Inselmann, M. Blank and K. Baumann

Department of Cell Physiology, Institute of Physiology, University of Hamburg, Grindelallee 117, D-2000 Hamburg 13, FRG

INTRODUCTION

Nephrotoxicity is the most important side effect of cyclosporine A (CsA) treatment and has been well documented in patients and experimental animals (1). The nature of CsA-induced renal damage is complex and the precise mechanism is still unclear. Some possible pathogenetic mechanisms have already been investigated. There is convincing evidence that a direct CsA effect on tubular cell could also contribute to CsA nephrotoxicity (2). CsA is taken up by isolated proximal tubule segments in a rapid, time-dependent and saturable manner (3). A saturable binding of CsA to isolated rat renal brush border membranes was also shown. This binding may be best explained by a partitioning process of the lipophilic CsA into the phospholipid phase of the cell membrane rather than binding to a specific membrane component. These findings demonstrate that CsA has the ability to interact with renal tubular cell membranes, even at low concentrations, and therefore has a distinct potential for toxic effects on renal cells. The aim of the present study was to investigate in vitro whether or not CsA induces lipid peroxidation in isolated rat renal microsomes and moreover to evaluate the influence of CsA on glucose uptake by rat renal brush border membrane vesicles. To the best of our knowledge there appeared only one report regarding to CsA-induced nephrotoxicity and lipid peroxidation. In vivo studies (4) have shown that treatment of male Wistar rats with CsA leads to a high levels of malondialdehyde in renal tissue compared to kidneys of non-treated rats. Long-term CsA treatment leads to high blood glucose concentrations and severe glucosuria indicating that CsA possesses a diabetogenic effect which is likely to be responsible for glycogen accumulation in renal tubular cells (5,6).

METHODS

Male Wistar rats were killed by decapitation. The kidneys were removed and subsequently homogenized in a sucrose-Tris buffer for microsome preparation (7,8). Microsomes, about 350 ug protein per ml for each sample of 2 ml medium, were either incubated in a CsA containing medium (1.5 mg/ml) for 0.5, 1, 2 or 3 h or with different CsA concentrations: 0.035, 0.075, 0.15, 0.25, 0.75, 1.5 or 3 mg/ml for 3 h. The incubation buffer was composed as follows: 96.7 mM NaCl, 7.4 mM sodium phosphate buffer, 40 mM KCl, 0.74 mM $CaCl_2$ and 10 mM lactic acid, pH 7.4. The incubations were carried out by using a metabolic shaker at $37^{\circ}C$ in a pure oxygen atmosphere. Control values were obtained by incubating the renal microsomes under the same conditions in the described medium but without CsA. Microsomal lipid peroxidation was monitored by measuring the production of malondialdehyde (MDA) by the thiobarbituric acid assay (9). Inhibition of CsA-induced lipid peroxidation in renal microsomes was investigated using the radical scavenger alpha-tocopherol, final concentration 1 mM (10).

To test the effect of CSA on glucose uptake by renal brush border membrane vesicles, renal cortical slices were incubated for 1 or 3 h in the same medium (11) used for microsomes, at $37^{\circ}C$, pH 7.4 and CsA concentration 1.5 mg/ml. From these incubated renal cortical slices brush border membrane vesicles were prepared by a Mg^{2+} precipitation method (12). Control values were obtained by using the same procedure but without CSA added. To evaluate the quality of the brush border membrane preparation the specific activity of the marker enzymes alkaline phosphatase and Na^+/K^+-stimulated ATPase was measured. Under all experimental conditions we found an enrichment factor of 10.2 for alkaline phosphatase and 1.2 for Na^+/K^+-stimulated ATPase. D-glucose uptake by the brush border membrane vesicles were assesed by equilibrated in a buffered solution by applying an initial sodium or potassium gradient of 100 mM outside, 0 mM inside. To obtain the kinetic data of the sodium-dependent D-glucose uptake various D-glucose concentrations were used in the incubation medium. The uptake of ^3H-labelled D-glucose was measured by using a slightly modified rapid filtration method (13). ^{14}C-labelled L-glucose was also used to measure the passive glucose influx in the presence of an initial potassium gradient of 100 mM. Initial glucose uptake velocities were calculated based on the assumption of first order kinetics. For the active D-glucose influx the values of affinity and maximal velocity and for the passive L-glucose influx the passive influx constants were obtained by least square analysis of the Michaelis-Menten equation and first order kinetic, respectively.

CSA (100 mg CSA/ml Of a 12.6% ethanolic solution, Sandimmun$^{(R)}$ from Sandoz, Basel, Switzerland) was dissolved in the incubation medium by ultrasonication diluting the ethanol to a final concentration of 0.4%. The precipitation of CsA was prevented by a short period of warming. Control experiments were performed by incubating renal microsomes or renal cortical slices under the same experimental conditions in a CsA-free, but the same concentration of ethanol containing medium, respectively.

RESULTS

Incubation of renal microsomes with different cyclosporine concentration for 3 h led to a concentration-dependent production of MDA. At the highest CSA concentration a 7-fold net increase of lipid peroxidation was observed in comparison to control incubations. MDA production raised from 0.73 nmol/mg protein in control incubations to 5.85 nmol/mg protein at the highest CsA concentration (Fig. 1). To optimize the incubation conditions regarding MDA determination higher microsomal protein concentrations were used in preliminary experiments. Up to now MDA production increased significantly at a lower CsA concentration of 3 ug/ml as compared to control incubations (data not shown). When isolated renal microsomes were incubated for different periods of time with CsA (1.5 mg/ml) MDA production increased in a time-dependent manner (data not shown). After a 3 h incubation a net increase of lipid peroxidation products of 200% occurred. The radical scavenger alpha-tocopherol (1 mM) reduced the CsA-induced MDA production for about 50% after 3 h of incubation (data not shown). All experiments were repeated with heat denaturated microsomes production of MDA did not show any significant difference when compared to MDA production in native microsomes.

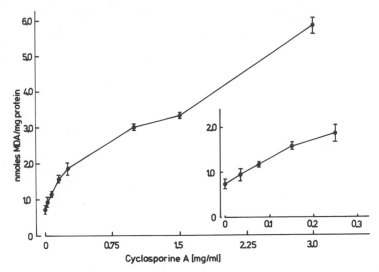

Fig. 1. Cyclosporine A-induced concentration-dependent production of malondialdehyde (MDA) in isolated renal microsomes. Renal microsomes (about 350 ug/1ml protein for each sample of 2 ml) were incubated in a medium with different CsA concentrations for 3 h, at 37°C, pH 7.4, in a pure oxygen atmosphere. All values are significantly different as compared to the control value, within the series all values are significantly different between each other (p < 0.05). Inset: CsA concentration from 0 to 0.25 mg/ml.

The effect of CsA on D-glucose uptake by renal brush border membrane vesicles was assessed in the presence of sodium where the curve of the D-glucose overshoot was almost identical from vesicles prepared from fresh control slices and those prepared after 1 h incubation. Compared to the corresponding control curve the incubation of renal cortical slices with CsA for 1 h depressed the D-glucose overshoot in subsequently prepared brush border membrane vesicles as shown for a typical experiment (Fig. 2, left panel). In the presence of potassium the vesicular passive D-glucose uptake is enhanced after 1 h CsA as compared to 1 h slice incubation without CsA. There was no difference in final steady-state distribution of D-glucose nor maximal L-glucose uptake values after 120 min in membrane preparations from CsA incubated or control slices, indicating that all vesicle preparations possessed the same intravesicular space. The right panel of Fig. 2 summarizes the calculated transport parameters of the active D-glucose uptake and the passive L-glucose uptake by vesicle preparations from 1 and 3 h incubated slices in the absence and presence of CsA. In agreement with the results of the D-glucose experiments in the presence of potassium the influx constants of L-glucose were enhanced after the incubation of slices with CsA as compared to the corresponding control values. The glucose transporter of renal brush border membranes prepared from CsA incubated slices had a lower affinity (higher apparent K_t value) for D-glucose than those from control incubated slices. After incubation of slices with CsA the maximal uptake rates (V_{max}) of D-glucose decreased in comparison to the corresponding control values. The 1 h and 3 h control values of the various transport parameters were not statistically different. Compared to the corresponding control values the extent of change of the various transport parameters was more pronounced after 3 h than after 1 h incubation of slices with CsA.

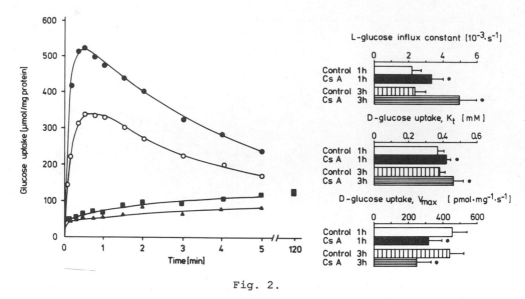

Fig. 2.

Left panel: Effect of cyclosporine A on D-glucose uptake at a D-glucose concentation of 1 mM by renal brush border membrane vesicles in the presence of sodium or potassium. Vesicles were prepared from renal cortical slices which were incubated for 1 h with CsA (1.5 mg/ml) or without CsA (control) in a pure oxygen atmosphere at $37^{O}C$, pH 7.4.

    (●) Without CSA in the presence of sodium
    (○) with CSA in the presence of sodium
    (▨) with CsA in the presence of potassium
    (▲) CsA in the presence of potassium

Right panel: Transport parameters of sodium-dependent D-glucose uptake (apparent K_t and V_{max} values) and influx constants of L-glucose int brush border membrane vesicles prepared from control and CSA (1.5 mg/ml) incubated renal cortical slices (incubation time 1 or 3 h, $37^{O}C$, pH 7.4). *All values (mean ± S.D.) in the presence of CSA are significantly different as compared to the corresponding control values (p < 0.05).

DISCUSSION

It is well known that cyclosporine A treatment causes functional and morphological damage to renal cells. Treatment of rats with CsA were correlated with dilatation of smooth and rough endoplasmic reticulum and more-over with structural damage to the proximal tubule of the kidney (14). Recently Aso et al. (4) reported that treatment of rats with CsA increases the concentration of lipid peroxidation products in renal tissue with correlated alteration of kidney function. These data are in good agreement with results of the present study. As shown CsA caused in vitro a time- and concentration-dependent induction of malondialdehyde production in renal microsomes which was reduced by the radical scavenger alpha-tocopherol, thus indicating indirectly that generation of free radicals and subsequent lipid peroxidation may participate, at least in part, in inducing CsA nephrotoxicity. CsA-induced a non-enzymatic lipid peroxidation since native and heat denaturated microsomes revealed the same increase in MDA production. These results are consistent with the view that the parent compound is the toxic species, although the generation of a toxic metabolite or toxic metabolites in our subcellular kidney fragments cannot be excluded. Lipid peroxidation is accompanied by a functional membrane injury as shown by alterations of the active and passive glucose uptake by brush border membrane vesicles prepared from CsA incubated renal cortical slices. CsA led to an enhanced leakiness of the vesicular membrane for small non-electrolytes such as L- and D-glucose. If we assume that CsA also induces an increase in membrane leakiness to sodium ions than, at least in part, the decrease of the sodium-gradient induced maximal D-glucose uptake rate could be explained in a simple manner. An enhanced sodium leak would lead to a faster dissipation of the initial sodium gradient, thus reducing the driving force for the sodium-dependent D-glucose uptake. On the other hand a decrease in D-glucose affinity to the D-glucose transport sites would mean that the glucose carrier must either be structurally altered or their environment is so changed that their glucose binding site is less available.

REFERENCES

1.   R.Y. Calne, S. Thiru, P. McMaster, G.N. Craddock, D.J.G. White, D.B. Evans, D.C. Dunn, B.D. Pentlow and K. Rolles, Cyclosporin A in patients receiving renal allografts from cadaver donors. Lancet, 2:1323 (1978).

2.   C. Cunningham, M. Gavin, P.H. Whiting, M.D. Burke, F. Macintyre, A.W. Thomson and J.G. Simpson, Serum cyclosporin levels, hepatic drug metabolism and renal tubulotoxicity. Biochem. Pharmacol., 33:2857 (1984).

3.   N.M. Jackson, R.P. O'Connor and H.D. Humes, Cyclosporine (Cs) interactions with renal proximal tubule cells (PTC) and subcellular membranes. Clin. Res., 33:487A (1985).

4.   Y. Aso, A. Tajima, K. Suzuki, Y. Ohtawara, N. Ohta, M. Hata and T. Tsukada, Nephrotoxicity in rats receiving cyclosporine. Biochemical and morphological study. Nippon Hinyokika Gakkai Zasshi, 76:1454 (1985).

5.   B. Ryffel, P. Donatsch, M. Madorin, B.E. Matter, G. Ruttimann, H. Schon, R. Stoll and J. Wilson, Toxicological evaluation of cyclosporin A. Arch. Toxicol., 53:107 (1983).

6.   T. Bertani, N. Perico, M. Abbate, C. Battaglia and G. Remuzzi, Renal injury induced by long-term administration of cyclosporin A to rats. Am. J. Pathol., 127:569 (1987).

7.   C. De Duve, B.C. Pressman, R. Gianetto, R. Wattiaux and F. Appelmans, Tissue fractionation studies. 6. Intracellular distribution patterns of enzymes in rat liver tissue. Biochem. J., 60:604 (1955).

8.   B. Sedgwick and G. Hubscher, Metabolism of Phospholipids IX. Phosphatidate phosphohydrolase in rat liver. Biochim. Biophys. Acta, 106:63 (1965).

9.   J.A. Buege and S.D. Aust, Microsomal lipid peroxidation. Methods Enzymol., 52:302 (1978).

10. C. Cojocel, K.H. Laeschke, G. Inselmann and K. Baumann, Inhibition of cephaloridine-induced lipid peroxidation. Toxicology, 35:295 (1985).

11. R.J. Cross and J.V. Taggart, Renal tubular transport. Accumulation of p-aminohippurate by rabbit kidney slices. Am. J. Physiol., 161:181 (1950).

12. J. Bibez, B. Stieger, W. Haase and H. Murer, A high yield preparation

for rat kidney brush border membranes. Different behaviour of lysosomal markers. <u>Biochim. Biophys. Acta</u>, 647:169 (1981).

13. M.E. Blank, F. Bode, E. Huland, D.F. Diedrich and K. Baumann, Kinetic studies of D-glucose transport in renal brush border membrane vesicles of streptozotocin-induced diabetic rats. <u>Biochim. Biophys. Acta</u>, 844:314 (1985).

14. P.H. Whiting, A.W. Thomson, J.T. Blair and J.G. Simpson, Experimental cyclosporine A nephrotoxicity. <u>Br. J. Exp. Path</u>., 63:88 (1982).

CHRONIC RENAL TUBULAR DAMAGE CAUSED BY CYCLOSPORIN A

P.H. Whiting*, N.J. Saunders, K.J. Thomson, and J.G. Simpson

*Departments of Chemical Pathology and Pathology, University of Aberdeen, Foresterhill, Aberdeen AB9 2ZD, UK

INTRODUCTION

Some degree of renal dysfunction occurs in virtually all patients receiving the immunosuppressant cyclosporin A (CsA) and a variety of animal models have been employed to study this process. Although the rat model has been relatively successful in mimicking the functional aspects of CsA nephrotoxicity (Blair et al., 1982; Thomson et al., 1984; Mihatsch et al., 1986), there has been less correspondence between the renal structural effects of CsA in man and experimental animals.

Clinically, there appear to be three main types of structural damage associated with CsA (Mihatsch et al., 1985). None of these are specific, but all are present more commonly after CsA than in other situations. In patients with prolonged oliguria or anuria following renal transplantation, the kidneys may show diffuse interstitial fibrosis (interactive toxicity). Acute toxicity, which is dose-related and less common now that lower initial and tampering doses of CsA are employed, may be accompanied by a toxic proximal tubulopathy. The third type of CsA-induced renal lesion is chronic toxicity, associated with either striped (i.e. radial) interstitial fibrosis or an arteriolopathy or both.

Virtually all of the animal model studies of CsA-nephrotoxicity in which renal morphology has been studied have shown the acute toxicity, first described in this laboratory (Simpson et al., 1981) and consisting, as in man, of proximal tubular damage. This dose-related lesion is, however, reversible and apparently non-progressive. The present study was designed to examine whether or not CsA was capable of inducing chronic renal damage experimentally.

MATERIALS AND METHODS

<u>Animals</u>. Male Sprague-Dawley rats (mean weight 280g), were used throughout. They were housed in a temperature-controlled environment and allowed free access to food (Oxoid pasteurised rat and mouse breeding diet) and water.

<u>Cyclosporin</u>. Cyclosporin A (Sandoz Ltd., Basle, Switzerland) was provided in powdered form and dissolved initially at $20^{\circ}C$ in absolute alcohol. Conscious animals received either CsA or its vehicle (10% ethanol in olive

oil) daily by oral gavage using a No 4 fine gauge intravenous cannula (Portex Ltd., Hythe, UK).

Experimental Protocol. Four groups of animals were employed. The control group consisted of 8 rats treated only with the vehicle for 12 weeks. Two test groups of animals received CsA at a dose of either 10 or 20 mg/kg/24hr; from each of these two groups 6 animals were killed at 4, 7 and 10 days and then 2, 4, 8 and 12 weeks. (All the controls were killed at 12 weeks.) The fourth group consisted of 6 animals treated daily with CsA (10mg/kg) for 4 weeks and then left untreated for a further 4 weeks before sacrifice. Blood and urine sampling, serum and urine biochemistry, estimation of renal function, CsA measurement, and renal structural and statistical analyses were all performed as described previously (Duncan et al., 1986).

RESULTS

All animals, whether control or CsA treated, demonstrated a progressive weight gain over the experimental course. This weight gain was approximately 70, 45 and 15% at 12 weeks for control animals and those treated with CsA at 10 and 20mg/kg respectively compared to pretreatment values. Glycosuria and urinary flow rate (UFR), unchanged in the control group over the experimental course, were also progressively increased in both CsA treatment groups from pretreatment values of 0.53±0.31mmol/mmol urinary creatinine and 0.76±0.15ml/hr (mean±SD) to values of 149.26±108.92 and 2.31±10.6 at week 12, respectively. Although the magnitude of these changes was similar in both CsA groups, increased glycosuria and UFR occurred earlier in the 20mg/kg group (days 7 and 14 respectively) than in the lower dose groups (days 10 and 28).

Compared to control values, which remained relatively constant over the experimental course, both CsA groups demonstrated a 30% decrease in creatinine clearance rates by day 14 (Fig. 1). This reduction was maintained in the high treatment group until day 70, with a slight improvement observed on day 84, but in the low CsA dose group an increase was noted, from day 82 onwards, to levels intermediate between those demonstrated by control animal and those treated with the higher CsA dose, until day 70. On day 84, although observed mean creatinine clearance values were CsA dose-related, there was no significant difference between the experimental groups.

NAG enzymuria (Fig. 1) was increased over the experimental course following treatment with both CsA doses. Although urinary enzyme release in both CsA groups was similar, peak activities were noted on days 56 and 84 for the low and high dose groups respectively. In addition, CsA at 10mg/kg caused a progressive increase in enzymuria, while treatment at the higher dose was associated with a slight reduction in activities after day 56.

CsA, administered at 10mg/kg for 28 days, produced values for urine flow rate, glycosuria and NAG enzymuria of 1.19±0.49mg/hr, 78.5±48.0mmol/mmol and 123±25IU/mmol (mean±SD) respectively, compared to control values of 0.56±0.22, 0.47±0.33 and 77±21 (all p<0.01), but without a significant reduction in creatinine clearance (327±45ml/hr/kg). All the above values returned to within normal limits following the withdrawal of treatment for a further 28 days.

The trough serum CsA concentrations, observed following drug treatment at either 20 or 10mg/kg, were both dose-related and relatively constant over the experimental period. Levels averaged 1.627 and 0.938 mg/l in the 20 and 10mg/kg CsA groups respectively.

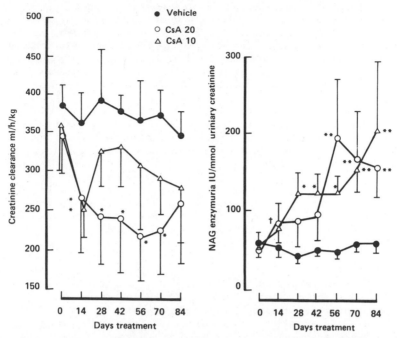

Fig. 1 The effect of CsA on creatinine clearance and NAG enzymuria. Results are expressed as the mean±1SD of 6 determinations. CsA and vehicle treated groups compared at each time point by analysis of variance: (†), p < 0.5; *, p < 0.01; **, p < 0.001.

No structural abnormalities were observed in the control group, but following CsA treatment tubular and interstitial changes were noted which fell into two distinct categories. First to appear, by day 4 and only with CsA at 20mg/kg, was an acute tubular toxicity involving the proximal tubule. The change, which was present in most animals killed up to 2 weeks, but only one animals (8 weeks) after that, was most pronounced in the proximal straight tubule as a course isometric vacuolation due to dilatation of the endoplasmic reticulum. Individual cells were affected uniformly, but the number of involved cells per tubular profile and the proportion of profiles involved varied. Occasionally necrotic cells were noted. Accompanying the vacuolation was a more general proximal tubular disturbance, with lysosomal enlargement, mitochondrial damage with giant mitochondria formation, and focal lipid disposition, all most pronounced in the proximal convoluted segment.

The other lesion, chronic tubular damage, appeared rather later and was progressive. It was first seen in 3 of the day 7 animals treated with CsA at 20mg/kg, and in one of the animals treated with CsA at 10mg/kg on day 10. At this early stage, the abnormality was only notable in the superficial cortex, especially in the immediate subcapsular area. It consisted of wedge-shaped foci of tubular atrophy. Affected tubules, which were of the proximal convoluted type, were either dilated or narrowed and showed epithelial simplification and basement membrane thickening. Often there was an associated interstitial infiltrate of mature lymphocytes. With time the number of animals involved increased as did the severity of the chronic damage, which was well established by 4 weeks in the 20mg/kg CsA group. By this time, foci of tubular atrophy had also appeared deeper in the cortex (never below the corticomedullary junction), joined to the subcapsular lesions in a radial fashion; the degree of proximal tubular (convoluted and straight segments) dilatation or atrophy, even as far as tubular collapse, had increased, although the intervening cortex was normal. As the study progressed, particularly with the higher CsA dose, the radial stripes of tubular atrophy increased in number and thickness, the latter due to interstitial fibrosis; even in animals treated with only 10mg/kg, the lesions were prominent by 12 weeks.

Glomeruli caught up in the radial lesions showed periglomerular fibrosis, but no intrinsic abnormality, and the arteries, arterioles and pelvicalyceal system were all normal. The chronic tubular damage was, however, associated with calcification at the corticomedullary junction which by 4 weeks was striking.

In the group of animals treated with CsA at 10mg/kg for 4 weeks, but left for a further 4 weeks before being killed, there was chronic tubular damage of similar severity to that seen in animals treated with CsA at the same dose for 4 weeks and killed immediately thereafter.

DISCUSSION

This study has demonstrated that CsA given at relatively low doses to intact animals causes consistent abnormalities in renal function as well as two types of renal damage. The trough CsA levels produced were moderate when compared to the clinical therapeutic range. Renal dysfunction was characterised by elevated NAG enzymuria, glycosuria and urine flow rate in both groups. However, only in the high CsA dose group were consistent significant reduction in creatinine clearance rates noted: although, numerically, rates were also lower in the low dose group, they were not significantly different from values observed in either the control or high dose CsA groups. Although a clear relationship between CsA dose and reduction in the rate of creatinine clearance has been demonstrated, no such relationship was established for any other parameter. The lack of a dose-relationship for the glycosuria in particular raises doubts as to the value of this parameter as an indicator of nephrotoxicity, as has been suggested by Chan et al., (1987), especially when CsA has also been shown to be diabetogenic (Helmchen et al., 1984; Laube and Hahn, 1985; Thomson et al., 1986). Similar alterations in creatinine clearance rates and enzymuria have also been observed in experimental and clinical CsA nephrotoxicity (Whiting et al., 1982; Myers et al., 1984; Duncan et al., 1986; Kotanko et al., 1986).

The acute toxicity, seen only with the higher dose of CsA and then only early on in the study, has been noted in most other experimental studies as well as clinically. It is species, strain and dose-related, as well as being reversible both experimentally and clinically (Mihatsch et al., 1985). The acute lesion and the renal function abnormalities associated with CsA occur experimentally and clinically, but the lack of a more chronic structural lesion in animal models has led to doubt as to the relevance of such studies for the clinical situation. The present study does now show, however, that CsA can cause a chronic and progressive dose-related scarring process with tubular atrophy in the intact rat. That this lesion has not previously been observed probably reflects the short-term, high dose nature of most animal studies, where the chronic lesion may also have been obscured by the more severe and generalised nature of the acute damage. At least one other group has now also seen chronic CsA renal damage in the rat (Dieperink et al., personal communication). The chronic lesion involved individual nephrons in a more generalised fashion than the acute tubulopathy, but still predominantly in the proximal segment. The cause of these CsA-induced lesions is not clear, although there is a striking association between chronic tubular damage and calcification at the corticomedullar junction.

Chronic tubular damage as seen in this model is similar to the striped interstitial fibrosis with tubular atrophy first described by Thiru et al. (1983). Although it is not specific for CsA, Mihatsch et al. (1985) consider the lesion to be the primary structural equivalent of chronic CsA nephrotoxicity in man. In the current study, renal function was normal 4 weeks after cessation of CsA administration. There was, however, continuing structural chronic tubular damage in the kidney. The long-term significance of this lesion as regards renal function is unclear.

The results of this study suggest that the Sprague-Dawley rat is a suitable animal to study the chronic nephrotoxicity associated with CsA administration. Such studies may be of considerable importance if CsA is to achieve its full clinical potential in areas other than organ transplantation.

REFERENCES

Blair, J.T., Thomson, A.W., Whiting, P.H., Davidson, R.J.L., and Simpson, J.G., 1982, Toxicity of the immune suppressant cyclosporin A in the rat, J. Pathol., 138:163.

Chan, P., Chapman, J.R., and Morris, P.J., 1987, Glycosuria: an index of cyclosporine nephrotoxicity, Transplant. Proc., 19:1780.

Duncan, J.I., Thomson, A.W., Simpson, J.G., and Whiting, P.H., 1986, A comparative toxicological study of cyclosporine and Nva^2-cyclosporine in Sprague-Dawley rats, Transplantation, 42:395.

Kotanko, P., Keiler, R., Knabl, L., Aulitzky, W., Margreiter, R., Gstraunthaler, G., and Pfaller, W., 1986, Urinary enzyme analysis in renal allograft transplantation., Clin. Chim. Acta, 160:37.

Helmchen, U., Schmidt, W.E., Siegl, E.G., and Creutzfeldt, W., 1984, Morphological and functional changes of pancreatic beta-cells in cyclosporin A-treated rats, Diabetologia, 27:416.

Laube, F., and Hahn, J.H., 1985, Effect of cyclosporin A on insulin secretion in vitro, Horm. Metabol. Res., 17:43.

Mihatsch, M.J., Ryffel, B., Hermle, M., Brunner, F.P., and Thiel, G., 1986, Morphology of cyclosporine nephrotoxicity in the rat, Clin. Nephrol., 25 (suppl.1):92.

Mihatsch, M.J., Thiel, G., Basler, V., Ryffel, B., Landmann, J., von Overbeck, J., and Zollinger, H.U., 1985, Morphologic patterns in cyclosporin-treated renal transplant recipients, Transplant. Proc., 17 (suppl. 1):101.

Myers, B.D., Ross, J., Newton, K., Luetscher, J., and Perloth, M., 1984, Cyclosporine-associated chronic nephropathy, New Engl. J. Med., 311:699.

Simpson, J.G., Blair, J.T., Whiting, P.H., and Thomson, A.W., 1981, Cyclosporin A-induced renal proximal tubular damage, IRCS Med. Sci., 9:562.

Thiru, S., Maher, E.R., Hamilton, D.V., Evans, D.B., and Calne, R.Y., 1983, Tubular changes in renal transplant recipients on cyclosporine, Transplant. Proc., 15 (suppl. 1):2846.

Thomson, A.W., Whiting, P.H., and Simpson, J.G., 1984: Cyclosporine: immunology, toxicity and pharmacology in experimental animals, <u>Agents and Actions</u>, 15:306.

Thomson, K.J., Saunders, N.J., Simpson, J.G., and Whiting, P.H., 1987, The effects of cyclosporin A on glucose homeostasis, <u>Nephrology, Dialysis and Transplantation</u>, 12:62.

Whiting, P.H., Thomson, A.W., Blair, J.T., and Simpson, J.G., 1982, Experimental cyclosporin nephrotoxicity, <u>Br. J. Exp. Pathol</u>. 63:88.

EFFECTS OF ACUTE AND CHRONIC CYCLOSPORINE ADMINISTRATION ON GLOMERULAR HAEMODYNAMICS IN RATS

Elvino J.G.Barros, Mirian A.Boim, Luiz A.R.Moura, Oswaldo L. Ramos and Nestor Schor

Nephrology Division, Escola Paulista de Medicina, Rua Botucatu, 740 04023 S O Paulo, SP, Brazil

INTRODUCTION

Cyclosporine (CsA) a potent immunosuppressive drug which has afforded benefit in transplantation and in the treatment of several immune-mediated diseases (1-3). However, a number of side effects have been observed, with nephrotoxicity being the most common and important (4-6). The impairment of glomerular filtration rate (GFR) and thus, acute renal failure (ARF) observed with CsA appears to be related with renal haemodynamic alterations (7,8). No significant glomerular lesions have been found (4).

It has been suggested that hormonal factors may participate in this acute nephrotoxicity. Both, activation of renin-angiotensin (RAS) and suppression of prostaglandin (PG) system have been observed (9). We have studied the renal microcirculation in response to acute CsA treatment.

MATERIALS AND METHODS.

Munich-Wistar rats were submitted to glomerular haemodynamic studies during two experimental periods. After surgery for micropuncture technique preparation (10) and the respective equilibration period, an initial control period was was followed by a second series of studies with the cyclosporine-vehicle, Cremophor (Sandoz, Basle-Switzerland), with 0.4 to 0.6ml, iv, in the control group. In CsA group, rats were treated with 50 mg/kg of CsA, iv, (Sandoz, Basle-Switzerland) in the second study period, after the control measurements. In order to evaluate hormonal factors in acute CsA toxicity, additional experimental groups were treated with calcium channel blocker, DI-Verapamil (Knoll, USA) 20ug/kg/min, iv, or Captopril (SQ 14.255, Squibb, NJ, USA), 2mg/kg/hr, iv, during both periods. Additional rats were treated with prostaglandin synthesis inhibitor, Indomethacin (Merck Sharp & Dhome Ltd., USA), 2mg/kg, iv, in bolus. The role of anti-diuretic hormone (ADH) in CsA nephrotoxicity was evaluated in Brattleboro rats, a genetic diabetes insipidus strain lacking endogenous vasopressin. In order to evaluate strain differences, heterozygote Brattleboro rats served as control group for the homozygote ones. For all these groups, CsA was given using the same protocol as described above.

The effect of chronic CsA treatment was further evaluated in Munich-Wistar rats, which received 9 daily doses of Cremophor, 0.4 to 0.6ml, IP (control) or CsA, 25mg/kg, IP.

RESULTS

Total glomerular filtration rate (GFR) and renal plasma flow, (RPF) were reduced by about 50% and 56% respectively (p < 0.05) after CsA administration alone. This was followed by an impressive increase on total renal vascular resistance, TRVR (230%). Partial protection in CsA-induced haemodynamic changes was observed during angiotensin I converting enzyme inhibition (Captopril) and also with Ca channel blocked (Verapamil), since both, lessened the GFR and RPF decreases and blunted the increase in TRVR (p < 0.05). Indomethacin failed to modify the GFR, RPF and TRVR alterations induced by CsA.

The micropuncture data obtained before and after CsA administration are shown in Figure 1. Mean single nephron GFR (SNGFR) and glomerular plasma flow (Q_A) were reduced after CsA, 27.90±3.39 to 14.02±3.49 nl/min (p < 0.02) and 100.99±17.09 to 44.37±13.37 nl/min (p < 0.01), respectively. Mean glomerular capillary hydraulic pressure (PGC) increased from 45±1 to 55±4mmHg (p < 0.02) after CsA infusion. Since mean tubular hydraulic pressure (P_T) did not change, the observed transcapillary glomerular hydraulic pressure difference (ΔP) increases were due to PGC elevations. Total renal arteriolar resistance (R_T) rose significantly (245%) due to increases in both, afferent (R_A) and efferent arteriolar resistance (R_E) of 185% and 360% respectively.

Reduced values of glomerular ultrafiltration coefficient (K_f) were found after CsA, averaging from 0.096±0.030 to 0.031±0.010nl/(sec.mmHg), p < 0.05. Acute CsA infusion in Brattleboro heterozygote rats induced marked falls in GFR and RPF with an increase of TRVR (Table 1).

Table 1 - Summary of whole kidney function in Brattleboro rats before and after acute CsA administration.

		GFR	RPF	TRVR
		..... ml/min		mmHg.min/ml
HOMOZYGOTE	BEFORE	0.88a	2.76	38
		±0.04	0.20	3
	AFTER	0.69*	1.91*	55*
		±0.06	0.13	4
HETEROZYGOTE	BEFORE	0.99	2.67	51
		±0.06	0.26	4
	AFTER	0.42*	0.94*	147*
		±0.06	0.12	21

a $\overline{X}$±SE, *p < 0.05 after vs before CsA

These changes were similar to those observed in Munich-Wistar rats. However, in Brattleboro homozygote rats, the renal function parameters were significantly less affected than observed for CsA in heterozygote and in Munich-Wistar rats.

Figure 2 summarizes the micropuncture data obtained from groups chronically treated with Cremaphor or CsA. Mean SNGFR and Q_A were reduced from 38.69±4.25 to 20.38±2.31 nl/min and 114.69±9.52 to 53.87±6.31 nl/min (p < 0.01), respectively. Differently from acute infusion, after chronic CsA treatment, PGC decreased from 44±1 to 34±1 mmHg (p < 0.01)

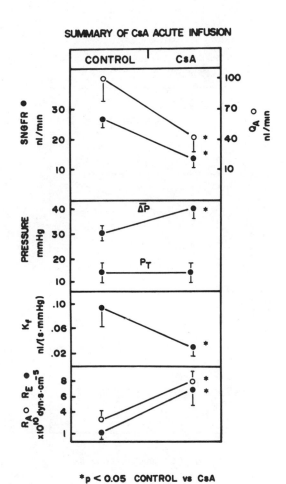

SUMMARY OF CsA ACUTE INFUSION

*p < 0.05 CONTROL vs CsA

Figure 1 - Summary of glomerular haemodynamic data before and after acute CsA administration.

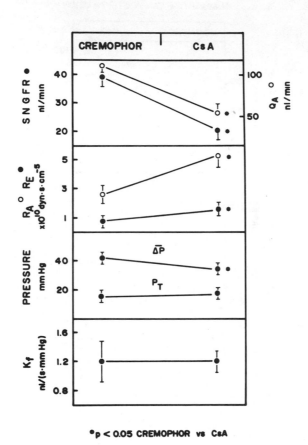

°p < 0.05 CREMOPHOR vs CsA

Figure 2 - Summary of glomerular haemodynamic data after vehicle (Cremophor) or CsA chronic treated rats.

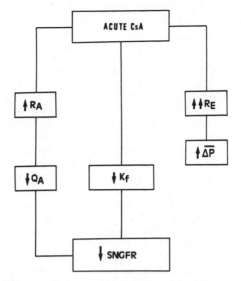

Figure 3 - Possible pathways of acute CsA effects on glomerular function

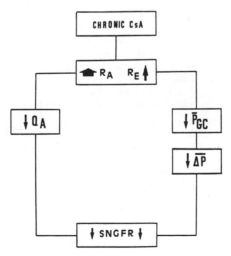

Figure 4 - Possible pathways of chronic CsA effects on glomerular function

and PT did not change, thus ΔP decreased. R_T was elevated, however, in this case (chronic CsA), R_T elevation was due to mainly R_A increases (Figure 2). Mean K_f after 9 days of CsA was not different from values obtained with CsA vehicle, Cremophor. Figures 3 and 4 summarize the effects of acute and chronic CsA, respectively.

DISCUSSION

In the present experimental protocol of acute CsA treatment, we observed an increase on both arteriolar resistances and, despite the observed increase in mean ΔP, SNGFR was reduced. The vasoconstriction caused a fall of mean Q_A. Nevertheless, the fall of Q_A was not the only factor responsible for the decline in SNGFR. Our data indicate that SNGFR was also decreased due to a significant fall in K_f. The decline on K_f was also suggested in man by Myers et al (11) in patients after heart transplantation. Moreover, they also deduced by indirect methodology an increase in ΔP, similar to the observed by direct micropuncture data in rats in the present study. Taken together findings on glomerular haemodynamics resemble those produced by endogenous or exogenous angiotensin II (AII). In fact, AII is capable to reduce K_f (12,13). Moreover, it has been suggested that renal functional changes induced by CsA on total renal blood flow and glomerular filtration rate observed in rats may be caused by stimulation of the renin-angiotensin system (9,14). CsA has been shown to stimulate the renin-angiotensin system both in vitro and in vivo (9,14,15). Captopril completely abolished the renal vasoconstriction induced by CsA was and the fall in GFR and reduced the fall in RPF. These findings suggest that AII may play an important role on the pathogenesis of renal vasoconstriction produced by acute CsA administration. AII could have altered renal function in this model of nephrotoxicity by several mechanisms. One of them was through a stimulation of tubuloglomerular feedback mechanism, leading to an increase in renin and AII production.

Another possibility could have been the direct action of AII in decreasing K_f. The benefical effects of captopril in rats receiving CsA infusion could also be due to stimulation of kallikrein-kinin and/or on PG system (16). On the other hand, Murray et al (7) found no effect of Captopril on CsA induced fall in RPF despite the fact that an increase on plasma renin activity was observed. The relationship between the stimulation of the RAS and the observed functional abnormalities is not clear. Gerken et al (17) showed that high salt intake protects from CsA nephrotoxicity while low Na intake increases it. The stimulation of renin by CsA may increase renal PGs and thereby modulate CsA nephrotoxicity. Several studies have suggested that renal PGs are depressed by CsA (10,14,18). However, Paller and Murray (19) observed that CsA administration is associated with a stimulation of renal PG synthesis. Inhibition of PG synthesis by Indomethacin or Meclofenamate led to an increase in CsA renal toxicity (7,19). Recently it was suggested that PGs affect CsA toxicity by blocking intestinal absorption of this drug (20). Thus, the conflicting and inconclusive studies do not permit a definite statement to be made concerning the role of PGs on CsA nephrotoxicity. In the present experimental model, however, the use of Indomethacin maintained essentially the same results as found with CsA alone, implying that the PG system has a minor (if any) effect in impairing glomerular haemodynamics during acute CsA treatment. It is possible that CsA has a PG inhibition-like effect and thus, simultaneous treatment with Indomethacin and CsA did not enhance the nephrotoxicity.

Since it is clear that CsA caused an increase in resistances, it became important to evaluate the effect of a vasodilator Ca-channel blocker drug. Iaina et al (21), observed that CsA plus ischaemia produces ARF which can be attenuated by the use of Verapamil. Verapamil reduces the severity of renal insufficiency as well as histological damage. In the present study, Verapamil attenuated CsA effects on TRVR and RPF leading to an improvement of GFR. This protective action could be explained either by arteriolar vasodilatation and/or by interaction with the RAS.

Antidiuretic hormone (ADH) is another vasoactive substance which is capable of influencing the process of glomerular ultrafiltration, mainly by reducing K_f (12). In the present study, acute CsA administration in Brattleboro rats produced a decline in GFR and RPF of only 22% and 31%, respectively, when compared with the observed reductions of 51% and 55% seen in Munich-Wistar rats. Perhaps, different sensitivities of these rat strains could explain our findings. To test this possibility, we studied heterozygote Brattleboro rats, from which the data were not different from Munich-Wistar rats. This supports the idea that strain differences did not account for the difference in nephrotoxicity. Therefore, we can postulate that the presence of ADH is in some way necessary for that full nephrotoxic action of CsA in the rat kidney. It is also clear that in the absence of this hormone it is still possible to observe significant nephrotoxic action of this drug. It is possible that ADH participates in this pathophysiology either by its vasoconstrictor effect or reducing K_f. The mechanism of the ADH-associated fall in K_f is independent of a pathway involving AII since both act selective and independent on K_f, via mesangial cell contraction (12).

After chronic CsA treatment, decreased mean GFR, RPF and increased mean TRVR, were observed. However, the micropuncture data showed that the vasoconstriction was mainly due to a preferential increase on R_A that caused both declines of Q_A and ΔP. In contrast to the acute study, no significant alteration on K_f was found, but the variance of this data and for the P_T measurement was abnormally large, and statistical analysis did not detected any significant differences. The presence of tubules with a very low hydraulic pressures, possible non-filtering nephrons and others with very high values with obstructions, suggest a heterogeneous effect of chronic CsA on cortical area. Thus, it is possible that mean K_f was not found to be altered because of this increased heterogeneous effect.

Thus, during acute CsA administration a predominant increase on mean R_E was observed, the increase on mean PGC was not sufficient to offset the decline on mean Q_A and K_f and therefore, a reduction on SNGFR occurred. By contrast, during chronic CsA administration the most predominant effect was rising mean R_A and thus, a decline on mean PGC was observed. In this situation, a decrease on SNGFR was due mainly to a decline on ΔP and Q_A.

REFERENCES

1. B.D. Kahan, Cyclosporine: the agent and its actions, Transplant. Proc. 17:5 (1985).

2. A.W. Thompson, P.H. Whiting and J.G. Simpson, Cyclosporine: immunology, toxicity and pharmacology in experimental animals, Agents. Actions. 15:306 (1984).

3. J.F. Borel, Cyclosporine A present experimental status, Transplant. Proc. 13:344 (1981).

4. S.O. Bohman, G. Klintmalm, O. Ringden, B. Sundelin and H. Welzek, Interstitial fibrosis in human kidney grafts after 12 to 46 months of cyclosporine therapy, Transplant. Proc. 17:1168 (1985).

5. S.M. Flechner, G. Van Buren, R.H. Herman and B. D. Kahan, The nephrotoxicity of cyclosporine in renal transplant recipients, Transplant. Proc. 15:2689 (1983).

6. J.M. Hows, J.M. Smith, A. Bughn and E.C. Gordon-Smith, Nephrotoxicity in marrow graft recipients treated with cyclosporine, Transplant. Proc. 15:2708 (1983).

7. B.M. Murray, M.S. Paller and T.F. Ferris, Effect of cyclosporine administration on renal hemodynamics in conscious rats, Kidney Int. 28:767 (1985).

8. B.M. Murray and. M.S. Paller, Beneficial effects of renal denervation and prazosin on GFR and renal blood flow after cyclosporine in rats, Clin. Nephrol. 25:537 (1986).

9. N. Perico, A. Benigni, E. Bosco, M. Possini, S. Orisio, F. Ghilardi, A. Piccinelli and G. Remuzzi, Acute cyclosporine nephrotoxicity in rats: which role for renin-angiotensin system and glomerular prostaglandin?, Clin. Nephrol. 25:583 (1986).

10. N. Schor, I. Ichikawa, H.G. Rennke, J.L. Troy and B.M. Brenner, Pathophysiology of altered glomerular function in aminoglycoside-treated rats, Kidney Int. 19:288 (1981).

11. B.D. Myers, J. Ross, L. Newton, J. Luetscher and M. Pelroth, Cyclosporine associated chronic nephropathy, N. Engl. J. Med. 311:699 (1984).

12. N. Schor, I. Ichikawa and B.M. Brenner, Mechanism of action of various hormones and vasoactive substances on glomerular ultrafiltration in the rat, Kidney Int. 20:442 (1981).

13. R.C. Blantz, K.S. Konnen and B.J. Tucker, Angiotensin II effect upon the glomerular microcirculation and ultrafiltration coefficient on the rat, J. Clin. Invest. 57:419 (1976).

14. H. Siegel, B. Ryffel, P. Petric, P. Shoemaker, A. Muller, P. Donatsch and M. Mihatsch, Cyclosporine, the renin-angiotensin system, and renal adverse reactions, Transplant. Proc. 15:2719 (1983).

15. C.R. Baxter, G.G. Duggin, B.M. Hall, J.S. Harvath and D.J. Tiller, Stimulation of renin release from rat renal cortical slices by cyclosporine A, Res. Com. Chem. Pathol. Pharmacol. 43:417 (1984).

16. R.E. McCaa, J.E. Hall and C.S. McCaa, The effects of angiotensin I converting enzyme inhibition on arterial blood pressure and urinary sodium excretion. Role of the renal renin-angiotensin and kallikrein-kinin system, Circ. Res. 43:132 (1978).

17. J.F. Gerken, S.B. Bhgwandeen, P.J. Dosen and A.J. Smith, The effect of salt intake on cyclosporine-induced impairment of renal function in rats, Transplantation 38:412 (1984).

18. D. Adu, C.J. Lote, J. Michael, J. H. Turney and P. McMaster, Does cyclosporine inhibit renal prostaglandin synthesis? Proc. EDTA-ERA 21:969 (1984).

19. M.S. Paller and B.M. Murray, Renal dysfunction in animal model of cyclosporine toxicity, Transplant. Proc. 17:155 (1985).

20. B. Ryffel, P. Dontsch, P. Hiestand and M. J. Mihatsch, PGE2 reduces nephrotoxicity and immunosupression of cyclosporine in rats, Clin. Nephrol. 21:595 (1986).

21. A. Iaina, D. Herzog, D. Cohen, S. Gavendo, S. Kapuler, I. Serban, G. Schiby and H.E. Eliahou, Calcium entry-blockade with verapamil in cyclosporine A plus ischemia-induced acute renal failure in rats, Clin. Nephrol. 25:S168 (1986).

INTRACELLULAR LOCALIZATION OF CYCLOSPORIN A IN THE RAT KIDNEY

Miloslav Dobrota and Julian R. Louis

Robens Institute of Industrial and Environmental Health and Safety, University of Surrey, Guildford, Surrey, GU2 5XH

INTRODUCTION

Cyclosporin A (CyA), a most potent and clinically useful immuno-suppressive agent, also produces a number of side-effects in man and experimental animals. Nephrotoxicity, characterised by the formation of numerous large vacuoles in the straight proximal tubules in the corticomedullary region or the S3 (P3) segment of the nephron (1), is the most notable side effect of CyA. There are indications that the S3 region may also accumulate the greatest proportion of CyA (2). The biochemical changes associated with the nephrotoxicity are consistent with tubular damage and include elevated urinary excretion of lysosomal and brush border enzymes (3). The heterogeneous range of vacuoles appear to be of lysosomal, mitochondrial and possibly of endoplasmic reticulum origin. However, the positive localization of acid phosphatase within many of the vacuoles (4) suggest that the majority might be of lysosomal origin. What remains unknown is whether these vacuoles form as a result of accumulation of cyclosporin or as an indirect effect of more complex secondary factors. The aim of the study described here was to investigate the intracellular localization of CyA in the kidney and to determine whether the vacuoles accumulate and contain CyA.

EXPERIMENTAL PROCEDURES

Animals. ^{3}HCyA was administered by gavage, to Wistar Albino male rats, as six daily doses each containing 20mg CyA (100mg/kg), 8.98uCi ^{3}H in a volume of 0.5ml. Control animals were dosed with six daily doses (0.5ml) of the ethanol/olive oil vehicle. At 24h after the sixth dose samples of blood and various tissues (kidney, liver, heart, lungs, thymus, fat, etc.) were taken for determination of radioactivity.

Tissues. The kidneys were removed and pieces were immediately fixed for histology and electron microscopy. Kidney cortices were carefully excised and placed in ice cold 0.25M sucrose containing 5mM Tris-HCl, pH 7.4. The medullas were also placed in ice cold sucrose.

Subcellular Fractionation. The kidney cortices were homogenised and fractionated by differential pelleting into nuclear (N), mitochondria/lysosomes (ML), microsomal (MIC) fractions and cytosol (SUP). The ML fraction was further subfractionated to resolve the lysosomal populations, mitochondria, brush border membranes, peroxisomes and ER, by rate zonal sedimentation. All these procedures were carried out exactly as described previously (5).

The 'N' pellet was resuspended in cold 0.25M sucrose and layered (1.5ml) over a linear sucrose gradient (30ml ranging from 0.35 to 1.9M) and a cushion (3ml) of 2M sucrose. The tubes, containing sample and gradient, were placed in a TST 28.38 Kontron rotor and spin at 6,000 rev/min for 25min in a Centrikon ultracentrifuge (Kontron, Zurich, Switzerland). The gradient was finally displaced and collected as 20 x 1.5ml fractions.

Assays. Isotope counting, protein and enzymes. Aqueous samples of tissue homogenates of kidney cortex in 0.25M sucrose and liver, heart, lung, thymus, medulla and various subcellular fractions were added directly to Pico-Fluor 30 (Packard) scintillant. The fat was homogenised directly in the Pico-Fluor 30 scintillant. The radioactivity was measured with an LKB-Wallac 1219 Rackbeta 'Spectral' liquid scintillation counter and automatically corrected to DPM. Protein was measured by the Bio-Rad reagent kit. Marker enzymes, acid phosphatase (lysosomes), succinic dehydrogenase (mitochondria), catalase (peroxisomes), glucose-6-phosphatase (endoplasmic reticulum), 5'-nucleotidase and alkaline phosphatase (plasma membrane) were assayed as described in ref (5).

Chromatography. The cytosol from the ^{3}HCyA treated animals was fractionated by Sephadex G-75 gel exclusion chromatography using a 25x1cm column and 0.015M Ammonium formate, pH 8.0 as the eluting buffer. The column was precalibrated with a range of molecular weight markers.

RESULTS

Morphology. Histopathology of the rat kidneys, examined by light microscopy (not illustrated) showed the typical lesion caused by CyA with extensive vocalization of the straight proximal tubules in the cortico-medullary region and in a few medullary rays extending into the cortex.

The ultrastructure of the kidney cortex (Fig 1) shows three distinct features: tubule cell with numerous large vacuoles which appear to be almost empty and resemble fat droplets (panel a), a number of tubule cells with extremely large irregular shaped lysosomes (panel b) and tubule cells with numerous swollen, damaged mitochondria (panel c).

Tissue Distribution of ^{3}H-CyA. The proportion (%) of the administered dose of ^{3}HCyA in the various tissues (Table 1), indicates firstly the relatively low uptake retention of ^{3}HCyA in most of the tissues except for fat and confirms the rapid excretion. Indeed the 'high' proportion in the liver is consistent with the major route of excretion being via bile. After fat and liver it is the kidney which contains the highest proportion of ^{3}HCyA on the basis of percent of dose and also per gram of tissue.

TABLE 1. Distribution of ^{3}HCyA in the tissues of the rat given as % recovery of total dose (Mean of 2 experiments, 12 animals).

TISSUE	^{3}HuCi/g OF TISSUE	RECOVERY (%) OF DOSE IN TISSUE
Kidney	40.5	0.14
Lung	27.0	0.07
Heart	18.0	0.02
Thymus	27.0	0.02
Liver	72.1	0.91
Fat	252.2	–
Blood	4.5	0.02

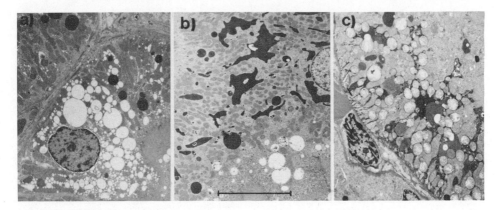

Fig. 1. Morphology of the kidney cortex after CyA treatment showing proximal tubules with a) large vacuoles, b) giant irregular lysosomes, c) damaged mitochondria.

Subcellular Distribution of ^{3}H-CyA.   The distribution of ^{3}HCyA in the classical subfractions of the kidney cortex (Table 2) shows that a major proportion of CyA is present in the supernatant fraction (see Discussion) with the ML, at 21.1% being the highest of the particulate fractions. Comparison with the distributions of marker enzymes amongst these classical fractions do not indicate any clear cut association of CyA with any specific subcellular structures. The distributions of marker enzymes amongst the subfractions of normal (control) kidney cortex are not illustrated because they are essentially the same as those in Table 2. The specific activities of these enzymes are also not illustrated since there is little difference between experimental and control values which in turn are consistent with previously published values (5).

TABLE 2.   Percent distribution (recovery) of ^{3}HCYA, protein and marker enzymes in the classical subfractions of the rat kidney cortex of CYA treated animals.

	N	ML	MIC	SUP	TOTAL
^{3}HCyA	7.3	21.1	11.1	61.1	100.6
Protein	11.0	18.3	17.1	31.8	78.2
Acid Phosphatase	8.4	38.8	23.4	24.9	94.5
Succinic dehydrogenase	9.1	52.2	74.1	1.5	77.2
Catalase	4.0	18.3	17.7	40.1	80.1
Glucose-6-phosphatase	11.9	17.8	49.3	9.3	88.4
5' Nucleotidase	13.0	12.0	50.4	11.8	87.4
Alkaline Phosphatase	13.7	26.6	22.4	17.7	80.4

Subfractionation of the ML by rate zonal sedimentation (Fig 2) resolves this fraction into five major regions (peaks), which are identified in the legend to Fig. 2. The most important feature of the ^{3}HCyA distribution in this complex profile is that it closely follows that of the lysosomal marker acid phosphatase. The distributions of all the marker enzymes in Fig. 2 are the same as obtained with the ML fraction from control animals (5), despite the structural changes induced by CyA.

The rate sedimentation of the 'N' fraction, was carried out in order to establish if the large vacuoles, lysosomes and mitochondria, induced by

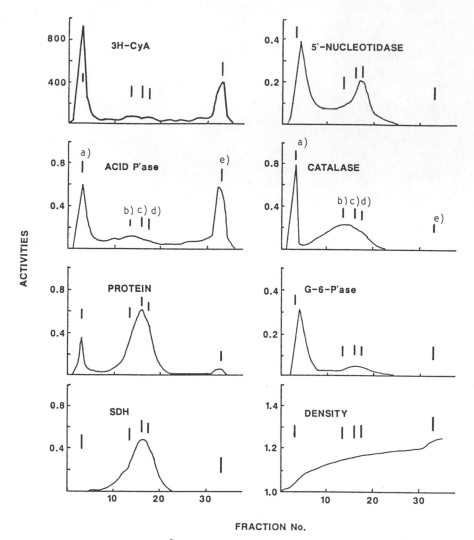

Fig 2. Distribution of [3]HCyA radiolabel (DPM), protein (mg) and marker
enzymes (uM/min) after rate zonal sedimentation of the cortical 'ML'
fraction. Details of gradient and conditions are as described elsewhere
(5). Regions marked represent, a) sample position (unsedimentable
material), b) small lysosomes and peroxisomes, c) mitochondria, d) brush
border membranes, e) large lysosomes.

CyA can be resolved and identified amongst the large particulates normally
present in this fraction. The profile of the subfractionated 'N' fraction
(Fig. 3) indicates, like that of the ML fraction, that the distribution of
[3]HCyA is very similar to that of the lysosomal marker, acid phosphatase,
whilst, all the other market enzymes exhibit quite different
distributions. The single peak of radioactivity at fraction 18 (the peak
at fraction 1 is not relevant as it represents the initial sample
position) coincides with the single peak of acid phosphatase and the major
peak of protein, whilst the dual peaks of succinic dehydrogenase and
alkaline phosphatase indicate that CyA is not likely to be associated with
mitochondria or plasma membranes.

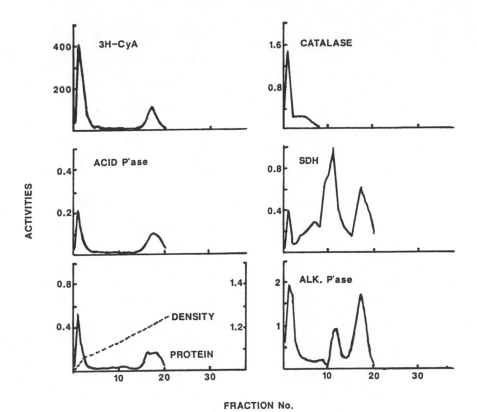

FRACTION No.

Fig 3. Distribution of ^{3}HCyA radiolabel (DPM), protein (mg) and marker enzymes (uM/min) after rate sedimentation of the cortical 'N' fraction. The method is described in detail in the Experimental Procedures.

The high proportion of ^{3}HCyA in the 'SUP' fraction was investigated further by gel exclusion chromatography to examine the range of cytosolic macromolecules which may be associated with the CyA. The separation of the 'SUP' by Sephadex G-75 chromatography (not illustrated) indicates that the ^{3}H-label is present in two distinct peaks, which correspond to molecular weights of 6,500 and 11,000 daltons. This would initially suggest that ^{3}HCyA is associated with a low molecular weight protein and possibly its dimer. However, the elution of authentic ^{3}HCyA at a position coincident with 6,000 daltons suggest that CyA either behaves atypically because of its chemistry (e.g. lipophilicity) or possibly elutes as a tetramer.

DISCUSSION

The structural changes induced by CyA and the tissue distributions are consistent with the literature on CyA (1,4) and confirm the formation of various large vacuoles at the corticomedullary junction of the kidney.

Whilst the distributions and specific activities of marker enzymes in the various subfractions examined are very similar to those found with the control rat kidney, significant changes were observed with catalase (reduced in the 'SUP' increased in the 'ML') and alkaline phosphatase (reduced in the 'MIC'). These changes suggest a possible effects of CyA on peroxisomes and on brush border membranes, although neither of these appear to be structurally altered.

The distribution of CyA amongst classical subfractions suggests a predominantly cytosolic localization but this may be elevated as a

329

significant proportion of this 61% may be due to CyA released from the large and thus fragile vacuoles which are disrupted during homogenization. This would suggest that if CyA is present in the vacuoles, which most likely represent giant endocytic vacuoles, it is in the soluble form. The two distinct molecular size forms of ^{3}HCyA present in the supernatant fraction may indeed represent CyA of the cytosol location and CyA originating from intra-vacuole contents. The relatively low proportion of ^{3}HCyA associated with membraneous particulates is rather surprising although it is consistent with relatively low in vitro binding of CyA to subcellular fractions (2). It is possible that CyA during uptake binds to a receptor protein and the subsequent CyA-receptor complex remains soluble.

The differences between particulate and cytosolic CyA may also represent very different mechanisms of uptake in the different regions of the nephron with the cytosolic perhaps originating from the S3 segment and the particulate being attributable to the proximal convolute tubule. The clear association of CyA with the lysosomal populations of the 'N' and 'ML' fractions strongly suggests that the uptake mechanism occurs via the endocytic pathway with CyA being processed like other oligopeptides. This association with lysosomes also supports the idea that a proportion of CyA is taken up into the proximal convoluted tubule since it is this region of the nephron that contains most of the lysosomes and indeed the largest lysosomes (protein droplets). The uptake of CyA into the S3 region of the nephron (with relatively few lysosomes) may occur via a different mechanism, possibly by a basolateral route, as it is difficult to envisage why CyA present in the lumen is not reabsorbed efficiently in the upper regions of the nephron.

The localization of CyA in the kidney and in the intracellular compartments is an important aspect of understanding the lesion induced by CyA. Whilst this study has demonstrated the association of CyA with lysosomes of the proximal convoluted tubule the question of the vacuoles in the S3 segment needs further investigation. Are the uptake, distribution and intracellular processing of CyA altered if the vacuole formation is largely abolished by high salt intake (6)?

REFERENCES

1. M.J. Mihatsch., B. Ryffel, M. Hermle., F.P. Brunner and G. Thiel (1986). Morphology of cyclosporin nephrotoxicity in the rat. Clin. Nephrol. 25 (Suppl 1): 52-58.

2. B. Ryffel., J. Wilson., R. Maurer., F. Gudat and Mihatsch. (1986). Problems of cyclosporine localisation in the renal tissue. Clin. Nephrol 25 (Suppl 1): 534-536.

3. P.H. Whiting., A.W. Thompson and Simpson, J.G. (1986). Cyclosporine and renal enzyme excretion. Clin. Nephrol. 25 (Suppl 1): 5100-5104.

4. G.A. Verpooten., I. Wybo., V.M. Pattyn., P.G. Hendrix., R.A. Guiliano., E.J. Nouwen, E.J., F. Roels and M.E. DeBroe (1986). Cyclosporin nephrotoxicity: Comparative cytochemical study of rat kidney and human allograft biopsies. Clin. Nephrol. 25 (Suppl 1): 518-522.

5. K.J. Andersen., H.J. Haga and M. Dobrota. (1987). Lysosomes of the renal cortex: Heterogeneity and role in protein handling, Kid Internat. 31: 886-897.

6. F.J. Gerkens., S.B. Bhagwandeen., P.J. Dosen. and A.J. Smith, (1984). The effect of salt intake on cyclosporine-induced impairment of renal function in rats. Transplantation, 38: 412-423.

330

DISTRIBUTION OF PLATINUM AMONGST THE SUBCELLULAR ORGANELLES OF THE RAT KIDNEY AFTER ORAL ADMINISTRATION OF CISPLATIN

S.P. Binks and M. Dobrota

Robens Institute of Industrial and Environmental Health and Safety, University of Surrey, Guildford, Surrey, GU2 5XH

INTRODUCTION

Cisplatin is an effective anticancer agent when administered i.v. to experimental animals and man (1). Its use, however is limited by its toxicity to a number of organs including the kidney (2). These side effects can be modulated by the use of second generation analogues such as carboplatin (3) and alternative routes of administration. Recent studies have demonstrated that cisplatin is orally absorbed, that the nephro-toxicity associated with the compound could be significantly reduced using this route and that oral cisplatin is effective against several murine tumours (4). We have previously reported that oral cisplatin (in rats) could potentiate its hepatotoxicity, although the greatest proportion of the absorbed Pt is still associated with the kidney (5). In this study we have examined the uptake and subcellular localization of platinum in the rat kidney cortex following oral administration of cisplatin with the aim of identifying the sites of Pt accumulation and relating this to the nephrotoxicity.

MATERIALS AND METHODS

Subcellular Fractionation. Male albino wistar rats (200-250g) were administered Cisplatin by gavage either as a bolus dose (57mg/kg) suspended in a tragacanth mucilage or daily (2mg/kg) for 28 days, dissolved in 0.9% saline. Twenty four hours after dosing the animals were killed and the kidneys were quickly removed and placed in ice-cold 0.25M sucrose/5mM Tris-HCl, pH7.4. Entire cortices were carefully dissected free and homogenised in the 0.25M sucrose using a Potter Elvehjem homogeniser rotated at 1000 rev/min. The 10% (w/v) homogenate was then filtered through a coarse sieve and classical subfractions, Nuclear (N), Mitochondrial (ML), Microsomal (MIC) and cytosolic (SUP) were prepared by differential pelleting (6). The 'ML' fraction was resuspended in the 0.25M sucrose and further subfractionations by rate sedimentation in an high speed zonal rotor (MSE Scientific Instruments, Crawley, Sussex, UK). All these procedures were carried out exactly as described previously (6).

Chemical and Enzyme Assays. Protein (PROT) and marker enzymes, Glucose-6-phosphatase (G-6-P'), 5'-Nucleotidase (AMP'), succinate dehydrogenase (SDH), acid phosphatase (Acid P') and catalase (CAT) were assayed in the various fractions as described by Andersen et al (6) For the analysis of platinum, tissue homogenates and subcellular fractions were digested in nitric acid at $200^{\circ}C$, taken to dryness and resuspended in 1% HCl. Samples were then analysed for platinum by electrothermal atomic absorption spectrometry on a Pye Unican SP9090 spectrophotometer.

Electron Microprobe Analysis. Cisplatin (1mg/kg) in 0.9% saline was administered by gavage daily for 35 days. Control animals received an equivalent volume of saline. After killing the animals, small pieces of kidney cortex, were fixed in ice-cold glutaraldehyde solution (4%) buffered with 0.1M cacodylate buffer, pH 7.4 for 2 hr. The samples were then washed in cacodylate buffer, and one half of the samples counterfixed in 2% osmic acid whilst the rest were put into 25% alcohol. After dehydration in the alcohol both sets of specimens were embedded in Epon 812 resin (TAAB Labs, Reading, UK). Ultra-thin sections were examined on a Phillips 400T analytical transmission electron microscope at 80Kv. The samples fixed only with glutaraldehyde were mounted on aluminium grids and either left unstained or counterstained with uranyl acetate. In order to resolve the platinum peaks by X-ray microprobe analysis it was necessary to take these precautions since osmium, copper and lead show prominent peaks which interfere with the platinum profile.

RESULTS

Homogeneity of Subcellular Fractions. Table 1 lists the percentage recoveries of marker enzymes, and protein found in the classical fractions of the kidney cortex. The highest proportion of succinate dehydrogenase and acid phosphatase were found in the 'ML' fraction, glucose-6-phosphatase and 5'-nucleotidase in the microsomal fraction and catalase in the cytosolic fraction. These relative proportions of marker enzymes and protein in the classical subfractions are similar to distributions observed with normal untreated kidney cortex (6).

TABLE 1. Percent recoveries of protein and marker enzymes in the classical subfractions of rat kidney cortex after oral administration of Cis-Pt, a) Bolus dose, 57 mg/kg, b) Daily (x28), 2 mg/kg.

	FRACTION	SDH	ACID P'	AMP'	G-6-P'	CAT	PROT
a)	'N'	12.1	9.93	16.33	19.8	3.71	14.9
	'ML'	68.1	42.42	18.39	17.23	10.80	27.5
	'MIC'	11.9	14.57	39.8	41.4	8.44	16.6
	'SUP'	1.58	21.70	8.50	4.60	78.70	30.9
a)	'N'	6.71	5.4	8.09	14.49	6.8	13.24
	'ML'	49.7	29.0	17.7	19.32	24.4	23.7
	'MIC'	20.3	15.16	43.53	46.7	15.6	16.09
	'SUP'	5.9	28.8	10.56	8.9	59.0	37.70

Rate Sedimentation of Cortical Lysosomes. Following the rate zonal sedimentation of the 'ML' fraction the distribution patterns of protein and acid phosphatase shown in Figure 1, indicate three main regions which are identified by marker enzymes. Although these enzymes are not illustrated in Fig. 1 (see Fig. 2 article), the positions of the various subcellular organelles are marked and are described in the Fig. 1 legend.

Localization of Cis-Pt Identified by Fractionation. The distribution of platinum among the subcellular fractions after either a single bolus dose

(57 mg/kg) or a daily dose (2 mg/kg) of cisplatin shows (Table 2) that the greatest proportion of platinum is associated with the 'ML' fraction (45-60%) although multiple dosing resulted in an increased proportion of platinum in the cytosolic fraction. The nuclear fraction contained the lowest concentrations of platinum after both dosage regimes. Further subfractionation of the 'ML' fraction by rate zonal sedimentation showed that the platinum was localized primarily in fractions 1-4, 13-18 and 29-30 (Fig 1). This distribution closely follows the acid phosphatase indicating a close association with the various population of lysosomes which is consistently obtained with the single and multiple doses.

TABLE 2. Distribution of platinum in subcellular fractions of the rat kidney cortex 24h after oral administration of cisplatin (cortices of six animals were pooled prior to fractionation).

FRACTION	bolus 57mg/kg Cis-Pt		daily 2mg/kg Cis-Pt	
	% recovery	Pt. conc ng/g protein	% recovery	Pt. conc ng/mg protein
Homog	–	83.05	–	64.95
'N'	9.5	53.26	8.7	43.04
'ML'	59.0	176.36	45.7	131.0
'MIC'	11.39	56.8	12.10	49.1
'SUP'	23.5	53.22	37.2	67.04

Localization of Cis-Pt Identified by X-ray Probe Analysis. Examination of kidney cortices by transmission electron microscopy revealed an abundance of lysosomes with electron dense deposits in the proximal tubules (Fig 2a). X-ray microprobe analysis of these deposits in osmium fixed samples showed that they contained a large quantity of iron but no platinum peaks could be discerned due to a masking effect by the osmium. These large iron containing lysosomes were also identified in the cortex of control animals. However, unosmicated sections of cortex, from cisplatin treated animals, also contained electron dense deposits within lysosomal-like structures (Fig 2).

By means of microprobe analysis platinum (Lα9.44 Kev, Lβ11.06 Kev), iron and also sulphur (Kα2.31 Kev), phosphorus (Kα2.01 Kev) and chlorine (2.62 Kev), were detected (Fig 3a) within these electron dense deposits, at levels higher than in the neighbouring cytosol (cell background, Fig 3b). No such platinum deposits were identified in kidney sections from control animals. X-ray microprobe analysis thus confirmed the observations of the subcellular studies that, after oral administration of cisplatin, platinum appears to be localized in lysosomes in the kidney cortex. Platinum was not detectable in mitochondria, nuclei or plasma membranes of the kidney cortical cells.

DISCUSSION

Although such an association has not been identified previously, it is clear, from the results presented here, that the kidney lysosomes are important intracellular targets after cisplatin administration. High concentrations of Pt in the 'ML' fraction of the kidney have been reported after Cis-Pt administration (9). It is not clear if the accumulation of Pt in renal lysosomes is similar to that of other metals (7). In the case

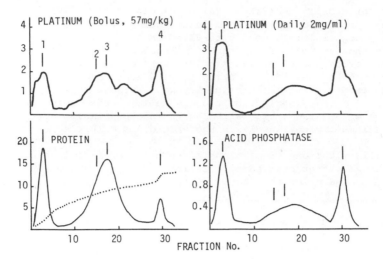

Fig. 1. Distributions of protein (mg), Acid phosphatase (um/min) and Pt (ug) after rate sedimentation of the cortical 'ML' fraction, from animals dosed with 2mg/kg Cis-Pt daily. The bolus dose pattern of Pt is from a different experiment, with virtually identical distribution of marker enzymes. The regions indicated are: 1. Sample position (unsedimentable material), 2. Peroxisomes, 3. Mitochondria, Small lysosomes, brush border membranes, 4. Large lysosomes.

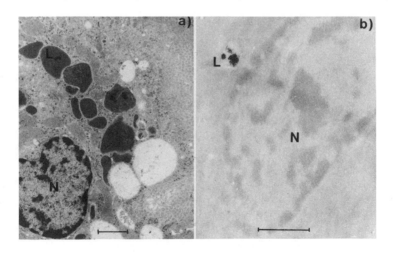

Fig. 2. Electron micrographs of kidney after multiple dosing of Cis-Pt. a) osmium fixed, counterstained section showing detailed morphology. b) section fixed only with glutaraldehyde and counterstained with uranyl acetate, showing lysosome (L) containing electron dense deposits which were analysed by electron microprobe analysis (EDX), See Fig 3a. N = Nucleus. The bar represents 1u.

of cisplatin, the association of Pt with both sulphur and phosphorus in large lysosomes may indicate mechanism of uptake which is similar to that of uranyl salts. The significance of iron in platinum rich lysosomes is unclear, but it may be irrelevant since high levels of iron were also found in kidney lysosomes of control animals.

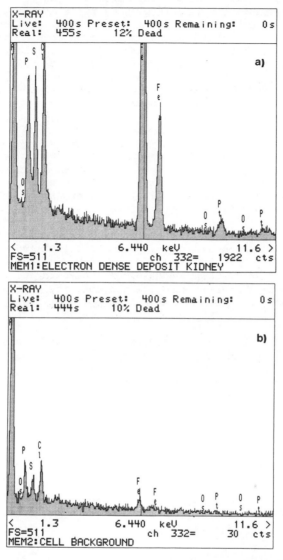

Fig. 3. EDX spectra of a) electron dense deposits found in lysosomes of rat kidney proximal tubule cells, b) cell cytoplasm adjacent to lysosomes. Spectra show element peaks at Kev values : Al; $K\alpha 1.49$ (specimen grid), P; $K\alpha 2.01$, S; $K\alpha 2.31$, Cl; $K\alpha 2.67$, Fe; $K\alpha 6.40$, Fe; $K\alpha 7.05$, Pt; $L\alpha 9.44$, Pt; $L\beta 11.06$.

It is generally accepted that the corticomedullary junction (S3 region) is the major site of both accumulation of Pt and the most prominent damage in the rat kidney (2). Since this region contains relatively few lysosomes it is possible that the deposition of Pt in lysosomes, which originate mainly from the S1 and S2 regions of the nephron, is not an important event in the nephrotoxicity and may even represent 'inactivation' of platinum. Whilst it is plausible that the association of Pt with lysosomes is not representable of the whole kidney under the experimental conditions chosen, this is not likely because the cortex (the starting material used in these studies) includes the deep cortex and thus would include most of the S3 region.

The apparent redistribution of platinum from the 'ML' to the supernatant with time (comparison of single dose with multiple dosing) could be due to induction of a cytosolic binding protein such as metallothionein. Platinum in the form of cisplatin has been shown to bind to this protein (9) although it probably does not induce its synthesis per se but may induce it by perturbing the homeostasis of zinc. Alternatively, the apparent increase in cytosolic platinum after multiple dosing could be artefactual due to the release of Pt from endosomal/lysosomal compartment whose fragility is increased by the platinum.

REFERENCES

1. Prestayko, A., D'Aoust, J., Issell, B. and Crooke, S. (1979). Cisplatin (cis-diamino-dichloroplatinum II). Cancer Treat Rev 5: 17-39.

2. Goldstein, R. and Mayor G. (1983). The nephrotoxicity of cisplatin Life Sciences 32: 685-690.

3. Barnard, C., Cleare, M. and Hydes, P. (1986). Second generation anticancer platinum compounds. Chem. Brit. 22 : 1001-1004.

4. Siddik, Z., Boxall, F., Goddard, P., Barnard, C. and Harrap, K. (1984). Antitumour, Pharmacokinetic and toxicity studies with orally administered cisplatin, CBDC and CHIP. Proc Amer Assoc Cancer Res 25: 369.

5. Binks, S. and Dobrota, M. (1986). Comparative study of cisplatin toxicity and route of administration. Biochem. Soc. Trans, 14: 694-695.

6. Andersen, K.J., Haga, H.J. and Dobrota, M. (1987). Lysosomes of the renal cortex: Heterogeneity and role in protein handling, Kidney Internat. 31: 886-897.

7. Galle, P. (1983). The role of lysosomes in the renal concentration of mineral elements. In: "Advances in Nephrology", Vol 12, eds. Hamburger, J., Crosnier, J., Grunfeld, J.P. and Maxwell, M.H. Year Book Medical Publishers, Chicago.

8. Ghadially, F.N., Lalonde, J.M.A. and Yang-Steppuhn, S. (1982). Uraniosomes produced in cultured rabbit kidney cells by uranyl acetate. Virchows Arch (Cell Pathol) 39: 21-30.

9. Sharma, R.P. and Edwards, I.R. (1983). Cis-Platinum: Subcellular distribution and binding to cytosolic ligands. Biochem. Pharmacol 32: 2665-2669.

ALPHA-METHYLGLUCOSE UPTAKE BY ISOLATED RAT KIDNEY PROXIMAL TUBULAR CELLS AS A PARAMETER FOR CELL INTEGRITY IN VITRO

P.J. Boogaard, G.J. Mulder, and J.F. Nagelkerke

Division of Toxicology, Center for Bio-Pharmaceutical Sciences, University of Leiden, P.O.Box 9503, Leiden, The Netherlands

INTRODUCTION

A large number of nephrotoxins cause damage to the proximal tubule in vivo. Many typical in vivo tubular cell functions are conserved in freshly isolated rat kidney cells (Ormstad et al., 1981; Jones et al., 1979). An advantage of the use of isolated cells as compared to the in vivo experiment is that it permits a defined quantitatively and qualitatively cellular environment, which allows study of the relationship between the concentration of a nephrotoxin, exposure time and effect. Extra-renal effects can also be excluded, thus isolated tubular cells are very suitable to study the effects of nephrotoxins which exert their effect directly at the tubular site.

One of the functions of the proximal tubular cell is the transport of solutes between blood and urine, and an early indicator of proximal tubular damage, is the excretion of glucose into the urine. We have therefore chosen glucose transport as a parameter by which damage to the proximal tubular cells may be sensitively and easily assessed. However, glucose is normally transported both into the cell at the apical side, and out again at the basolateral side; therefore it is not suitable for determination of transport in single cells.

Alpha-methylglucose (a-MG, 1-O-methyl-alpha-D-glucopyranoside) is a non-metabolizable glucose analogue, which is a substrate for the carrier for active Na^+-dependent glucose uptake at the apical membrane of the proximal tubule, but not for the carrier for facilitated transport at the basolateral site (Silvermann, 1986; Ullrich, 1986). Thus, after uptake the sugar is trapped within the cell, which allows measurement of glucose-carrier mediated transport in isolated cells.

In this paper we report the characterization of the a-MG transport in isolated renal epithelial cells, the effect of Nycodens (the density medium used in isolation of these cells) and the effects of the oncolytic agent cis-diamminedichloroplatinum (II) (CDDP) and its non-cytostatic congener trans-diamminedichloroplatinum (II) (TDDP) on a-MG transport.

METHODS AND MATERIALS

<u>Analysis and chemicals</u>.   Intracellular ATP concentrations were determined

by luciferineluciferase bio-luminescence (Kimmich et al., 1975) and protein by the method of Lowry et al. (1951).

Collagenase (from Closteridium histolyticum) was purchased from Boehringer, [U-^{14}C]-a-MG (150 mCi/mmole) and [6,6'(n)-^{3}H]- sucrose (6 Ci/mmole) from Amersham. CDDP (Cisplatin) was a gift from Dr. D. de Vos (Pharmachemie B.V.). TDDP was synthesised by the group of Dr. J. Reedijk (Dept. Inorg. Chem., Univ. of Leiden), purity was greater than 98% as determined by elemental analysis and IR- and UV-spectroscopy. Phloridzin dihydrate was purchased from Aldrich Chemical Company.

Cell Isolation.   Kidney tubular cells were isolated from male Wistar rats (250 g body weight), that had free access to food and water, by collagenase perfusion, essentially as described by Jones et al. (1979). Kidneys were perfused with 150 ml calcium-free Hanks' buffer (pH = 7.4) containing 0.5 mM EGTA and 25 mM HEPES but no albumin. The initial flow was about 12 ml/min; when all blood was removed, normally within a minute, flow rate was reduced to 7.5 ml/min. After perfusion with an additional 25 ml of this buffer, but now without EGTA, the kidneys were perfused with the same buffer containing 4 mM Ca^{2+} and 0.12 % w/v collagenase for 15 min. Following this perfusion the capsule was removed, the tissue dispersed in Hanks'-HEPES-buffer and the mixture filtered through several layers of nylon-gauze (80 mesh). After washing three times with buffer and pelleting (3 min, 85xg) the cell pellet was resuspended in 4 ml of buffer and mixed with 4 ml of a solution containing 34 % w/v Nycodens, dissolved in 6.70 mM KCl, 1.22 mM CaCl$_2$, 10.0 mM HEPES and approximately 5 mM NaOH to adjust pH to 7.40. This cell suspension (final density 1.06 g/ml, osmolality 295 mOsm/kg, pH = 7.40) was divided over 2 tubes; 1 ml incubation medium was added on top of the Nycodens layer in each tube. This was spun for 5 min at 500xg. The cells which accumulated in a small band on top of the Nycodens were carefully removed with a capillary pipette and transferred into the incubation medium.

Incubations.   The cells were (in a concentration of about 3 million cells/ml), incubated in Hanks' buffer (pH = 7.40) supplemented with 25 mM HEPES, 2.5% w/v albumin (fraction V), the same amino acids as in minimal essential medium, 11.2 mM alanine as carbon source, but no glucose, at 37°C under 95% O$_2$/5% CO$_2$, on a rotatory shaker (150 cycles/min).The cells were preincubated for 15 min, after which phloridzin, CDDP or TDDP, dissolved in the incubation buffer were added. A-MG uptake was determined after 10 min incubation in the case of phloridzin and after different times of incubation in the case of CDDP and TDDP.

Alpha-methylglucose Uptake.   In order to determine a-MG uptake 700 ìl of the incubations (about 2 million cells) were transferred into vials containing 200 ul buffer (carbogen saturated, 37°C) containing [^{14}C]-a-MG (25 uCi/mmole) and [^{3}H]-sucrose (56 uCi/mmole); the final concentrations of both sugars was 5 mM. After 2 min incubation aliquots were pipetted into 10 volumes of ice-cold Krebs-Henseleit-bicarbonate buffer and cells were separated from the medium by rapid centrifugation. They were washed three times with 10 volumes ice-cold buffer. The cells were lysed in 500 ul distilled water and the samples deproteinated by centrifugation after addition of 500 ul trichloroacetic acid (10 % w/v final concentration). The supernatant was mixed with Emulsifier Safe (Packard) and the radioactivity determined by liquid scintillation counting.

RESULTS AND DISCUSSION

Cell Isolation.   The initial cell suspension obtained after sieving and washing, was fractionated by isopycnic centrifugation using Nycodens, which is marketed as a low osmolar, non-toxic, high density medium. Dead

338

cells, debris and small fragments of undigested tissue which had passed
through the 80 mesh filter were adequately removed. Nycodens is not only
used as a low osmolar density medium but also as a renographic contrast
medium (iohexol, Omnipaque). The non-ionogenic contrast media are believed
to give no renal function impairment in contrast to the ionic (e.g.
Diatrizoate), and are in common clinical use now (Albrechtsson et al.,
1985). However recently it was shown that iohexol could impair renal
function and could, when administered i.v. to rats, cause glucosuria. We
found however that a-MG uptake was completely unaffected by Nycodens (see
below). Moreover, intracellular ATP concentrations were the same and
transmission electron microscopy did not show the typical vacuolization of
the proximal tubular cells reported after in vivo treatment with high
doses iohexol. Therefore we conclude that the use of Nycodens in
fractionating by isopycnic centrifugation is suitable for isolating rat
kidney proximal tubular cells.

Routinely, the yield was about 30 million cells per kidney. The cells had
an initial viability, as determined by Trypan blue exclusion, of 95±5%;
10±8% of the total lactate dehydrogenase initially present in the freshly
isolated cells had leaked out. The percentage of cells of proximal tubular
origin, as counted after staining for gamma-glutamyltranspeptidase
(Rutenberg et al., 1969), was greater than 80 %. After a 30 min period to
recover from isolation stress the intracellular ATP concentration
had increased from initially approximately 6 nmole/mg protein to 8±1
nmole/mg protein, which is comparable to the concentration found in intact
kidney (Soltoff, 1986). ATP remained essentially constant for at least 3
hr.

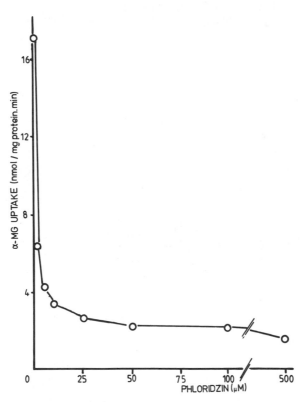

Fig. 1. Effect of phloridzin on a-MG uptake. Cells were preincubated for
10 min with the inhibitor before a-MG uptake was determined.

A-MG Uptake.   As shown in Fig. 1 a-MG uptake could be inhibited by a 10 min preincubation with phloridzin. Phloridzin is a very specific and potent competitive inhibitor of Na$^+$-dependent glucose transport (Ullrich, 1986; Silvermann, 1986); it inhibited a-MG uptake by 63$\pm$2% at a concentration of 1.0 uM and by 87$\pm$1% at 50 uM, indicating that the observed uptake is mediated by the glucose transporter. In all experiments passive diffusion was determined by including [^{3}H]-sucrose in the same incubations in order to assess the extent of non-carrier mediated uptake. The small percentage a-MG uptake which could not be inhibited by phloridzin is probably due to passive diffusion into the cells.

a-MG uptake was time and concentration dependent. Uptake was linear for at least 2 min. Apparent V_{max} and K_m were obtained by Lineweaver-Burke plots from the values measured when cells were incubated with a wide range of different concentrations a-MG. V_{max} was 4.26$\pm$0.01 nmole/mg protein/min and K_m 5.4$\pm$0.7 mM; the latter is comparable to the value obtained for the low affinity-high capacity glucose transporter in vivo (Silvermann, 1976).

a-MG uptake was not altered by the use of Nycodens. In cells isolated without further purification after washing, apparent V_{max} and K_m were 3.9$\pm$0.5 nmole/mg protein/min and 4.6$\pm$1.2 mM repectively, which do not differ significantly from values obtained with cells isolated by using Nycodens. A possible explanation for this lack of Nycodens toxicity as it was reported to occur in vivo, in our in vitro incubations might be that the cells do not take up enough of the iohexol at 4°C during the 5 min isopycnic centrifugation that we used.

To test whether a-MG uptake in isolated cells is a sensitive parameter for assessing nephrotoxicity, we used the nephrotoxic agent CDDP and its congener TDDP. As shown in Fig. 2. A and B both CDDP and TDDP inhibited a-MG uptake and decreased ATP in a time and concentration dependent

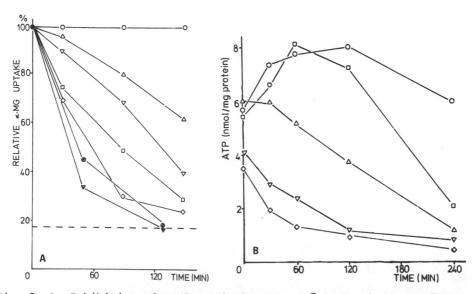

Fig. 2. A. Inhibition of a-MG uptake by CDDP (○ 0 uM, △ 100 uM, ▽ 250 uM, 500 □ uM and ◇ 1000 uM) and TDDP (● 100 uM and ▼ 500 uM). Dashed line represents passive diffusion of sucrose into the cells. Absolute a-MG uptake decreases about 20% in 2.5 hours. B. Depletion of intracellular ATP by CDDP (□ 100 uM and △ 500 uM) and TDDP (▽ 100 uM and ◇ 500 uM) compared to control (○). DDP's were added to cell suspension after 15 min preincubation.

manner. TDDP appears to be more toxic than CDDP which contrasts with in vivo observations. As trans-platinum (II) compounds generally are more reactive than the corresponding cis-isomers (Howe-Grant and Lippard, 1980), due to a smaller labilizing trans-effect of the NH_3-ligand as compared to the Cl^--ligand, TDDP binds more avidly to nucleophiles. Thus TDDP inhibits different enzymes in vitro more rapidly than does CDDP (Aull et al., 1977; McGuire et al., 1984). However, in vivo, non-specific binding to non-essential macromolecules, already in blood, may protect from toxicity. Probably our in vitro observations reflect this high reactivity of TDDP compared to CDDP. While both CDDP and TDDP are claimed not to be hepatotoxic in vivo (Leonard et al., 1971; Von Hoff et al., 1979), we found that in isolated hepatocytes TDDP (100 and 500 uM) was highly toxic as measured by lactate dehydrogenase leakage, too, while CDDP in the same concentrations showed no effect (data not shown).

CONCLUSIONS

Rat kidney tubular cells of predominant proximal origin can be isolated in high yield. These cells show active a-MG uptake which can be used as a parameter to assess cell integrity. The low-osmolar, high density medium Nycodens, also in use as renographic contrast medium, did not alter cell integrity as measured by a-MG uptake and intracellular ATP, although in vivo, renal function impairment due to this compound is reported. The nephrotoxic cytostatic agent CDDP decreased a-MG uptake in a time and concentration dependent manner.

REFERENCES

Albrechtsson U., Hultberg B., Lárusdóttir H. and Norgren L., 1985, Nephrotoxicity of ionic and non-ionic contrast media in aortofemoral angiography, Acta Radiol. Diagnosis, 26, 615-618

Aull J.L., Rice C. and Tebbets L.A., 1977, Interactions of platinum complexes with the essential and non-essential sulfhydryl groups of thymidylate synthetase, Biochemistry, 16, 672-677

Howe-Grant M.E. and Lippard S.J., 1980, Aqueous platinum (II) chemistry; binding to biological molecules. In: "Metal ions in Biological systems", Vol.11: "Metal complexes as anticancer agents", Sigel H. ed., Marcel Dekker, New York

Jones D.P., Sundby G.-B., Ormstad K. and Orrenius S., 1979, Use of isolated kidney cells for study of drug metabolism, Biochem. Pharmacol., 29, 929-935

Kimmich G.A., Randles J. and Brand J.S., 1975, Assay of picomole amounts of ATP, ADP, and AMP using the luciferase enzyme system, Anal. Biochem., 69, 187-206

Leonard B.J., Eccleston E., Jones D., Todd P. and Walpole A., 1979, Antileukemic and nephrotoxic properties of platinum compounds, Nature, 234, 43-45

Lowry O.H., Rosebrough N.J., Farr A.L. and Randau R.J., 1951, Protein measurement with the Folin phenol reagent, J. Biol. Chem., 193, 265-275

McGuire J.P., Friedmann M.E. and McAuliffe C.A., 1984, Studies of enzyme inhibition. The interaction of some platinum (II) complexes with fumarase and malate dehydrogenase, Inorg. Chim. Acta, 91, 161–165

Ormstad K., Orrenius S. and Jones D.P., 1981, Preparation and characteristics of isolated kidney cells, Meth. Enz., 77, 137–146

Rutenberg A.M., Kim H., Fishbein J.W., Hanker J.S., Wasserberg H.L. and Seligman A.M., 1969, Histochemical and structural demonstration of gamma-glutamyltranspeptidase activity, J. Histochem. Cytochem, 17, 517–525

Silvermann M., 1976, Glucose transport in the kidney, Biochem. Biophys. Acta. 457, 303–351

Silvermann M., 1986, Comparison of glucose transport mechanisms at opposing surfaces of the renal proximal tubular cell, Biochem. Cell. Biol., 64, 1092–1098

Soltoff S.P., 1986, ATP and the regulation of renal cell function, Ann. Rev. Phys., 48, 9–31

Ullrich K.J., 1986, Polarity of the proximal tubular cell: comparison of luminal and contraluminal transport systems for hexoses, dicarboxylates and sulfate, In: "Endocrine regulation electrolyte balance," Krueck F. and Thurau K. eds. p.28–35, Springer Verlag, Heidelberg

Von Hoff D.D., Schilsky R., Reichert C.M., Reddick R.L., Rozencweig M., Young R.C. and Muggis F.M., 1979, Toxic effects of cis-dichlorodiammine-platinum (II) in man, Canc. Tr. Rep., 63, 1527–1531

LIPID PEROXIDATION AS A MECHANISM OF CISPLATIN-INDUCED NEPHROTOXICITY

J. Hannemann and K. Baumann

Department of Cell Physiology, Institute of Physiology, University of Hamburg, Gzindelallee 117, D-2000 Hamburg 13, FRG

INTRODUCTION

Cisplatin (cis-platinum-II-diammine dichloride, CP), an antitumour agent against many solid tumours (1), causes as a major side-effect nephro-toxicity (2). Nephrotoxicity has an occurrence of 25-75% in humans (3), depending on single or multiple course therapy. The mechanism of the CP-induced nephrotoxicity is not well known. The administration of antioxidants or radical scavengers reduces the CP-induced nephrotoxicity in vivo (4-6). Increased in vivo production of the lipid peroxidation product malondialdehyde in the kidney after CP-treatment of the rat, has been shown very recently (5). In the present in vitro study, the effect of CP, and the combined effect of CP and antioxidants or radical scavengers on lipid peroxidation and pyruvate-stimulated gluconeogenesis in rat renal cortical slices were investigated. It has been shown that rat renal cortical slices accumulated CP manifold above the concentration in the incubation medium, involving an interaction with the organic base carrier system at the basolateral side of proximal tubular cells (7). Transport into the tubular cells across the luminal membrane seems not to be a prerequisite of CP-induced nephrotoxicity, since nonfiltering kidneys developed toxicity after CP-treatment (8), and recovery of radiolabelled CP in the urine after microinjection into early segments of proximal tubules was 94% (9). The kidney has the ability to biotransform CP intracellularly (7), but CP-metabolites have not been characterized.

METHODS

Renal cortical slices (80-120 mg), prepared from untreated male Wistar rats (220-250g) were used for in vitro incubations in a medium under 100%-O_2-atmosphere. Slices were either incubated in a 1 mg/ml CP-containing medium for different periods of time (7.5 - 300 min) or at different CP-concentrations for 3 h. In another series of experiments antioxidants and radical scavengers, (alpha-tocopherol, (+)-cyanidanol-3 or N,N'-diphenyl-p-phenylenediamine) of various concentrations were added to the CP-containing incubation medium. The medium used for control slices was free of CP in all series of experiments. Lipid peroxidation was monitored by measuring the production of malondialdehyde (MDA) in renal cortical slices, using the thiobarbituric acid (TBA)-assay (10). The MDA-concentration of the sample was calculated using an extinction coefficient of 1.56×10^{-5} M^{-1} $.cm^{-1}$. Following the incubation in the described CP-medium, pyruvate-stimulated gluconeogenesis was measured as glucose-production in a pyruvate-containing (11), CP-free medium after a subsequent 60 min incubation of the slices. Glucose was determined by using the Glucoquantest (Boehringer Mannheim, Mannheim, FRG).

RESULTS

Incubation in a medium containing 1 mg/ml cisplatin (CP) led to a time-dependent increase of MDA-production in renal cortical slices (Fig. 1), reaching a maximum of about twice as much as observed in control slices after an incubation of 300 min. More than twice as much MDA-production as observed in corresponding control slices was induced by a CP-concentration of 1.5 mg/ml in the incubation medium after 180 min (data not shown). CP led to a time-dependent decrease of pyruvate-stimulated gluconeogenesis (Fig. 2). The decrease of pyruvate-stimulated gluconeogenesis occurred after shorter periods of incubation time than the increase of MDA-production did. Incubation of renal cortical slices, using various concentrations of CP, led to a concentration-dependent increase in MDA-production and a concentration-dependent decrease in gluconeogenesis (data not shown). Anti-oxidants and radical scavengers reduced CP-induced MDA-production in a concentration-dependent manner (Fig. 3). N,N'-diphenyl-p-phenylenediamine (DPPD) was the most effective inhibitor. Alpha-Tocopherol was less effective than DPPD or (+)-cyanidanol-3. Antioxidants and radical scavengers did not reverse the CP-induced decrease of gluconeogenesis (data not shown).

DISCUSSION

Generation of free radicals and lipid peroxidation have been proposed as a mechanism of toxicity of different agents such as cephaloridine (12,13) carbon tetrachloride or paraquat. The mechanism of the nephrotoxicity of CP has been the subject of many studies, but has not been elucidated. Previous studies (4,5) have shown that administration of antioxidants or radical scavengers prior to CP administration reduces nephrotoxicity. The results of the present study show enhanced MDA-production, as a parameter of lipid peroxidation, in renal cortical slices after incubation in a CP-containing medium. Inhibition of CP-induced MDA-production by the radical scavengers and anti-oxidants alpha-tocopherol, (+)-cyanidanol-3 or DPPD suggests indirectly that CP, respectively its metabolites, induces lipid peroxidation by generation of free radicals in renal cortical slices in vitro. These results are in good agreement with data showing that in vivo MDA-production in rat kidneys by CP, can be reduced by DPPD and, less effective, by alpha-tocopherol (5).

Many different parameters of cell function have been investigated after CP-administration in vitro and in vivo, showing some contradictionary results. CP reduced tetraethylammonium (TEA)- and p-aminohippurate (PAH)-accumulation in renal cortical slices in vitro, but in vivo results of the same study did not show an effect of CP os TEA- or PAH-transport (14). In contrast another in vivo study showed a decrease of PAH-transport in renal cortical slices, isolated from CP-treated rats. The i.p. administration of CP to male F344 rats 1, 3, 5, 8, or 15 days before preparing kidney slices, did not decrease gluconeogenesis (15). In the present in vitro study under different conditions (male Wistar rats, different CP-dose directly added to the slice incubation medium) pyruvate-stimulated gluconeogenesis was investigated as a parameter of cell function. Gluconeogenesis was significantly depressed after an incubation in a CP-containing medium after a minimal incubation time of 7.5 min. CP-induced decrease of gluconeogenesis could not be altered by radical scavengers and antioxidants, indicating that there might be more than one mechanism Of CP-induced nephrotxoicity. Recent in vitro data (16) is comparable to our results, where CP-induced MDA-production and which were inhibited by radical scavengers and anti-oxidants in renal

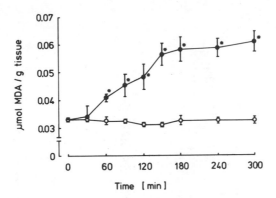

Fig. 1. Time-dependent effect of cisplatin on MDA-production. Renal cortical slices were incubated in a CP-containing medium (1 mg/ml) for different periods of time at 37°C. Symbols represent mean ± S.D, n > 4. *Significantly different (p < 0.05) from corresponding control values. (○) control (●) cisplatin 1 mg/ml.

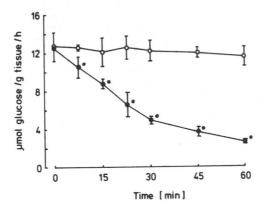

Fig. 2. Time-dependent effect of cisplatin on pyruvate-stimulated gluconeogenesis. Renal cortical slices were incubated in a CP-containing medium (1 mg/ml) for different periods of time at 37°C. Symbols represent mean ± S.D, n > 4. *Significantly different (p < 0.05) from corresponding control values. (○) control (●) cisplatin 1 mg/ml.

cortical slices. In vitro, PAH-transport (used as a parameter of cell function) recovered after i.p. injection of antioxidants prior to CP-administration (16). Preliminary in vitro results of our laboratory indicate only a slight effect of radical scavengers and anti-oxidants on CP-induced decrease of TEA- or PAH-transport in renal cortical slices. Thus, somewhat different in vitro incubation conditions seem to be the cause of partially different results in similar experiments. The determination of more than one parameter of cell function might be useful to evaluate the CP-induced nephrotoxicity under in vitro and in vivo conditions.

In conclusion, the results of the present study indicate that generation of free radicals and subsequent lipid peroxidation may participate in inducing CP-nephrotoxicity. Since the decrease of gluconeogenesis occurred earlier than the increase of MDA-production and since radical

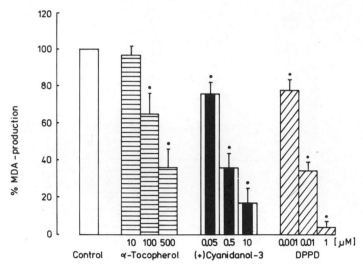

Fig. 3. Effects of antioxidants and radical scavengers on CP-induced MDA-production. Renal cortical slices were incubated for 3 h at 37°C in a medium, containing CP (1 mg/ml) in the presence and absence of one of the antioxidants or radical scavengers such as d-tocopherol, (+)-cyanidanol-3 or DPPD (N,N'-diphenyl-p-phenylenediamine) at various concentrations. The difference between the value observed after 3 h incubation in a CP-free medium and the value observed after 3 h incubation in a 1 mg/ml CP-containing medium represents the CP-induced MDA-production. This Value was used as 100% (control) to calculate the percentage of MDA-production in the presence of CP and one of the antioxidants or radical scavengers. Symbols represent mean $\pm$ S.D, n > 4. *Significantly different (p < 0.05) from corresponding control values.

scavengers and antioxidants could not inhibit CP-induced decrease of pyruvate-stimulated gluconeogenesis, the alteration of gluconeogenesis might be independent of the occurrence of lipid peroxidation.

REFERENCES

1.   L.H. Einhorn, Combination chemotherapy with cis-dichlordiammine-platinum (II) in disseminated testicular cancer. Cancer Treat. Rep., 63:1659 (1979).

2.   D.D. Choie, D.S. Longnecker and A.A. del Campo, Acute and chronic cis-platin nephropathy in rats. Lab. Invest., 44:397 (1981).

3.   R.S. Goldstein and G.H. Mayor, Minireview: The nephrotoxicity of cis-platin. Life Sci., 32:685 (1983).

4.   J.E. McGinness, P.H. Proctor, H.B. Demopoulos, J.A. Hokanson and D.S. Kirkpatrick, Amelioration of cis-platinum nephrotoxicity by orgotein (superoxide dismutase). Physiol. Chem. Physics, 10:867 (1978).

5.   K. Sugihara, S. Nakano, M. Koda, K. Tanaka, N. Fukuishi and M. Gemba, Stimulatory effect of cisplatin on production of lipid peroxidation in renal tissues. Japan. J. Pharmacol., 43:247 (1987).

6.   D.C. Dobyan, J.M. Bull, F.R. Strebel, B.A. Sunderland and R.E. Bulger, Protective effects of O-(ß-hydroxyethyl)-rutoside on cis-platinum-

induced acute renal failure in the rat. <u>Lab. Invest</u>., 55:557 (1986).

7.   R. Safirstein, P. Miller and J.B. Guttenplan, Uptake and metabolism of cisplatin by rat kidney. <u>Kidney Int</u>., 25:753 (1984).

8.   K. Miura, R.S. Goldstein, D.A. Pasino and J.B. Hook, Cisplatin nephrotoxicity: Role of filtration and tubular transport of cisplatin in isolated perfused kidneys. <u>Toxicology</u>, 44:147 (1987).

9.   R. Safirstein, J. Winston, D. Moel, S. Dikman and J. Guttenplan, Cis-platin nephrotoxicity: Insights into mechanism. <u>Int. J. Androl</u>., 10:325 (1987).

10. J.A. Buege and S.D. Aust, Microsomal lipid peroxidation. <u>Meth</u>. <u>Enzymol</u>., 52:302 (1978).

11.   A. Roobol and G.A.O. Alleyne, Control of renal cortex ammoniagenesis and its relationship to renal cortex gluconeogenesis. <u>Biochim. Biophys</u>. <u>Acta</u>, 362:83 (1974).

12.   C. Cojocel, J. Hannemann and K. Baumann, Cephaloridine-induced lipid peroxidation initiated by reactive oxygen species as a possible mechanism of cephaloridine nephrotoxicity. <u>Biochim. Biophys. Acta</u>, 834:402 (1985).

13. C. Cojocel, K.H. Laeschke, G. Inselmann and K. Baumann, Inhibition of cephaloridine-induced lipid peroxidation. <u>Toxicology</u>, 35:295 (1985).

14.   R.S. Goldstein, B. Noozdewier, J.T. Bond, J.B. Hook and G.H. Mayor, Cis-dichlorodiammineplatinum nephrotoxicity: Time course and dose response of renal functional impairment. <u>Toxicol. Appl. Pharmacol</u>., 60: 163 (1981).

15.   C.L. Litterst, M.A. Smith, J.H. Smith, M. Copley and J. Uozumi, Sensitivity of in vitro renal function tests as indicators of cis-platin-induced renal toxicity. Third International Symposium on Nephrotoxicity, Guildford, UK, 1987 (Abstract).

16.   K. Sugihara, S. Nakano and M. Gemba, Effect of cisplatin on in vitro production of lipid peroxides in rat kidney cortex. <u>Japan. J. Pharmacol</u>., 44:71 (1987).

RENAL TOXICITY OF CIS-DICHLORODIAMMINE PLATINUM IN RATS

Mirian A. Boim, Elvino J.G. Barros, Luiz A.R. Moura, Oswaldo L. Ramos and
Nestor Schor

Nephrology Division, Escola Paulista de Medicina, Rua Botucatu, 740 04023
S O Paulo, SP, Brazil

INTRODUCTION

Cis-Dichlorodiammine Platinum (DDP) is an effective anticancer agent that
changes the natural history of many tumours, especially testicular
carcinoma. However, its use in the treatment of several kinds of solid
tumours has been restricted by a high renal toxicity incidence (1-3).
Acute or chronic DDP administration in experimental models have shown an
important reduction on glomerular filtration rate but, the pathophysiological mechanism of this acute renal failure (ARF) is unclear.

The present study was undertaken to evaluate the glomerular haemodynamics
during a single dose of DDP and better characterize possible mechanisms of
ARF. A single dose of DDP (6mg/kg, ip, Bristol Laboratory, Brazil) was
given to 9 adult Munich-Wistar rats given or vehicle (n = 6). After four
days (standard diet and water ad lib.), surgery was undertaken after
inactin anaesthesia (100mg/kg, ip). The animals were placed on a
temperature regulated table and following traqueostomy, the left femoral
artery was catheterized (PE50) to measure mean arterial pressure (AP)
(Gould-Recorder-2200, Ohio, USA) and blood sampling. PE50 catheters were
also inserted into left and right jugular veins for the infusion of 10%
inulin and 2% PAH solutions and rat serum for euvolaemic conditions (4).
The left ureter was catheterized (PE10) for urine sampling and flow rate
determinations and the left kidney was prepared for micropuncture studies.

After a 45 min equilibration period, appropriate measurements and
collections for total renal function studies were performed.
Simultaneously, glomerular haemodynamics were evaluated by micropuncture
technique (4). In summary, fluid samples were obtained from surface
proximal tubules during 1-3 min from at least three nephrons. At the same
time blood was obtained from femoral artery for plasma inulin
determination by the anthrone method (5). The fluid tubular volume was
measured and the inulin concentration was determined (6), in order to
obtain the single nephron glomerular filtration rate (SNGFR). Colloid
osmotic pressure (π) of plasma pre and pos glomerular was estimated by
determination of protein concentration in afferent (C_A) and efferent (C_E)
arteriolar blood plasma, as described previously (7). With these
estimates, single nephron filtration fraction (SNFF), glomerular plasma
flow rate (Q_A), afferent (R_A), efferent (R_E), total (R_T) arteriolar
resistances and glomerular capillary ultrafiltration coefficient (K_f),
were obtained by using equations given elsewhere (8).

Hydraulic pressures were measured in superficial renal micro- structures, by a continuous recording servonull micropipette transducer system (IPM Inc, San Diego, CA, USA). Direct measurements were obtained from glomerular capillaries (PGC), proximal tubules (P_T), efferent arterioles (PEA) and peritubular capillaries (PC)

STATISTICAL ANALYSIS

Was performed by the student unpaired test. Statistical significance was defined as $p < 0.05$. All data were reported as mean$\pm$SEM.

RESULTS AND DISCUSSION.

Whole kidney function data obtained with DDP treatment using this protocol are summarized in Table 1. Both mean total glomerular filtration rate (GFR) and renal plasma flow rate (RPF) declined from 0.96 ± 0.05 to 0.33 ± 0.04 ml/min and 3.02 ± 0.34 to 0.86 ± 0.27 ml/min ($p < 0.05$), respectively with an impressive increase on total renal vascular resistance (TRVR) from 20.48 ± 2.66 to 93.25 ± 12.50 mmHg.min/ml ($p < 0.05$). Taken together with an approximate four fold increase on urinary flow rate (V'), the present protocol characterizes a non-oliguric ARF.

Table 1 - Whole kidney function data

	GFR	RPF	TRVR	V'
	...... ml/min		mmHg.min/ml	ul/min
VEHICLE	0.96[a]	3.02	20.48	3.33
	±0.05	0.34	2.66	0.32
DDP	0.33*	0.86*	93.25*	12.37*
	±0.04	0.27	12.50	2.23

a $\overline{X} \pm$ SE, *$p < 0.05$: DDP vs Vehicle group

Table 2 - Summary of glomerular haemodynamic data

	SNGFR	Q_A	SNFF	PGC	P_T	ΔP	R_A	R_E	R_T	K_f
	..nl/min..		%	..mmHg..			$\times 10^{10}$dyn.sec.cm^{-5}			nl/(s.mmHg)
VEHICLE	34[a]	106	34	46	15	31	2.5	1.3	3.8	.094
	±2	9	1	1	1	1	0.2	0.1	0.2	.010
DDP	20*	61*	33	41*	14	28*	4.7*	2.3*	7.0*	.063
	±2	6	3	1	2	1	0.5	0.3	0.4	.016

a $\overline{X} \pm$ SE, *$p < 0.05$: DDP vs Vehicle group

The glomerular haemodynamics data are depicted in Table 2. Similar to whole GFR and RPF, SNGFR and glomerular plasma flow rate (Q_A) declined from 34 ± 2 to 20 ± 2 nl/min and from 106 ± 9 to 61 ± 6 nl/min ($p < 0.05$), respectively. However, total renal function declined by 65% and single nephron data (superficial nephron) by 40%.

Since mean tubular hydraulic pressure (P_T) did not change (Table 2) and mean glomerular capillary hydraulic pressure (PGC) decreased from 46 ± 1 to 41 ± 1 mmHg (p < 0.05) and the mean transcapillary hydraulic pressure difference (ΔP) also declined. Afferent (R_A), efferent (R_E) and total arteriolar resistances (R_T) increased, mainly R_A. Although a decline in 30% on mean glomerular ultrafiltration coefficient (K_f) was observed, no statistical significance was achieved.

Haemodynamic data shows a predominant increase in mean R_A which led to a reduction on both Q_A and PGC. Since P_T was stable, no significant tubular obstruction was observed and, mean K_f was maintained. Thus, a decline on mean single nephron GFR was due to a reduction on Q_A and ΔP. Finally, since total renal function was more affected than superficial nephrons, a higher juxtamedullary nephron injury is suggested.

ACKNOWLEDGEMENTS

This work was supported by grants from FAPESP, CNPq, CAPES and IPEPENHI. The authors thank Ms. Marina Andre' da Silva for secretarial assistance.

REFERENCES

1. P.P. Choie, D.S. Longnecker and A.A. Delcampo, Acute and chronic cisplatin nephropathy in rats, Lab. Invest. 44:397 (1981).

2. P.J. Loehrer and L.H. Eihorn, Cisplatin, Ann. Intern. Med. 100:704 (1984).

3. N.E. Madias and J.T. Harrington, Platinum Nephrotoxicity, Am. J. Med. 68:307 (1978).

4. N. Schor, I. Ichikawa and B.M. Brenner, Mechanisms of action of various hormones and vasoactive substances on glomerular ultrafiltration in the rat, Kidney Int. 20:442 (1981).

5. J. Fuhr, J. Kaczmarczyk and C.D. Kruettgen, Eine eunfache colorimetrische methode zur inulinbestmung for nierenclearance-untersuchungen bei stoffwechselgesunden und diabetikern, Klin. Wochenschr, 33:729 (1955).

6. G.G. Vurek and S.E. Pegran, Fluorimetric method for the determination of nanogram quantities of inulin, Anal. Biochem. 16:409 (1966).

7. J.W. Viets, W.M. Deen, J.L. Troy and B.M. Brenner, Determination of serum protein concentration in nanoliter blood samples using fluorescamine or O-phthaladehyde, Anal. Biochem. 8:513 (1978).

8. W.M. Deen, C.R. Robertson and B.M. Brenner, A model of glomerular ultrafiltration in the rat, Am. J. Physiol. 223:1178 (1972).

UPTAKE OF CISPLATIN (^{195m}Pt) INTO LLCPK$_1$ CELLS IN THE PRESENCE OF DIETHYLDITHIOCARBAMATE (DDTC), MERCAPTOETHANESULPHATE (MESNA) AND AMILORIDE

B. Casey (1), S. McGuinness (1), I. Pratt (1), M.P. Ryan (1), C.A. McAuliffe (2) H.L. Sharma (3) and N.D. Tinker (2,3)

(1) Department of Pharmacology, University College Dublin, Ireland. (2) Chemistry Dept., University of Manchester, Institute of Science and Technology, Manchester, (3) University of Manchester, Manchester, England

INTRODUCTION

Cisplatin a platinum-containing co-ordination complex, is an effective antineoplastic agent used in the treatment of a variety of human malignancies including ovarian, testicular and small cell lung tumours. The clinical use of cisplatin (CP) is limited chiefly by dose-related-cumulative nephrotoxicity which is characterised by necrosis of the S3 segment of the proximal tubule. While CP is known to accumulate in the kidney (1), the mechanism of renal cellular accumulation is unclear although it has been suggested (2) that the drug may interact with the organic transport system in the kidney. The pars recta is notably a major site of active transport which is further support for this theory.

Non-specific protection against nephrotoxicity has been achieved in patients by vigorous hydration and diuresis before, during and after cisplatin administration leading to a reduction in the incidence and severity of nephrotoxicity (3). However, more specific agents for ameliorating CP nephrotoxicity have been reported including diethyl-dithiocarbamate (DDTC) (4), mercaptoethanesulphate (MESNA) (5) and furosemide (6). These agents may prevent the interaction of the drug with critical subcellular targets or may alter transport in to or out of kidney cells.

The aims of this study were to:-

1. Characterize the process of accumulation of ^{195m}Pt radiolabelled CP in an established renal epithelial cell line, LLCPK$_1$, derived from pig kidney which manifests transport properties of the proximal tubule (7).

2. Investigate the effects of DDTC, MESNA, and the diuretic amiloride in combination with CP in this cell culture system with a view to assessing the cytoprotective effect of these agents in vitro.

MATERIALS AND METHODS

LLCPK$_1$ cells were obtained form Flow Laboratories (Irvine, Scotland), cultured in Dulbecco's modified Eagles medium (DMEM) supplemented with 10% foetal calf serum and glutamine 2 mM (Flow, Laboratories) and maintained in an atmosphere of 9% CO_2/91% air at 37°C. Parallel experiments were performed in the absence of foetal calf serum. ^{195m}Pt-CP was a gift from Dr. H. Sharma and co-workers, University of Manchester Institute of Science and Technology, Manchester, U.K. DDTC and MESNA were obtained form Sigma Chemical Co., Poole, Dorset, U.K., while amiloride was obtained from Merck, Sharpe & Dohme Ltd., Hoddesdon, Herts., U.K.

LLCPK$_1$ cells were seeded at a density of 2×10^4 cells/well in 24-well plates. On reaching confluency (4 days) the cells were exposed to ^{195m}Pt cisplatin (5 ug/ml and 40 nCi/ml) with or without the concomitant addition of DDTC (1 mM), MESNA (5 mM) or amiloride (0.1 mM). At specified time intervals over a 48 hr time course the medium was removed and the cells washed briefly three times with a buffered salts solution. The cells were solubilised with detergent (2% SDS, 1 ml) and the samples counted in a 1282-Computagamma LKB gamma counter. Cell number per well was counted using a crystal violet stain for cell nuclei and results were expressed as CPM x 10^6.

RESULTS

Cisplatin was progressively accumulated by LLCPK$_1$ cells maintained in a serum-free medium over a 48 hr period (Table 1). Uptake of the drug was lower in the presence of serum-containing medium, a gradual increase was found over the first 8 hr, but drug accumulation levelled off thereafter in serum-containing medium (Table 1).

Table 1. Uptake of ^{195m}Pt cisplatin into LLCPK$_1$ cells in the presence and absence of serum.

^{195m}Pt uptake (cpm/10^6 cells)

TIME [hr]	Serum-containing medium	Serum-free medium
2	540±36	893±130**
4	629±32	1051±83*
8	847±100	1762±123**
12	800±112	2500±615
24	797±47	2738±941
48	833±72	4581±745*

The results shown are mean values±s.e.m. * = $p < 0.01$; ** = $p < 0.005$. Asterisks indicate significant difference from uptake in serum-containing medium.

DDTC markedly stimulated the uptake of CP in serum-free and, to a lesser extent, in serum-containing medium (Table 2). Levels of CP in cells in the presence of DDTC were 10-fold (serum-containing medium) to 40-fold (serum-free medium) those found in the absence of DDTC.

Although CP levels in the cells in the presence of MESNA increased over 48 hr in serum-free medium the uptake was lower than that found in the absence of MESNA (Table 2). Uptake of CP was essentially unaltered by the inclusion of MESNA in serum-containing medium. Amiloride had little effect (on the uptake of CP over a 2 hr period (data not shown). At longer time intervals (12-48 hr) accumulation of CP occurred in the presence of amiloride in both serum-containing and serum-free medium. This accumulation was significantly higher· than with CP alone in serum-containing medium, but markedly reduced in serum-free medium (Table 2).

Cell replication in the presence of MESNA and CP at 24 hr was essentially similar to that in controls, was 75% of control in the presence of DDTC and CP and 65% of control in the presence of amiloride. Similar results were obtained at 48 hr, although the cytoprotective effects of MESNA and

Table 2. Uptake of ^{195m}Pt-cisplatin into $LLCPK_1$ cells after a 48 hour exposure period in the presence or absence of cytoprotectants.

^{195m}Pt uptake (CPM/10^6 cells)

Medium	CP (5ug/ml)	DDTC (1 mM)	MESNA (5 mM)	Amiloride (0.1 mM)
Serum (a) containing	833±72	8828±475*	882±43	1292±165*
Serum (b) free	4581±745	14998±1407**	1481±43*	1744±103*

The results showm are mean values± s.e.m.
* = p < 0.05; ** = p < 0.01. Asterisks indicate significant difference from CP alone.

DDTC were less marked and amiloride had no protective effect (Table 3). The addition of metabolic inhibitors (KCN/iodoacetate) did not reduce the uptake of CP over a 2 hr period (data not presented), and appreciable cell death did not occur over this period (Table 3).

Table 3. Effect of cisplatin on replication of $LLCPK_1$ cells in the presence or absence of cytoprotectants in serum-containing medium.

Cell number x 10^6/well

Time (hours)	Control	CP (5ug/ml)	DDTC (1 mM)	MESNA (5 mM)	Amiloride (0.1 mM)
24	80.8+2.1	24.0±1.2**	61.8±7.2*	74.0±9.4	52.6±7.0*
48	90.4±3.1	25.2±3.1**	54.1±3.6*	62.4±2.9	36.2±3.9

The results shown are mean values±s.e.m.
* p = < 0.05; ** p = <0.01. Asterisks indicate significant difference from control.

DISCUSSION

CP uptake into $LLCPK_1$ cells appeared to occur by passive diffusion as evidenced by a gradual increase in drug uptake which continued in the presence of metabolic inhibitors. The presence of serum in the culture medium reduced the cellular uptake of CP in vitro, which agrees with in vivo observations that CP binds extensively to a variety of plasma proteins (8).

DDTC reduced the antimitotic effect of CP on $LLCPK_1$ cells in culture although it did not reduce the accumulation of CP. DDTC has proven to afford protection against CP nephrotoxicity in experimental animals (4), but from our study it appears not to exert its cytoprotective effect in culture by decreasing cellular uptake. This suggests an alternative mechanism of action which remains to be elucidated further.

MESNA also reduced the antimitotic effect of CP on $LLCPK_1$ cells in culture which could be attributed to the reduction of CP accumulation in the cells. This observed decrease may be due to chelation of the heavy metal complex CP with this sulphydryl-containing compound. Renal damage has been (5) prevented in experimental animals using this highly reactive thio compound .

Although amiloride reduced the accumulation of CP in serum-free medium a
similar reduction was not observed in serum-containing medium and only a
very slight reduction in the antimitotic effect of CP on LLCPK$_1$ cells in
culture was observed. Amiloride therefore did not exert a cytoprotective
effect on LLCPK$_1$ cells exposed to CP and this correlates with our
observations that amiloride does not reduce CP nephrotoxicity in vivo
despite its diuretic action (9).

ACKNOWLEDGEMENTS

This work was supported by a grant from the St. Luke's Hospital Cancer
Research Fund.

REFERENCES

1. Litterst, C.L., 1981, Alterations in the toxicity of cisdichloro-
diammine platinum II and in tissue localization of platinum as a function
of NaCl concentration in the vehicle of administration. Toxicol. Appl.
Pharmacol., 61:99-108.

2. Safirstein, R., Miller, P. and Guttenplan, J.B., 1984, Uptake and
metabolism of cisplatin by rat kidney. Kidney Int., 25:753-758.

3. Hayes, D.M., Cvitkovic, E., Golbey, R.B., Scheiner, E., Helson, L.,
Krakoff, I.H., 1977, High dose cisplatinum diammine dichloride. Cancer,
39:1372.

4. Borch, R.F., Pleasants, M.E., 1979, Inhibition of nephrotoxicity by
diethyldithiocarbamate rescue in a rat model. Proc. Natl. Acad. Sci. USA.,
76:12:6611-6614.

5. Kempf, S.R., Ivankovic, S., Wiessler, M., Schmahl, D., 1985, Effective
prevention of the nephrotoxicity of cisplatin (CDDP) by administration of
sodium 2-mercaptoethane-sulfonate (MESNA) in rats. Br. J. Cancer., 52:937-
939.

6. Ward, J.M., Crabin, M.E., Berlin, E., Young, D.M., 1977, Prevention of
renal failure in rats receiving cisdiamminedichloroplatinum (II) by
administration of furosemide. Cancer Res., 37:1238-1240.

7. Rabito, C.A., 1986, Occluding junctions in a renal cell line (LLCPK$_1$)
with characteristics of proximal tubular cells., Am. J. Physiol. 250:F734-
F743.

8. De Conti, R.C., Toftness, B.R., Lange, R.C., Creasey, W.A., 1973,
Clinical and pharmacological studies with cisdiamminedichloroplatinum
(II). Cancer Res., 33:1310-1315.

9. Ormond, T., McGuinness, S., Pratt, I., Ryan, M.P., McAuliffe, C.A.,
Sharma, H.L., Tinker, N.D., The effect of amiloride on cisplatin induced
nephrotoxicity and the renal uptake of (^{195m}Pt) cisplatin in male Wistar
rats (this volume).

THE EFFECT OF AMILORIDE ON CISPLATIN INDUCED NEPHROTOXICITY AND THE RENAL UPTAKE OF (^{195m}Pt) CISPLATIN IN MALE WISTAR RATS

T. Ormond (1), S. McGuinness (1), I. Pratt (1), M.P. Ryan (1), C.A. McAuliffe (2), H.L. Sharma (3) and N.D. Tinker (2,3). (1) Department of Pharmacology, University College Dublin, Ireland, (2) Chemistry Department, University of Manchester, Institute of Science and Technology, Manchester, and (3) University of Manchester, Manchester, England

INTRODUCTION

Cisplatin is an effective antineoplastic agent. Its clinical use is complicated by nephrotoxicity, (Goldstein et al., 1981) hypomagnesaemia and inappropriate renal magnesium wasting (Shilsky et al., 1979). Co-administration of diuretics decreases the general nephrotoxicity, but may exacerbate the magnesium wasting. Amiloride is a potassium and magnesium sparing diuretic (Devane and Ryan, 1983) which theoretically may overcome the cisplatin induced nephrotoxicity and magnesium loss. The purpose of this study was to evaluate the effect of amiloride on:-

i) cisplatin induced nephrotoxicity and
ii) renal, hepatic, plasma and urinary concentrations of (^{195m}Pt) cisplatin in male Wistar rats.

METHODS

A) In order to assess the effect of amiloride on cisplatin-induced nephrotoxicity rats received a single dose of cisplatin (CP, 6 mg/kg i.p., Sigma Chemical Co., Poole, Dorset). Amiloride (2.5 mg/kg i.p., Merck, Sharpe & Dohme Ltd.) was given 1 hr prior and 24 hr after CP, and animals were killed on day 5 after dosing. Indices of nephrotoxicity included blood urea nitrogen, kidney:body weight ratio and in vitro uptake of tetraethylammonium bromide (TEA) into slices of renal cortex from treated rats.

B) Two separate studies on the distribution of ^{195m}Pt-CP in rat tissues were carried out; one at 24 hr (n = 6 per group) and the other at 96 hr (n = 4 per group) after dosing. Radiolabelled CP (a gift from Dr. H.L. Sharma, Department of Medical Biophysics, UMIST, Manchester, U.K.) was given as a single i.p. injection (6 mg/kg) to all rats and one group at each time interval also received amiloride (2.5 mg/kg) one hr prior to CP. Animals were housed in metabolism cages and urine was taken at 6 and 12 hr intervals. Animals were killed at 24 or 96 hr. Samples of urine, plasma, liver and one kidney cortex from each rat were analysed for radioactivity in a 1282-Compugamma universal gamma counter to determine distribution of ^{195m}Pt-cisplatin. The remaining kidney cortex was processed to determine the amount of ^{195m}Pt-CP covalently bound in the kidney. Results for tissue distribution studies are expressed as cpm x 10^4/g tissue wet weight and covalently-bound CP is expressed as cpm/mg protein.

357

RESULTS

A) The nephrotoxicity of cisplatin was evidenced by significant increases in blood urea nitrogen ($p < 0.01$) and increased kidney:body weight ratios ($p < 0.01$) (Table 1). Amiloride treatment did not lessen the nephrotoxicity as measured by these indices (Table 1), and in the case of ^{14}C-TEA uptake into renal slices there was an indication of increased nephrotoxicity in the cisplatin and amiloride-treated group (Table 1).

Table 1. The effect of amiloride on cisplatin-induced nephrotoxicity

Index	Control	Cisplatin	Amiloride	Amiloride+Cisplat
Blood urea nitrogen (mg/dl)	59.7±12.1	255.0±13.4**	62.6±9.9	250.0±8.0**
Kidney wt: Body wt ratio (x10^{-3})	8.9±0.1	11.5±0.3**	9.3±0.4	12.6±0.5**
^{14}C-TEA uptake slice:medium ratio	15.9±2.4	11.5±1.6	N.D.	9.8±1.2*

* $p < 0.05$; ** $p < 0.005$; N.D. not determined.

B) Levels of ^{195m}Pt-cisplatin were significantly higher ($p < 0.01$) in the kidneys and plasma of amiloride co-treated animals compared with those in animals receiving CP alone, 24 hr after dosing. There was no significant difference in the levels of CP in liver tissue in the two groups (Table 2).

Table 2. The effect of amiloride on plasma, hepatic and renal ^{195m}Pt cisplatin and on the covalent binding of ^{195m}Pt in the renal cortex at 24 hours.

Treatment	Plasma (cpm/ml)	Liver	Renal cortex (cpm x 10^4/g)	Covalently bound (cpm/mg protein)
Cisplatin (6 mg/kg)	10543±364	7.16±0.31	23.7±0.5	1016±112
Cisplatin (6 mg/kg) and Amiloride (2.5 mg/kg)	12076±160	7.96±0.25	27.0±0.8	1078±111
	P<.01	N.S.	P<.01	N.S.

At 96 hr and following a second booster dose of amiloride, the levels of ^{195m}Pt-cisplatin were still higher in the kidneys of rats co-treated with amiloride compared with those in rats receiving CP alone ($p < 0.02$) (Table 3). The levels in plasma were also higher ($p < 0.01$; Table 3) and there was an increase in covalently bound ^{195m}Pt-cisplatin in the renal cortex of amiloride co-treated rats ($p < 0.05$, Table 3). As with the 24 hr study, there was no significant difference in the levels of CP in the liver.

CONCLUSIONS

It has been suggested that cisplatin accumulation by the kidney may

Table 3. The effect of amiloride on plasma, hepatic and renal ^{195m}Pt cisplatin and on the covalent binding of ^{195m}Pt in the renal cortex at 4 days.

Treatment	Plasma (cpm/ml)	Liver (cpm x 10^4/g)	Renal cortex	Covalently bound (cpm/mg protein)
Cisplatin (6 mg/kg)	3268±167	5.83±0.16	15.8±0.11	729±42
Cisplatin (6 mg/kg) and Amiloride (2.5 mg/kg)	4271±126	6.36±0.13	18.4±0.76	1025±112
	$P < 0.01$	N.S.	$P < 0.02$	$P < 0.05$

involve a specific interaction with the organic base transport system (Safirstein et al., 1984). Amiloride is a magnesium sparing diuretic that is secreted into the proximal tubule via the organic base transport system (Baer, et al., 1967). By virtue of these two facts and because it is a diuretic it seemed likely that amiloride might prevent the cisplatin induced nephrotoxicity by reducing the renal accumulation of the drug. These data however suggest that the converse is true and that:-

1) co-administration of amiloride does not prevent cisplatin nephrotoxicity in rats;
2) amiloride co-treatment leads to prolonged retention of cisplatin in the kidney and
3) competition between cisplatin and amiloride for transport from the proximal renal cell into the tubular lumen could lead to prolonged renal retention of cisplatin resulting in increased nephrotoxicity.

ACKNOWLEDGEMENTS

This work was supported by the Health Research Board of Ireland.

REFERENCES

Baer, J.E., Jones, C.B., Spitzer, S.A. and Russo, H.F. (1967). The potassium-sparing and natriuretic activity of N-amidino-3-5-diamino-6-chloropyrazinecarboxamide hydrochloride dihydrate (amiloride hydro-chloride). J. Pharmacol. Exp. Ther. 157:472-485.

Devane, J. and Ryan, M.P. (1983). Evidence for a magnesium-sparing action by amiloride during renal clearance studies in rats. Br. J. Pharmac., 79:891-896.

Goldstein, R.S., Noordewier, B., Bond, J.T., Hook, J. and Mayor, G.H. (1981). cis-Dichlorodiammineplatinum nephrotoxicity time course and dose response of renal functional impairment. Toxicol. Appl. Pharmacol., 60:163-175.

Safirstein, R., Miller, P., and Guttenplan, J.B. (1984). Uptake and metabolism of cisplatin by rat kidney. Kidney Int. 25:753-758.

Schilsky, R.L. and Anderson, T. (1979). Hypomagnesemia and renal magnesium wasting in patients receiving cisplatin. Ann. Int. Med., 90:929-931.

THE RESPONSE OF THE PIG KIDNEY TO A COMBINATION OF CISPLATIN AND IRRADIATION

M.E.C. Robbins, M. Robinson, M. Rezvani and J.W. Hopewell

CRC Normal Tissue Radiobiology Research Group, (University of Oxford) Research Institute, Churchill Hospital, Headington, Oxford OX3 7LJ, UK

INTRODUCTION

Cis-dichlorodiammine platinum II, or cisplatin (c-DDP), has become one of the principal chemotherapeutic agents in the treatment of some solid tumours, particularly testicular (1) and ovarian cancers (2). A primary factor limiting its use is the associated nephrotoxicity (3). The majority of patients with advance ovarian carcinoma who enter remission after treatment with cisplatin only maintain this state for a relatively short period of time. This appears to be a result of the presence of residual micro-metastic disease. Radiotherapy treatment involving the irradiation of the whole abdomen might increase the prospects of cure in these patients, but might also result in increased nephrotoxicity.

Increase renal damage following c-DDP administration combined with renal irradiation has been reported in the mouse (4). However, there is a need for additional experimental systems to define further the interaction between c-DDP and radiation on renal function. The effects of single and fractionated doses of radiation on the pig kidney have been well documented (5,6) and the effects of c-DDP on the pig kidney have also been reported (7). In the present study the response of the pig kideny to c-DDP followed by irradiation was investigation.

MATERIALS AND METHODS

Twelve mature female Large White pigs, approximately 10 months of age, were used. Of these, seven received c-DDP four weeks prior to the irradiation of the right kidney while the remaining five animals received irradiation alone. Prior to the infusion of single dose of c-DDP (2.5 mg/kg body weight) pigs were hydrated with two litres of saline, administered via an ear vein. c-DDP was then given mixed with one litre of saline to which an anti-emetic agent (Maxolon, 100 mg) had been added. A further litre of saline was subsequently administered i.v.

Prior to, and four weeks after c-DDP administration, individual kidney glomerular filtration rate (GFR) and effective renal plasma flow (ERPF) was assessed using ^{99m}Tc-DTPA diethylene triamine-penta-acetic acid) and ^{131}I-hippuran renography (6). Over this period weekly blood samples were taken from 3 of the pigs. These samples were analysed to determine the haematocrit (Hct), haemoglobin (Hb) and the total red blood cell count (RBC).

The right kidney was irradiated with a single dose of 11.9Gy of ^{60}Co gamma-rays at a dose-rate of 0.7Gy/min (SSD 72cm). All experimental studies were carried out under anaesthesia, maintained with a gas mixture of 2-3% halothane, 30% nitrous oxide and 70% oxygen. At intervals of 2, 4, 6, 8, 12, 16, 20 and 24 weeks following irradiation renal function was determined by ^{99m}Tc-DTPA and ^{131}I-hippuran renography.

RESULTS

Effects of c-DDP on renal function. Although the majority of pigs appeared to tolerate c-DDP administration reasonably well, two animals appeared unwell 4 days after drug treatement; both of these animals died within 9 days. The exact cause of death was not determined. The percentage changes in total renal haemodynamics in the 5 surviving animals four weeks after c-DDP treatment are shown in Fig. 1. Most animals showed a reduction in both GFR and ERPF; the mean reduction in GFR (36.2 ± 18.9%) was more pronounced than for ERPF (12.6 ± 19.4%), but this difference was not significant ($p > 0.55$). In three pigs the Hct, HB and RBC count was determined at weekly intervals after the infusion of c-DDP. Changes in the haematological status of these animals are shown in Table 1. Fourteen days after the infusion of c-DDP the Hct, HB and RBC counts were reduced and despite some evidence for recovery at 21 days all three haematological parameters were still reduced four weeks after c-DDP administration.

Effect of irradiation on renal function. The time-related changes in individuals kidney GFR and ERPF in animals receiving c-DDP followed by 11.9Gy to the right kidney and those pigs receiving c-DDP prior to irradiation had a reduced renal function relative to those receiving irradiation alone, changes in individuals kidney GFR and ERPF after irradiation were expressed as a percentage of the pre-irradiation values. Pigs in which only the right kidney was irradiated showed a marked increase in GFR on both the irradiated and the contralateral unirradiated kidney after 2 weeks. By 4 weeks after irradiation irradiated kidney GFR had fallen below the pre-irradiated value and there was little significant change in renal function between then and 20 weeks. There was a suggestion of some recovery in function at 24 weeks, but this did not prove to be statistically significant ($p > 0.1$).

Table 1. Time-related changes in haematocrit (Hct), haemoglobin (HB) and red blood cell counts (RBC) in oigs receiving a single dose of 2.5 mg/kg body weight of c-DDP. (* S.E.; PT = pre-treatment).

Time after drug (days)	Hct (%)	Hb (g/dl)	RBC ($\times 10^{12}$/l)
PT	31.90 ± 0.79*	11.07 ± 0.63	5.85 ± 0.13
7	31.84 ± 0.85	11.13 ± 0.59	5.90 ± 0.10
14	27.97 ± 1.04	9.57 ± 0.43	4.99 ± 0.16
21	30.57 ± 2.66	10.13 ± 0.73	5.14 ± 0.72
28	23.90 ± 0.95	8.30 ± 0.64	4.29 ± 0.29

In pigs receiving c-DDP prior to irradiation there was no hyperaemic response 2 weeks after irradiation; moreover, irradiated kidney GFR fell markedly between 2 and 4 weeks to values significantly lower ($p < 0.05$) than those seen in pigs receiving irradiation alone. This increase in the severity of damage in c-DDP treated animals was maintained until 24 weeks after irradiation. From 4-24 weeks after irradiation GFR in the unirradiated kidneys increased linearly with time. The GFR in the

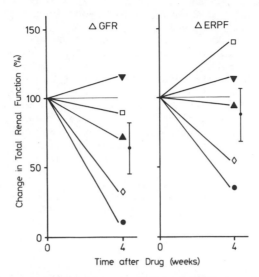

Figure 1. Percentage modification in GFR and ERPF in pigs (n = 5) 4 weeks after the infusion of c-DDP (2.5 mg/kg body weight). Each animal is represented by a separate symbol. Error bar represents mean percentage change ± S.E.

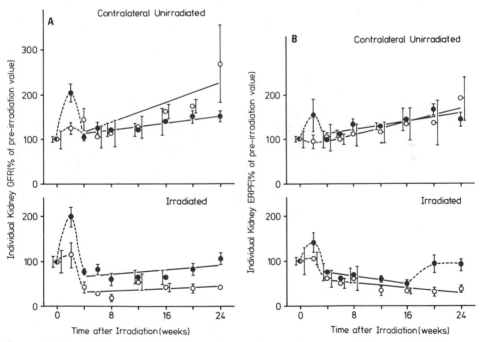

Figure 2. Time-related changes in individual kidney GFR and ERPF in pigs receiving c-DDP followed by 11.9Gy of gamma-rays (o) or 11.9Gy of gamma-rays along (●) to the right kidney (lower panel). The corresponding values for the unirradiated kidneys in the same animals are also given (upper panel). The solid lines represent data points fitted by linear regression analysis. Error bars represent mean ± S.E.

unirradiated kidney of c-DDP treated animals increased at a greater rate than in those pigs which did not received c-DDP (p < 0.05).

The changes observed in individual kidney ERPF were similar to those described for GFP. In pigs receiving irradiation along there was a 50% increase in ERPF in both kidneys 2 weeks after irradiation. This was followed by a decrease in irradiated kidney ERPF at 4 weeks, declining to 50% of the pre-irradiation value by 16 weeks. At 20-24 weeks after irradiation there appeared to be some significant recovery in function (p < 0.05). Animals that received c-DDP before irradiation exhibited no increase in ERPF 2 weeks after irradiation. Moreover, ERPF declined progressively between 4 and 24 weeks after irradiation, with no evidence of any recovery in function. In the contralateral unirradiated kidney the ERPF increased linearly with time from four weeks after irradiation of the other kidney. However, there appeared to be no significant difference (p > 0.1) in the rate of increase irrespective of whether or not the pigs had received c-DDP before irradiation of the right kidney.

DISCUSSION

The results of the present study indicate that a single dose of 2.5mg/kg body weight of c-DDP produced a reduction in total GFR and ERPF in the Large White pig, although the severity of this effect was variable. A c-DDP dose of 2.5mg/kg has previously been reported to be a 'Pharmacological dose' in the Landrace pig (7). However, as two out of the seven pigs in the present study died after this dose. The Large White pig would seem to be more sensitive to the effects of c-DDP than pigs of the Landrace strain.

Although the exact cause of death in the above two pigs was not determined, both showed a marked reduction in their RBC, Hb and Hct levels, and there was evidence of gastrointestinal haemorrhage at post-mortem. A significant reduction in the RBC count, Hb and Hct was also found in a small representative group of the surviving animals. Similar cisplatin-induced haematological toxicity has been reported in the rat (8), and leucopenia, anaemia and thrombocytopenia are commonly associated with c-DDP toxicity in patients. The underlying cause of c-DDP-induced anaemia dose not appear to be the lysis of erythrocytes, as assessed from osmotic fragility test on the RBC's of the rat (8). Furthermore, a depression of erythropoietic activity is unlikely to account for the severe anaemia since this would develop more slowly because of the relatively long mean life span of red blood cells (42 days) in the pig. Siddik (8) concluded that thrombocytopenia was the most probable cause of platinum compound-induced anaemia, which would arise as a result of internal haemorrhaging. It is interesting to note that both pigs which died following c-DDP treatment exhibited evidence of internal haemorrhage, suggesting that the mechanisms of cisplatin-induced anaemia may be similar in the pig. Thus c-DDP appears to have similar biological properties in differing animal systems. Further support for this suggestion is the finding that the reduction in renal haemodynamics observed after c-DDP was quantitatively greater in terms of GFR and ERPF. A similar result was obtained for the rat (9).

The time-course for the changes in renal function following the administration of c-DDP have been investigated in both clinical and experimental studies. Patients treated with a single dose of c-DDP (3-5mg/kg) showed a transient increase in serum creatinine levels up to approximately seven days after infusion, followed by a return to pre-treatment levels by 16-20 days (10). Gonzales-Vitale (11) reported similar findings in patients who received several courses of drug treatment, in that in six out of seven patients, an elevation of blood urea nitrogen and serum creatinine levels occurred with a peak evident at six days after each treatment. A similar time-course of c-DDP-induced reduction in renal function has been reported in the dog (12). A limitation of all these studies was the use of relatively insensitive parameters for measuring decrements in renal function. More extensive studies in rodents (4,9), using radionuclide techniques to determine changes in both GFR and ERPF, have confirmed the earlier findings. However, these more recent studies have suggested that the time required for renal function to return to 'control level' appears to be longer than was originally believed. Stewart (4) have reported that after low doses of c-DDP recovery of function can take up to 10 weeks. Thus it can be concluded that the maximum reduction in renal function elicited by c-DDP occurs within the first week of treatment; this is followed by a dose-dependent recovery which can take several weeks. Although there is as yet no information with regard to this in the pig, it seems likely that the time-course for changes in renal function will be similar.

Thus prior treatment with c-DDP enhanced the radiation-induced reduction in individual kidney GFR and ERPF. The reduction in renal haemodynamics in the irradiated kidney of pigs which received c-DDP prior to irradiation appeared greater than that found in pigs receiving irradiation alone. This finding was supported by the observation that the compensatory increase in GFR noted in the contralateral unirradiated kidney of c-DDP treated pigs was greater than that found in the unirradiated kidneys of animals which did not receive c-DDP. The question raised by these observation is whether or not this enhanced reduction in renal function is the result of an additive or a supra-additive toxicity. In order to answer this question comprehensively it would be necessary to have information on the effects of c-DDP on renal function over a time-period similar to that used in the post-irradiation study i.e. 24 weeks. This information is not available. However, in view of the results from other studies in which the time-course of c-DDP treated pigs had occurred in the four week interval allowed between administration of the drug and the subsequent irradiation of the right kidney. If this was the case, then the enhanced reduction in renal haemodynamics in the c-DDP treated pigs had occurred in the four week interval allowed between administration of the drug and the subsequent irradiation of the right kidney. If this was the case, then the enhanced reduction in renal haemodynamics following irradiation of the right kidney is indicative of supra-additive toxicity. These findings contradict results of investigations in the mouse, where additive rather than supra-additive renal injury following irradiation of c-DDP treated kidneys was reported (4). More information is required from experimental studies before this question of additive versus supra-additive toxicity can be resolved. These initial findings suggest that the pig may be a useful model in which to investigate the nephrotoxicity of c-DDP in combination with radiation.

REFERENCES

1. L.H. Einhorn and J. Donohue, Cis-diammineodichloroplatinum, vinblastine and bleomycin combination chemotherapy in disseminated testibular cancer, Ann. Intern. Med. 87:293 (1977).

2. E. Wiltshaw and T. Kroner, Phase II study of cis-dichlorodiammine-platinum (II) in advanced adenocarcinoma of the ovary, Cancer Treat. Rep. 60:55 (1976).

3. A.H. Calvert, Clinical applications of platinum metal complexes, In: "Biochemical Mechanisms of Platinum Antitumor Drugs", eds. D.C.H. McBrien and T.F. Slater, IRL Press, Oxford (1986).

4.   F. Stewart, S. Bohlken, A. Begg and H. Bartelink, Renal damage in mice after treatment with cisplatinum alone or in combination with X-irradiation, Int. J. Radiat. Oncol. Biol. Phys. 1:61 (1975).

6.   M.E.C. Robbins, J.W. Hopewell and Y. Gunn, Effects of single doses of X-rays on renal function in unilaterally irradiated pigs, Radiother. Oncol. 4:143 (1985).

7.   A.M. Cupak and J. Vorlicek, Isotope nephrography in the study of cisplatin nephrotoxicity in pigs. Vet. Med. Praha. 27:541 (1982).

8.   Z.H. Siddik, F.E. Boxall and K.R. Harrap, Haematological toxicity of carboplatin in rats, Brit. J. Cancer 55:375 (1987).

9.   H.T.M. Jongejan, A.P. Provoost, E.D. Woolf and J.C. Molenaar, Nephrotoxicity of cis-platin comparing young and adult rats, Ped. Res. 20:9 (1986).

10. D.M. Hayes, E. Cvitokovic, R.B. Golbey, E. Scheiner, L. Helson and I.H. Krakoff, High-dose cis-platinum diammine dichloride, Cancer 39:1372 (1977).

11. J.C. Gonzalez-Vitale, D.M. Hayes, E. Cvitokovic and S. Sternberg, The renal pathology in clinical trials of cis-platinum (II) diammine dichloride, Cancer 39:1362 (1977).

12. E. Cvitokovic, J. Spaulding, V. Bethune, J. Martin and W.F. Whitmore, Improvement of cis-dichlorodiamminediplatinum (NSC-119875) : Therapeutic index in an animal model, Cancer 39:1357 (1977)

THE EFFECT OF ACETAZOLAMIDE AND FUROSEMIDE ON LITHIUM CLEARANCE AND CISPLATIN NEPHROTOXICITY IN THE RAT

H. T. Heidemann, L. Gjessing, K.-H. Brune, and E.E. Ohnhaus

I. Medizinische Klinik der Christian-Albrechts-Universitat, D-2300 Kiel 1, Federal Republic of Germany

INTRODUCTION

The clinical use of cisplatin is limited because of its potential nephro-toxicity. Diuretics such as acetazolamide or furosemide are known to decrease cisplatin nephrotoxicity (Osman et al., 1984; Heidemann et al., 1985). Since mannitol 5% and glucose 30% also have beneficial effects on cisplatin-induced kidney failure (Pera et al., 1979; Heidemann, unpublished data) the question arose whether intratubular dilution of cisplatin in the proximal tubules might contribute to the observed protection. It was therefore the aim of this study to compare the lithium clearance during diuretic treatment at the time of cisplatin administration with the kidney function after 5 days.

METHODS

The bladder of Wistar rats (230-280g) were cannulated with silastic tubing under Nembutal anaesthesia (60 mg/kg ip) 3 days before the experiment. At the time of the experiment all rats were kept in individual metabolic cages to collect urine. The animals were divided into three groups and received the following treatments:

```
Vehicle (saline)             + cisplatin (5 mg/kg iv)
Acetazolamide (25 mg/kg iv)  + cisplatin (5 mg/kg iv)
Furosemide (10 mg/kg iv)     + cisplatin (5 mg/kg iv)
```

After administration of lithium (0.6 mmol/kg orally) a glucose 5% infusion (6 ml/hr) was started. After 1 hr of equilibrium two 1-hr urine samples were collected and a blood sample was taken in the middle of the collecting periods to measure haematocrit, sodium, potassium, creatinine, BUN and lithium. Acetazolamide, furosemide or vehicle were injected after the first hour of urine sampling, 5 min before the cisplatin. Thereafter the urine was collected for another 1 hr. On day 4/5 after the cisplatin administration the animals again were housed in metabolic cages to collect 24-hr urines. Blood samples were taken in the middle of the collecting periods. Sodium, potassium, creatinine, BUN and haematocrit were measured in the serum and sodium, potassium and creatinine in the urine. Student's t-test for unpaired data was used to compare the groups, where $p < 0.05$ was considered significant.

RESULTS

Cisplatin nephrotoxicity could be observed 5 days after the drug administration. The serum creatinine concentrations were significantly elevated (Fig. 1) and creatinine clearances were significantly reduced compared to the vehicle treated rats (0.14±0.04 versus 0.55±0.04 ml/min/100g). Pre-treatment with either acetazolamide or furosemide significantly decreased cisplatin nephrotoxicity (Fig. 1).
The creatinine clearance was 0.28±0.05 ml/min/100g in the acetazolamide group and 0.17±0.03 ml/min/100g in the furosemide group. The pre-treatment serum concentrations of creatinine, BUN, sodium and potassium as well as the haematocrit are shown in Table 1. They were all within the normal range and no differences existed between the different groups. Acetazolamide and furosemide significantly increased urine volume and sodium excretion (Table 1). Cisplatin had no effect on the lithium clearance (Table 2). Acetazolamide and furosemide caused an increase of the lithium clearance (Table 2). The delta-lithium clearance of the rats treated with acetazolamide was significantly higher than in the animals treated with furosemide (Fig. 1). The correlation factor of the reciprocal of the serum creatinine concentrations 5 days after the cisplatin administration and the delta-lithium clearance at the time of cisplatin administration was 0.62 (p < 0.01).

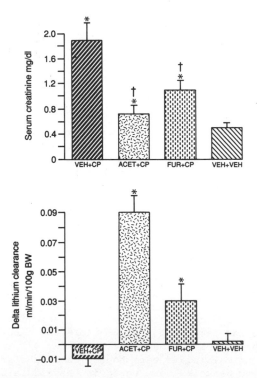

Fig. 1. The effect of acetazolamide, furosemide and vehicle on cisplatin nephrotoxicity measured as serum creatinine. The effect of acetazolamide, furosemide and vehicle on lithium clearance at the time of cisplatin administration (* = p < 0.05 compared to VEH+VEH, * = p < 0.05 compared to VEH+CP; X±SEM).

Table 1. Serum concentrations of sodium, potassium, creatinine, BUN and haematocrit before cisplatin (CP) administration (X±SEM).

	S_{Na} mmol/l	S_K mmol/l	S_{Cr} mg/dl	S_{BUN} mg/dl	HKT %
VEH+CP[a]	150.5±2.1	4.2±0.2	0.49±0.05	15.4±1.1	41.3±1.6
ACET+CP	151.5±2.0	4.6±0.2	0.46±0.04	14.5±0.8	39.5±1.6
FUR+CP	149.5±2.9	4.6±0.3	0.49±0.06	14.9±0.8	41.6±1.7
VEH+VEH	148.7±1.5	4.2±0.3	0.47±0.06	15.8±0.8	42.7±1.5

[a] VEH = vehicle, ACET = acetazolamide, FUR = furosemide

Table 2. Urine volume, sodium excretion and lithium clearance 1 hr before and after the cisplatin (CP administration (* = $p < 0.05$ in comparison to its own control; X±SEM)

	U_{Vol} ml 1 hr	2 hr	U_{Na} mmol/l 1 hr	2 hr	Cl_{Li} ml/min/100g 1 hr	2 hr
VEH+CP[a]	4.6±0.3	5.3±0.6	13.1±2.8	8.4±2.5	0.19±0.03	0.18±0.03
ACET+CP	4.8±1.0	10.6±0.7*	15.6±8.7	52.5±5.2*	0.17±0.01	0.26±0.03*
FUR+CP	4.5±0.6	11.4±0.6*	14.0±5.2	80.3±8.1*	0.23±0.05	0.26±0.04
VEH+VEH	3.4±1.0	3.5±0.5	13.8±5.4	13.0±2.9	0.18±0.03	0.18±0.03

[a] VEH = vehicle, ACET = acetazolamide, FUR = furosemide

DISCUSSION

Cisplatin induces renal failure in the rat, as shown by the elevated serum creatinine concentration is and decreased creatinine clearance 5 days after a single intravenous dose of cisplatin. Nephrotoxicity of cisplatin can be decreased in humans and laboratory animals by diuretics such as acetazolamide and furosemide (Heidemann et al., 1985). The mechanism by which the drug damage and diuretic protects the kidneys are not yet known. Furosemide has been shown to be protective in other models of acute renal failure (Mason et al., 1981), where the effect may be due to either prevention of tubular obstruction or by dilution of the nephrotoxic compound. Prevention of tubular obstruction by diuretics is rather unlikely for cisplatin, since this drug has no effect on renal blood blow and GFR within the first 24-48 hr (Safirstein et al., 1987) and diuretics are only protective when administered prior to the cisplatin.

Mannitol (5%) also decreases cisplatin nephrotoxicity (Pera et al., 1979) and we have shown that the same effect can be achieved by osmotic diuresis with 30% glucose (Heidemann, unpublished data). Possible mechanisms for this protective effect are increased tubular flow rate and prevention of tubular swelling by the toxic compound (Flores et al., 1972).

Cisplatin is excreted into the urine by filtration and by active secretion (Safirstein et al., 1987). The drug preferentially damages the S_3-segment of the proximal tubules. Assuming that acetazolamide, furosemide, mannitol-5% and glucose-30% are protective by the same mechanisms, intra-tubular dilution of cisplatin in the proximal tubules is a possible explanation. Acetazolamide acts on the proximal tubules by inhibition of the carbonic anhydrase, furosemide is a loop diuretic but also acts on the proximal tubules. The weaker action of furosemide on the proximal tubules could be the explanation for the effect that this drug is less protective than acetazolamide, although it is the more potent diuretic.

The lithium clearance is a measurement of the flow rate to the distal tubules. Our results show that acetazolamide has more effect on the lithium clearance and is more protective than furosemide. This result agrees with the diuretic actions of these drugs on the different parts of the nephrons. The good correlation of the change in lithium clearance at the time of cisplatin administration, and the kidney function 5 days later, is regarded as evidence that the diuretic induced nephro-protection is in part due to intratubular dilution. In terms of the clinical use of cisplatin a comparative study should show whether acetazolamide can further decrease the hazardous effects of cisplatin on the kidney.

REFERENCES

Flores, J., Diborra, D.R., Beck, C.H., Leaf, A. The role of cell swelling in ischemic renal damage and the protective effect of hypertonic solute. J. Clin. Invest.: 51, 118-222 (1972).

Heidemann, H.Th., Gerkens, J.F., Jackson, E.K., Branch, R.A. Attenuation of cisplatinum induced nephrotoxicity in the rat by high salt diet, furosemide and acetazolamide. Naunyn-Schmiedeberg's Arch. Pharmacol.: 329, 201-205 (1985).

Mason, J., Kain, H., Welsch, J., Schnermann, J. The early phase of experimental acute renal failure VI. The influence of furosemide. Pflugers Arch.: 392, 125-133 (1981).

Osman, N.M., Copley, M.P., Litterst, C.L. Amelioration of cisplatin-induced nephrotoxicity by the diuretic acetazolamide in F 344 rats. Cancer Treat. Rep.: 68, 999-1004 (1984).

Pera, M.F., Zook, B.C., Harder, H.C. Effects of mannitol of furosemide diuresis on the nephrotoxicity and physiological disposition of cis-dichloro-diammineplatinum-(II) in rats. Cancer Res.: 39, 1278-1279 (1979).

Safirstein, R., Winston, J., Moel, D., Dikman, S., Guttenplan, J. Cisplatin nephrotoxicity: insights into mechanism. Int. J. Andrology: 10, 325-346 (1987).

SENSITIVITY OF IN VITRO ION ACCUMULATION, GLUCONEOGENESIS AND OTHER PARAMETERS AS INDICATORS OF CISPLATIN-INDUCED RENAL TOXICITY

Charles Litterst, Jacqueline H. Smith, Mary Ann Smith, Marion Copley and Jiro Uozumi

Division of Cancer Treatment, National Cancer Institute, NIH, Bethesda, MD, 20892, USA

INTRODUCTION

The kidney is a complex organ which controls the fluid and salt balance, and the homeostasis of numerous other organs. Consequently, the functional integrity of the kidney is of paramount importance in maintaining health. Because of its central role in excretion, the kidney is exposed to high and often prolonged concentrations of most xenobiotics that enter the body. Adverse effects on renal function are produced by a large number of these chemicals, including heavy metals such as mercury and cadmium, and drugs such as aminoglycoside antibiotics and antineoplastic agents. One widely used antineoplastic agent whose dose limiting toxicity is to the kidney is cis-diamminedichloroplatinum-II (cisplatin, cisPt). This drug is a square planar molecule which undergoes a complex spontaneous hydrolysis to yield several uncharacterized metabolites, several of which have the potential of being the ultimate toxicant.

Because of the importance of the kidney in maintaining homeostasis, accurate monitoring of renal function in experimental toxicity testing is essential. However, many of the clinical parameters commonly used to assess functional status of the kidney are relatively insensitive. Thus BUN or creatinine rarely show significant elevations until glomerular filtration is decreased by 50-75%. Toxicologists, therefore, are continually searching for sensitive methods to evaluate renal function. Extensive studies of urinary enzymes, however, have previously demonstrated that these parameters are not significantly more sensitive for detecting cisPt nephrotoxicity than traditional urinary parameters such as protein and glucose (1). In a continuing effort to evaluate parameters of renal function for their suitability as sensitive early aids in diagnosing renal malfunction, we have investigated the effect of cisPt on organic ion transport and on gluconeogenesis when these parameters are measured in fresh slices of kidneys from experimental animals treated with the drug. These results were then compared to results of standard urinalysis evaluations.

METHODS

Adult (9-10 weeks of age) male Fisher 344 rats (Animal Genetics and Production Branch, NCI) were injected iv with 2,4,8,16 mg/kg of cisPt

371

freshly prepared in 0.9% NaCl. At 1,3,5,8,15 days after injection groups of rats (n = 4) were killed by exsanguination after ether anaesthesia.

Blood was collected from the vena cava and used for determination of BUN, creatinine, and total platinum levels. Kidneys were immediately removed and fresh slices prepared by hand for determination of gluconeogenesis and accumulation of the organic ions p-aminohippurate (PAH) and tetra-ethylammonium (TEA). Sections of kidneys were placed in 10% buffered formalin and subsequently stained with hematoxylin and eosin for histologic evaluation. One group of animals was kept in metabolic cages and urine collected on ice daily for determination of glucose, protein, and the activity of N-acetylglucosaminidase (NAG), gamma-glutamyltranspeptidase (GGT), and alanine aminopeptidase (AAP). Fresh kidney slices were incubated in buffer at room temperature under an atmosphere of 100% oxygen. After 90 minutes, glucose production from pyruvate was determined in the medium and the accumulation of the organic ions was determined in the tissue slices. Organic ion accumulation was expressed as slice to medium ratio (S/M ratio) and gluconeogenesis as nmol glucose produced/g tissue wet weight/minute. Details of methods can be found elsewhere (2,3). Data from the experimental groups were compared to data from control groups killed and analysed on the same days. Results in this manuscript are expressed as percent of control, with mean control values provided in the tables. Statistically significant differences between experimental and control values were determined by Dunnett's t-test.

RESULTS

The rate of increase in body weight of animals injected with 2 mg/kg cisPt was less than controls between days 3-15 after treatment. At 4 mg/kg cisPt, treated groups lost weight for the first five days after treatment and then gained weight similarly to controls (Data not presented). Renal concentration of platinum in the 2 mg/kg group declined by 36% throughout the 15 day observation period (day 1, 6.1 ± 1.0 ug/g; day 8, 5.1 ± 0.3; day 15, 3.9 ± 0.2 ug/g). At 4 mg/kg the rate of loss of platinum during the first week was greater (day 1, 12.6 ± 2.9; day 8, 7.5 ± 1.4; day 15, 6.9 ug/g), although the total decrease in platinum concentration was similar (36% vs 45%). At 4 mg/kg diarrhoea was evident, and distended stomachs and gas- or liquid-filled intestines were observed at necropsy.

Neither PAH nor TEA accumulation in fresh kidney slices from rats treated with cisPt were altered by the 2 mg/kg dose at any time during the study (Table 1). At 4 mg/kg, only sporadic and inconsistent changes in these two parameters occurred. At 8 mg/kg significant decreases occurred in both parameters at all times when surviving animals were analysed (16 mg/kg, data not shown). Animal deaths occurred at 8 mg/kg between the 8th and 15th study days, so changes in ion transport observed at that dose probably reflect secondary effects of a primary lesion elsewhere in the cell rather than a primary effect on these cell membrane transport functions.

Gluconeogenesis was unaffected by cisPt at any dose shown, except for a single time (Table 1). Thus both gluconeogenesis and ion transport appear to be ineffective in defining cisPt renal toxicity at doses below 4 mg/kg.

The lowest dose of cisPt, however, did produce alterations in urinary parameters of renal function (Table 2). Thus both NAG and GGT were significantly elevated on Day 1 at 2 mg/kg, and nearly all urinary parameters were elevated by Day 3. Similarly, protein and glucose were significantly increased by the lowest dose, although statistically significant increases were not observed until day 3.

Table 1. Organic ion accumulation and gluconeognesis in fresh kidney slices from rats treated with cisPt. Data are percent of control+.

Days Post-injection

		1	3	5	8	15
PAH	2 mg/kg	108	91	93	102	101
	4 mg/kg	86*	96	90	96	74*
	8 mg/kg	73*	80	60*	59*	NS
TEA	2 mg/kg	101	87	94	93	99
	4 mg/kg	84	87	75*	93	88
	8 mg/kg	80*	81*	57*	36*	NS
GLUCONEO.	2 mg/kg	100	90	95	111	119
	4 mg/kg	89	105	100	89	85
	8 mg/kg	80*	108	101	89	NS

+   Mean control values ($X \pm SD$; n = 13): PAH, 20.9 ± 1.8 S/M ratio; TEA, 27.1 ± 3.3 S/M ratio; gluconeogenesis, 420 ± 43 nmol glucose/g/minute. Day 1 control values not included in calculation.

*   Statistically significant difference at $p < 0.05$
NS = No survivors

Histologic changes in the kidney following 2 mg/kg cisPt were not evident until day 5, at which time there was minimal multifocal necrosis present in the proximal tubules, with cell debris and dilated tubules. Giant cells with various pyknotic nuclear changes also were seen. A similar histologic picture also was observed on day 8, with widespread resolution by day 15, when the only evidence of tubular damage was the presence of dilated tubules. At higher doses, similar changes were observed earlier and were more prevalent and severe.

Table 2. Urinalysis results from rats injected with cisPt. Data are percent of control+.

Days Post-injection

		1	3	5	8	15
Protein	2 mg/kg	223	950*	712*	240	543
	4 mg/kg	95	645*	926*	121	103
Glucose	2 mg/kg	160	1275*	950*	250	240*
	4 mg/kg	138	3750*	2667*	182	100
NAG	2 mg/kg	124*	222*	126	213*	250*
	4 mg/kg	88	236*	448	108	130
GGT	2 mg/kg	215*	267*	101	95	274
	4 mg/kg	149	148	221	57	29
AAP	2 mg/kg	108	218*	85	70	325
	4 mg/kg	90	328*	287	82	61

+ Mean control values ($X \pm SD$, n = 10): protein, 0.9 ± 0.5 mg/da; glucose 1.4 ± 0.8 mg/da; NAG, 49 ± 20 IU/24 hr; GGT, 2.18 ± 1.32 IU/24 hr; AAP, 0.14 ± 0.09 IU/24 hr.

* Statistically significant difference at $p < 0.05$.

373

DISCUSSION

The observations of cisPt-induced renal toxicity recorded in this study are consistent with previous reports of cisPt renal toxicity. In addition, the changes in urinary parameters also are similar to previously published results (1). However in most previous studies organic ion accumulation was utilized as a tool for evaluating mechanism of renal handling of cisPt, and cellular metabolism was used to help define cellular sites of action, rather than as potential early indicators of renal damage. Our results, however, suggest that these parameters may not be as sensitive as those parameters traditionally used to detect renal toxicity, such as urinalysis.

It is of interest to note that histopathologic signs of toxicity were not evident until day 5 at the lowest cisPt dose, even though there were consistent changes in all urinary parameters of renal function by day 3, including 10-fold increases in urinary levels of both glucose and protein, and greater than 2-fold increases in activities of urinary enzymes. There were, however, no changes in renal slice parameters of kidney function.

The lack of sensitivity of renal slice parameters is disappointing from the perspective of predictive toxicology, particularly because previous work has shown transport of both TEA and PAH to be inhibited following treatment of chickens with cisPt (4). However, when ion transport was studied in kidney slices from rats treated with cisPt, no change in accumulation was observed (5), which is consistent with the present results. When cisPt was added to kidney slices from control rats, however, an inhibition of transport of both PAH and TEA was observed (5). A similar effect was seen with mouse kidney slices, but extremely high cisPt concentrations (10 mM) were necessary for inhibition (6). Similarly, organic ion accumulation in both basolateral and brush border membrane vesicles from rat kidney have been shown to be sensitive to cisPt when incubated in vitro (7). These studies, along with the results of the present communication, suggest that the concentration of cisPt achieved in the kidney following parenteral administration to animals may be below the level required to produce inhibition of ion transport. Alternatively, cisPt may be sequestered within the cell and not available for reaction at the basolateral membrane. Similar findings have been reported for ATPase, which has been shown to be inhibited only by extremely high concentrations of cisPt in vitro (8-10), but which is not affected in vivo (11).

Although gluconeogenesis has not been studied following cisPt administration, cell respiration measured by calcium ion release from isolated mitochondria and by oxygen consumption have been evaluated. CisPt alone at concentrations up to 0.5 mM had no effect on either parameter (12), which is consistent with the lack of effect on gluconeogenesis shown in the present study.

These results do provide information on the likely early site of action of cisPt. It appears as if basolateral membrane transport of organic ions is not affected at doses of drug that cause increases in urinary parameters of renal toxicity and ultimate histologic lesions. Similarly the lack of effect on gluconeogenesis suggests that basic intracellular energy production is not initially altered following cisPt administration, even though ultrastructural studies show dramatic changes in mitochondrial appearance soon after cisPt administration (12).

In conclusion, organic ion accumulation and gluconeogenesis in renal cortical slices were poor indicators of early toxic effects to the kidney resulting from cisPt administration because these parameters are not

affected except at high doses.   Traditional urinalysis parameters appear
to be as sensitive, or more sensitive, than histology in defining early
renal toxicity from cisPt.   The poor sensitivity and delayed response of
renal slice parameters indicate that membrane function and cell metabolism
may not be early targets of cisPt at the cellular level.

REFERENCES

1. Litterst, CL, JH Smith, MA Smith, J Uozumi, M Copley, Sensitivity of
urinary enzymes as indicators of renal toxicity of the anticancer drug
cisplatin, <u>Uremia Invest</u>. 9:111 (1985)

2. Smith, JH, MA Smith, CL Litterst, MP Copley, J Uozumi, MR Boyd,
Comparative toxicity and renal distribution of the platinum analogs
tetraplatin, CHIP and cisplatin at equimolar doses in the Fischer 344 rat,
<u>Fund. Appl. Tox</u>., In Press (1987).

3. Smith, MA, JH Smith, CL Litterst, MP Copley, J Uozumi, MR Boyd, In vivo
biochemical indices of nephrotoxicity of platinum analogs tetraplatin,
CHIP, and cisplatin in the F-344 rat, <u>Fund. Appl. Tox</u>. In Press, (1987).

4. Bird, JE, MM Walser, AJ Quebbemann, Protective effect of organic cation
transport   inhibitors   on   cis-diamminedichloroplatinum-induced
nephrotoxicity, <u>J. Pharmacol. Exptl. Therap</u>. 231 :752 (1984).

5. Goldstein, RS, B Noordewier, JT Bond, JB Hook, GH Mayor, cis-Dichlorodiammineplatinum nephrotoxicity: time course and dose response of renal
functional impairment, <u>Tox. Appl. Pharmacol</u>. 60:163 (1981).

6. Nelson, JA, G Santos, BH Herbert, Mechanisms for the renal secretion of
cisplatin, <u>Cancer Treat. Rep</u>. 68:849 (1984).

7. Williams, PD, GH Hottendorf, Effect of cisplatin on organic ion
transport in membrane vesicles from rat kidney cortex, <u>Cancer Treat. Rep</u>.
69:875 (1985).

8. Guarino, AM, DS Miller, ST Arnold, JB Pritchard, RD Davis, MA Urbanek,
TJ Miller, CL Litterst, Platinate toxicity: past, present, and prospects,
<u>Cancer Treat. Rep</u>. 63:1475 (1979).

9. Daley-Yates, PT, DCH McBrien, Inhibition of renal ATPase by cisplatin
and some biotransformation products, <u>Chem.-Biol. Interact</u>. 40:325 (1982).

10. Nechay, BR, SL Neldon, Characteristics of inhibition of human renal
adenosine triphosphatases by cisplatin and chloroplatinic acid, <u>Cancer
Treat. Rep</u>. 68:1135 (1984).

11. Uozumi, J, CL Litterst, Effect of cisplatin on renal ATPase activity
in vivo and in vitro, <u>Cancer Chemother. Pharmacol</u>. 15:93 (1985).

12. Aggarwal, SK, MW Whitehouse, C Ramachandran, Ultrastructural effects
of cisplatin, <u>In</u>: Cisplatin: Current Status and New Developments (AW
Prestayko, ST Crooke, SK Carter, eds), Academic Press, NY, p. 79, 1980.

ASSESSMENT OF NEPHROTOXICITY BY ANALYSIS OF A RANDOMIZED MULTI-CENTRE COMPARATIVE STUDY REGARDING THE PREVIOUS EXTEND OF KIDNEY DAMAGE

A. Werner Mondorf, Wolfgang Mondorf and Anita Klingen

Zentrum der Inneren Medizin der Universitatskliniken Frankfurt, Theodor-Stern-Kai 7, D-6000 Frankfurt 70, FRG

INTRODUCTION

For the assessment of nephrotoxicity we need to differentiate between kidney alteration, kidney lesion and kidney necrosis. Any toxic agent may first alter kidney structures by means of reversible effects on kidney cells without cellular destruction and no functional impairment. More toxic agents may then lead to lesions of kidney structures by means of cellular destruction with compensate functional for the impairment of the kidney. Toxic agents leading subsequently to kidney necrosis show cellular destruction and not compensated functional impairment of the kidney damage (Table 1). The main parameters of nephrotoxicity in clinical use, such as creatinine in serum, creatinine-clearance and protein in urine are functional parameters shown to be sensitive for kidney necrosis, poorly sensitive for kidney lesions and not sensitive for kidney alteration. Concerning kidney damage they have therefore to be evaluated as late phase parameters. Every drug related nephrotoxicity begins with alteration of the kidney before leading subsequently to lesions and necrosis. It is of importance to detect nephrotoxicity in their early stages of alteration before cell destruction and consequently functional impairment occurs.

Table 1.   Assessment of nephrotoxicity

Stage I	Alteration	no cell destruction	reversible	no functional impairment
Stage II	Lesion	cell destruction	reversible	functional impairment compensated
Stage III	Necrosis	cell destruction	irreversible	functional impairment not compensated

A major target of drug nephrotoxicity is the proximal tubular cell. Alteration in brush-border membrane results in increased turnover processes in the kidney cortex followed by a corresponding increased excretion of alanine-aminopeptidase (AAP) from the surface of the proximal tubular cell, long before glomerular or tubular function are disturbed.

377

AAP excretion is directly correlated with the strength and duration of toxic alteration of the proximal tubules (1-6).

MATERIALS AND METHODS

In a randomized multi-centre comparative study a total of 164 patients suffering from infectious diseases received either ceftazidime 2x2g/d (CAZ, n = 88) or the combination of cefotaxime 3x2g/d and tobramycin 1 x 3mg/kg/d (CTX+TOB, n = 76). Urinalysis and AAP excretion in 24hr urines and serum-creatinine were determined. The kinetic activity of AAP was determined in untreated urine specimens. L-Alanine-p-nitranilide was used as the substrate (Merck, Darmstadt) for AAP in phosphate buffer at pH 7.6. In the test batch, 0.2 ml of a $1.66x10^{-2}$ M solution of L-alanine-p-nitranilide was used, into which 0.4 ml untreated urine was pipetted and made up to a final volume of 2 ml with 0.1 M phosphate buffer, 1.4 ml. The measurement was carried out in a spectrophotometer at 405 nm and 25°C. All enzyme activities as measured were converted to 24hr excretion. All samples were stored in glycerol (1:10) for preservation of the enzymes at -20°C (7).

RESULTS AND DISCUSSION

AAP elimination differed highly on pretreatment days. Therefore we formed three groups:-

1. Patients with normal AAP activity in urines up to 4,500 mU/24hr (n = 47).
2. Moderately elevated AAP activity between 4,500 and 10,000 mU/24hr (n = 48) and
3. Strongly elevated AAP activity above 10,000 mU/24hr (n = 69), (table 2).

Table 2

AAP-Activity in 24-hour urine on pre-treatment day

	Group 1 n=47	Group 2 n=48	Group 3 n=69
A A P (mU/24h)	< 4 500	4 500–10 000	> 10 000
	NORMAL	MILD ALTERATION	SEVERE ALTERATION

Characterization of Group Members. The three groups were characterized as follows. Their average age was slightly below and in group 2 and 3 slightly above 50 years. The mean was 48 years in group one. In group 2 with mild injury 56 years and in group 3 with severe injury 52 years. Within all three groups no difference of age could be seen between patients treated either with ceftazidime or the combination cefotaxime + tobramycin. Sex of patients showed a higher percentage of female (75%) in group 1 and a higher, percentage of male (60%) in group 3. These results count for both medications. In group 2 a higher percentage of females were treated with the combination (70%) and a high percentage of males (60%) with ceftazidime.

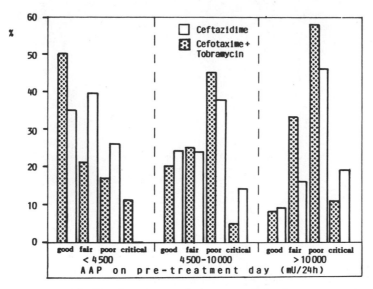

Figure 1.   General Status of Health

In group 3 patients general status of health was evaluated mostly as poor, whereas in group 1 patients were generally in good health. Patients in group 2 showed a tendency towards poor general status of health compared with group 1 (Figure 1). Nearly all patients in group 3 had acute infections (95%) with an average duration of six days. Similar results in group 2 with 80% acute, 10% chronic and 5% recurrent infections. Average duration was 12 days. The longest duration of infection was found in group 1 with 16 days and the highest percentage of chronic infections (30%). Of these patients 70% had acute and 2% recurrent infections. Patients with septicaemia were almost equally present in all three groups (18-22%). These result count for both medications.

Although the exclusion criteria of the study was patients with serum creatinine of less than 136 nmol/l a tendency towards higher creatinine in serum was seen in group 3 compared with group 1 (Figure 2). Four patients of group 3 in the cefotaxime+tobramycin collective exceeded above 136 nmol/l and only two in the ceftazidime collective of which one belonged to group 3 and one to group 2. A remarkable difference was evident regarding the previous application of antibiotics (Figure 3). While 35% to 39% of group 3 were previously treated with antibiotics in group 1, only 8% in the ceftazidime and none in the cefotaxime+tobramycin collective had previous mediaction.

Behaviour of AAP during Treatment with Different Antibiotics. A total of 76 patients were treated with the combination cefotaxime plus tobramycin and 88 patients with ceftazidime as a single drug over a maximum of ten days. The behaviour of AAP activity in 24hr urine before (0), during (2-10) on immediately post (ipost) and post treatment days demonstrates Figure 4. In all three groups a different increase of AAP elimination could be observed when treated with cefotaxime+tobramycin. The higher the pretreatment value the higher the increase of AAP activity during treatment. After one day of treatment a marked decrease of AAP elimination could be observed in all three groups. The results differed tremendously in the ceftazidime collective. No AAP increase in group one, no distinct increase in group 2 and even a decrease in group 3. In contrast to the findings with the combination therapy the AAP showed an increase in the days after treatment.

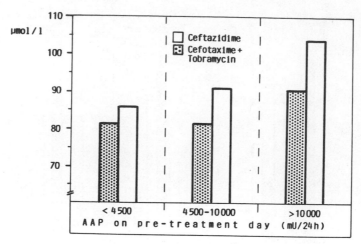

Figure 2. Creatinine in Serum

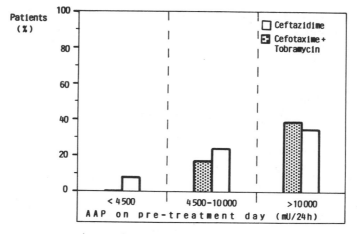

Figure 3. Previous Antibiotics

In all three groups the average value of creatinine in serum did not change. As shows in table 3 four patients in the combination collective and two patients in the ceftazidime collective showed an increase of serum creatinine from normal values before treatment to values above 136 nmol/l.

CONCLUSION

This study could show that AAP elimination in urine reflects toxic alteration of the kidney cortex by antibiotics with different toxic potential. The combination of cefotaxime with tobramycin causes a distinct alteration of the tubular cells Whilst by treatment with ceftazidime alone no toxic effects could be demonstrated. The extend of kidney alteration during treatment depends upon the extend of kidney alteration before treatment. Previous administration of antibiotics seems to be the main factor for elevated AAP activity in urine and consequent alteration of the kidney cortex.

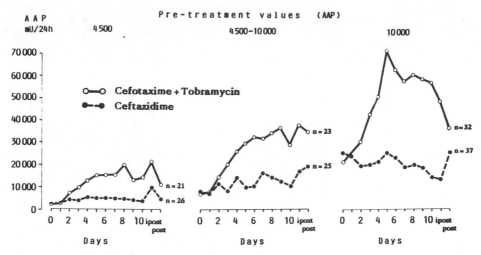

Figure 4. AAP changes following different regimens, compared by pre-treatment values

Table 3. Patients with an Increase of Creatinine in Serum (> 136 umol/l)

Pat.	AAP(0)	AAP(T)	Cr(0)	Cr(3)	Cr(ipost)
CEFOTAXIME + TOBRAMYCIN					
U.D.	5 264	17 796	62	160	136
B.L.	4 758	17 298	106	141	
T.J.	1 155	14 617	46	196	39
S.B.		12 389	119	161	76
CEFTAZIDIME					
V.S.	10 724	9 379	71	148	150
K.L.	7 017	14 436	133	309	186

AAP(0)   AAP on pre-treatment day (mU/24h)
AAP(T)   AAP mean value of treatment days (mU/24h)

Cr(0)   Creatinine in serum on pre-treatment day (μmol/l)
Cr(3)   Creatinine in serum third day of treatment (μmol/l)
Cr(ipost) Creatinine in serum on immediately post treatment day (μmol/l)

REFERENCES

1. U. Burchardt, G. Schinkothe, K. Meinel, D. Anton, I. Krebbel and L. Neef, Aminoglykosidnephropathie, Z. Gesamte Inn. Med. 37: 388-392 (1982).

2. A.W. Mondorf, J. Breier, J. Hendus, J.E. Scherberich, G. Mackenrodt, P.M. Shah, W. Stille and W. Schoeppe, Effect of aminoglycosides on proximal tubular membranes of the human kidney, Europ. J. Clin. Pharmacol. 13: 133-142 (1978).

3. A.W. Mondorf, W. Schoeppe, Is the potential nephrotoxicity of drugs predictible? Experiences with a volunteer model. Contr. Nephrol. 42:93-99 (1984).

4. G. Heinert, J. Wyrobnik and J. Scherberich, Quantitative computer histophotometry of membrane-integrated and lysosomal enzymes indicating inductive and alternative affects of aminoglycosides. Current Chemotherapy & Imnunotherapy, Proc.12th Internatll. Congr. of Chemotherapy, Florence, Italy, 852-854 (1981).

5. F.W. Falkenberg, U. Mondorf, D. Pierard, C. Gauhl, A.W. Mondorf, U. Mai, G. Kantwerk, U. Meier, A. Rindhage, M. Rohracker, Identification of fragments of proximal and distal tubular cells in the urine of patients under cytostatic treatment by immunoelectron microscopy with monoclonal antibodies, Am. J. Kid. Dis., 9:129-137 (1987).

6. R.G. Price, Urinary enzymes, nephrotoxicity and renal disease, Toxicol., 23: 99-134 (1982).

7. M. Nakamura, T. Itoh, K. Miyata, T. Uchisaka, T. Tanabe, M. Aono and K. Kimura, Protection by glycerol of urinary L-alanine aminopeptidase activity from freezing and thawing inactivation, Toxicol. Lett., 21: 321-324 (1984).

DRUG PHARMACOKINETICS IN RENAL FAILURE - INFLUENCE OF DISEASE TYPE

Amor Maiza and Peter T. Daley-Yates

Department of Pharmacy, University of Manchester, Manchester M13 9PL, UK

INTRODUCTION

For many drugs the major route of elimination from the body is renal excretion. Therefore, a loss of renal function will lead to excessive accumulation of the drug or its metabolites in the body, unless the drug dosage is reduced. The problem is particularly acute for drugs that have a narrow therapeutic index intended for patients with severe renal insufficiency. A failure to appropriately adjust dosage can lead to toxicity, which for some drugs may be life-threatening.

The most widely used methods for reducing drug dosage in patients with renal insufficiency is to assume a direct proportionality between the renal clearance of the drug and creatinine clearance, itself taken as a measure of glomerular filtration rate (GFR). This assumption is embedded in the many nomograms, equations and pharmacokinetic models (with or without feedback via plasma concentration measurements) that are currently available (1,2). However, in patients with severe renal impairment these methods often fail to predict accurately the dosage regimen needed to achieve a therapeutic plasma concentration of the drug (3). One reason for this lack of accuracy is the complication that renal disease may alter the non-renal disposition of certain drugs, or that the pharmacokinetic analysis used assumes a simple one compartment model, when a more complicated model is more appropriate. Another possible reason is the consistent neglect of the type of renal disease, which can be characterised according to the site of damage along the nephron, e.g. glomerulonephritis, proximal tubular necrosis, medullary or papillary necrosis. That is, the assumption is made that there is only one type of renal disease and that changes in GFR adequately describe the extent of the disease for the purposes of dose adjustment (2,4). This assumption is based on the "intact nephron hypothesis" (5,6) which proposes that damage to either the renal tubules or glomeruli results in the complete loss of function for the nephron affected. For drugs that are handled by the kidney in the same way as creatinine (i.e. mainly by glomerular filtration) the "intact nephron hypothesis" is probably valid. This hypothesis predicts that even when tubular secretion is a major component, the clearance of the drug still parallels the GFR (1). However, several sets of circumstances call this hypothesis into question:-

(i) where predominantly glomerular disease exists (glomerulonephritis) and the drug is eliminated principally by tubular secretion (7,8);

(ii) where the renal tubule is damaged (tubular and interstitial disease) thereby significantly affecting the ability of the renal tubule to secrete or reabsorb drugs, but without greatly influencing GFR. Under these conditions a markedly different renal clearance for the drug compared to that predicted by current methods may result (9,10,11). For drugs where tubular transport is a predominant process in their disposition the extent of validity of the "Intact nephron hypothesis" has not been established.

In contrast to previous studies in this area we have induced experimental renal failure with chemicals known to produce well localized damage such as proximal tubular necrosis, papillary necrosis and glomerulonephritis in rats.

The aims of the present study are:-

i) To assess the significance that the type of renal damage has in determining the renal clearance of drugs in renal failure, and,

ii) To test the extent of validity of the "Intact nephron hypothesis".

To this end we are attempting to correlate the changes in the renal clearance of drugs and model compounds and the type of renal failure. Here we present preliminary results for four models of experimental renal failure.

METHODS

Induction of Experimental Renal Failure. Male sprague-Dawley rats (250 to 350g) were used for the induction of site specific renal damage using protocols previously demonstrated to induce the following lesions: proximal tubular necrosis, induced by a single i.p. injection of cisplatin (5 mg/kg or 3 mg/kg) (12). Four days were allowed for the development of the lesion. A single i.v. injection of 2-bromoethanamine-hydrobromide (150 mg/kg) was used to induce renal papillary necrosis (13) within 24h. Glomerulonephritis was produced by 6 weekly i.m. injections of sodium aurothiomalate (0.05 mg/kg) (14). Proteinuria was measured every week to follow the induction of the glomerular damage. Glomerulonephritis was also induced by 6 daily i.p. injections (7mg/kg) of puromycin aminonucleoside (15). Proteinuria was measured daily after the last injection, 15 days were necessary for the lesion to develop.

These animals were then used for the measurement of renal clearance, see below. At the end of the experiment the rat was killed and the left kidney removed, cut in half and fixed for 24h in a solution of 5% formaldehyde in phosphate buffered saline. The tissue was then processed for embedding in paraffin and following sectioning stained with H&E prior to histological examination.

Clearance Measurements. Clearance measurements were carried out on rats with experimental renal failure induced as described above or on control animals, they were anaesthetised with pentobarbital 50 mg/kg i.p. Both the jugular vein and carotid artery were cannulated with a PE50 catheter. A PE90 catheter was inserted into the bladder for collection of urine. The venous catheter was used for constant infusion of inulin and p-aminohippurate (PAH). The arterial catheter was used to sample blood. Urine was collected into preweighed tubes. The exact volume of urine was determined by weighing. A priming dose of inulin and PAH (10 mg and 1.5 mg respectively in 0.2 ml) was first injected via the venous catheter followed by a constant infusion of inulin (50 mg/ml) and PAH (18 mg/ml) at

384

a rate of 1.2 ml/hr (16). Forty five minutes was allowed after beginning
the infusion for equilibrium to be attained before starting three urine
collection periods of 20 min each. At the middle of each period a blood
sample was taken. Renal clearance (Clx) was calculated using the equation
Clx = Ux/Px.V where Ux and Px are respectively the urine and plasma
concentrations (mg/ml) and V the urine flow (ml/min). The secretory
clearance of PAH (Cl SC PAH) was calculated by substracting the GFR (Cl
INULIN) from Cl PAH.

Assessment of Renal Function.   To assess the renal function the following
parameters were measured.   GFR (using the clearance of inulin); plasma
creatinine, blood urea nitrogen and urinary proteins; PAH (as an indicator
of the tubular secretory capacity) and urinary glucose (to assess tubular
reabsorption).

RESULTS

Morphological observations.   There was close agreement between the
morphological changes we found and those which have been reported
previously (11-14).   In the case of cisplatin the lesion was confined to
the pars recta of the proximal tubule.   Aurothiomalate produced changes
which appeared to be confined to thickening of the glomerular basement
membrane.   Bromoethanamine   caused a characteristic papillary necrosis.
Only minimal glomerular changes were induced by puromycin aminonucleoside.

Functional Changes.   The protocols employed did not produce large
elevations in blood urea nitrogen or plasma creatinine.   Glucosuria was
highest in cisplatin treated animals which correlates with the tubular
damaged found.   Surprisingly proteinuria was highest in bromoethanamine
treated animals despite the absence of an obvious lesion in the glomerulus
or proximal tubule (Table 1).

Table 1. Effect of different models of experimental renal failure on
renal function in the rat.

	GFR	Cl PAH	Cl SC PAH	Plasma creat.	Urinary glucose	Urinary protein	BUN
		ml/min/100g		mg/100ml	mg/24h	mg/24h	mg/100ml
CONTROL (n = 10)							
	0.51	1.78	1.28	0.49	< 0.1	58	19
	±0.11	±0.49	±0.43	±0.095		±12	±3
CISPLATIN (n = 11)							
	0.063	0.11	0.049	1.83	218	135	52
	±0.048	±0.09	±0.063	±1.18	±92	±39	±15
2-BROMOETHANAMINE (n = 8)							
	0.118	0.62	0.51	1.29	15	409	45
	±0.05	±0.32	±0.28	±0.1	±5	±88	±5
PUROMYCIN AMINONUCLEOSIDE (n = 4)							
	0.19	1.12	0.89	0.96	0.42	98	33
	±0.11	±0.59	±0.50	±0.03	±0.17	±8	±5
AUROTHIOMALATE (n = 8)							
	0.31	1.18	0.92	0.66	0.45	109	35
	±0.08	±0.39	±0.41	±0.08	±0.13	±27	±3

Values are mean ± S.D. and n = Number of animals.

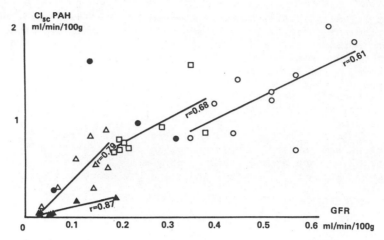

Figure 1. Relationship between GFR and Cl $_{SC\ PAH}$: following renal damage with cisplatin (▲), 2-bromoethanamine hydrobromide (△) puromycin aminonucleoside (●) and sodium aurothiomalate (◻) compared to Control (○). Each point represents a mean of three clearance measurements from the same rat. The lines were drawn using the method of least squares, where r = the correlation coefficient.

In general, for all the models of ERF used we did not find a parallel decrease in glomerular and tubular function except for aurothiomalate where tubular and glomerular function decreased approximately in parallel (Figure 1). The preliminary results for puromycin aminonucleoside show a greater decrease in GFR than tubular function (Cl $_{SC\ PAH}$). Only cisplatin reduced the Cl $_{SC\ PAH}$ to a value below that of the GFR. Animals treated with bromoethanamine showed only small changes in both GFR and Cl SC PAH, however, a marked polyuria was evident 24h following dosing.

DISCUSSION

Since 1960 there has been considerable controversy in the literature concerning changes in morphology and kidney function in renal disease. The "intact nephron hypothesis" expounded by Bricker et al (5,6) states that irrespective of the type of renal disease the end result is the same degree of functional impairment. That is to say, there is no correlation between the various morphological changes seen and the resultant renal dysfunction. Bricker's reasoning was that any damaged nephron becomes completely nonfunctioning. Or if the damage is focal the remaining undamaged part decreases its function in parallel.

A counter argument has been developed by Biber et al (17). They used dichromate and mercury to induce kidney damage. In contrast to Bricker's assertion they found that despite proximal tubular damage glomerular function did not fall in parallel and the nephron still contributed to the urine formation. Therefore they concluded that a close agreement exists between morphological and functional changes in their models of experimental renal failure.

We have used well known nephrotoxic agents at well studied doses and developed site specific models of experimental renal failure for proximal tubular necrosis, papillary necrosis and glomerulonephritis. In the light of our findings there is a good correlation between morphological and functional impairment. In other words, except for aurothiomalate the models of ERF we have used do not produce the same pattern of functional impairment.

In many circumstances creatinine clearance or plasma creatinine have poor predictive value as estimators of kidney function. The GFR gives no information about the tubular function of the nephron. Ideally, a direct measurement of the secretory capacity of the nephron, such as the measurement of endogenous 1-N-methyl-nicotinamide clearance should also be undertaken.

Our observations may have implications for drug therapy in patients with renal impairment. However much more work is required to assess the significance of the type of renal disease in determining interpatient variability in pharmacokinetics.

REFERENCES

1.   Fabre, J. and Balant, L. Renal failure, drug pharmacokinetics and drug action. Clin. Pharmacol., 1:99-120 (1976).

2.   Dettli, L. Drug dosage in renal disease. Clin. Pharmacol., 1:126-134 (1976).

3.   Burton, M.W., Vasko, M.R. and Brattier, D.C. Comparison of drug dosing methods. Clin. Pharmacol., 10:1-37 (1985).

4.   Welling, P.G., Craig, W.A. and Kunin, M.C. Prediction of drug dosage in patients with renal failure using data derived from normal subjects. Clin. Pharmacol. Therap., 18:45-52 (1975).

5.   Bricker, N.S., Morrin, P.A.F. and Kime, S.W. The pathologic physiology of chronic Bright's disease. Am. J. Med., 28:77-98 (1960).

6.   Bricker, N.S. Klahr, S., Lubowitz, H. and Rieselbach, R.E. Renal function in chronic renal disease. Medicine 44:263-288 (1965).

7.   Cottier, P. and Haldemann, G. De l'emploi d'un Sulfamide   (Ro - 4393) a duree d'action prolongee dans le traitement de la pyelonephrite chronique. J. d'Urol. Nephrol., 70:797-809 (1964).

8.   Williams, O.M., Wimpenny, J. and Asscher, A.W. Renal clearance of sodium sulphadimidine in normal and uraemic subjects. Lancet 2:1058-1060 (1968).

9.   Petipierre, B., Perrin, L., Rudhardt, M., Herrera, A. and Fabre, J. Behaviour of chlorpropamide in renal insufficiency and under the effect of associated drug therapy. Int. J. Clin. Pharmacol., 6:120 (1972).

10.   Shim, C.K., Sawada, Y., Iga, T. and Hanano, M. Estimation of renal secretory function for organic cations by endogenous N-methylnicotinamide in rats with experimental renal failure. J. Pharmaco. Biopharm., 12:23-42 (1984).

11.   Giacomini, K.M., Roberts, S.M. and Levy, G. Evaluation of methods for producing renal dysfunction in rats. J. Pharm. Sci., 70:117-121 (1981)

12. Daley-Yates, P.T. and McBrien, D.C.H. Cisplatin nephrotoxicity. In: Nephrotoxicity, Assessment and Pathogenesis (eds. P.H. Bach, F.W. Bonner,

J.W. Bridges and E.A. Lock), pp 358-370. John Wiley & Sons, Chichester (1982).

13. Hill, G.S., Willye, R.G., Miller, M. and Heptinstall, R.M. Experimental papillary necrosis of the kidney. Am. J. Pathol. 68:213 (1972).

14. Nagi, A.H., Alexander, F. and Barabas, A.Z. Gold nephropathy in rats - Light and electron microscopic studies. Exp. Mol. Pathol., 15:354 (1971).

15. Fiegelson, E.B., Drake, J.W. and Recant, L., Experimental aminonucleoside nephrosis in rats. J. Lab. Clin. Med. 50:437 (1957).

16. Stitzer, S.O. and Maldonado M.M., Clearance methods in the rat. In: Methods in Pharmacology, Vol 2 (ed. M.M. Maldonado), pp 23-40. Plenum Press, New York (1978).

17. Biber, T.U.L., Mylle, M., Baines, A.D., Gottschalk, C.W., Oliver, J.R. and MacDowell, M.C. A study by micropuncture and microdissection of acute renal damage in rats. Amer. J. Med. 44:664-705 (1968).

ANALGESIC RELATED RENAL INJURY IN MAN

M.M. Elseviers and M.E. De Broe

Department of Nephrology, University of Antwerp, Universiteitsplein 1, B - 2610 Wilrijk, Belgium

INTRODUCTION

It was first reported in the 1950's, that the ingestion of large amounts of some pain-relieving drugs, consumed over prolonged periods, was associated with the development of kidney disease and renal failure (13). It also became clear that prolonged abuse of analgesics increased the risk of these patients developing urothelial tumours, particularly in the renal pelvis and the upper ureter. More than 30 years later, analgesic nephropathy still remains a controversial issue; where the causal relationship between abuse of analgesics and renal damage and upper urothelial carcinoma is still a matter of debate (12). The diagnosis of the disease remains difficult because the criteria are not well established, the clinical signs are non-specific and abusers tend to deny their analgesic habituation. The key chronic lesion that develops as a result of analgesic abuse is papillary necrosis, but the precise mechanism that underlies this lesion is still unclear and the factors that relate to the progression of renal degenerative changes and malignancy are also a matter of speculation (1). As yet, no adequate answer can be given to the questions of which of the nephrotoxic effects are caused by each of the different components in mixed analgesics, the amount of which analgesic(s) have to be ingestion (over what period of time) to cause renal damage, nor the relative risk and possible predisposing factors in the development of analgesic nephropathy (9).

PREVALENCE OF ANALGESIC NEPHROPATHY

Analgesic-associated terminal renal failure has been reported in a number of different places throughout the world, but the prevalence shows important geographical variations. In those countries where the highest incidence of analgesic nephropathy was first reported there has been a striking decrease in the number of new case due to appropriate measures such as public and physician awareness programmes, legislation to limit the sale of these products and reduce the availability of mixed analgesics (2,15), but in other countries (6,8,10) analgesic abuse related kidney disease still remains one of the main causes of end-stage renal failure (table 1).

Table 1.   International prevalence of analgesic nephropathy in patients with end-stage renal failure (12)

Country	Year	Percentage	Reference
Australia	1985	15	Nanra, 1987*
Belgium	1984	18	Elseviers, 1987
Canada	1976	3	Gault, 1978*
France	1979	2	Brynger, 1980
F.R. Germany	1983	13	Pommer, 1986
Great Britain	1979	1	Brynger, 1980
Italy	1979	1	Brynger, 1980
Scandinavia	1979	3	Brynger, 1980*
Spain	1979	1	Brynger, 1980
Switzerland	1980	20	Mihatsch, 1987

* Declined prevalence due to analgesic legislation in Australia (1978-80), Canada (1973) and Scandinavia (1961).

In several European countries the occurrence of this disease seems to be underestimated. In a recent study undertaken in the Federal Republic of Germany a 13% prevalence of analgesic nephropathy was found in dialysis patients, while the appropriate data of the European Dialysis and Transplant Association (EDTA) was never more than 6%. As shown in figure 1, the proportion of nephropathies of unknown aetiology reported in the EDTA registry for the dialysis population of the European countries (1980-1984) may also be indicative of the underestimation of analgesic nephropathy. This proportion, which showed an inverse correlation with the prevalence of analgesic nephropathy, was low in Switzerland and Belgium, was more than 10% in the Federal Republic of Germany, France and Italy, and was more than 20% in Portugal were analgesic nephropathy per se is rarely, if ever, reported (3).

ANALGESIC NEPHROPATHY IN BELGIUM

In Belgium analgesic nephropathy is a common disease. In 1983 we started an investigation on analgesic nephropathy, aimed at establishing information on the sales of these medicines, their use and abuse, the kind of products actually abused (tables versus powders; and if there was a preference for any one brand name, etc), to relate the renal degenerative effects with the level of analgesic abuse and any other factors affecting or contributing to the renal failure or urothelial carcinoma (4,6).

Prevalence of analgesic nephropathy in Belgium

A survey on the prevalence of analgesic nephropathy among the Belgian population with end-stage renal disease was undertaken by a short questionnaire sent to all dialysis centres (n = 54), to ascertain the total number of adult patients and those who were known analgesic abusers, and the age and sex distribution for each group. Data from 53 dialysis units showed that there were 17.9% who had analgesic nephropathy (in 1984) compared to 18.4% (in 1979) where the data came from 46 dialysis centres (14).

There was a striking geographical difference in the prevalence of this disease within Belgium. The epicentre was situated in a small area in the north and involved 3 dialysis units, where the maximum frequency was 51%. In the southern part of the country analgesic nephropathy was present at a markedly lower level (figure 2).

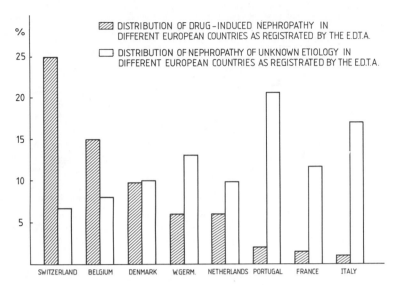

Figure 1. Drug-induced nephropathy and nephropathy of unknown aetiology in different European countries as reported by the EDTA

Sales of analgesics in Belgium

An analysis of the sales figures of analgesics, showed that in 1983 the total volume of sales in Belgium amounted to 26 million packages. On average this represents 2.6 packages or approximately 25g per capita per year. Analgesic mixtures constituted 63% of the total sales of analgesics, three out of four of these products contained caffeine, a product that may be important in the development of the abusive use of the mixtures. The overall sales of analgesics in 1983 was approximately the same in the north and south of the country (figure 3). A striking difference was, however, observe in the kind of products sold. Single analgesics were sold mostly in the south, analgesic mixtures formulated as tablets were sold almost equally all over the country, and more importantly powdered analgesic mixtures were the most commonly abused product, especially in the north of the country (figure 4).

Use and abuse of analgesics in Belgium

An investigative survey on the use of analgesics by the general population was undertaken in three areas of the north of Belgium where there were markedly different prevalences of analgesic nephropathy. A stratified random sample of the population included individuals from urban to rural areas. Persons were randomly picked from voters lists, thus limiting the study population to those over 18 years, and a total of 855 subjects were interviewed at home, with a structured questionnaire.

The results of this investigation showed that analgesic products were commonly used in the population, 83% of the investigated subjects had minimal one of the twelve most popular products in their home medicine chests (table 3). The vast majority of the investigated population had single analgesics at home (64%). Single analgesics however, shared only 37% of the national market. We noticed a daily consumption of analgesics in 28 subjects, 18 of them fulfilled the

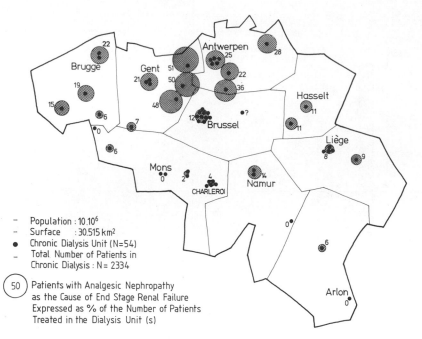

Figure 2.   Prevalence of analgesic nephropathy   as a cause of end-stage renal   failure   in Belgium   (December 1984).

Reprinted with   permission of Nephr.   Dial. Transpl..

Table 2.   Analgesics   at the home medicine chests (population survey n = 855)

                                        Percentage patients

No analgesics at home	17
Analgesics at home for occasional use	51
Analgesics at home for monthly use	24.5
Analgesics at home for weekly use	4.5
Analgesics at home for daily use	3.1

criteria   for abuse.   The mean   age of these   abusers was   52.3   years, 72% were female,   analgesic mixtures were   mostly consumed.

Retrospective study of patients with documented analgesic nephropathy.

All patients   with documented analgesic nephropathy from 7 nephrology units, where they had either   been under dialysis treatment for   less than two years (n = 33) or were   seen at the outpatient   clinics less than two years ago   (n = 104)   were included.   They were investigated with a structured   questionnaire and a standard psychological   test.   The results showed that patients with documented analgesic nephropathy were mostly females of the lower socio-economic   classes.   Complaints of headache occurred in   60% of the cases, but most of the subjects admitted that their analgesic abuse had become a habit where the stimulating effect of analgesics was an important factor. As shown in table   4, there is a large variation in the period over which analgesics were abused and total amount taken. All of these patients (except 2) abused analgesic

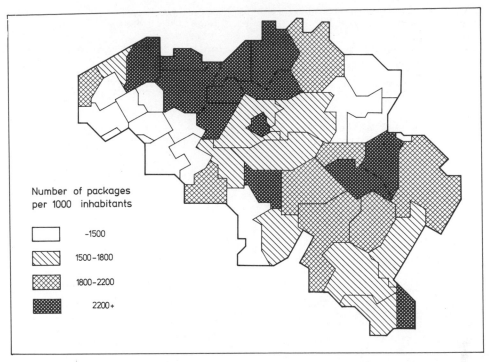

Figure 3 .   Sales   of analgesics   in Belgium,   1983

Number of packages
per 1000 inhabitants

	-1500
	1500–1800
	1800–2200
	2200+

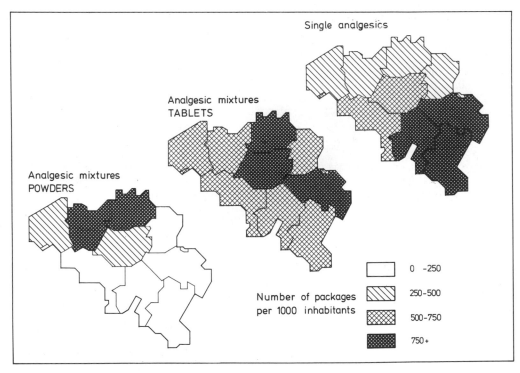

Single analgesics

Analgesic mixtures
TABLETS

Analgesic mixtures
POWDERS

Number of packages
per 1000 inhabitants

	0 -250
	250–500
	500–750
	750+

Figure   4.   Sales of different kinds of analgesics   in Belgium,
1983.   Reprinted with permission of Nephr. Dial. Transpl

mixtures. Dialysis patients reached the end-stage of renal failure after an average ingestion of 21 years (range 4-56 years).

Table 3. Analgesic consumption by patients with documented analgesic - nephropathy

	Outpatients	Dialysis patients
Age of the start of abuse (year)		
minimal	10	14
maximal	60	58
mean	33	31
Number of years of abuse		
minimal	1	4
maximal	66	56
mean	24	21
Total number of units		
minimal	1100	6000
maximal	222000	190000
mean	43500	42200

Prospective study of active analgesic abusers and controls

Active analgesic abusers (defined as those daily users of analgesics for at least 1 year with a minimum intake of 1000 units) were referred to the research team by family doctors, pharmacists and each other. For every subject out of the study group, a matched control was randomly picked from voters lists. The case/control pairs were matched for age, sex, professional status and living environment. Cases and controls were questioned with a structured questionnaire and a standard psychological test. Subjects are contacted once a year during five years for a blood and urine sample, weight and blood pressure measurements. Results of these part of the study will be available in 1990.

THE MISCONCEPTION OF PHENACETIN-INDUCED RENAL DAMAGE

In the initial reports on analgesic nephropathy, it was found that phenacetin was present in most of the analgesic mixtures abused. This generated the oversimplified conclusion that phenacetin was the nephrotoxic agent. However, the removal of phenacetin from non-prescription analgesics has not been followed by the expected fall in end-stage renal failure from analgesic nephropathy. In Australia the incidence of analgesic nephropathy was increasing in the 1970's, despite the restriction of phenacetin. In an overview concerning the role of phenacetin, Prescott stated that in the past, insufficient attention has been given to the higher, at least experimental nephro-toxic potential of the other analgesic components. He concluded that phenacetin was unlikely to be the primary cause of analgesic nephropathy (11).

The sale of phenacetin containing analgesics in Belgium has declined since 1972. In that year the composition of the most popular analgesic powder "Witte Kruis" was modified. Phenacetin was removed and replaced by antipyrine. Subjects who abused this product before 1972 sustained their habit. In the retrospective study (11 cases) as well as in the prospective study (3 cases), we could observe that

394

the daily consumption of the modified drug also can cause renal damage. During the last decade the pharmaceutical industry spontaneously banned phenacetin from several other analgesic mixtures. Since 1972 the sales of phenacetin containing analgesics reduced to 21% (in 1976), 9% (in 1983) and less than 3% in 1987. Nevertheless, the prevalence of analgesic nephropathy in dialysis patients in Belgium remained at the same level between 1979 and 1984. These data strongly support the concept that phenacetin was not the most important aetiological criteria in the genesis of the lesion.

CONCLUSION

Analgesic nephropathy still remains a serious problem in several European countries and may also be under-diagnosed in those countries where there is apparently a low incidence. Nevertheless, it is one of the few renal diseases currently suitable for primary prevention. Several countries (Sweden, Canada, Australia) have been successful in the elimination or significant decrease this nephropathy by restricting the availability of analgesic mixtures and limiting over-the-counter medication to single analgesics.

A number of questions concerning this kind of renal disease are still unsolved. There is a need to develop more sensitive diagnostic criteria and to adequately define stages in the development of renal papillary necrosis and its progression to end-stage renal failure and upper urothelial carcinoma. The determination of the molecular pathogenesis of renal papillary necrosis is an important goal for experimental research and understanding how the lesion can be modulated in human analgesic abusers. Furthermore, additional epidemiologic investigations and long-term prospective studies are needed to clearly define risk and how best to clinically conrol the primary condition and its secondary consequences.

REFERENCES

1. Bach P.H. and Bridges J.W., 1985, Chemically induced renal papillary necrosis and upper urothelial carcinoma, CRC Crit. Rev. Toxicol., 15:217.

2. Bengtsson U., 1979, Prevention of renal disease, Proc. Eur. Dial. Transplant. Assoc., 466.

3. Buccianti G., De Broe M.E. and Challah S., 1987, Combined European study on Analgesic Nephropathy, In: "Prevention in Nephrology", G. Buccianti, ed., Masson, Milano.

4. Elseviers M.M. and De Broe M.E., 1986, 25 Jaar analgetica nefropathie in Belgie, Tijdschr. Geneeskd., 42:819.

5. Elseviers M.M. and De Broe M.E., 1987, Wurde das Problem der Analgetika-Nephropathie durch die Entfernung des Phenacetins aus analgetischen Mischpraparaten gelost?, Mitt. Klin. Nephrologie, 16:187.

6. Elseviers M.M. and De Broe M.E., 1987, Is analgesic nephropathy still a problem in Belgium?, Nephr. Dial. Transpl. (in press).

7. Kincaid-Smith P., 1986, Effects of non-narcotic analgesics on the kidney, Drugs, 32:109.

8. Mihatsch M.J., Hofer H.O., Gutzwiler F., Brunner F.P. and Zollinger H.U., 1980, Phenacetinabusus, Schweiz. Med. Wschr., 110:108.

9.   National Institutes   of Health.   Consensus   Conference,   1984,
Analgesic-associated   kidney disease,   JAMA, 251:3123.

10.   Pommer W.,   Glaeske G. and Molzahn M.,   1986, The analgesic problem
in the Federal Republic of Germany: analgesic   consumption,   frequency of
analgesic nephropathy and regional   differences, Clin. Nephrol.,   26:273.

11.   Prescott L.F.,   1982, Analgesic nephropathy: A reassessment of the
role of phenacetin and other analgesics, Drugs, 23:75.

12.   Schwarz A.,   1987,   Analgesic-associated   nephropathy,   Klin.
Wochenschr., 65:1.

13. Spuhler O. and Zollinger H.U., 1953, Die Chronische Interstitielle
Nephritis, Z. Klin. Med.,   151:1.

14.   Vanherweghem J.L. and Even-Adin D.,   1982, Epidemiology of analgesic
nephropathy in Belgium, Clin. Nephrol.,   17:129.

15.   Wilson D.R.   and Gault H.H., 1982,   Declining incidence of analgesic
nephropathy in Canada, Can. Med. Assoc. J., 127:500.

PROGRESSION OF RENAL FAILURE IN ANALGESIC ASSOCIATED NEPHROPATHY

A. Schwarz, U. Kunzendorf, and G. Offermann

Klinikum Steglitz, University Hospital, Hindenburgdamm 30, D-1000 Berlin 45, FRG

INTRODUCTION

No more than 5% of analgesic abusers develop analgesic nephropathy (AN), but it remains uncertain whether analgesics or other factors are the only predisposing or causal factor (Buckalew and Schey 1986, Schwarz 1987). In a clinical study, we tried to find out which factors influence further progression of AN once it has developed.

METHODS

In a cross-sectional study, we investigated all patients of our outpatient clinic (n = 127). Paracetamol (acetaminophen) is metabolized to N-acetyl-p-aminophenol (APAP) and its presence in the urine indicates the ingestion of paracetamol or phenacetin containing analgesics in the preceding 24 hours. Urine specimens were tested 1 to 4 times for APAP using a specrophotometric method (Welch and Conney, 1965). The change of renal clearance during observation of the patients in the outpatient clinic was evaluated by the 1/crea method. The slope of clearance decline was calculated by linear regression analysis, and progression of renal failure was expressed as clearance loss per year. Three groups of patient were formed: analgesic abuser with a regularly positive APAP test (who were taken as active analgesic abusers), patients with a negative APAP test (abusers who had stopped the habit), and patients with other kidney diseases (controls). Progression of renal failure in these three groups was compared. Beside non-parametric statistics (Chi-square-distribution test, Wilcoxon U-test), all variables were tested by a multivariate analysis using table Statistical Package for the Social Sciences (SPSS) computer program. In the patients with AN, the diagnostic signs were papillary necrosis (46%), cumulative intake of more than 1000 tablets (80%), roentgenological evidence of irregular kidney shrinkage with papillary cavities (26%), chronic interstitial nephritis in renal biopsy (19%), tubular syndrome (14%), urinary tract infections (33%), and uroepithelial carcinoma (5%). In most cases, diagnosis was confirmed by more than one technique (95%). The roentgenological, sonographic, or clinical evidence of papillary necrosis after exclusion of diabetes mellitus, vesico-ureteral reflux, or sickle cell anaemia were considered to be pathognomonic for AN. In the absence of papillary necrosis, at least two other signs were required to establish the diagnosis of AN.

RESULTS

AN was the most frequent kidney disease in our renal outpatient clinic
(44%). The APAP test was positive in 13/57 of the analgesic patients and
2/70 of the patients with other kidney diseases (21% vs. 3%, p = 0.0001).
There was no significant difference in age or the percentage of women
among the three groups (Tables 1 and 2), nor in the time of observation
(AN with continued abuse 52 months, AN in those who stopped abuse 60
months, other kidney diseases 55 months). The creatinine level at the
beginning of the observation period was significantly higher in the
analgesic group than in the other patient group (Table 1). AN patients
with continued abuse had a more rapid decline of renal function than those
who stopped the abuse (Fig. 1), but the difference was not statistically
significant (Table 2). Analgesic patients with continued abuse showed
no improvement of renal function during the observation time. Compared
to AN patients who stopped their abuse, this was on the border of
statistical significance (0% vs. 21%, p = 0.056). The analgesic
patients had urinary tract infections and a lower body mass index more
frequently than patients with other renal diseases (Table 1). There was
no significant difference in hypertension between the groups. However,
severe hypertension requiring more than one antihypertensive drug was more
frequent in the analgesic group (60% vs. 41%, p = 0.04). Significantly
more patients in the analgesic group than in the group of patients with

Table 1. AAN patients compared to patients with other kidney disease

	Univariate Statistics			Multivariate Statistics	
	AAN (n=57)	Other Kidney Diseases (n=70)	Statistical Significance	Discriminant proportion	Statistical Significance
Loss of clearance per year (ml/min; $\bar{x} \pm$ SD)	4.8 ± 10	5.1 ± 14.9	n.s.	0%	n.s.
Initial creatinine (µmol/l; $\bar{x} \pm$ SD)	247 ± 144	159 ± 125	p=0.0004	21%	p=0.0001
Age (years; $\bar{x} \pm$ SD)	57 ± 11	52 ± 15	n.s.	0%	n.s.
Sex (% women)	65	61	n.s.	0%	n.s.
Papillary necrosis (%)	46	0	p<0.0001	30%	p<0.0001
Urinary tract infection (%)	26	6	p=0.0001	22%	p<0.0001
Hypertension (number of) antihypertensives; $\bar{x} \pm$ SD)	2.7 ± 1.3	2.5 ± 1.3	n.s.	8%	n.s.
Body weight (kg; $\bar{x} \pm$ SD)	63 ± 13	68 ± 14	p=0.02	0%	n.s.
Body mass index ($\bar{x} \pm$ SD)	23 ± 4	25 ± 4	p=0.03	0%	n.s.
Weight change (% body weight; $\bar{x} \pm$ SD)	-1.0 ± 7	0.8 ± 6.3	n.s.	12%	p=0.01
Death during investigation period (%)	18	3	p=0.005	7%	n.s.

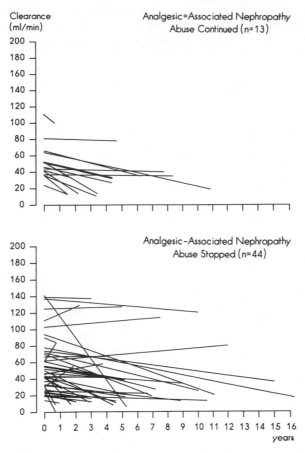

Fig. 1. Clearance loss in analgesic patients with continued abuse compared to those who stopped abuse (x± SD = 6.9±5.5 vs. 4.1±11, n.s. using the Wilcoxon U-test).

other kidney diseases died during the 18 months of investigation (Table 1). The ages or the patients who died were not significantly different in either group (62 vs. 59 years.). The causes of death in the analgesic group were coronary heart disease (n = 3), acute cardiac death (n = 1), stroke (n = 2), hypokalaemia (n = 2); ovarian carcinoma (n = 1), and peritonitis following cholecystectomy (n = 1). The causes of death in the patients with other kidney diseases were acute cardiac death (n = 1) and colon carcinoma (n = 1). In multivariate statistics, significant differences between patients with AN and those with other kidney diseases were the presence of papillary necrosis, the higher initial creatinine level, and more frequent urinary tract infections in the analgesic group (Table 1). Significant differences between analgesic patients with continued abuse and those who stopped abuse were the more rapid clearance loss per year and the higher percentage of women in the analgesic group with continued abuse (Table 2).

DISCUSSION

Compared to patients with other renal diseases, analgesic abuse have papillary necrosis and urinary tract infections more frequently, have more advanced renal insufficiency, more severe hypertension, lower body weight and lose more weight during progression of renal failure and have a higher mortality.

Table 2. AAN patients with a positive NAPAP test (abuse continues) compared to AAN patients with a negative one (abuse stopped).

	Univariate Statistics			Multivariate Statistics	
	AAN Abuse Continued (n=13)	AAN Abuse Stopped (n=44)	Statistical Significance	Discriminant proportion	Statistical Significance
Loss of clearance per year (ml/min; $\bar{x} \pm SD$)	6.9 ± 5.5	4.1 ± 11	n.s.	26%	p=0.04
Initial creatinine (μmol/l; $\bar{x} \pm SD$)	222 ± 96	253 ± 156	n.s.	16%	n.s.
Age (years; $\bar{x} \pm SD$)	52 ± 6	58 ± 12	n.s.	15%	n.s.
Sex (% women)	85	59	n.s.	19%	p=0.04
Papillary necrosis (%)	39	46	n.s.	0%	n.s.
Urinary tract infection (%)	31	19	n.s.	11%	n.s.
Hypertension (number of antihypertensives; $\bar{x} \pm SD$)	2.6 ± 1.5	2.7 ± 1.3	n.s.	0%	n.s.
Body weight (kg; $\bar{x} \pm SD$)	56 ± 12	65 ± 12	p=0.02	0%	n.s.
Body mass index ($\bar{x} \pm SD$)	21 ± 5	24 ± 4	p=0.02	12%	n.s.
Weight change (% body weight; $\bar{x} \pm SD$)	-4.1 ± 9.9	-0.1 ± 5.7	n.s.	0%	n.s.
Death during investigation period (%)	15	18	n.s.	0%	n.s.

When compared to those analgesic patients who stopped taking the offending drugs the active abuser has a more rapid decline of renal function with no improvement, a lower body weight and the group consisted of more women.

The analgesic patients continue their abuse of paracetamol and phenacetin in 212 of the cases despite renal insufficiency and the strict medical advice not to take any more drugs. Our study shows that further analgesic abuse does promote the progression of renal insufficiency and that there is no improvement of renal function without stopping analgesic abuse. The clearance loss calculated by the l/crea method is even more marked regarding the weight loss of analgesic patients. However, patients who stopped their abuse may also have a steady progression of renal failure. This means that there must be another factor, beside analgesic abuse, that promotes renal insufficiency. From our study, we can not conclude which factor(s) are involved, but our data suggests that it is not urinary tract infection, hypertension, or hyperalimentation.

REFERENCES.

Buckalew VM, Schey HM. Renal disease from habitual antipyretic analgesic consumption: an assessment of the epidemiologic evidence. Medicine, 11:291-303, 1986.

Schwarz A. Analgesic-associated nephropathy. Klin Wochenschr., 65:1-16, 1987.

Welch RM, Conney AH. A simple method for the quantitative determination of N-acetyl-p-aminophenol (APAP) in urine. Clin Chem., 12:1064-1067, 1965.

THE RENAL RESPONSE OF A NONHUMAN PRIMATE (BABOON) TO CERTAIN NONSTEROIDAL ANTI-INFLAMMATORY DRUGS

Paul N. Skelton-Stroud

Ciba-Geigy Pharmaceuticals, Stamford Lodge, Altrincham Road, Wilmslow, Cheshire, SK9 4LY, UK

INTRODUCTION

Renal papillary necrosis (RPN) in man can follow the abuse of non narcotic analgesics or nonsteroidal anti-inflammatory drugs (NSAIDs). Secondary cortical interstitial nephritis may also occur. In extreme cases affected kidneys can progress to end-stage renal failure (ESRF) or upper urothelial carcinoma (UUC).

In predictive toxicological investigations the regulatory authorities require compounds for intended use in man to be tested in both rodent and nonrodent laboratory animals. Data is presented from the experimental administration of two NSAIDs of the oxicam class, piroxicam (Feldene [R], Pfizer) and CGP 13 214 D, to a nonrodent species (baboons). The results confirm the pronounced variability of significant changes in laboratory animals and the need for utmost caution in the extrapolation and comparison with similar changes in man.

MATERIALS AND METHODS

Animals of East African origin were obtained from an accredited supply agency following two months quarantine isolation and thorough veterinary examination. They were tested for tuberculosis and treated for parasites. Upon arrival in the unit they were individually housed and maintained within the experimental area for not less than two months before the start of the study. Veterinary examinations and preventive medicine procedures were repeated. They were fed a proprietary diet for nonhuman primates supplemented with fruit and ascorbic acid tablets, and water was available ad libitum.

Haematological and urine samples were analysed pretest and at regular intervals throughout the study. The compounds were administered by oral gavage, daily for three months. The oral route was chosen since that was the most common route of administration for such anti-inflammatory compounds in man. Test compounds were prepared freshly each day and suspended in a solution of 1% (m/v) Methocel vehicle (methyl cellulose-400, Ciba-Geigy), and given at a rate of 5 ml/kg body weight. Piroxicam was given at doses of 20 mg/kg and 6 mg/kg, and the Ciba-Geigy compound at 6 mg/kg and 2 mg/kg.

Comprehensive necropsies were performed and a wide range of tissues were sampled for subsequent microscopy. Tissues were fixed in Bouin's fluid, routinely processed, sectioned at 5um and stained with haematoxylin and eosin (HE). Additional sections of selected kidneys were stained by the Sudan IV method to identify lipids, by a trichrome-PAS method to identify polysaccharides, and by an alizarin red-S method to identify calcium salts. Some unstained sections were examined by scanning electron microscopy and X-ray diffraction to identify crystals. Reserve samples of most tissues were placed into 10% neutral phosphate buffered formalin.

RESULTS

A range of lesions was seen in the kidneys. At 20 mg/kg piroxicam, a discrete focus of papillary necrosis, was seen unilaterally in a male animal that had been necropsied before schedule (Fig. 1). Pale yellow crystals were also present, more clearly visible under polarized light (Fig. 2). Epithelial hyperplasia at the papilla tip was characterised by small basophilic cells in papillary projections (Fig. 2). Some of the cells were vacuolated. In the interstitium at the edge of the lesion basophilic material surrounded tubules near the papilla tip. Interstitial necrosis was present immediately at the edge of the mineralised areas, but was also present in smaller foci higher in the papilla. Epithelial hyperplasia was present in papillary collecting ducts with occasional mitotic figures. A moderate tubulo-interstitial nephritis was present in the cortex. In the other kidney of the same animal similar changes were found but without RPN. A few crystals were present in the papilla interstitium immediately below the epithelium (Fig. 3). All crystals stained positive for calcium and oxalate constituents with alizarin red-S at specific pH values when compared with acetic and hydrochloric acid controls. SEM and X-ray diffraction data supported this analysis. Within the same dose group moderate papilla interstitial hyperaemia and haemorrhage with minimal epithelial hyperplasia and mitotic figures were noted in a female animal (Fig. 4). Similar but lesser changes were seen in a second female. The kidneys of the remaining animals at this dose rate were comparable to controls.

At 6 mg/kg piroxicam a minute focus of unilateral RPN was found, in a single female animal, and epithelial hyperplasia, interstitial haemorrhage and crystal deposition occurred unilaterally in another individual female. The remaining female showed some epithelial hyperplasia and mitotic figures. Males were comparable to controls.

Variation in the severity of lesions between kidneys of the same animal also occurred at 6 mg/kg CGP 13 214 D. Crystals were found in the interstitium of only one kidney in a male animal, yet both kidneys displayed interstitial haemorrhage, interstitial basophilic material and epithelial hyperplasia. A few small intratubular crystals were seen in another male. A combination of tubulointerstitial nephritis, subepithelial interstitial mineralisation and papilla epithelial hyperplasia were seen in a female animal.

At the lower dose of 2 mg/kg CGP 13 214 D male animal kidneys were comparable to control with a single exception. This animal showed unilateral papilla interstitial necrosis with papillitis and epithelial hyperplasia. Papilla hyperplasia and crystals, plus focal subacute interstitial nephritis containing a solutary crystal were seen in the cortex of one kidney in a female animal.

Control animal kidneys showed the normal range of naturally occurring lesions but one female displayed a very low grade focal hyperplasia of the papilla tip epithelium.

Sections stained for lipids from animals representative of all groups showed no notable histological changes.

Overall the clinical chemistry changes were very minor and generally nonspecific in regard to renal injury except for alterations in urea levels. Slight increases in urea were noted at a low incidence in the majority treated with 20 mg/kg piroxicam. Levels were not consistently raised and occurred only in the middle of the study. Similarly slight

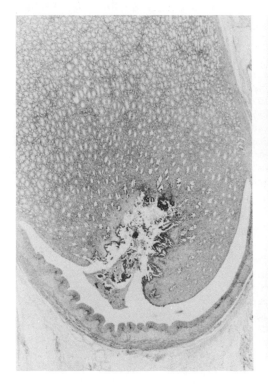

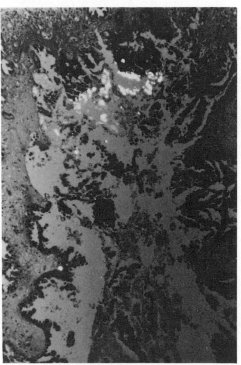

Fig. 1.   Unilateral RPN at
20 mg/kg (x5)

Fig. 2. RPN shows crystals and
epithelial hyperplasia (x50)

increases were noted in one animal at 6 mg/kg piroxicam and in two animals at 6 mg/kg CGP 13 214 D. Urinalysis showed a moderate haemoglobinuria in two females at 20 mg/kg piroxicam early in the study. It persisted in one animal. These animals showed microscopic papilla interstitial haemorrhage. No crystalluria was noted in any of the animals which displayed crystals at subsequent microscopy.

Evidence of varying degrees of gastrointestinal irritation was seen in treated animals, but was more obvious at the highest dose of 20 mg/kg piroxicam. Haematological data showed a tendency towards raised leukocyte counts in such animals.

DISCUSSION

Most of the published literature on NSAID investigations in nonhuman primates have described metabolic studies. Such studies in different species of laboratory animals have shown that piroxicam at 20 mg/kg has a plasma half-life of 2-9 hours in the rhesus monkey (Hobbs and Twomey, 1981) when compared to the much longer 45 hours in man (Hobbs and Twomey, 1979). Some 22% of the dose was recorded as unchanged drug in faeces after oral dosing. It was reduced to 6% following parenteral administration. CGP 13 214 D is also an oxicam. A plasma half-life of 26 hr in baboons has been shown after oral dosing thereby resulting in higher systemic exposure to the unchanged compound.

There are only few published reports on toxicological studies with anti-inflammatory agents in nonhuman primates. A chronic two year oral study in rhesus monkeys (Emerson, 1976) showed a varied dose-dependent toxicity with individual responses to treatment, and no specific reference to renal lesions. Similarly, no kidney pathology was found in a six month study with parsalmide (Parsal [R], Midy, Mazue et al, 1976). In a one month oral study with bucloxic acid (Esfar [R], Midy) in baboons at doses of 1200, 600, 300 and 150 mg/kg/day, pale areas were seen on the kidney surfaces at necropsy at all dose levels. These were found to be foci of dilated tubules with interstitial lymphoid infiltrates. But in the six month oral study at doses of 250, 100 or 40 mg/kg/day also in baboons, no kidney changes were found (Mazue et al, 1974). Combined gastrointestinal and renal lesions are not uncommon in laboratory animals experimentally treated with NSAIDs. Such a combination was found in monkeys treated with mefenamic acid, flufenamic acid and meclofenamic acid (Kaump, 1966). The kidney changes comprised dilated collecting tubules, pyelonephritic scars and pyelonephritis, respectively. A combination of lesions also occurred in this particular study.

The hypothesis suggested to explain the mechanisms of RPN are diverse. They include the immunological effects of NSAIDs, disturbed renal inter-mediary metabolism, hypoxia and vasoconstriction, and the counter-current theory, yet there is conflicting evidence to support some of these (Bach and Bridges, 1974). Data from rheumatoid arthritis studies in man using piroxicam, indomethacin and carprofen have suggested significant reductions in immunoglobulin can be achieved without affecting cell viability, and the effects can be reversed with low levels of prostaglandin E2 (Goodwin, 1984). Whilst baboons show lymphocytic infiltrates in many tissues, including the kidneys, it is doubtful that an immunological basis for RPN could be seriously considered. Medullary ischaemia has long been held to be the predisposing change in RPN. The medulla is particularly susceptible to hypoxia and it is thought that prostaglandin synthesised within the medullary interstitium facilitates vasodilation as part of the normal kidney function in this region. This is then countered by the inhibitory action of many NSAIDs causing disturbed medullary blood flow and ischaemia. Certainly the interstitial hyperaemia and haemorrhage seen in some animals in this study would lend support to this theory. However a reasonable counter argument could be offered on the basis that the vascular changes and prostaglandin alterations are too simple a combination to conveniently lead to RPN, and technical limitations prevent the proper testing of the role of prostaglandin alterations.

The reproducibility of RPN experimentally is fraught with difficulty (Kaump, 1966; Bokelman et al, 1971; Rosner, 1976; Bach and Bridges, 1982) and the potential nephrotoxicity of some individual analgesics is yet uncertain (Bach and Hardy, 1985). A complicating factor with some NSAIDs is their tendency to produce gastrointestinal lesions so severe as to preclude significant renal changes (Emerson et al, 1973). Yet gastro-intestinal lesions causing significant fluid loss can promote RPN. In this study the animal at 20 mg/kg piroxicam with RPN was sacrificed before schedule with gastrointestinal changes.

The most common change in the kidneys in this study was papilla epithelial hyperplasia. This could have been a result of the passage of acidic urine since most NSAIDs are acidic in solution. Deposition of oxalate crystals in the interstitium being found both with RPN and independent of RPN emphasizes the role of the interstitial cells and matrix in the pathogenesis of RPN. Crystals have been reported in horses with RPN (Gunson, 1983) and in rats (Bach, personal communication). Since urine is a supersaturated solution it is thought that pH alterations caused by excreted NSAID administration, then calcium is precipitated and combines with oxalate and phosphate forming crystals. This could explain the identification of both crystals and of areas of basophilic mineral deposition.

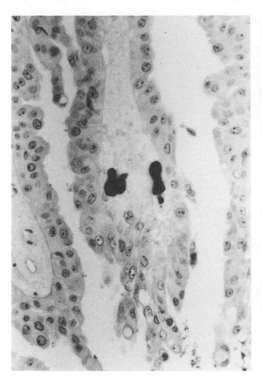 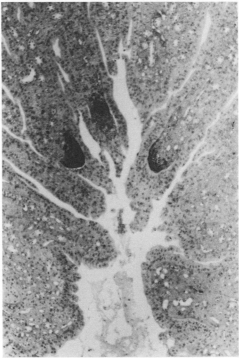

Fig. 3.   Crystals present in the papilla interstitium (x102)

Fig. 4. Interstitial hyperaemia and haemorrhage (x25)

The renal data derived from this study have shown that a spectrum of lesions can follow NSAID administration in a nonhuman primate species. The lesions may be compared to those in man following NSAID abuse or to chemically-induced RPN in other laboratory animals. Overall the lesions in the baboon were less severe than in man. In man RPN is usually bilateral, but in baboons it was unilateral. In man and some experimental animals RPN affects a large area of the papilla but in the baboon, it was discrete. Inflammatory infiltrates were not a major component of RPN in the baboon, nor were they common in the cortex. Crystals were seen in the baboon but have not been reported in man. No incidences of end-stage kidneys nor urothelial carcinoma have been reported in the nonhuman primate literature following NSAID administration and this reflects the duration of such studies which seldom exceeding twelve months. Although spontaneous RPN has not been recorded in baboons (Skelton-Stroud, unpublished results) the variability of the data within this study confirm the need for caution in extrapolation of such experimentally derived results to similar changes in man.

Further investigations need to clarify the role of the interstitial cell and interstitial matrix in the early phases of the pathogenesis of RPN, and to determine why interstitial cells have a poor regenerative capacity to insult, and their role in local medullary prostaglandin function.

REFERENCES

Bach, P.H., Bridges, J.W. Chemical associated renal papillary necrosis. In: Nephrotoxicity: Assessment and Pathogenesis. eds: P.H. Bach, F.W. Bonner, J.W. Bridges, E.A. Lock. pp 437-459 John Wiley, Chichester, 1982.

Bach, P.H., Bridges, J.W. The role of metabolic activation of analgesics and nonsteroidal anti-inflammatory drugs in the development of renal papillary necrosis and upper urothelial carcinoma. Prostagland Leuk Med 15:251-274, 1984.

Bach, P.H., Hardy, T.L. Relevance of animal models to analgesic-associated renal papillary necrosis in humans. Kidney Int 28:605-613, 1985.

Bokelman, D.L., Bagdon, W.J., Mattis, P.A., Stonier, P.F. Strain-dependent renal toxicity of a nonsteroid anti-inflammatory agent. Toxicol Appl Pharmacol 19:111-124, 1971.

Emerson, J.L., Gibson, W.R., Pierce, E.C., Todd, G.E. Pre-clinical toxicology of fenoprofen. Toxicol Appl Pharmacol 25:444 Abstract, 1973.

Emerson, J.L. Chronic oral toxicity of a nonsteroidal anti-inflammatory reagent in rhesus monkeys. Toxicol Appl Pharmacol 37:184, 1976.

Goodwin, J.W. Immunologic effects of nonsteroidal anti-inflammatory drugs. Amer J Med 77:7-15, 1984.

Gunson, D.E. Renal papillary necrosis in horses. J Am Med Ass 182:263-266, 1983.

Hobbs, D.C., Twomey, T.M. Piroxicam pharmacokinetics in man: aspirin and antacid studies. J Clin Pharmacol 19:270-281, 1979.

Hobbs D.C., Twomey, T.M. Metabolism of piroxicam by laboratory animals. Drugs Metab Disp 9:114-118, 1981.

Kaump, D.H. Pharmacology of the fenamates II. Toxicology in animals. Ann Physiol Med (Suppl) pp 16-23, 1966.

Mazue, G., Vallee, E., Genet, P., Navorro, J., Brunaud, M. Studies of Buxcloxic acid (804 CB). Arzneim-Forsch (Drug Res) 9a:1398-1413, 1974.

Mazue, G., Berthe, J., Richer, G., Vallee, E. Parsalmide: A new anti-inflammatory agent. Note IX: Toxicological study of parsalmide; oral toxicity study in baboons. Boll Clin Farma 115:216-229, 1976.

Rosner, I. Experimental analgesic nephropathy. CRC Crit Rev Toxicol 4:331-352, 1976.

MORPHOLOGICAL CHANGES IN THE PIG KIDNEY ASSOCIATED WITH AN ACUTELY INDUCED RENAL PAPILLARY NECROSIS

N.J. Gregg, M.E.C. Robbins[*], J.W. Hopewell[*] and P.H. Bach

Nephrotoxicity Research Group, Robens Institute, University of Surrey, Guildford, Surrey and [*] CRC Radiobiology Research Group, Churchill Hospital, Oxford, UK

INTRODUCTION

Analgesic abuse leads to the development of renal papillary necrosis (RPN) and may cause upper urothelial carcinoma in man. Animal models offer a potentially important means by which to define the underlying pathogenesis of RPN. Moreover, their use could improve early diagnosis, allowing the identification of which analgesic has the greatest papillotoxic potential and define what factors exacerbate this lesion (1). Many analgesics induce gastro-intestinal toxicity in rats which limits the use of this species for studying analgesic-induced RPN (2). The use of the non-analgesic papillotoxic chemical 2-bromoethanamine (BEA) hydrobromide, has helped define the mechanistic basis of RPN, particularly because this compound targets selectively for the medulla and causes a lesion in rodents within 24-48 hr (1). The BEA-induced RPN in the Wistar rat shows most of the pathological changes described in human analgesic abusers (3). The primary choice of rodents for nephrotoxicity studies reflects their low cost, ready availability, ease of handling and the considerable base-line data on renal function and toxicity. However, the extrapolation of nephrotoxicity data from rodents to man is complicated by the marked renal anatomical and functional differences between the two species. In contrast the human and pig kidney are remarkably similar in terms of physiological and anatomical characteristics (Table I).

Table 1. Comparison of some morphological and functional parameters in kidneys of man and pig.

Species	GFR[a]	Glomeruli		Proximal tubule		Maximal	% Long
		Number[b]	Radius[c]	Length[d]	Radius[c]	Osmolality	loops
Man	75	2×10^6	100	16	36	1400	14
Pig	72	2×10^6	83	30	35	1080	3

a = ml/min/m^2 b = in both kidneys   c = um   d = mm   e = mOsmol/kg

Data from (5) & (6).

Both man and the pig are multipapillate, produce urine of similar osmolality, and have GFR values, numbers of glomeruli per kidney and nephron dimensions that are comparable (4-6). The pig is thus an attractive model to study clinically important nephrotoxicity, particularly RPN. These preliminary findings show that BEA causes a RPN in the pig kidney, which is morphologically similar to that in the Wistar rat.

METHODS

Four female Large White pigs, six months old (weight 50 kg), were given freshly prepared 2-bromoethanamine (BEA) hydrobromide (BDH, Poole, Dorset, UK) by a slow iv infusion (over 2-3 minutes) while anaesthetised with a mixture of 2-3% halothane, $\pm 30\%$ nitrous oxide plus $\pm 70\%$ oxygen. BEA was given at dose levels of 50 (n = 2) or 100mg/kg (n = 2). The animals were allowed access to food and water and monitored daily for any obvious signs of distress.

After 7 days the animals (n = 3) were killed after an overdose of halothane anaesthesia and autopsied. The kidneys, ureters and bladder were removed intact. The kidneys were then bisected longitudinally along the lateral border through the hilus. All tissues were fixed in calcium: formaldehyde (4°C) for 72 hr. Control kidneys and bladder were obtained from abattoir material.

The cut interior surfaces of the kidneys were examined macroscopically and tissue blocks of renal pyramids were prepared to include the papilla tip as described by Lomax-Smith and Seymour (7). Together with pieces of ureter and bladder, the blocks were processed and embedded in glycol-methacrylate resin (JB-4, Polysciences, Northampton, UK). Semi-thin sections (1um) were routinely stained with Haematoxylin and Eosin, Giemsa and Toluidine Blue, using modified standard methods (8).

RESULTS

General observations. Neither animal given 50 mg/kg BEA showed any signs of distress, but those receiving 100 mg/kg had an emetic response 15 min after recovering from the anaesthetic. This lasted for several hr, and 1 animal died (from unknown causes) approximately 24 hr later.

Macroscopic changes. There were prominent casts in the medullary rays, and dark areas at the papilla tips from which the epithelium covering had exfoliated in pigs given the high dose. There were no pronounced changes apparent in the pigs given 50 mg/kg BEA.

Microscopic changes. Interstitial cells, the interstitial cell matrix and columnar collecting duct epithelium in control papillae showed no abnormal histology (Figure 1). Morphological changes that were concomitant with the onset of early RPN were present after dosing with 50 and 100 mg/kg BEA (Figure 2 a-d). These included disruption of interstitial matrix (Figures 2a,b), focal interstitial cell necrosis (Figures 2b,d), exfoliation of the papilla covering epithelium (Figure 2c), and necrosis of collecting duct epithelial cells (Figure 2c,d). These changes were more pronounced in the animals given 100 mg/kg BEA.

DISCUSSION

This study shows that BEA causes a dose related RPN in the pig. The morphological changes observed were essentially the same as in the rat and included foci of interstitial cell necrosis together with disruption of

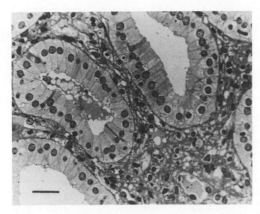

Figure 1   Semi-thin section of control papilla tip showing intact interstitial matrix and collecting ducts. Giemsa. Bar = 40 um.

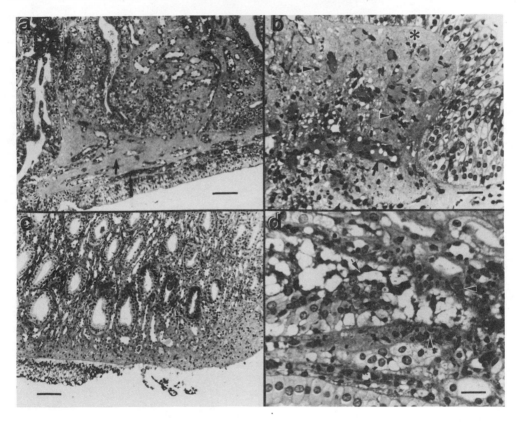

Figure 2 **a** Papilla tip from pig kidney 7 days after single iv dose BEA (100 mg/kg) showing disruption of interstitial matrix (arrowhead) with a decrease in staining. Giemsa. Bar = 100um. **b** Focal interstitial cell necrosis (arrowheads) together with disrupted interstitial matrix (*) and necrotic collecting ducts (arrows) in papilla tip, 7 days after single iv dose of BEA (100 mg/kg).   Giemsa. Bar = 40um. **c** Papilla tip, 7 days after single iv dose BEA 50 mg/kg showing exfoliated covering epithelium and necrotic collecting duct cells with basophilic nuclei. Giemsa. Bar = 100 um.   **d** Focal interstitial cell necrosis (arrowheads) and necrotic collecting duct epithelial cells (arrow) in papilla, 7 days after single iv dose BEA (100 mg/kg). Giemsa. Bar = 25 um.

the extra-cellular matrix, loss of the covering epithelia and necrosis of the collecting ducts. In the rat these anatomical elements are also the earliest to show degenerative changes, but the lesion was less pronounced in the pig compared to Wistar rats given the same dose.

The decreased effects of BEA on the pig medulla may be due to a number of causes. The multipapillate anatomy of the pig kidney may be less prone to the papillotoxic effects because BEA is not "concentrated" in a single papillae as it is in the rat, or because the urine concentrating capacity of the pig is less than that of the rat (5). Alternatively, both the hepatic and renal metabolism of several chemicals differs in rats and pigs (9,10). These and other factors may account for the reduced severity of the renal lesion in the pig and serves to illustrate marked species differences in the renal handling of nephrotoxic compounds in the multi-papillate kidney. Thus in conclusion BEA is less papillotoxic to the pig, but there is a greater systemic toxicity at high doses.

REFERENCES

1. Bach, P.H. and Bridges, J.W. (1985) Chemically induced renal papillary necrosis and upper urothelial carcinoma. CRC Crit. Rev. Toxicol. 15, 217-439.

2. Bach, P.H. and Hardy, T.L. (1985) The relevance of animal models to the study of analgesic associated renal papillary necrosis in man. Kidney Int. 28, 605-613.

3. Gregg, N.J., Courtauld, E.A. and Bach, P.H. (1988) High resolution light microscope enzyme histochemical changes in an acutely induced renal papillary necrosis. Tox. Pathol. Submitted.

4. Terris, J.M. (1986) Swine as a model in renal physiology and nephrology: an overview. In: Swine in Biomedical Research, Vol III. Ed. Tumbleson, M.E. Plenum Press, New York and London.

5. Stolte, H. and Alt, J.M. (1982) The choice of animals for nephrotoxic investigations. In: Nephrotoxicity; Assessment and Pathogenesis. Eds. Bach, P.H., Bonner, F.W., Bridges, J.W. and Lock, E.A. John Wiley & Sons.

6. Mudge, G.H. (1982) Comparative pharmacology of the kidney: Implications for drug-induced renal failure. In: Nephrotoxicity; Assessment and Pathogenesis. Eds. Bach, P.H., Bonner, F.W., Bridges, J.W. and Lock, E.A. John Wiley & Sons.

7. Lomax-Smith, J. and Seymour, A.E. (1980) Unsuspected analgesic nephro-pathy in transitional cell carcinoma of the upper urinary tract: a morphological study. Histopathology 4, 255-269.

8. Bancroft, J.B. and Stevens, A. (1982). Theory and Practice of Histological Technique. 2nd Edition. Churchill Livingstone.

9. Shimada, A., Iizuka, H. and Tomoji, Y. (1986). Pharmacodynamic study on drug susceptibility in Gottingen miniature pigs. In: Swine in Biomedical Research, Vol I. Ed. Tumbleson, M.E. Plenum Press, New York and London.

10. Fujimori, K., Takahashi, A., Numata, H. and Takanaka, A. (1986). Drug metabolism enzyme system of Gottingen miniature pigs. In: Swine in Biomedical Research, Vol I. Ed. Tumbleson, M.E. Plenum Press, New York and

UPPER UROTHELIAL CARCINOMA, USING N-BUTYL-N-(4-HYDROXYBUTYL)-NITROSAMINE

AND AN ACUTE PAPILLARY NECROSIS

N.J. Gregg, P. Ijomah, E.A. Courtauld and P.H. Bach

Nephrotoxicity Research Group, Robens Institute, University of Surrey, Guildford, Surrey, GU2 5XH, UK

INTRODUCTION

Upper urothelial carcinoma (UUC) in analgesic abusers has been closely associated with renal papillary necrosis (RPN) since it was first reported (1). UUC has only rarely been induced in animals using analgesics (2), thus a "cause-and-effect" relationship has not been established (3). The underlying mechanism of RPN is not fully understood and animal models of analgesic-induced lesion are difficult to study because of the:-

i) long latent induction time of the lesion using analgesics
ii) large biological variation in extent of the lesion, and
iii) extra-renal toxicity e.g. gastric ulceration and perforation associated with the prolonged inappropriately high non-clinical doses of analgesics.

In view of these limitations, a rapidly induced model of RPN would be useful to help elucidate and identify factors contributing to secondary renal changes, the association between RPN and UUC and the pathomechanism of UUC. 2-Bromoethanamine (BEA) hydrobromide has no structural relationship to the analgesics, but it is an ideal model probe that induces an acute, dose-related RPN within 24-48 hr after a single injection. This lesion has been widely studied (see 3) and one of its secondary consequences is a simple hyperplasia localised to the pelvis, ureter and the epithelium covering the papilla, but this change does not progress to carcinoma (4).

Previous research using a 2-stage initiation-promotion model has established that bladder hyperplasia may develop into tumours (5). We have developed such a model by initiating the urothelium with a urothelial specific carcinogen; N-butyl-N-(4-hydroxybutyl)-nitrosamine (BBN) and then "promoted" urothelial cell proliferation by inducing RPN with BEA. BBN was chosen as the carcinogen to facilitate controlled oral dosing (6), to reduce the exposure risk to personnel and because of its greater specificity with no benign extra-urothelial tumours induced.

METHODS

Two groups of male Wistar rats (University of Surrey strain) weighing 120g were oral dosed twice weekly for 5 weeks with BBN (MRI, Kansas City,

411

Missouri, USA) to a total dose of 800 mg. Each dose was administered in a 0.5 ml volume of a 20:80 ethanol:water (6). After one weeks respite, one of these groups was injected ip with a single dose of freshly prepared BEA (Aldrich, Poole, Dorset, UK) at 100 mg/kg (7) in physiological saline. A control group received a 0.5 ml volume of the ethanol:water solution twice weekly for 5 weeks, and then after one weeks respite received a single ip dose of BEA.

Animals were allowed food and water ad libitum, monitored daily and groups of animals (n = 3) were sacrificed periodically up to 40 weeks after BEA. Kidney, bladder and ureter tissues were dissected and fixed for 24 hr at 4 $^{\circ}$C in 4% (v/v) formaldehyde:1% (w/v) calcium chloride fixative.

Transverse slices of the kidney containing the papilla tip, bladder and the upper 2 cm portion of the ureter were embedded in glycolmethacrylate resin (JB-4, Polysciences, Northampton, UK). Semi-thin sections (1 um) were stained with Haematoxylin and Eosin (H&E), Giemsa, Toluidine blue, or PAS (4). RPN and urothelial changes were graded according to Burry (8), and Mostofi (9) respectively.

RESULTS

Control urothelium epithelial layer is typically 2-4 cells thick (Fig. 1a). Six weeks after BBN/BEA treatment there was papillary and nodular hyperplasia in the ureter (Fig. 1b) and aggregates of mast cells within the lamina propria. Within the superficial layer of epithelium dysplastic cells with basophilic nuclei were present.

Thirteen weeks after BBN/BEA both papillary and nodular hyperplasia was present along the entire length of the ureter (Fig. 2a), together with foci of nodular hyperplasia that appeared to invade the lamina propria and with multinucleated cells in the superficial layer (Fig. 2b). Dysplasia and "invasive" P2 foci were in the lamina propria and approaching the muscularis layer (Fig. 2c).

Thirty-four weeks after BBN/BEA treatment dysplastic changes were more frequent, extensive and advanced and a large tumourous mass was found in the pelvis, adjacent to the truncated papilla stump of one kidney (Fig. 2d). This tumour arose from the pelvic wall in which there were numerous mitotic figures.

Forty weeks after BBN/BEA treatment dysplasia in the pelvis and ureter was more advanced and another kidney had a nodular tumourous mass filling the upper ureter and extending into the pelvis. The tumour was dysplastic, with the loss of cellular polarity and it was extremely difficult to differentiate between the laminae propria and muscularis, suggesting an "invasive" stage.

Bladder tumours were present in the BBN/BEA treated animals, after 21 weeks, but not in BBN only (up to 30 weeks) or BEA only treated animals (up to 40 weeks).

DISCUSSION

Compared to the BEA only and BBN only control groups, animals from the BBN/BEA group had more severe urothelial abnormalities. Tumours in the renal pelvis and upper ureter were only found in the BBN/BEA treated animals, and bladder tumours appeared earlier and were usually larger with more dysplasia and cellular atypia than in the BBN only. The finding in this study that "nodular" invasive hyperplasia and nodular tumour tissue lacks any positive staining for this enzyme suggests the existence

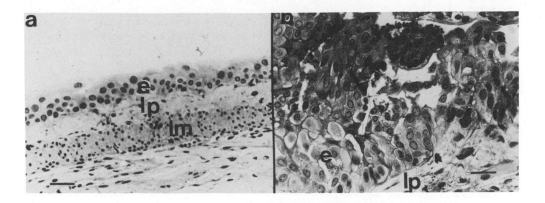

Figure 1. **a** Control urothelium from Wistar rat showing three distinct layers; e = epithelium, lp = lamina propria, lm = lamina muscularis. Giemsa stain. Bar = 40 um. **b** Nodular and papillary hyperplasia in ureter from animal 6 weeks after BBN initiation and BEA promotion (BBN/BEA). Many areas are dysplastic with extremely basophilic nuclei sloughing into lumen. Giemsa. Bar = 25 um.

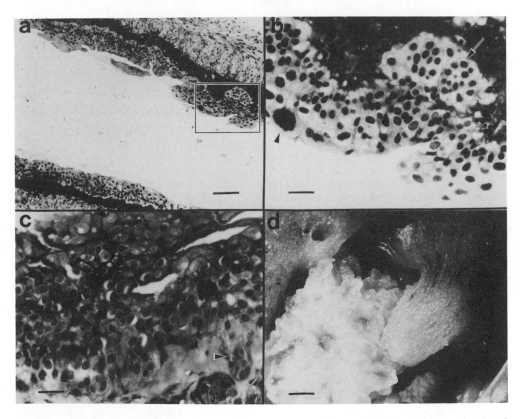

Figure 2 **a**. Disorganised hyperplastic ureteric urothelium from animal 13 weeks after BBN/BEA treatment. Giemsa. Bar = 80 um. Inset **b** shows nodular 'invasive' area (arrow) and large multinucleated cells (arrow-head). Giemsa. Bar = 20 um. **c**. Papillary and nodular hyperplasia in ureter, 13 weeks after BBN/BEA treatment. Toluidine blue. Bar = 20 um. **d**. Macroscopic photograph of tumour found in pelvis 40 weeks after BBN/BEA treatment. Bar = 1 mm.

of premalignant and malignant cell populations within the urothelium of animals that had been initiated before an acute RPN was induced. These data suggest that a BBN initiated urothelium can be promoted to preneoplastic and neoplastic cells by an acute RPN. This classical 2-stage process suggests that analgesic-associated RPN may be a key factor in producing a proliferative population in a pelvic or ureteric epithelial cells that had already been initiated. These proliferating cells could then progress to localized upper urothelial dysplastic foci and with time a carcinoma. It is presently uncertain how valid a 2-stage model is for human analgesic abusers. Many of these patients have, however, been exposed to potential urothelial initiating agents by a high incidence of cigarette smoking which has been associated with an increased incidence of urothelial malignancies and carcinomas (10).

REFERENCES

1. Hultengren, N., Lagergren, C. and Ljungquivst, A. Carcinoma of the renal pelvis in renal papillary necrosis. Acta. Chir. Scand. 130, 314-320, 1965.

2. Isaka, H., Yoshii, H., Otsuji, A., Koike, M., Nagai, Y., Koura, M., Sugiyasu, K. and Kanabayashi, T. Tumors of Sprague-Dawley rats induced by long-term feeding of phenacetin. Gann 70, 29-36, 1979.

3. Bach, P.H. and Bridges, J.W. Chemically induced renal papillary necrosis and upper urothelial carcinoma. CRC Crit. Rev. Tox. 15, 217-439, 1985.

4. Gregg, N.J., Courtauld, E.A. and Bach, P.H. High resolution light microscope enzyme histochemical changes in an acutely induced renal papillary necrosis. Tox. Pathol. Submitted. 1987.

5. Cohen, S.M. Pathology of experimental bladder cancer in rodents. In: The Pathology of Bladder Cancer VII. Eds. Bryan, G.T. and Cohen, S.M. CRC Press, Boca Raton, Florida, 1983.

6. Becci, P.J., Thompson, H.J., Grubbs, C.J. and Moon, R.C. A quantitative dosing schedule for the induction of transitional cell carcinomas in female F344 rats with the use of N-butyl-N-(4-hydroxybutyl)nitrosamine. JCNI. 62, 187-191, 1979.

7. Bach, P.H., Grasso, P., Molland, E.A. and Bridges, J.W. Changes in medullary glycosaminoglycan histochemistry and microvascular filling during the development of 2-Bromoethanamine hydrobromide-induced renal papillary necrosis. Tox. Appl. Pharmacol. 69, 333-344, 1983.

8. Burry, A., Cross, R. and Axelsen, R. Analgesic nephropathy and the renal concentrating mechanism. Pathol. Ann. 12, 1-31, 1977.

9. Mostofi, F.K., Sobin, L-H. and Torloni, H. Histological typing of urinary bladder tumours. International histological classification of tumours. 10, WHO, Geneva, 1973.

10. McCredie, M., Stewart, J.H. and Ford, J.M. Analgesics and tobacco as risk factors for cancer of the ureter and renal pelvis. J. Urol. 130, 28-30, 1983.

were cut.   Serial semi-thin (1um) sections were cut to include the papilla tip, mouth of the ureter and the cortex and of the bladder using glass "Ralph" knives.

Sections were stained for with haematoxylin and eosin (H & E), Giemsa's stain, Toludine Blue and PAS.   Enzyme histochemistry was performed to show the distribution of alkaline phosphatase (Alk Phos), acid phosphatase (Acid Phos), gamma-glutamyl transpeptidase (GGT) and adenosine triphosphatase (ATPase) using methods modified by Burnett (4).

RESULTS

Morphology and enzyme histochemistry results are summarised in Tables I and II.

Table I. Time course of morphological changes

Time Point   Morphological Changes

Control   Normal with papilla interstitial matrix increasing in volume towards tip.   Urothelium 2-4 cells thick, paler superficial layer which is PAS positive.

2 hr   No changes discernible.

4 hr Medullary interstitial cell nuclei becoming acutely irregular and pyknotic (Fig. 1a).

6 hr   Mild hyperplasia of papilla covering epithelium to 2-3 cells thick.

8 hr   Marked pyknosis of interstitial cell nuclei, sloughing of hyper-plastic covering epithelium.   Platelets adhering to endothelium dilated distal tubular profiles.

12 hr   Leading edge of sloughing covering epithelium showing mild 2-3 cell thick hyperplasia.   Degenerative changes in tubular elements in papilla.   Hyperplasia in upper ureteric urothelium.

18 hr   50% of papilla affected by RPN. Cytoplasmic granules in necrotic collecting duct cells, mitotic figures present.   Hyperplasia of pelvic urothelium opposite leading edge of covering epithelium (Fig. 1b).

24 hr   Medulla affected by necrosis, loss of tissue integrity with cellular debris and proteinaceous casts in papilla.   Casts in dilated distal tubules in cortex.   Fornix area of urothelium, hyperplastic, mitotic figures present.

48 hr   Covering epithelium leading edge 5 cells thick, cells very irregular nuclei, cytoplasmic granules present. General hyperplasia of pelvic and ureteric urothelium (Fig. 1c).

72 hr   75% denudation of papilla covering epithelium.   Tubular necrosis extending to outer medulla.   Marked dilatation of proximal and distal tubules.

144 hr   100% loss of covering epithelium, papilla is a mass of necrotic tubules, (Fig. 1d) lymphocytic infiltration.   Sloughing of pelvic and ureteric urothelium, bladder urothelial superficial layer becoming increasingly basophilic.   Numerous granules in proximal tubule segments.

HIGH RESOLUTION MICROSCOPIC CHANGES IN AN ACUTELY INDUCED RENAL PAPILLARY NECROSIS: MORPHOLOGY AND ENZYME HISTOCHEMISTRY

N.J. Gregg,   E.A. Courtauld and P.H. Bach

Nephrotoxicity Research Group, Robens Institute, University of Surrey, Guildford, GU2 5XH, UK

INTRODUCTION

Renal papillary necrosis (RPN) has been associated with an excessive consumption of analgesics and nonsteroidal anti-inflammatory drugs (1). The course of development of this lesion in man has been documented from post mortem tissue, where autolysis, other diseases and marked variability in the extent of lesion have made it difficult to determine the progression of pathological changes. There is some evidence to suggest that the renal medullary interstitial cells are the primary site of toxic injury and that microvascular, collecting duct and tubular degeneration are secondary changes. 2-Bromoethanamine (BEA) hydrobromide is a chemical which induces RPN rapidly and has allowed the progression of RPN to be studied. There are marked similarities between this acute BEA induced lesion and changes that have been reported in animals dosed chronically with analgesics and non-steroidal anti-inflammatory drugs, and also the clinical condition in human analgesic abusers (1,2).

We have re-evaluated the detailed time-course of an acute papillary necrosis using semi-thin glycolmethacrylate embedded sections to provide detailed pathological changes. Furthermore, the ability to combine "routine" staining with selective enzyme histochemistry on serial semi thin (1um) sections enhances the ability to inter-relate changes in different cell types during the course of the development of degenerative processes that lead to RPN.

MATERIALS AND METHODS

Male Wistar rats, University of Surrey strain, were injected ip with a single dose of BEA 100 mg/kg body weight (BDH, Poole, Dorset, UK) freshly prepared in physiological saline (3) and control animals injected with vehicle only.

Animals were sacrificed by cervical dislocation in groups of 3 at 2, 8, 12, 18, 24, 48, 72 and 144 hr and pairs of control animals similarly sacrificed at 12, 48 and 144 hr. All tissue processing performed at $4^{\circ}C$. The right kidney, ureter and the inflated bladder immersion fixed in formal calcium fixative (4% v/v formaldehyde, calcium chloride). After 24 hr fixation 1-2 mm thick slices cut including the papilla tip, cortex, and a longitudinal slice of

Table II. Time course of histochemical changes

Time point	Histochemical changes

Control   Occasion PAS positive granules in urothelium Alk Phos and ATPase enzyme staining in proximal tubule brush borders (also GGT), intermediate and basal layer of urothelium with superficial layer devoid of stain (Fig. 2a).

2 hr   No changes discernible.

4 hr   Increase in interstitial matrix staining with Giemsa.   Slight increase in ATPase staining around pyknotic nuclei.

6 hr   Slight decrease in Alk Phos and GGT proximal tubule brush border staining.

8 hr Increase in Alk Phos staining in pelvic urothelium opposite denuded covering epithelium (Fig. 2b). Acid Phos increase staining in the S1 and S2 proximal tubule segments.

12 hr Increase interstitial matrix staining at papilla tip.   Hyperplastic urothelium has increased apical Alk Phos staining and increased ATPase staining of endothelium sub-urothelial capillaries.

18 hr   Mosaic pattern of Alk Phos and ATPase staining in hyperplastic urothelium (Fig. 2c). ATPase endothelial staining increase, moderate Acid Phos staining of interstitial cells in medulla.

24 hr   Decreased interstitial matrix staining, loss of proximal tubular brush border enzymes Alk Phos, ATPase and GGT coincide with an increase of these enzymes in proteinaceous casts in the necrotic papilla. Loss of Acid Phos staining from S2 proximal tubule segment.

48 hr   PAS positive staining material in proteinaceous casts. Continued loss of Alk Phos, ATPase and GGT from proximal tubule brush borders, also loss of Alk Phos and ATPase to slight degree from pelvic and ureteric urothelium.

72 hr   Variable enzyme staining in proteinaceous casts, GGT most pronounced.   Urothelial staining in ureter reduced to few Alk Phos positive cells, no bladder staining at all. Sub- urothelial capillary ATPase staining increased (Fig. 2d).

144 hr   Granular Alk Phos and GGT staining in interstitium adjacent to hyperplastic fornix urothelium. Increased Acid Phos lysosomal staining in proximal tubule segments. Sub-urothelial capillary ATPase endothelial staining increase in quantity to occlude lumen.

DISCUSSION

The renal medullary interstitial cells are the first morphological feature to be affected in the cascade of degenerative changes that leads to RPN. These are followed by loss of the mucopolysaccharide matrix and degeneration of the endothelium, distal tubules, collecting ducts and loops of Henle.

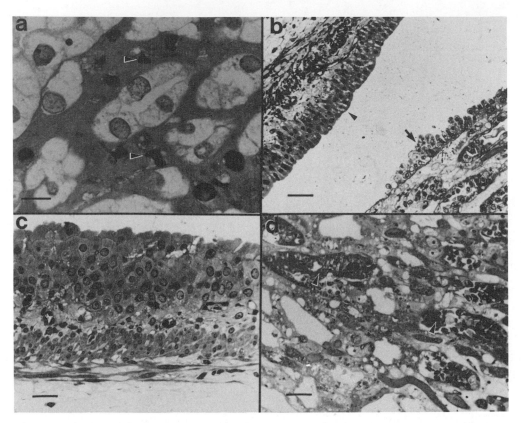

Figure 1   **a**. Medullary interstitial cell nuclei (arrowheads) becoming acutely irregular and pyknotic 4 hr after BEA (100mg/Kg). Giemsa. Bar = 10 um.   **b**. Hyperplasia of pelvic urothelium (arrowhead) opposite leading edge of covering epithelium (arrow) 18 hr after BEA. Toluidine blue. Bar = 100um.   **c**. Hyperplastic pelvic urothelium , 72 hours after BEA (100 mg/kg). Giemsa. Bar = 40 um.   **d**. Papilla tip is a mass of necrotic tissue, with casts in loops of Henle and collecting ducts consisting of exfoliated cell debris. Giemsa. Bar = 25 um.

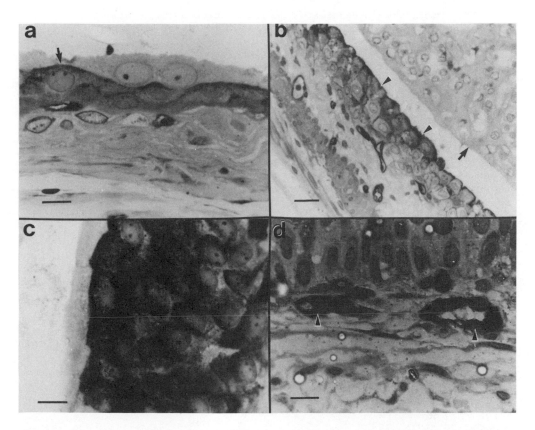

Figure 2 **a.** Alkaline phosphatase (Alk. Phos.) staining in control bladder urothelium (arrow). Superficial "umbrella" cell layer devoid of stain. Bar = 10um. **b.** Increased Alk. Phos. staining in pelvic urothelium (arrowheads) opposite denuded covering epithelium (arrow) 8 hr after BEA. Bar = 20 um. **c.** Mosaic pattern of Alk. Phos. staining in hyperplastic urothelium, 18 hr after BEA. Bar = 10 um. **d.** Sub-urothelial capillary endothelium stained with ATPase, thickness increasing to occlude lumen (arrowheads). Bar = 10 um.

The sensitivity of the medullary interstitial cells to BEA may be due to one or more of the following:-

- The interstitial cells are rich in prostaglandin hydroperoxidase and other peroxidases, which have the potential to produced biologically reactive intermediates (5).

- The medulla has very low levels of glutathione and therefore once generated and reactive intermediates would not readily be inactivated (5).

- The medullary interstitial cells contain a large amount of lipid droplets which are very rich in polyunsaturated fatty acids (5).

Thus the consequence of generating a reactive intermediate could be that of a sustained lipid peroxidation that was localized to the target cells, but also affected adjacent anatomical elements of the medulla. The interstitial cells synthesise the mucopolysaccharide ground substance that serves to support the delicate elements (loops of Henle and capillaries) in the medulla and also acts as a matrix that controls the availability and movement of liquid, ions and other molecules between the different compartments. Thus an early loss of the mucopolysaccharide matrix will drastically affect renal function and morphology, and play an important role in the cascade of degenerative changes that follows. Furthermore, where as epithelial cells have a significant regenerative capacity, the medullary interstitial cells do not undergo proliferative changes when damaged, nor is there a stem cell population from which to replace "lost or damaged" cells (1).

The subtle degenerative changes in the proximal tubule do not appear to be central to the development of the papillary lesion. Exfoliated brush border enzymes and cells are ,however, important components of the proteinaceous casts in the distal nephron.

Hyperplasia, the formation of distal tubular casts and then the proximal and distal tubular dilatation all appear to be secondary consequences of papillary necrosis, and the delayed increase in Alk Phos staining in urothelium support this. The increased ATPase staining of sub-urothelial capillary endothelium suggests that there is a progressive microangiopathy similar to that described in human analgesic abusers with RPN (6).

ACKNOWLEDGEMENTS

This research is supported by the Cancer Research Campaign of Great Britain, International Agency for Research on Cancer and Wellcome Trust.

REFERENCES

1. Bach, P.H. and Bridges, J.W. (1985), Chemically induced Renal Papillary Necrosis and Upper Urothelial Carcinoma, CRC Crit. Rev. Tox. 15, 217-439

2. Bach, P.H. and Hardy, T.L.(1985) The relevance of animal models to the study of analgesic associated renal papillary necrosis in man. Kidney Int. 28, 605-613.

3. Bach, P.H., Grasso, P., Molland, E.A. and Bridges, J.W. (1983), Changes in Medullary Glycosaminoglycan Histochemistry and Microvascular filling during the development of 2-Bromoethanamine Hydrobromide-induced Renal Papillary Necrosis. Toxicol App. Pharm. 69, 333-344

4.   Burnett, R. (1982) A study of Enzymatic and structural Renal damage induced by Nephrotoxic Agents in the rat.   M.Phil.   Thesis, University of Nottingham.

5.   Bach, P.H. and Bridges, J.W. (1984) The role of metabolic activation of   analgesics   and non- steroidal anti-inflammatory drugs   in   the development of renal papillary necrosis and upper   urothelial   carcinoma. Prost. Leuk. Med. 15 :251-274.

6.   Mihatsch, M.J., Hofer, H.O., Gudat, F., Knusli, C., Torhorst, J. and Zollinger, U. (1984) Capillary sclerosis and analgesic nephropathy. Clin. Nephrol. 20:285-301.

CANNULATION OF THE BILE DUCT PROTECTS AGAINST PARA-AMINOPHENOL-INDUCED NEPHROTOXICITY IN THE FISCHER 344 RAT

K. P. R. Gartland (1), C. T. Eason (2), F. W. Bonner (2) and J. K. Nicholson (1)

(1) Department of Chemistry, Birkbeck College, University of London, Malet Street, London WC1E 7HX, and (2) Department of Toxicology, Sterling-Winthrop Research Centre, Alnwick, Northumberland NE66 2JH, U.K.

INTRODUCTION

Para-aminophenol (PAP) produces necrosis of proximal convoluted tubules acutely in the rat after a single injection (1), and has been demonstrated to be a minor metabolite of paracetamol in the Fischer 344 (F344) rat and Fischer-derived isolated perfused kidney (2). Examination of urine from PAP-treated rats by high resolution proton nuclear magnetic resonance (NMR) spectroscopy revealed dose-related elevations in the urinary excretion of glucose, amino acids, and lactic acid (3,4) while conventional methods showed enzymuria (4).

Paracetamol (APAP; N-acetyl-p-aminophenol) is structurally closely related to PAP, and metabolites of APAP have been shown to be excreted by the biliary route in rats (5,6) and mice (7). These metabolites are the glucuronic acid and sulphate conjugates (5,6), in addition to the glutathione conjugate (8). Hinson et al successfully isolated and purified the glutathione conjugate of APAP 3-(glutathion-S-yl)-paracetamol, from rat bile and, employing the ^{1}H and ^{13}C NMR spectra, succeeded in structurally characterizing this adduct.

Toxicity arising from PAP has been previously suggested to result from a dose-related depletion kidney reduced glutathione (GSH) and covalent binding to essential renal macromolecules (9). However, results obtained from experiments in which GSH was depleted by buthionine sulphoximine (BSO) strongly suggest a role for a toxic GSH conjugate, or breakdown product of a GSH conjugate in the mechanism of toxicity of PAP (10). In addition, findings from experiments in which rats were pretreated with aminooxyacetic acid (AOA), a ß-lyase inhibitor, support a role for this enzyme in the mechanism of toxicity of PAP (11).

Since the GSH conjugate of APAP is excreted in bile, and PAP is a structural analogue of APAP, we chose to examine the role of the liver in PAP-induced nephrotoxicity by treating animals in which the bile duct had been cannulated to divert hepatic metabolites away from the systemic system.

EXPERIMENTAL

Animals and Treatments. Male Fischer 344 rats were allocated to 4 groups

of 3 rats each, 2 control and 2 treated groups. The bile ducts of 6 rats
(2 groups) were cannulated by the method of Tomlinson et al (12) and
immediately after surgery, were housed in glass metabolism cages and
allowed to recover for a period of 24 hr prior to treatment. Animals
received a single i.p. injection of either saline (control), or a 50 mg/ml
solution of p-aminophenol hydrochloride in saline equivalent to a dose
of 100 mg/kg body weight.

Sample Collection and Conventional Methodology. Bile and urine were
collected over ice for 24 hr prior to, and at 8 and 24 hr after dosing.
Gamma-glutamyl transpeptidase (GGT) and N-acetyl-ß-D-glucosaminidase
(NAG) were measured in desalted urine (Sephadex G25M) by the methods of
Naftalin et al (13)and Maruhn (14) respectively. Urine glucose was
measured by the hexokinase method employing a Sigma diagnostic kit (cat.
16-UV). Animals were killed 24 hr after dosing and blood removed for
measurement of plasma urea (Beckman kit). Renal histopathology was also
examined at this time, and 7 um wax sections were tissue stained with
haematoxylin and eosin.

^{1}H NMR Urinalysis. Samples were examined either non-lyophilized or
after lyophilization (to correct for any increase in urine flow rate) by
high resolution proton NMR Spectroscopy at a field strength of 9.4 Tesla
equivalent to a frequency of 400 MHz for the 1H nucleus. Urine (0.45 ml)
was diluted with 0.05 ml ^{2}H$_2$O (field frequency lock) containing sodium 3-
(tri-methylsilyl)-(2,2,3,3,-^{2}H)1-1-propionate as an internal shift
reference (0 ppm). Single pulse experiments were employed with the
following conditions: 64 free induction decays (FIDs) were collected into
16,384 computer points using 38° pulses, acquisition time 1.7 seconds. A
further delay of 2.0 seconds between pulses was added to ensure that the
spectra were fully T$_1$ relaxed. A continuous secondary irradiation field
was applied at the resonance frequency of water to suppress the intense
water signal.

RESULTS

Conventional Urinalysis. Figures 1-4 display the effect of prior biliary
cannulation on PAP-induced polyuria (Fig. 1), enzymuria (Figs. 2 and 3)
and glycosuria (Fig. 4). While the elevations seen in all of these
urinary parameters following PAP are considerably reduced by biliary
cannulation, they are not prevented. Elevations in urinary enzymes and
glucose are still very apparent following biliary cannulation.

Plasma Urea Nitrogen (Table 1). When measured, the urea nitrogen
concentration of plasma was found to be elevated after biliary
cannulation alone. Consequently, urea nitrogen was not employed in these
studies as an index of nephrotoxicity.

Table 1. Blood Urea Nitrogen   mean ± SE (n)

BUN   (mg/100ml)

Control	(NC)	15.77±0.74(3)
Treated	(NC)	37.63±2.99(3)
Control	(C)	22.61±1.24(2)
Treated	(C)	25.51±1.89(3)

Proton NMR Urinalysis. Shown in figures 5 and 6 are the proton NMR
spectra of urine from control (bottom trace), non-cannulated (NC) animals
(middle trace), and cannulated (C) animals (top trace) collected 8

424

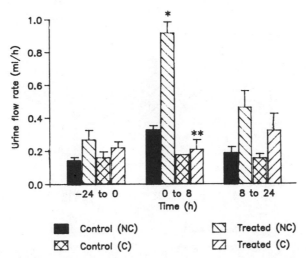

Figure 1.   The effect of biliary cannulation on PAP-induced polyuria. NC
= non-cannulated; C = cannulated.   Treated rats received 100 mg/kg PAP in
saline. Statistics (t-test) * p < 0.001   when compared to control (NC); **
p < 0.001 when compared to treated (NCl;   ***. p < 0.1 when compared to
control (C).

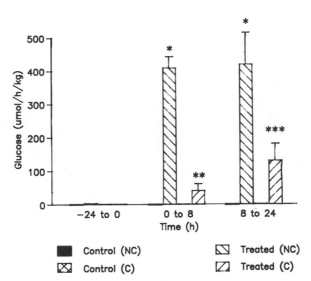

Figure 2.   The effect of biliary cannulation on PAP-induced glycosuria.
NC = non-cannulated; C = cannulated.   Treated rats received 100 mg/kg PAP
in saline. Statistics (t-test) * p < 0.001   when compared to control (NC);
** p < 0.001 when compared to treated (NC);   ***. p < 0.1 when compared to
control (C).

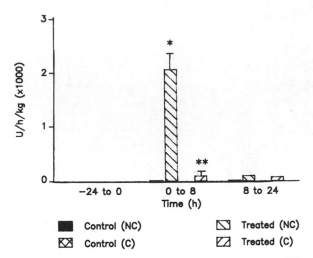

Figure 3.   The effect of biliary cannulation on PAP-induced enzymuria: Gamma-glutamyl Transpeptidase (GGT).   NC = non-cannulated; C = cannulated. Treated rats received 100mg/kg PAP in saline. * p < 0.001 when compared to control   (NC);   ** p < 0.001 when compared to treated (NC);   *** p < 0.002 when compared to treated (NC).

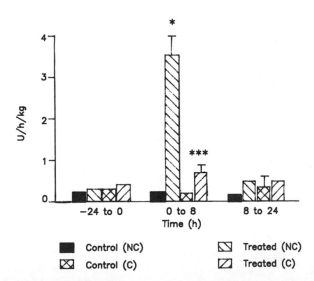

Figure 4.   The effect of biliary cannulation on PAP-induced enzymuria: N-acetyl-ß-D-glucosaminidase   (NAG).   NC = non-cannulated;   C = cannulated. Treated rats received 100mg/kg PAP in saline.   *:   p < 0.001 when compared to control (NC); ** p < 0.001 when compared to treated (NC); *** p < 0.002 when compared to treated (NC).

(Fig. 5) and 24 hr (Fig. 6) after treatment. The lower trace of both figures represents the normal proton NMR profile of rat urine. The principle features of the middle trace are glycosuria, lactic aciduria and aminoaciduria (alanine, glutamine, valine). These abnormalities are partially prevented by cannulation of the common bile duct.

Renal Histopathology. Both micrographs are from animals treated with PAP. Fig. 7a shows the lesion produced in the cortex of a non-cannulated animal by a 100 mg/kg dose of PAP. Necrosis of proximal tubules in the mid- and deep cortex together with intermittent zones of radial necrosis are apparent. The micrograph shown in Figure 7b is from a cannulated animal. No overall signs of tubular necrosis are apparent except in the mid-cortex where occasional tubules have become necrotic and fragmented.

DISCUSSION

In the present study we have shown that cannulation of the common bile duct partially protects against p-aminophenol-induced nephrotoxicity in the Fischer 344 rat. This is supported by results obtained from measurements of urinary enzymes (GGT and NAG) and urine glucose, together with ^{1}H NMR urinalysis and renal histopathology. This finding strongly implicates the liver in the mechanism of toxicity of PAP and suggests that a hepatic metabolite is generated, excreted in the bile, to the small intestine, reabsorbed into the blood and transported to the kidneys where the toxic effects are manifest. Previous experiments in which GSH was depleted in vivo by buthionine sulphoximine treatment strongly suggest that this metabolite is the GSH conjugate of treatment strongly suggest that this metabolite is the GSH conjugate of p-amino-phenol (10). he renal selectivity of the GSH conjugate has been attributed to the processing of the conjugates by GGT and cysteinylglycine dipeptidase (CGD) which convert glutathione conjugates to cysteine conjugates (15). These peptidases are present in the lumenal and baso-lateral membranes of the proximal tubule (16) and also in the villous tips of the small intestine (17).

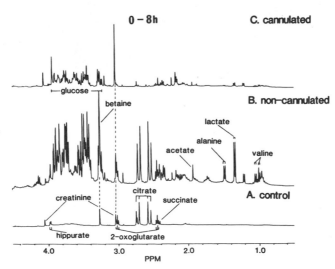

Figure 5. 400 MHZ proton NMR Spectra 8 hr after treatment; urine collected from A = control, B = non-cannulated and C = cannulated rats.

427

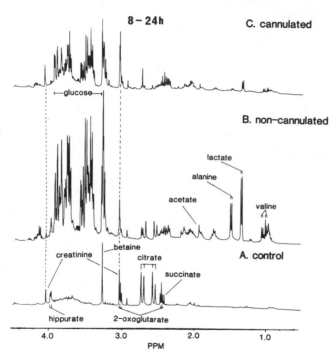

Figure 6.   400 MHZ proton NMR Spectra 16 hr (8-24h) after treatment; urine collected from A = control, B = non-cannulated and C = cannulated rats.

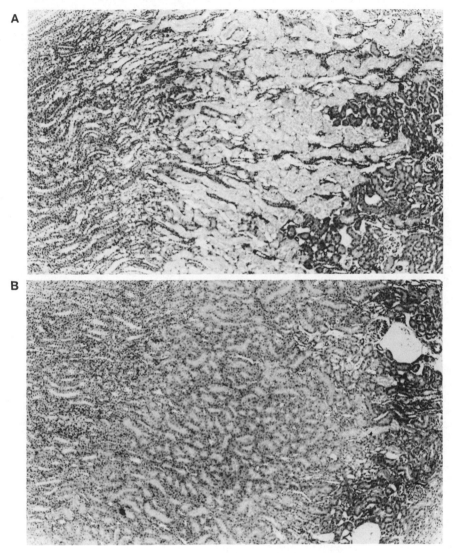

Figure 7. Light micrographs of kidneys from rats 24 hr after treatment with PAP. A) Kidneys from non-cannulated animals show a radial cortico-medullary necrosis. B) Kidneys from bile duct cannulated animals show occasional mid-cortical necrosis.

A number of studies have examined the metabolism of the biliary GSH conjugate of paracetamol - a drug closely related structurally to PAP. There appears to be two major sites of metabolism of the glutathione conjugate of paracetamol i.e. the small intestine and the kidney. This conjugate has been shown to be degraded to the cysteine conjugate by the kidney in vivo (5) and in vitro (18), and also by the epithelial ells of the small intestine in vivo (7), and in vitro (17).

Grafstrom et al (17) have proposed that, because of the luminal position of GGT and CGD in the proximal tubule and small intestine action of these enzymes on a GSH conjugate would probably occur before absorption of the cysteine conjugate. Fischer et al (7) noted a high tissue-to-plasma ratio of the cysteine conjugate of paracetamol in the kidney, and following nephrectomy, a 40% reduction in the amount of this conjugate present in the animal 1 hr after APAP, suggesting a major role for the kidney in the formation of the cysteine conjugate. This group further reported high concentrations of the cysteine conjugate in the intestine of mice following excretion of the glutathione conjugate in bile indicating that this tissue also plays a major role in APAP-cysteine formation. Thus both the small intestine and kidney make a substantial contribution to the total amount of cysteine conjugate generated from the glutathione adduct of paracetamol. In the case of the PAP-GSH adduct, however, although both small intestine and kidney have the capacity to generate cysteine conjugates, the exact contribution of each remains a matter for speculation.

The finding of only partial protection by biliary cannulation against the nephrotoxic effects of PAP implies that a portion of the PAP-GSH adduct is being excreted from the liver by the sinusoidal route into the blood to travel directly to the kidney. Alternatively, an extrahepatic component may exist - such as generation of a toxic species by some other mechanism within the kidney itself.

Cannulation of the bile duct produced a 10% protection on comparison of data from clinical chemistry. Therefore, we may in fact have succeeded in separating two contributing pathways of excretion of the PAP-GSH adduct from the liver. That is, it is possible that, under normal circumstances, 70% of the total amount of PAP-GSH generated in the liver is excreted in the bile, while a much smaller amount (30%) is excreted by the sinusoidal route. All of the PAP-GSH leaving the liver by the sinusoidal route would then be degraded by GGT and CGD in the proximal tubule, while that proportion excreted in the bile would, in theory, be exposed to both tissues. Alternatively, this smaller component of toxicity may represent unchanged PAP bypassing the liver and travelling directly to the kidney. The recent finding by Lash et al (19) of ß-lyase activity on the outer membrane of mitochondria from rat renal cortex is notable, since a role for this enzyme in the mechanism of toxicity of PAP has been suggested (11). Indeed, Crowe et al (20) demonstrated that, whereas oxidative phosphorylation and respiratory control were significantly reduced in mitochondria isolated from PAP-treated rats, when added directly to mitochondria from naive rats, PAP failed to alter respiratory activity suggesting that PAP itself does not have a direct effect on mitochondria. This group go on to suggest that a metabolite of PAP, possibly formed in the liver, may be responsible for the mitochondrial damage. This is in agreement with the findings of the present study. These findings suggest that the toxic species is being generated on the outer mitochondrial membrane and damaging the mitochondrion directly.

Therefore, in summary, we propose that p-aminophenol is nephrotoxic via a GSH conjugate, generated in the liver which is predominantly excreted in

430

bile. Subsequent metabolism of this adduct by GGT and CGD located in the proximal tubule and intestinal epithelium, generates a cysteine conjugate. Following uptake by the proximal tubular cell, this conjugate is cleaved by mitochondrial ß-lyase to produce pyruvate, ammonia and a thiol, the reactive species which produces damage to the mitochondrion. This will lead ultimately to depletion of cellular ATP and cell death.

REFERENCES

1. C.R. Green, K.N. Ham and J.D. Tange, Kidney lesions induced in rats by p-aminophenol, B.M.J., 1:162-164 (1969).

2. J.F. Newton, C.H. Kuo, M.W. Gemborys, G.H. Mudge and J.B. Hook, Nephro-toxicity of p-aminophenol: a metabolite of acetaminophen in the Fischer 344 rat, Tox. Appl. Pharmacol., 65:336-344 (1982).

3. J.K. Nicholson and K.P.R. Gartland, In: Cells, Membranes and Disease, including Renal, ed. E. Reid, G.M.W. Cook and J.P. Luzio, Methodological Surveys in Biochemistry and Analysis Vol. 17, pp 397-408, Plenum Press, New York (1987).

4. K.P.R. Gartland, J.K. Nicholson, J.A. Timbrell and F.W. Bonner, Detection and assessment of p-aminophenol-induced nephrotoxic lesions by proton NMR spectroscopy, Human Tox., 5:122-123 (1986).

5. C.-P. Siegers, K. Roznan and C.D. Klaassen, Biliary excretion and enterohepatic circulation of paracetamol in the rat, Xenobiotica, 13: 591-596 (1983).

6. C.-P. Siegers and C.D. Klaassen Biliary excretion of acetaminophen in ureter-ligated rats, Pharmacology, 28:177-180 (1984).

7. L.J. Fischer, M.D. Green and A.W. Harman. Studies on the fate of the glutathione and cysteine conjugates of acetaminophen in mice, Drug Metab. Disp., 13:121-126 (1985).

8. J.A. Hinson, T.T. Monks, M. Hong, R.J. Highet and L.R. Pohl, 3-(glutathion-S-yl)acetaminophen: a biliary metabolite of acetaminophen, Drug Metab. Disp., 10:47-50 (1982).

9. C.A. Crowe, A.C. Yong, I.C. Calder, K.N. Ham and J.D. Tange, The nephrotoxicity of p-aminophenol. 1. The effect on microsomal cytochromes, glutathione and covalent binding in kidney and liver, Chem. Biol. Interact. 27:235-243 (1979).

10. K.P.R. Gartland, F.W. Bonner and J.K. Nicholson, The effect of buthionine sulphoximine on p-aminophenol-induced nephrotoxicity in the F344 rat, Human Tox. (in press).

11. K.P.R. Gartland, F.W. Bonner and J.K. Nicholson (unpublished observations) (1987).

12. P.W. Tomlinson, D.J. Jeffrey and C.W. Filer, A novel technique for assessment of biliary secretion and enterohepatic circulation in the unrestrained conscious rat, Xenobiotica, 11:863-870 (1981).

13. L.M. Naftalin, M. Sexton, J.F. Whitaker and D. Tracy, A routine procedure for estimating serum gamma-glutamyl transpeptidase activity, Clin. Chim. Acta, 26:293-296 (1969).

14. D. Maruhn, Rapid Colorimetric assay for ß-galactosidase and N-acetyl-

ß-D-glucosaminidase in human urine, <u>Clin. Chim. Acta</u>, 73:453-461 (1976).

15. A.A. Elfarra and M.W. Anders, Renal processing of glutathione conjugates. Role in nephrotoxicity, <u>Biochem. Pharmacol.</u>, 33:3729-3732 (1984).

16. P.D. Dass and T.C. Welbourne, Evidence for lumenal and anti-lumenal localization of gamma-glutamyl transpeptidase in rat kidney, <u>Life Sci.</u>, 355-360 (1981).

17. R. Grafstrom, K. Ormstad, P. Moldeus and S. Orrenius, Paracetamol metabolism in the isolated perfused rat liver with further metabolism of a biliary paracetamol conjugate by the small intestine, <u>Biochem. Pharmacol.</u>, 28:3573-3579 (1979).

18. J.F. Newton, D. Hoefle, M.W. Gemborys, G.H. Mudge and J.B. Hook, Metabolism and excretion of a glutathione conjugate of acetaminophen in the isolated perfused rat kidney, <u>J. Pharmacol. Exp. Ther.</u>, 237:519-524 (1986).

19. L.H. Lash, A.A. Elfarra and M.W. Anders, Renal cysteine conjugate ß-lyase. Bioactivation of nephrotoxic cysteine S-conjugates in mitochondrial outer membrane, <u>J. Biol. Chem.</u>, 261 : 5930-5935 (1986).

20. C.A. Crowe, I.C. Calder, N.P. Madsen, C.C. Funder, C.R. Green, K.N. Ham and J.D. Tange, An experimental model of analgesic-induced renal damage. Some effects of p-aminophenol on rat kidney mitochondria, <u>Xenobiotica</u>, 7:345-356 (1977).

EFFECTS OF ANTIDOTES ON THE HEPATO- AND NEPHROTOXICITY OF PARACETAMOL IN THE RAT

Walter Moller-Hartmann and Claus-Peter Siegers

Department of Toxicology, Medical University of Lubeck, D-2400 Lubeck (FRG)

INTRODUCTION

During intoxications with paracetamol hepatic and renal failure may develop, the latter also in the absence of liver damage (Boyer et al., 1971; Prescott et al., 1971; Cobden et al., 1982). Several antidotes are available for the treatment of severe paracetamol poisoning, these include mainly precursors of GSH-synthesis like methionine or N-acetylcysteine (Crome et al,. 1976; Prescott et al., 1977). In animal experiments diethyldithiocarbamate (dithiocarb) was shown to be an effective antidote against paracetamol-induced hepatotoxicity, due to its strong inhibitory influence on microsomal monooxygenases (Strubelt et al., 1974; Siegers et al., 1982). No experimental or clinical data, however, are available proving the efficacy of these antidotes in preventing paracetamol-induced renal damage. Moreover, it is still unclear, whether the metabolic pathways leading to hepatotoxic intermediates of paracetamol are the same for exerting nephrotoxic response.

METHODS

Male Wistar-rats (breeder: Winklemann, Borchen, FRG) weighing 300-400 g were used throughout. In the dose-finding-experiments the animals were fasted for 24 hr before receiving paracetamol; in all subsequent experiments fed rats were used.

Treatments: Paracetamol was suspended in a 1% tylose solution, controls received equal volumes (10 ml/kg) of tylose by gavage. L·methionine, N-acetylcysteine, indomethacin and dithiocarb were given simultaneously with paracetamol suspended in tylose; in the case of indomethacin an additional dose was given 24 hr after paracetamol. Blood was collected from the cut tip of the tail and plasma was obtained after addition of 20 ul heparin and centrifugation at 12000 rpm. Rats were placed in metabolic cages for 3-4 days which allowed a separate collection of urine and faeces and free access to food (Altromin [R] pellets) and tap water.

Biochemical determinations: Plasma enzyme activities (GPT, SDH), creatinine and urea concentrations in plasma as well as N-acetyl-ß-glucosaminidase (NAG) and gamma-glutamyltranspeptidase (GGT) activities in the urine were determined by using commercial reagent kits of Boehringer, Mannheim (FRG). Glutathione (GSH + 2GSSG) was estimated in liver and kidney tissue either by Ellman's method according to Sedlack and Lindsay (1968) or by a specific enzymic method according to Brehe and Burch (1976).

RESULTS AND CONCLUSIONS

The threshold dose of paracetamol evoking hepatotoxic and nephrotoxic effects was 1.0 g/kg po. Maximum increases of plasma enzyme activities indicating liver damage occurred 24 and 48 hr after treatment; concomitant increments of plasma creatinine and urea as well as urinary enzyme excretion (NAG, GGT) were observed (Figure 1). It is concluded that paracetamol-induced hepato- and nephrotoxicity show the same time-course.

As shown in figure 2 simultaneous treatment with 500 mg/kg methionine was only able to reduce paracetamol-induced hepatotoxicity at 24 hr, later on no hepatoprotection was observed. Methionine was not at all capable of protecting rats against the nephrotoxic effects of paracetamol. With the lower dose of methionine (150 mg/kg) no hepatoprotection was observed, and kidney damage even appeared to be enhanced by methionine (NAG, GGT, data not shown). With N-acetylcysteine (500 mg/kg) no hepatoprotection was seen, and nephrotoxicity was only reduced during the first 24 hr as evidenced by lower increments of NAG and GGT in the urine (data not shown).

Antidotal treatment with dithiocarb (200 mg/kg) proved to be effective in totally preventing paracetamol-induced hepatotoxicity and nephrotoxicity (Figure 3).

Treatment with indomethacin (2 x 10 mg/kg) did not influence the hepato-toxic effects of paracetamol, but potentiated the nephrotoxicity evoked by paracetamol as evidenced by stronger increments of plasma urea and urinary enzymes (data not shown).

Time course of GSH-levels in liver and kidney is depicted in Figure 4. In the liver paracetamol evoked a strong depletion of GSH (by 60%), whereas in the kidney no depletion was observed. Hepatic glutathione represents completely the nonprotein-bound sulfhydryls, whereas renal GSH accounts for only 3% of total SH-groups as evidenced by comparison of ELLMAN's method with the specific enzymic assay. It is concluded that paracetamol-induced hepatotoxicity is paralleled by a strong GSH-depletion indicating detoxification of reactive intermediates, which seems not to be the cast for the nephrotoxic response to paracetamol.

In summary, antidotes against paracetamol intoxication known as precursors of GSH-synthesis (methionine, N-acetylcysteine) neither provide complete protection against liver damage nor prevented renal injury. The lack of efficacy of indomethacin to influence liver or kidney damage during paracetamol-intoxication indicates, that prostaglandin synthetase are not involved in the bioactivation of paracetamol resulting in the formation of hepatotoxic and nephrotoxic intermediates. The efficacy of dithiocarb in completely protecting against paracetamol-induced hepato- and nephro-toxicity is explained by its inhibitory effects on microsomal mono-oxygenases known to catalyse the toxification of paracetamol. The absence of a depletion of GSH or other sulphydryls in the kidney indicates that bioactivation of paracetamol seems not be quantitatively important in this organ; this leads to the assumption that the further metabolism of paracetamol conjugates exported from the liver to the kidney might be responsible for the nephrotoxicity. In this respect, the C-S-lyase-mediated metabolic activation of cysteine-S-conjugates leading to nephrotoxic intermediates of paracetamol might be involved.

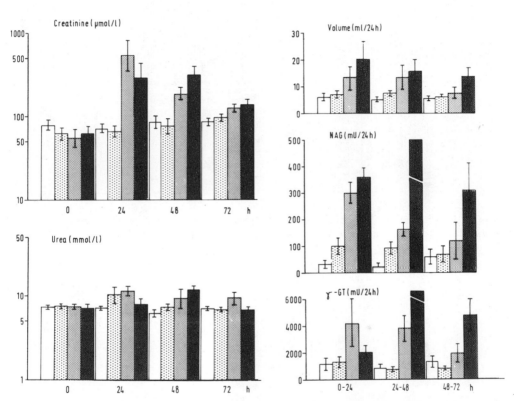

Figure 1. Dose-dependent effects of paracetamol (500-1000-15000 mg/kg po) on urea and creatinine concentrations, urine volume and enzymuria (NAG, GGT) in rats. Values represent geometric means (plasma parameters) or arithmetic means and standard errors out of 4-6 animals each. Open columns: controls receiving tylose po.

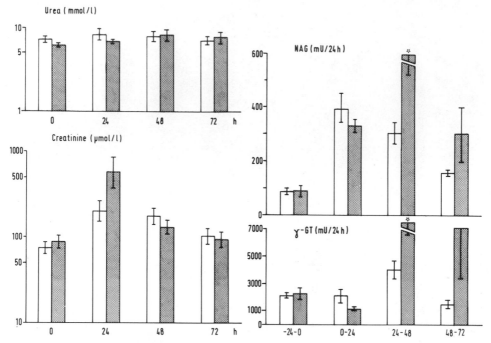

Figure 2. Influence of methionine (150 mg/kg po, hatched columns) on the nephrotoxicity induced by 1.5 g/kg paracetamol po * = p < 0.05.

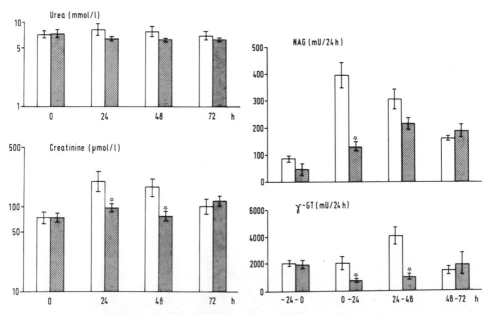

Figure 3. Influence of dithiocarb (200 mg/kg po, hatched columns) on the nephrotoxicity induced by 1.5 g/kg paracetamol po * = p < 0.05.

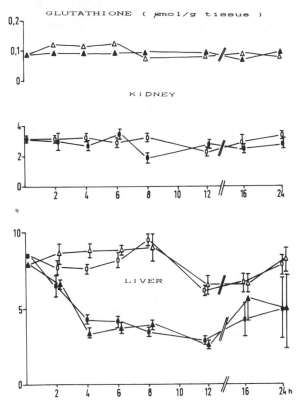

Figure 4. Effect of paracetamol (1.5 g/kg po) on liver and kidney glutathione levels, measured by Ellman's method (circles) and by a specific enzymatic method (triangles). Open symbols: controls. Filled symbols: paracetamol. Values represent arithmetic means and standard errors out of 3 animals each.

REFERENCES

Boyer, T.D. and Rouff, S.L. (1971). Acetaminophen-induced hepatic necrosis and renal failure. J. Am. Med. Assoc. 218, 440-441.

Brehe, J.E. and Burch, H.B. (1976). Enzymatic assay for glutathione. Anal. Biochem. 74, 189-197.

Cobden, I., Record, C.O., Ward, M.K. and Kerr, D.N.S. (1982). Paracetamol-induced acute renal failure in the absence of fulminant liver damage. Br. Med. J. 284, 21-22.

Crome, P., Vale, J.A., Volans, G.N., Widdup, B. and Goulding, R. (1976). Oral methionine in the treatment of severe paracetamol (acetaminophen) overdose. Lancet 2, 829-830.

Prescott, L.F., Wright, N., Roscoe, P. and Brown, S.S. (1971). Plasma-paracetamol half-life and hepatic necrosis in patients with paracetamol overdose. Lancet, 1, 519-522.

Prescott, L.F., Park, J., Ballantyne, A., Adriaenssens, P. and Proudfoot, A.T. (1977). Treatment of paracetamol (acetaminophen) poisoning with N-acetylcysteine. Lancet 2, 432-434.

Sedlack, J. and Lindsay, R.H. (1968). Estimation of total protein-bound and non protein sulfhydryl groups in tissue with Ellman's reagent. Anal. Biochem. 25, 192-205.

Siegers, C.-P., Larseille, J. and Younes, M. (1982). Effects of dithiocarb and (+)-catechin on microsomal enzyme activities of rat liver. Res. Commun. Chem. Pathol. Pharmacol. 36, 61-73.

Strubelt, O., Siegers, C.-P. and Schutt, A. (1974). The curative effects of cysteamine, cysteine and dithiocarb in experimental paracetamol poisoning, Arch. Toxicol. 33, 55-64.

CELIPTIUM INDUCED LIPID PEROXIDATION AND TOXICITY IN RAT RENAL CORTEX

G. Raguenez-Viotte, C. Dadoun, A.M. Van den Bossche, and J.P. Fillastre

INSERM U-295, Universite de Rouen. B.P.97 - 76 800 Saint Etienne du Rouvray - France

The antitumour drug Celiptium (N^2-methyl-9-hydroxyellipticinium) is an ellipticine derivative, effective in experimental tumours (1) and in man. Celiptium is metabolized in liver and excreted by the biliary tract (60%) and urine (30%). However, a renal metabolism occurs in both rats and humans treated with Celiptium, cysteine and N-acetylcysteine conjugates appear in the urine (2). Moreover, it was shown that isolated rat kidney cells metabolize Celiptium into the same conjugates which were found in rat or human urines whereas these compounds were not detected in bile (3).

Celiptium nephrotoxicity has been shown in man, but not in animals in previous studies (4). We have recently showed that the same type of nephrotoxicity occurs in Wistar rats. Celiptium causes a dose-dependent renal lesion characterized by tubular necrosis and tubulo-interstitial lesions (5).

Electron microscopy showed a lipid overload in proximal tubular cells of Celiptium treated rats; we reported now the effects of Celiptium on renal cortex lipids.

MATERIAL AND METHODS

Female Wistar rats, weighing about 200g, were allowed free access to water and received a single intravenous injection of Celiptium (N^2-methyl-9-hydroxyellipticinium acetate = 9-OH-NME) provided by the Sanofi Company (batch RD 6792).

Animals were sacrificed in groups of six at intervals of 2, 4 and 8 days after the injection. Animals were perfused via the aorta with a 0.1M phosphate buffer solution (pH 7.4).

Unfixed frozen sections (5um) were prepared with a cryostat. Total lipid accumulation were demonstrated with Oil Red O (ORO) (6). Ultrastructural studies were undertaken using conventional technique and sections were cut with a Reichert OM-U2 ultramicrotome, stained with uranyl acetate and lead citrate for examination under a Philips CM10 microscope.

Renal function was assessed by creatinine clearance. Kidney cortices were dissected and kept frozen at -20°C until analysis. Homogenates were made in distilled water (1:50, w/v). Proteins were measured by the method of Lowry (7). Lipids were extracted from 1-ml aliquots of renal cortex homogenates by the method of Bligh and Dyer (8). Total glycerol, cholesterol and free fatty acids were determined in lipid extracts enzymically with BioMerieux kits. Results were expressed as nanomoles/mg protein.

For determination of lipid peroxides, aliquots of lipid extracts were assayed iodometrically (9) and thiobarbituric acid (TBA) reactivity was measured in lipid extracts as described by OHKAWA (10). Data were expressed as micro- or nanoequivalents of lipid peroxides or MDA per mg of protein.

Phospholipids and neutral lipids were separated by silicic acid column chromatography. Phospholipids were separated by a two dimensional HPTLC system according to Skispski (11). The bands containing individual phospholipids were sprayed with iodine vapour, scraped from the plates and eluted with chloroform-methanol (2:1, v:v). The main phospholipids obtained were phosphatidylethanolamine (PE), -serine (PS), -choline (PC), -inositol (PI), diphosphatidylglycerol (DPG) and sphingomyelin (SM). Phospholipid classes and total phospholipid contents were quantitated by lipid phosphorus analysis according to Bartlett (12). Data were expressed as nanomoles of lipid phosphorus per mg of protein.

Fatty acids were determined by capillary gas-liquid chromatography (GLC). Fatty acid methyl esters (FAME) of total neutral lipids and total phospholipids were prepared according to Morrison (13). Chromatography was performed on a Perkin Elmer 8500 with a flame ionization detector. Glass columns RSL 500 (Alltech) were used. Methyl esters were identified by their retention times relative to standards. The amount of each ester was determined by an Shidmazu Integrator (CR3A). Fatty acids quantified were palmitic (16:0), stearic (18:0), oleic (18:1), linoleic (18:2), arachidonic (20:4), docosahexaenoic (22:6) acids. Fatty acid compositions were presented as weight percentages of total FAME. Means and standard deviations were calculated. Differences between the experimental control groups were compared using Student's t-test where * = $p < 5\%$, ** = $p < 1\%$ and *** = $p < 0.1\%$.

RESULTS

Morphological Studies. Histochemical analysis of kidney sections detected ORO-positive deposits in the renal cortex of Celiptium treated rats on day 8. These red-stained deposits were only seen in tubules whereas none was shown in glomeruli. Tubules and glomeruli of control kidneys did not contain any lipid material.

Electron microscopy showed no glomerular lesion in Celiptium treated rats while the presence of lipid-like deposits was noted in the cytoplasm of proximal tubular cells (Figure 1). These fatty deposits filled the still intact proximal tubular cell, but there were no alteration was seen in brush border, mitochondria, lysosomes and nuclei.

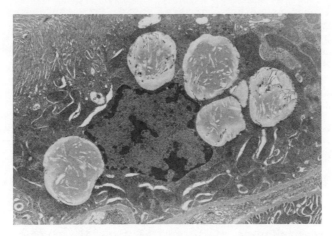

Figure 1.   Electron micrograph of 20mg/kg celiptum treated rats on day 8.
The proximal tubular cells are fill of fat deposits (x5200).

Renal Functional changes are shown in Table I.   Serum creatinine increased
on days 4 and 8 as creatinine clearance was significantly decreased.

Biochemical Study.   Total Neutral Lipids.   A single i.v. dose of 20
mg/kg Celiptium induced a significant increase of total neutral lipids in
renal cortex.   The total glycerol concentration increased 1.7-fold on
days 4 and 8,   while unesterified fatty acids levels increased 2-fold and
6-fold on days 2,   4 and 8 respectively.   Total cholesterol increased 1.4-
fold on day 8. (Table II)

Table I.   Renal Function in 20 mg/kg Celiptium treated rats

	Control	Day 2	Day 4	Day 8
Serum Creat.	9.29	60.49	88.22	66.33
(umole/l)	±13.52	±14.36	±43.49	±5.30
			*	***
Creat.Clearance	1.02	1.00	0.38	0.51
(ml/mn)	±0.05	±0.12	±0.18	±0.10
			***	***

Table II.   Effect of a single dose of 20mg/kg Celiptium on renal cortex
neutral lipids.

	Control	Day 2	Day 4	Day 8
Glycerol	10.40	12.33	13.68	16.92
(nmol/mg	±1.50	±1.87	±2.93	±3.15
protein)		ns	*	**
FFA	12.45	23.69	23.53	73.89
(nmol/mg	±2.30	±4.45	±3.47	±10.67
protein)		***	***	***
Cholesterol	30.00	45.20	32.38	42.02
(nmol/mg	±3.48	±5.15	±4.53	±8.81
protein)		***	ns	**

The fatty acid content of total neutral lipids from control and Celiptium
treated renal cortex showed a significant increase in linoleic (18:2),
arachidonic (20:4) and docosahexaenoic (22:6) acids (Figure 2a). The ratio
of unsaturated:saturated fatty acid increased 1.6-fold in treated rats on
days 4 and 8 (Table III).

Table III.   Ratio of unsaturated:saturated fatty acids

	Control	Day 2	Day 4	Day 8
Neutral Lipids	0.87	0.71	1.45	1.33
	±0.19	±0.073	±0.11	±0.23
		ns	***	**
Phospholipids	1.42	0.82	0.83	0.79
	±0.09	±0.31	±0.14	±0.13
		**	***	***

Phospholipids.   The renal cortical phospholipid content is analysed and
showed a 15% decrease in total phospholipids on days 4 and 8.   Analysis of
individual   phospholipids   showed   a decline   only in the   mass   of
phosphatidylethanolamine (PE) which represents 32% on day 2 and 49 to 50%
on days 4 and 8 (Table IV).

The fatty acid composition of total phospholipids showed that changes
occurred in arachidonic (20:4) and docosahexaenoic (22:6) acids as soon as
day 2 (Figure 2b).   The ratio of unsaturated:saturated fatty acids
decreased 1.7-fold on days 4 and 8 (Table III).

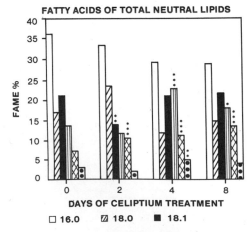

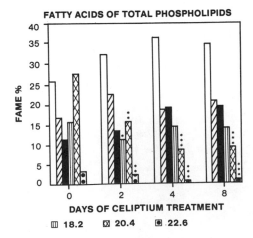

Figure 2.   Fatty acid composition in the renal cortex of Celiptium
treated rats (a) total neutral lipids, (b) total phospholipids.

442

Table IV.   Renal cortical Phospholipid Content (nanomoles/mg protein)

		Control	Day 2	Day 4	Day 8
Total Pi		273.26	237.06	233.17	246.41
		±15.55	±38.07	±16.56	±20.11
			ns	**	*
PC	%	30.80	32.41	33.03	34.41
		±1.63	±1.82	±3.28	±2.32
PE	%	29.95	23.46	18.04	18.74
		±2.66	±14.89	±6.31	±5.85
		**	***	***	
PI +PS	%	12.50	12.31	17.45	16.96
		±2.26	±1.53	±3.50	±2.60
SM	%	16.98	19.47	22.93	20.06
		±2.44	±1.89	±4.59	±4.66
DPG	%	7.88	10.98	9.18	9.40
		±1.92	±2.71	±2.10	±1.36

PC: phosphatidylcholine, PE: phosphatidylethanolamine, PI: phosphatidylinositol, PS: phosphatidyl-serine, SM: sphingomyelin, DPG: diphosphatidylglycerol.

Lipid Peroxides Analysis.   Lipid peroxides were measured in renal cortex
lipid extracts.   Measurements with the iodometric test revealed an
important increase in lipid hydroperoxides (7-fold on day 2, 8-fold on day
4 and 9-fold on day 8) in renal cortex from Celiptium treated rats as
compared to controls.   Thiobarbituric acid (TBA) reactivity values were
significantly (1.7-fold) higher in Celiptium than those of control rats
whatever the day after treatment (Table V).

Table V. Lipid Peroxides in 20 mg/kg Celiptium treated rats

	Control	Day 2	Day 4	Day 8
Lipid peroxides	2.58	18.86	20.56	23.88
(uequiv./mg prot.)	±1.82	±6.41	±2.59	±8.44
		**	***	***
TBA reactivity				
(nanoequiv.MDA	3.05	5.27	5.39	5.33
/mg protein.)	±0.48	±0.67	±0.58	±0.88
		***	***	***

DISCUSSION

Celiptium is an effective antitumoural agent with a very low hepatic and
medular toxicity. We have shown previously that Celiptium induced a dose-
dependent renal toxicity in Wistar rat.   The particular characteristics of
renal involvement are the occurrence of renal failure with tubulointerstital lesions, tubular necrosis and a lipid overload in proximal
tubular cells.   These changes are detectable at a dose of 10 mg/kg, but we
have choosen the single high dose of 20 mg/kg to study the effects of
Celiptium on renal cortical lipids.   The Oil Red O sections showed that
lipids overloading cells are hydrophobic lipids while total glycerol and
unesterified fatty acids levels increased in renal cortex.

These neutral lipids accumulate in the cytoplasm of proximal tubular cells as it may be seen under electron microscopy. The fatty acid composition of total neutral lipids showed a significant increase in polyunsaturated fatty acids of renal cortical treated rats. Analysis of phospholipids of renal cortex showed a decline of total phospholipids while a marked loss of phosphatidylethanolamine was noted as soon as day 2. The analysis of fatty acid composition showed an important decline of polyunsaturated fatty acids of renal cortical phospholipids. Changes occurred in arachidonic and docosahexaenoic acids. It is known that arachidonic acid is the most abundant polyunsaturated fatty acid present in renal cortical phospholipids and that polyunsaturated fatty acids are particularly susceptible to lipid peroxidation (14,15). Since it has been shown that in vitro autoxidation of hydroxyl derivatives of ellipticine leads to the formation of the reactive quinoneimine (16) and that a biooxidative activation of Celiptium occurs in the kidney with the appearance of highly electrophilic intermediates (17), we have measured the levels of lipid peroxides in renal cortex of Celiptium treated rats. This analysis showed the presence of hydroperoxides and TBA reactive material on days 2, 4 and 8.

Thus histochemistry and chemical analysis of lipids show that renal cortex contains peroxidized lipids, while it was noted a loss of polyunsaturated fatty acids in phospholipid fraction lead us to suppose that lipid peroxidation reactions occur in the pathogenesis of Celiptium nephrotoxicity.

REFERENCES

1.   C. Paoletti, J.B. Le Pecq, N. Dat Xuong, P. Juret, H. Garnier, J.L. Amiel, J. Rouesse, Antitumor activity, pharmacology and toxicity of ellipticines, ellipticinium and 9-hydroxy-derivatives: preliminary clinical trials of 2-methyl-9-hydroxy-ellipticinium (NSC-264-137). Recent Results Canc. Res., 74:107 (1980)

2.   B. Monsarrat, M. Maftouh, G. Meunier, B. Dugue, J. Bernadou, J.P. Armand, C. Picard-Fraire, B. Meunier, C. Paoletti, Human and rat urinary metabolites of the hydroxy methylellipticinium. Identification of cysteine conjugates supporting the bioxidative alkylation hypothesis. Biochem. Pharmacol., 32:3887 (1983)

3.   M. Maftouh, Y. Amiar, C.Picard-Fraire. Metabolism of the antitumor drug N2-methyl-9-hydroxyellipticinium acetate in isolated rat kidney cells. Biochem. Pharmacol., 34:427 (1985)

4.   P. Juret, A. Tanguy, A. Girard. L' acitate d' hydroxy-9-mithyl-2-ellipticinium. Etude toxicologique et thirapeutique chaz 100 cancereux. Nouv. Presse Med. 8:1494 (1978)

5.   G. Raguinez-Viotte, C. Dadoun, P. Buchet, T. Ducastelle, J.P. Fillastre. Renal toxicity of the antitumor drug N2-methyl-9-hydroxy-ellipticinium acetate in the Wistar rat. Submitted Arch Toxicology.

6.   O.B. Bayliss-High, Lipids In: Theory and practice of histological techniques, Bancroft, edited by J.D.Stevens, Melbourne-New York. p.217 (1982)

7.   O.H. Lowry, N.J. Rosebrough, A.L. Farr, R.J. Randall, Protein measurement with the Folin phenol reagent. J. Biol. Chem. 193:265 (1951)

8.   E.G. Bligh and W.J. Dyer. A rapid method of total lipid extraction and purification. Can. J. Biochem. Physiol. 37:911 (1959)

9.   J.A. Buege and S.D. Aust, Microsomal lipid peroxidation. Methods Enzymol. 52:302 (1978)

10.   H. Ohkawa, N. Ohishi, K. Yagi, Assay for lipid peroxides in animal tissues by thiobarbituric acid reaction. Anal. Biochem. 95:351 (1979)

11.   V.P. Skipski, R.F. Peterson, M. Barclay, Quantitative analysis of phospholipids by thin layer chromatography. Biochem. J. 90:374 (1964)

12. G.R. Bartlett, Phosphorus assay in column chromatography. J. Biol. Chem. 234:466 (1959)

13. W.R. Morrison and L.M. Smith, Preparation of fatty acid methyl esters and dimethylacetals from lipids with boron trifluoride-methanol. J. Lipid Res. 5:600 (1964)

14. A.L. Tappel, Lipid peroxidation damage to cell components. Fed. Proc. 32:1870 (1973)

15. H. Kappus, Lipid peroxidation: mechanisms, analysis, enzymology and biological relevance. In: "Oxidative stress" edited by H. Sies, Academic Press. p. 273 (1985)

16. C. Auclair, K. Hyland and C. Paoletti. Autooxidation of the antitumor drug 9-hydroxyellipticine and its derivatives. J. Med. Chem. 26:1438 (1983)

Lactate dehydrogenase = LDH (EC 1.1.1.27)
Alanine aminopeptidase = AAP (EC 3.4.11. -)
Gamma-glutamyltransferase = GGT (EC 2.3.2.2)
ß-Galactosidase = GAL (EC 3.2.1.30)
N-Acetyl-ß-D-glucosaminidase = NAG (EC 3.2.1.23)

Urine for the enzyme and protein determination was collected in 3h morning periods from 6 to 9 a.m. to obviate any influence of the circadian variation of urinary enzyme excretion. Immediately after the collection periods urine samples were prepared by gel filtration on Sephadex-G50 fine. Urinary enzyme excretion was calculated as mU/3h, correcting for the average adult body surface area of 1,73 m^2 (6) LDH is a cytoplasm enzyme, AAP and GGT are brush border membrane enzymes, NAG and GAL are localized in the lysosomes. Analysis of protein excretion was performed by SDS-PAGE-electrophoresis.

RESULTS

Three patients had a mild deterioration of their renal function, serum creatinine rose 1,0 mg/dl to 1,5 mg/dl, from 0,9 mg/dl to 1,4 mg/dl and from 0,8 mg/dl to 1,3 mg/dl. One patient developed mild proteinuria of 2 g/24h, in 3 patients severe proteinuria of 6-7 g/24h occurred. In these 4 patients SDS-PAGE-electrophoresis showed a non-selective glomerular and incomplete tubular proteinuria. Proteinuria started on day 3 or 4, deterioration or renal function on day 3. In all 11 patients pathological enzymuria was observed during application of chemotherapy (fig. 1 -5). Enzymuria started on day 2, reached its maximum on day 3 and persisted throughout the "hole period of chemotherapy. Data are presented as mean values ± SD. Three days after cessation of therapy all abnormal parameters returned to normal values.

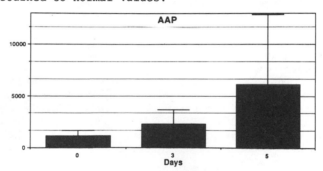

Fig. 1. Excretion of AAP during ifosfamide containing chemotherapy

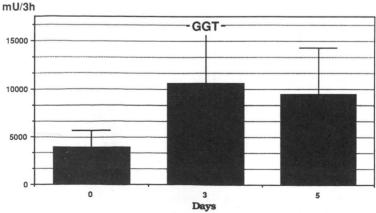

2. Excretion of GGT following ifosfamide containing chemotherapy

NEPHROTOXICITY OF IFOSFAMIDE IN COMBINATION CHEMOTHERAPY

Erhard Kurschel, and Ulrike Metz-Kurschel*

West German Tumour Centre and * Department of Renal and Hypertensive Diseases, University Medical School, Hufelandstr. 5S, D-4300 Essen, FRG

INTRODUCTION

Ifosfamide (Ifos) is a structural analogue of cyclophosphamide with a broad spectrum of antineoplastic activities both in solid tumours and haematological neoplasia. Its most important side effects are haemorrhagic cystitis, haematotoxicity, neurotoxicity and nephrotoxicity [1-4]. Haemorrhagic cystitis and to some extent nephrotoxicity can be ameliorated by concomitant administration of 2-mercaptoethane sulphonate sodium (Mesna R).

Monotherapy with ifosfamide is usually well tolerated without significa[nt] renal toxicity, but in combination therapy especially with other potent[ly] nephrotoxic agents like cis-Platinum or methotrexate patients are [at] increased risk of renal failure [5]. Data concerning nephrotoxicity mainly established in phase-I/II studies with ifosfamide, investiga[ted] in combination chemotherapy are scanty. This is especially important [for] the introduction of high-dose ifosfamide in combination therapy. [In the] present study we investigated the effects of ifosfamide in comb[ination] with etoposid or vindesine on renal function.

PATIENTS AND METHODS

We studied 11 male patients, age 19 - 63 years, median 56 [with] testicular and lung cancers. None had previous chemo- or radio[therapy].

Treatment regimens were:-

1) Ifosfamide $2g/m^2$, days 1-5,   Etoposid $120mg/m^2$ days 1-5

2) Ifosfamide $5g/m^2$ days 1-3,   Vindesine $3mg/m^2$ days 1-3

All patients received Mesna (20% of ifosfamide doses) i[n] hours after infusion of ifosfamide. Before the fir[st] chemotherapy all 11 patients had normal renal function nor proteinuria or enzymuria were detectable. Besides serum creatinine, BUN, protein excretion (Biur[et] analysis of the urinary sediment we determined t[he] following urinary enzymes:

Fig.

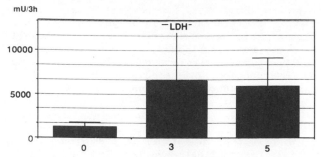

Fig. 3. Excretion of LDH following ifosfamide containing chemotherapy

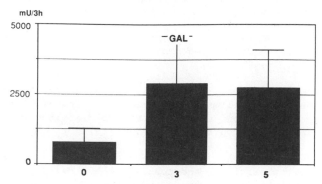

Fig. 4. Excretion of GAL following ifosfamide containing chemotherapy

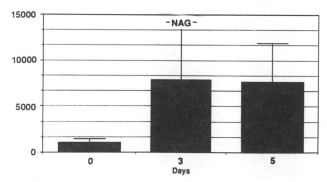

Fig. 5. Excretion of NAG following ifosfamide containing chemotherapy

DISCUSSION

Ifosfamide associated nephrotoxicity is commonly confined to the tubular epithelia, whereas glomerular injury is thought to be a rare complication. Our data (impairment of renal function, severe proteinuria, non-selective glomerular and incomplete tubular proteinuria in SDS-PAGE-electrophoresis, pathological enzymuria) show that glomerular and tubular toxicity is a common effect of ifosfamide in combination with etoposid or vindesine. There are no previous reports on nephrotoxic effects of etoposid or vindesine, so it is possible that in combination chemotherapy these two substances are able to potentiate the nephrotoxic potential of ifosfamide. Another explanation of our results which are contradictory to the majority of nephrotoxicity studies in the literature is that prior investigations have focused on tubular damage and glomerular function was analysed with rather insensitive methods. The biochemical basis of nephrotoxicity following ifosfamide administration is as yet unclear because of the complex metabolism of this oxazophorine, whether acrolein is involved in this process has to be established in our study the concomitant administration of Mesna prevented from haemorrhagic cystitis, but had no influence on renal dysfunction. This should be borne in mind as the use of ifosfamide containing chemotherapy regimens increases.

REFERENCES

1. W.P. Brade, K. Herdrich, M. Varini, Ifosfamide-pharmacology, safety, therapeutic potential, Cancer Treat Rev. 12 : 1-47 (1985)

2. J.J. Van Dyk, H.P. Falkson, A.M. Van der Merwe, G. Falkson, Unexpected toxicity in patients with iphosphamide, Cancer. 32: 921-924 (1972)

3. R.A. DeFronzo, M. Abeloff, H. Braine, R.L.Humphrey, P.J. Davis, Renal dysfunction dysfunction after treatment with ifosfamide, Chemother Rep. 58: 375-382 (1974)

4. C.B. Pratt, A.A. Green, M.E. Horowitz, W.H. Meyer, E. Douglass, F.A Hayes, E. Thompson, J. Wilimas, M. Igarashi, E. Kovnar, Central nervous system toxicity following treatment of pediatric patients with ifosfamide/mesna, J Clin Oncol.4: 1253-1261 (1986)

5. M.P. Goren, R.K. Wright, C.B. Pratt, Potentiation of ifosfamide neurotoxicity, hematotoxicity, and tubular nephrotoxicity by prior cis-Diamminedichloroplatinum(II) Therapy, Cancer Res. 47: 1457-1460 (1987)

6. D. Maruhn, I. Fuchs, G. Mues, K.D. Bock, Normal limits of urinary excretion of eleven enzymes, Clin Chem.22: 1567-1574 (1976)

RISK EVALUATION OF MUZOLIMINE AND FUROSEMIDE IN EXPERIMENTAL MODELS OF NEPHROTOXICITY

Claus-Peter Siegers and Britta Steffen

Department of Toxicology, Medical University of Lubeck, D-2400 Lubeck (FRG)

INTRODUCTION

Loop diuretics are assumed to be contraindicated in toxic renal failure, but there are little experimental and clinical data available to support or justify this assumption. Furosemide enhances the nephrotoxic response to both aminoglycoside and cephalosporine antibiotic in mice (James et al., 1975) and in dogs (Adelman et al., 1979), but this was not confirmed in patients (Smith and Lietman, 1983).

Muzolimine is a new loop diuretic which, in comparison to furosemide, has a prolonged diuretic effect and is believed to have a different mechanism of action (Davis et al., 1985). We have studied the effects of muzolimine or furosemide on the nephrotoxic response to Amanita phalloides, mercuric chloride, paracetamol, carbon tetrachloride, gentamycin and cephalothin.

MATERIALS AND METHODS

Male Wistar-rats (300-350 g) were kept for 3 days in metabolic cages with free access to food and tap water. The nephrotoxic agents were administered immediately after the first blood sample, the diuretics were given twice, 24 and 48 hr later.

Nephrotoxicity was monitored by daily measurements of plasma creatinine and urea concentrations and urinary enzyme excretion of N-acetyl-ß-glucos-aminidase (NAG) and gamma-glutamyltranspeptidase (GGT) activities using commercial reagent kits of Boehringer, Mannheim (FRG).

RESULTS AND DISCUSSION

Treatment of rats with lyophilized A. phalloides powder (40 mg/kg ip) led to significant increases of plasma creatinine and urea at 24 and 48 hr (Table 1). These effects were not augmented by the additional treatment with muzolimine (30 mg/kg po) or furosemide (40 mg/kg po) (data not shown).

Intravenous injection of mercuric chloride (1 mg/kg iv) was followed by a marked retention of creatinine and urea in plasma and strongly stimulated NAG-excretion (Table 1). The nephrotoxic effects of $HgCI_2$ were not

451

Table 1. Effects of diuretics or nephrotoxic agents 24 hr after treatment on creatinine and urea concentrations as well as N-acetyl-ß-glucosaminidase excretion in male rats. Values represent geometric means and their standard errors out of 6 rats each. * p < 0.05 as compared to controls (Dunnett's t-test).

Group/Treatment	Creatinine (umol/l)	Urea (mmol/l)	NAG (mU/24 h)
Controls	87.1 (77.6 - 97.8)	7.06 (6.68 - 7.47)	161 (135 - 193)
Muzolimine 30 mg/kg po	74.7 (63.3 - 88.1)	6.76 (6.52 - 7.02)	230 (280 - 255)
Furosemide 40 mg/kg po	69.3 (57.0 - 84.3)	6.31 (6.21 - 6.41)	183 (162 - 206)
A. phalloides 40 mg/kg/ ip	273* (232 - 320)	20.0* (16.1 - 24.8)	221 (209 - 233)
$HgCl_2$ 1 mg/kg iv	335 (316 - 355)	25.7* (24.5 - 26.9)	3697* (3301 - 4140)
Paracetamol 1.5 g/kg po	615* (328 - 1154)	8.12 (6.63 - 9.95)	322* (297 - 250)
CCl_4 0.5 ml/kg ip	371* (2992 - 473)	6.06 (5.84 - 6.29)	201 (172 - 236)
Gentamicin 500 mg/kg ip	80.4 (70.6 - 91.5)	7.92 (7.16 - 8.75)	297 (234 - 377)
Cephalothin 3 g/kg ip	87.4 (78.5 - 97.3)	5.87 (5.56 - 6.19)	160 (146 - 176)

potentiated by the administration of muzolimine or furosemide (data not shown).

Orally administered paracetamol (1.5 g/kg po) evoked significant elevations of creatinine and urea concentrations in plasma and a small increase in NAG excretion (Table 1). These nephrotoxic effects of paracetamol were not aggravated by muzolimine or furosemide (data not shown).

Following carbon tetrachloride administration (0.5 ml/kg ip) only an enhanced retention of plasma creatinine was observed (Table 1). Additional treatment with muzolimine led to significant enhancements of plasma urea and urinary enzyme excretion of NAG and GGT; the same effect was seen with furosemide (Figure 1).

Cephalothin (3 g/kg ip) alone did not cause any nephrotoxic effects, but in combination with the diuretics led to significant increases of NAG and GGT excretion, and, in the case of furosemide, creatinine (Figure 2).

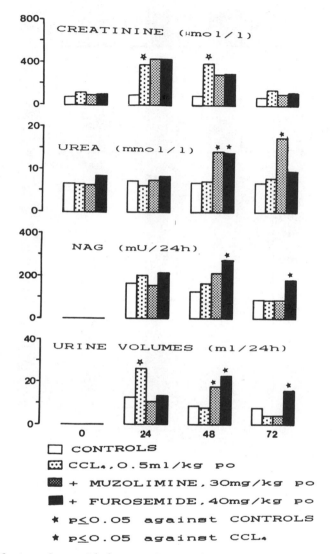

CREATININE (μmol/l)

UREA (mmol/l)

NAG (mU/24h)

URINE VOLUMES (ml/24h)

□ CONTROLS

▦ CCL₄,0.5ml/kg po

▦ + MUZOLIMINE,30mg/kg po

■ + FUROSEMIDE,40mg/kg po

☆ p≤0.05 against CONTROLS

★ p≤0.05 against CCL₄

Figure 1. Effects of muzolimine or furosemide on the nephrotoxic response to carbon tetrachloride in rats. Values represent geometric means of 6 rats.

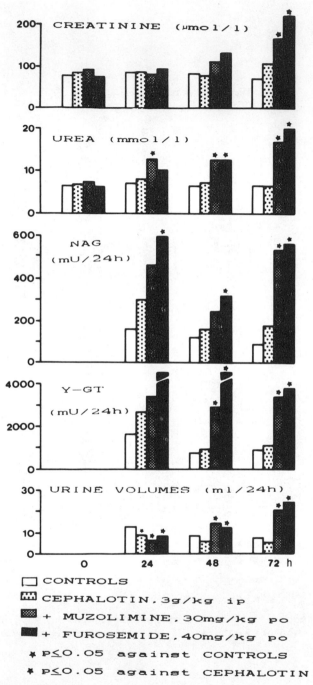

CREATININE (μmol/l)

UREA (mmol/l)

NAG (mU/24h)

Y-GT (mU/24h)

URINE VOLUMES (ml/24h)

0   24   48   72 h

☐ CONTROLS

▥ CEPHALOTIN, 3g/kg ip

▨ + MUZOLIMINE, 30mg/kg po

■ + FUROSEMIDE, 40mg/kg po

⁑ P≤0.05 against CONTROLS

✱ P≤0.05 against CEPHALOTIN

Figure 2. Effects of muzolimine or furosemide on the nephrotoxic response to cephalothin in rats. Values represent geometric means of 6 rats.

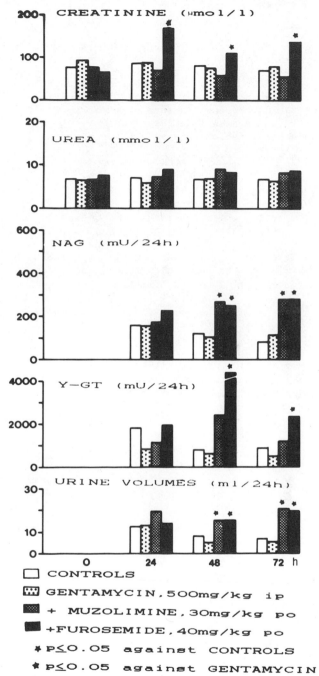

CREATININE (μmol/l)

UREA (mmol/l)

NAG (mU/24h)

Y—GT (mU/24h)

URINE VOLUMES (ml/24h)

☐ CONTROLS

▨ GENTAMYCIN,500mg/kg ip

▧ + MUZOLIMINE,30mg/kg po

■ +FUROSEMIDE,40mg/kg po

✳ P≤0.05 against CONTROLS

★ P≤0.05 against GENTAMYCIN

Figure 3. Effects of muzolimine or furosemide on the nephrotoxic
response to gentamicin in rats. Values represent geometric means of 6
rats.

Treatment of rats with gentamicin (500 mg/kg ip) only caused marginal nephrotoxic effects such as an insignificant increases of NAG (Table 1) or GGT. Together with muzolimine or furosemide, however, both plasma creatinine and urea were increased and there was a marked enzymuria (Figure 3).

Our experimental data with rats suggest that loop diuretics might be contraindicated in certain toxic nephropathy. We have shown that muzolimine and furosemide are able to potentiate the nephrotoxic response to gentamicin, cephalothin and carbon tetrachloride. This effect might be explained by a dehydration and reduction of the extracellular volume and thereby concentrating the toxic agents or their toxic intermediates in the renal cortex. During renal failure caused by <u>A. phalloides</u>, $HgCI_2$ or paracetamol neither diuretic aggravated the nephrotoxicity.

REFERENCES

Adelman, R.D., Spangler, W.L., Beason, F., Ishizaki, G. and Conzelman, G.M. (1979). Furosemide enhancement of experimental gentamycin nephrotoxicity. Comparison of functional and morphological changes with activities of urinary enzymes. <u>J. Infect. Dis</u>. 140, 342-352.

Davis, J.M., Takabatake, T., Thurau, K. and Haberle, D.A. (1985). The effect of muzolimine on the tubuloglomerular feedback mechanism in the rat kidney. <u>Z. Kardiol</u>. 72, Suppl.2, 161-165.

James, G., Smith, W., Bryant, H. and Balazs, T. (1975). Enhancement of antibiotic nephrotoxicity by furosemide: studies in mice. <u>Toxicol. Appl. Pharmacol</u>. 33, 199.

Smith, C.R. and Lietman, P.S. (1983). Effect of furosemide on aminoglycoside-induced nephrotoxicity and auditory toxicity in humans. <u>Antimicrob. Agent Chemother</u>. 23, 133-137.

THE ROLE OF OXIDATIVE STRESS IN CEPHALORIDINE NEPHROTOXICITY

Robin S. Goldstein, Randall S. Sozio, Joan B. Tarloff, and Jerry B. Hook

Smith Kline & French Laboratories, Department of Investigative Toxicology, P.O. Box 1539, King of Prussia, USA

INTRODUCTION

The cephalosporin antibiotic, cephaloridine (CPH), is nephrotoxic when administered in large dosages to humans and laboratory animals (1,2). In vivo, CPH nephrotoxicity is characterized histologically by acute proximal tubular necrosis and functionally by glycosuria, enzymuria, proteinuria and an impaired ability of renal cortical slices to accumulate organic ions (1-4). Previous studies have indicated that the nephrotoxicity of CPH is intimately related to its renal cortical accumulation and intracellular concentration (5). CPH is actively transported into the proximal tubule cell by an organic anion transport system (5,6). However, unlike many organic anions and cephalosporins, CPH undergoes only limited movement across the lumenal membrane into the tubular fluid. Consequently, high intracellular concentrations of CPH are attained in the proximal tubule which are critical to the development of nephrotoxicity (5).

Although the relationship between the tubular transport and toxicity of CPH has been well documented, the exact molecular mechanisms by which CPH induces toxicity are less well understood. Kuo et al. (7) have suggested that lipid peroxidation may play an important role. An involvement of peroxidative injury in CPH nephrotoxicity was suggested by the observation that renal cortical concentrations of conjugated dienes, products of lipid peroxidation, were increased shortly following in vivo administration of CPH to rats (7). Furthermore, CPH administration resulted in a dose-related depletion of renal cortical reduced glutathione (GSH) content accompanied by an increase in oxidized glutathione (GSSG) concentrations (7). Although these data suggested that lipid peroxidation was associated with CPH nephrotoxicity, it is difficult to determine whether lipid peroxidation was an initiating event mediating CPH nephrotoxicity or was secondary to cytotoxicity.

MATERIAL AND METHODS

To more definitively evaluate the role of lipid peroxidation in CPH nephrotoxicity, the time course of various biochemical events were evaluated in renal cortical slices exposed to CPH in vitro. Renal cortical slices from naive male Fischer-344 rats (200-250 g) were incubated at 37°C in a phosphate buffered medium containing 10 mM lactate with or without CPH. Slices were incubated for various periods of time

(30-180 min) and evaluated for accumulation of the organic anion, p-aminohippurate (PAH), malondialdehyde (MDA) production and GSH content.

RESULTS

Incubation of renal cortical slices with CPH resulted in a time-dependent alteration in PAH accumulation, MDA production and GSH content (Table 1). Furthermore, the onset of CPH-induced GSH depletion (30 min) preceded the earliest detectable increase in MDA production (90 min) which, in turn, preceded the earliest depression in PAH accumulation (120 min) (Table 1). These temporal data suggested a causal relationship between CPH-induced GSH depletion, lipid peroxidation and toxicity. More definitive evidence supporting a cause-effect relationship between CPH induced lipid peroxidation and toxicity is based on the observation that treatment of renal cortical slices with an antioxidant, such as N,N'-diphenyl-p-phenylenediamine (DPPD), blocked the effects of CPH on both lipid peroxidation and PAH accumulation (8). Furthermore, this antioxidant blocked CPH-induced loss in cell viability, reflected by preventing leakage of the cytosolic enzyme, lactate dehydrogenase (LDH), into incubation media (unpublished observations).

Table 1. Time Course of Biochemical Effects of CPH in Renal Cortical Slices [a,b]

Time (min)	CPH (mM)	PAH S/M	MDA (nmoles/g)	GSH (mmoles/g)
30	0	11.10[c]	35.94	1.64
	5	12.58	10.56	1.16[d]
60	0	11.60	37.21	1.41
	5	13.21	59.64	1.07[d]
90	0	11.82	40.64	1.49
	5	11.16	146.07[d]	0.80[d]
120	0	11.17	44.58	1.42
	5	4.83[d]	260.13[d]	0.65[d]
180	0	9.99	73.21	1.51
	5	1.30	355.19[d]	0.49[d]

a Data modified from Goldstein et al (8)
b Renal cortical slices from naive F-344 rats were incubated with or without 5 mM CPH.
c Values represent means of 4-6 experiments.
d Significantly different than controls ($p < 0.05$).

DISCUSSION

The mechanisms by which CPH induces lipid peroxidation in the intact cell are not entirely clear. However, anaerobic reduction of CPH by isolated renal cortical microsomes and the subsequent production of superoxide anion radicals and hydrogen peroxide has been reported (9), suggesting the possibility that CPH may undergo redox cycling. Both superoxide and hydrogen peroxide are known to react with transition metals, such as iron, to form very reactive oxygen free radicals which may initiate peroxidative reactions with membrane lipids. To determine if CPH toxicity is mediated by these iron-catalysed reactions, renal cortical slices were pretreated with the ferric iron-chelating agent, deferoxamine (20 mM). Indeed, deferoxamine completely blocked CPH-induced LDH leakage (Table 2), suggesting that CPH toxicity is dependent upon ferric iron and is presumably related to the catalytic role of iron in generating reactive oxygen free radicals (Figure 1).

Table 2. Modulation of CPH Nephrotoxicity[a]

	% LDH Leakage	
Treatment	Control	CPH
Control	24.8[b]	42.2[c]
Deferoxamine (20 mM)	25.5	28.5[d]
Control	25.8	44.7[c]
Aminotriazole (20 mM)	22.6	44.6[c]
Control	22.6	49.7[c]
BCNU (150 mM)	21.6	61.4[c,d]
Control	11.5	32.9[c]
Diethylmaleate (250 mM)	20.2	46.7[c,d]
Control	26.8	34.5[c]
Dithiothreitol (2 mM)	22.3	24.5[d]

a Renal cortical slices were incubated with 0 or 2.5 mM CPH for 120 min.
b Values represent means of 4-5 experiments.
c Significantly different than controls ($p < 0.05$).
d Significantly different than CPH treatment alone ($p < 0.05$).

In addition to bioactivation mechanisms involved in generating oxygen free radicals, the onset and severity of CPH nephrotoxicity may also be dependent on the ability of proximal tubular cells to detoxify oxygen radicals and hydrogen and/or lipid peroxides. Intracellular metabolism of peroxides is catalysed primarily by glutathione peroxidase and catalase. Catalase is a peroxisomal enzyme which catalyses the conversion of hydrogen peroxide to molecular oxygen and water. Previous studies have indicated that catalase is capable of blocking hydrogen peroxide evolution in CPH-treated microsomes (9).

To evaluate the role of catalase as a detoxification mechanism in CPH toxicity in the intact cell, renal cortical slices were pretreated with an inhibitor of catalase activity, aminotriazole (ATZ). Although ATZ decreased catalase activity by approximately 90%, no potentiation of CPH toxicity was observed (Table 2), suggesting that catalase may not be important in the detoxification of CPH-generated peroxides. The apparently minor role of catalase as a defence mechanism in CPH toxicity may relate to the inaccessibility of the peroxisomally contained catalase to CPH-induced peroxides formed in other subcellular sites.

In contrast to catalase, GSH peroxidase is both a cytosolic and mitochondrial enzyme and catalyses the conversion of hydrogen peroxide and lipid peroxides to the corresponding alcohols, using GSH as an electron donor. The product of this reaction, GSSG, can be reduced back to GSH via NADPH-dependent GSSG reductase. Thus, the GSH peroxidase-GSSG reductase complex is important not only in detoxification of peroxides, but also in maintaining intracellular thiol homeostasis. To evaluate the role of the glutathione redox cycle in CPH toxicity, renal cortical slices were preincubated with 150 mM 1,3-bis(2-chloroethyl)-1-nitrourea (BCNU), an

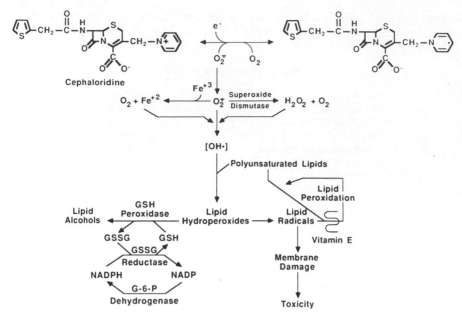

Figure 1.   Proposed biochemical mechanisms of CPH nephrotoxicity

inhibitor of GSSG reductase activity.   BCNU significantly potentiated CPH toxicity (Table 2), suggesting that GSSG reductase activity is an important defence mechanism against CPH toxicity.   Furthermore, treatment of renal cortical slices with the GSH depleting agent, diethylmaleate (DEM), also potentiated CPH toxicity (Table 2).   These data are consistent with the hypothesis that CPH toxicity is critically dependent on the ability of the cell to detoxify peroxides and maintain thiol homeostasis via the glutathione redox cycle.   Furthermore, the importance of intracellular thiol status in CPH toxicity is supported by the observation that the thiol reducing agent, dithiothreitol, completely prevented CPH toxicity in renal cortical slices (Table 2).   Maintenance of intracellular thiols in a reduced state also appears to be critical in preventing quinone-induced oxidative cellular injury.   Orrenius et al (11) have proposed that perturbation of thiol homeostasis during oxidative stress impairs calcium transport mechanisms, resulting in sustained increases in cytosolic free calcium, leading to cell death.   Similar mechanisms may be associated with CPH-induced oxidative stress and toxicity.

In summary, CPH may undergo cyclic one electron reduction-oxidation reactions, producing the superoxide anion radical (Figure 1).   Superoxide anion radicals can, in turn, be detoxified to hydrogen peroxide via superoxide dismutase.   These oxygen species may react with iron via the Fenton pathway, producing very reactive oxygen free radicals, which can react with polyunsaturated lipids forming lipid hydroperoxides.   The ability of the proximal tubular cell to combat CPH-induced oxidative stress and toxicity appears to be dependent, in part, on activity of the glutathione redox cycle.   Thus, susceptibility to CPH toxicity is dependent not only on those mechanisms generating oxygen free radicals but also on those mechanisms responsible for detoxifying oxygen radicals.

REFERENCES

1.   R.M. Atkinson, J.P. Currie, B. Davis, D.A.H. Pratt, H.M. Sharpe, and

E.G. Tomich, Acute toxicity of cephaloridine, an antibiotic derived from cephalosporin C, Toxicol. Appl. Pharmacol. 8:398 (1966).

2. R.D. Foord, Cephaloridine, cephalothin and the kidney, J. Antimicrob. Chemother. Suppl. 1:119 (1975).

3. J.S. Welles, W.R. Gibson, P.N. Harris, R.M. Small and R.C. Anderson, Toxicity, distribution and excretion of cephaloridine in laboratory animals, Antimicrob. Agents Chemother. 1965:863 (1965).

4. J.S. Wold, Cephalosporin Nephrotoxicity, In: "Toxicity of the Kidney", J.B. Hook, ed., Raven Press, New York (1981).

5. B. Tune, Relationship between the transport and toxicity of cephalosporins in the kidney, J. Infect Dis. 132:189 (1975).

6. K.J. Child and M.G. Dodds, Nephron transport and renal tubular effects of cephaloridine in animals, Brit. J. Pharmacol. Chemother. 30:354 (1967).

7. C.-H. Kuo, K. Maita, S.D. Sleight and J.B. Hook, Lipid peroxidation: A possible mechanism of cephaloridine-induced nephrotoxicity, Toxicol. Appl. Pharmacol. 67:78 (1983).

8. R.S. Goldstein, D.A. Pasino, W.R. Hewitt and J.B. Hook, Biochemical mechanisms of cephaloridine nephrotoxicity: time and concentration dependence of peroxidative injury, Toxicol. Appl. Pharmacol. 83:43 (1986).

9. C. Cojocel, J. Hannemann and K. Baumann, Cephaloridine-induced lipid peroxidation initiated by reactive oxygen species as a possible mechanism of cephaloridine nephrotoxicity, Biochem. Biophys. Acta 834:402 (1985).

10. D. DiMonte, G. Bellomo, H. Thor, P. Nicotera and S. Orrenius, Menadione-induced cytotoxicity is associated with protein thiol oxidation and alteration in intracellular Ca^{2+} homeostasis, Arch. Biochem. Biophys. 235:343 (1984).

STUDIES ON THE MECHANISM OF RADIOLOGICAL CONTRAST MEDIA INDUCED RENAL FAILURE

C.J. Powell, M. Dobrota (1), and E. Holtz (2)

DHSS Toxicology Department, St Bartholomew's Hospital Medical College, London EC1 7ED, (1) The Robens Institute, Surrey University Guildford, Surrey GU2 5XH and (2) Nycomed AS, Torshov, Oslo, Norway

INTRODUCTION

Radiological contrast media are usually derivatives of tri-iodobenzoic acid that are used to render soft tissues x-ray opaque for diagnostic imaging. The procedure routinely employed for x-ray imaging the urinary tract (urography) consists of intravenous administration of a contrast medium, which is then rapidly concentrated in the kidney and excreted in the urine. It is generally assumed that these compounds do not enter cells, but remain within the extracellular space and are filtered at the glomeruli, concentrated within the tubular lumen and then excreted. For this reason contrast media have been described as dyes rather than drugs and are considered to be metabolically and physiologically inert.

While the procedure is normally completely safe, a small proportion of patients subsequently experience a transient or, very rarely, a permanent decline in renal function (Cedgard et al, 1986). The patients at greatest risk are those, with pre-existing renal impairment, especially those with diabetic nephropathy or multiple myeloma nephropathy (Harkonen and Kjellstrand, 1981). Because this procedure is frequently used to investigate urinary tract abnormalities associated with impaired renal function and several million contrast procedures are performed annually, the number of patients at risk of developing contrast media related renal complications is significant.

Many of the problems associated with urographic contrast media have been attributed to their high osmolality. Therefore during the last few years a new class of low osmolar urographic contrast media have been introduced into clinical use. Some of the newer contrast media under development are actually isotonic with plasma. Because the mechanisms of contrast media related acute renal failure are poorly understood, the effect of these new low osmolar contrast media on renal structure and function deserve special attention.

Our initial approach was to develop an experimental model of contrast media induced nephrotoxicity, using the criteria that functional and structural alterations should be similar to those observed in the clinical setting. We found that when high doses of several contrast media were administered to male Wistar rats of 250g body weight, persistent nephrograms were observed at 48 hr. These were associated with iodine retention in the kidney (1-8.9mgI/g kidney) at 48 hr and structural alterations in the proximal tubules of the cortex (Powell et al, 1985). These features have been associated with the early pattern of contrast media related renal failure in patients (Older et al, 1976, Moreau et al, 1980).

Experiment 1.   Having established that features of human contrast media related renal impairment could be reproduced in an experimental model, we examined the effects of six structurally different contrast media on renal function and morphology. Thus, Iopamidol, Iopentol, Iohexol, Diatrizoate, Ioxaglate and Iodixanol (see Spataro 1984 for examples of structures) were administered intravenously to groups of six 250g male Wistar rats at one of 4 different dose levels: 1, 2, 5 or 10gI/kg. Eighteen control rats received intravenous saline injections in a similar manner. Albumin was measured in urine by immunoelectrophoresis using goat anti-rat serum albumin. Creatinine and urea were measured in plasma by conventional colourimetric methods. After 48 hr the kidneys were excised, fixed in formalin, embedded in paraffin wax and examined by light microscopy.

Measurement of urinary iodine showed that between 70 and 86% of the dose was excreted within the first 24 hr, with a further 2.5% in the next 24 hr. In rats which received the highest dose of the mono acidic and non-ionic dimeric contrast agents there was a substantially elevated albuminuria in the first 24 hr, but a return to control levels between 24 and 48 hr. Serum creatinine and urea levels measured at 48 hr were not significantly increased by any of the contrast media, even at the highest dose levels, Neither was there any alteration in 24 hr urinary volume.

Microscopic examination of the kidneys showed that 5 of the 6 contrast media caused a dose-related segmental vacuolation of proximal tubules (Fig 1 and 2). These lesions were most severe in animals which received the dimeric contrast agents, but were not induced by any dose of Diatrizoate: an ionic monomer. The vacuoles appeared empty, with the exception of those induced by Ioxaglate which contained small bright eosinophilic beads at the centre.

The demonstration that the severity of vacuolation was dose-related, but completely unrelated to the osmolality of the administered material, combined with the observation that some vacuoles contained proteinaceous material, tempts speculation that contrast media may be internalized within these cells and inhibit the reuptake or degradation of ultrafiltered proteins.

Experiment 2.   In order to examine whether the structural and functional changes caused by high doses of urographic contrast media were associated with intracellular localization of the material, a radiolabelled contrast medium was administered, and the intrarenal distribution was examined.

Accordingly, ^{14}C-Iodixanol was intravenously administered to 250g male Wistar rats. The level of radioactivity was measured in blood by sequential sampling and the excretion of radiolabel was measured in urine and faeces. At 24 hr the kidneys were excised, the cortices homogenised and then subfractioned by differential pelleting and rate zonal sedimentation, as described previously (Andersen et al, 1987). The distribution of radiolabel and several marker enzymes was examined in the four classical subcellular fractions: "Nuclear", "Mitochondrial/Lysosomal", "Microsomal" and "Supernatant or Cytosol". The kidneys of anaesthetised rats were also perfusion fixed for electron microscopy and processed for light microscopic autoradiography.

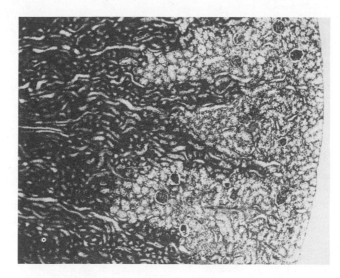

Figure 1. Extensive vacuolation of proximal convoluted tubules 48 hr after a single dose of 10gI/kg Iodixanol. Vacuolated areas interdigitate with medullary rays of proximal straight tubules. H&E staining, magnification x 48.

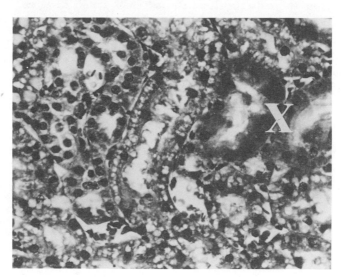

Figure 2. Detailed examination of vacuolated tubules shows empty vacuoles mostly located in the basal part of the cells, with a substantial degree of cellular disorganization, but no evidence of necrosis. Note that the adjacent proximal straight tubules (marked x) do not show structural abnormality. H&E staining, magnification x 250.

Iodixanol treatment did not alter the concentration of urine excreted over a 24 hr period, but urinary volume was slightly increased from 3-12 hr. As in our earlier experiments, most of the contrast medium was excreted within 24 hr and the levels of ^{14}C remaining in blood and urine were extremely low. However, approximately 1.5% of the administered dose was retained in the kidney at 24 hr (Table 1). Most of this material was localized in the cortex with less that 5% of the total in the medulla. Subcellular fractionation showed that approximately 56% of the radiolabel in the cortex was apparently located in the "Supernatant Cytosol" fraction, with a further 30% in the "Nuclear and Mitochondrial/Lysosomal", fractions very little activity was found in the "Microsomal" fraction.

Table 1. Recovery of ^{14}C label in the cortical and medulla homogenates and in the classical subfractions of the cortex 24 hr after i.v. administration of ^{14}C Iodixanol.

	Total uCi	% Cortical Homogenate	% Of Dose
Cortex homogenate	45.405	-	-
"Nuclear" fraction	6.414	14.1	-
Mitochondrial/Lysosomal, fraction	6.886	15.2	-
"Microsomal" fraction	1.261	2.8	-
Supernatant/Cytosol, fraction	25.581	56.3	-
Medulla homogenate	2.387	-	-
Total kidney	50.262	-	1.46%

Electron microscopic examination showed that the proximal convoluted tubules contained numerous membrane bound electron lucent vacuoles of varying size. Unlike the empty vacuoles found in immersion fixed kidneys, these vacuoles contained finely granular material and occasional membraneous inclusion bodies, suggesting that they were probably massively enlarged secondary lysosomes (Fig 3). This interpretation was reinforced by the lack of normal secondary lysosomes in these cells and a lack of degenerative changes in other organelles. Light microscopic autoradiography confirmed that most of the ^{14}C labelled Iodixanol was localized in the vacuolated region of proximal tubules.

These data unequivocally show that some radiological contrast media are internalized in the proximal tubular epithelium. Whether this results exclusively from reabsorption at the luminal face of the cells, or whether there is also some uptake from the basal face remains to be determined.

DISCUSSION

Lack of a suitable experimental model has been one of the greatest obstacles to understanding the mechanism of radiological contrast media nephrotoxicity. The persistent nephrograms which were present in this experimental model are one of the most consistent features of patients who subsequently develop contrast media associated renal impairment (Older et al, 1976). Vacuolation of proximal tubules has also been noted in patients following urographic investigation. (Moreau et al, 1980). These empty vacuoles, were observed in immersion fixed tissue and attempts to demonstrate that they contained contrast media were unsuccessful. This result accords with our experience that intracellular contrast media are prone to extraction from tissues during fixation and subsequent histological processing, and that perfusion fixation is necessary to retain the material.

In view of the marked alteration in renal albumin handling in our model, it is perhaps surprising that no change in plasma creatinine or urea was detected. However, our investigation was confined to one examination at 48 hr and the exact functional disturbances accompanying this model of nephrotoxicity are presently the subject of further study.

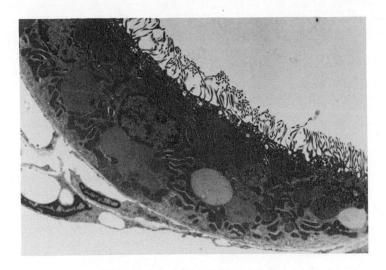

Figure 3. Large vacuoles distort the normal cytology of proximal convoluted tubules 24 hr after the administration of 3gI/kg Iodixanol. The number and size of these putative secondary lysosomes distorts the normal parallel arrangement of basal plasma membrane infoldings and mitochondria. Areas of endothelial cell detachment from the basal lamina of peritubular capillaries are also present. Magnification x 3000.

Renal morphological and functional changes developed irrespective of contrast media osmolality, and indeed were most markedly induced by low osmolar agents; clearly demonstrating that this was not an osmotic nephrosis. Moreover, in preliminary experiments we have observed that many vacuoles persist for up to two weeks following high doses of contrast agents. The localization of the vacuoles to the segment of the proximal tubule responsible for the reabsorption and catabolism of ultrafiltered proteins, combined with their electron microscopic appearance as enlarged secondary lysosomes, suggests that intracellular localization of contrast medium may be associated with the process of protein reabsorption. Furthermore, the autoradiographic localization of ^{14}C Iodixanol to the vacuolated cells suggests that contrast media may be contained within the vacuoles or associated with their membranes. Subcellular fractionation studies showed that 30% of the radiolabel was associated with the nuclear and mitochondrial/lysosomal fractions, providing firm evidence that Iodixanol was present within these organelles. However, it is probable that many of the large vacuoles ruptured during homogenization releasing their contents into the cytosol. The slightly higher recovery of the lysosomal marker enzyme: acid phosphatase, in the cytosol fraction of Iodixanol treated rats lends weight to this explanation. It is also possible that many larger vacuoles were equivalent in size to nuclei and therefore separated with this subcellular fraction, rather than the lysosomal fraction from which they probably originated.

The close correlation between persistent nephrograms, albuminuria, vacuole formation and intracellular localization of contrast media, indicates that these features may constitute the early phase of contrast media related renal failure. We have demonstrated that a small amount of urographic contrast media enters cells of the proximal tubule following high doses, and propose that it may interact with secondary lysosomes to perturb protein catabolism. In the normal kidney such a process would most probably be reversible, but in patients with a limited renal functional reserve, could lead to a more marked decline in renal function. The renal handling of radiological contrast media in animal models of reduced renal function is the subject of current investigation.

REFERENCES

Andersen, K.J., Haga, H.J. and Dobrota, M., 1987, Lysosomes of the renal cortex: Heterogeneity and role in protein handling. Kid. Int., 31:886.

Cedgard, S., Herlitz, H., Geterud, K., Altman, P.O. and Aurell. M. 1986, Acute renal insufficiency after administration of low osmolar contrast media. Lancet, Nov 29: 1281

Harkonen, S. and Kjellstrand, C., 1981. Contrast Nephropathy. Am. J. Nephrol., 1:69.

Moreau, J.F., Droz, D., Noel, L.H., Leibowitch, J., Jungers, P. and Michel, J.R., 1980. Tubular nephrotoxicity of water soluble iodinated contrast media. Invest. Radiol., 15:554.

Older, R.A., Miller, J.P., Jackson, D.C., Johnsrude, I.S. and Thompson, W.M., 1976. Angiographically induced renal failure and its radiographic detection. Am. J. Roentgenol., 126:1039.

Powell, C.J., Holtz, E. and Bridges, J.W. 1985. The nephrotoxicity of non-ionic and isosmotic dimeric radiological contrast media. J. Path., 146:276A.

Spataro, R., 1984, New contrast agents for urography. Radiol. Clin. N. America 22:239.

RADIOCONTRAST NEPHROTOXICITY IN DIABETES: CLINICAL CONSIDERATIONS AND

STUDIES IN THE DIABETIC RAT

C.A. Vaamonde, R. Papendick, W. Gouvea, R.T. Bier and H. Alpert

Medical and Research Services, Veterans Administration Medical Center and Department of Medicine, University of Miami School of Medicine, Miami, Florida 33125, USA

CLINICAL CONSIDERATIONS

Most drugs used in clinical practice have a low to very low incidence of renal toxicity. Nephrotoxicity tends to cluster around certain clinical circumstances or patient populations. Recognition of the risk factors for nephrotoxicity is, therefore, necessary for the understanding and prevention of renal damage (1).

A number of situations make the clinical evaluation of radiocontrast-induced nephrotoxicity difficult. Some of these include: the presence of more than one risk factor, the use of different criteria for the definition of nephrotoxicity, the patient populations, the type and route of administration of radiocontrast agent used, and the concomitant use of other nephrotoxicans. Although the safety of modern radiocontrast agents is often taken for granted, renal dysfunction can occur following the administration of virtually any intravascular radiocontrast. The current accepted frequency is about 10% of hospital-acquired acute renal failure (2). The specific interest of the investigators (radiologists vs nephrologists) may influence the assessment of the reported incidence.

It is generally thought that patients with diabetes mellitus are prone to the development of radiocontrast-induced acute renal failure. The diabetic state itself, pre-existing renal disease, dehydration, advanced age, nephrotic range proteinuria, and the dose of the radiocontrast agent administered, usually after repeated dosage (multiple radiographic studies) have been recognized (Table 1) as increasing the risk of nephrotoxicity in diabetic patients (3-6). Recent prospective studies, however, have indicated that diabetes per se was not a risk factor when patients were matched for pre-existing renal disease (4,5). Thus, it has become apparent that preexisting renal disease is a definite risk. Whereas other factors may act through prerenal- or disease-induced decreases in glomerular filtration rate (GFR) (Table 1).

EXPERIMENTAL RADIOCONTRAST NEPHROTOXICITY

Attempts to induce radiocontrast nephrotoxicity in non-diabetic animals have led to inconclusive or contradictory results (7-12). Intact hydrated rats with or without experimentally-induced acute renal failure do not develop radiocontrast nephrotoxicity (7-9). Transient reductions in glomerular filtration rate and renal blood flow have been reported

Table 1.   RISK FACTORS IN RADIOCONTRAST-INDUCED NEPHROTOXICITY

Pre-existing renal insufficiency *
Advanced age **

Dehydration ***

Congestive heart failure ***

Specific diseases ***
    Diabetes mellitus
    Multiple myeloma
    Vascular disease

Overdose (usually due to multiple exposure)

Hyperuricaemia, hyperuricosuria, proteinuria

Prior radiocontrast-induced acute renal failure

  * Definite risk factor.
 ** Overestimation of GFR resulting in overdosing.
*** Prerenal- or disease-induced decrease in GFR.

immediately following radiocontrast injection in rats and dogs (10-12),
but rarely has acute renal failure been studied or documented in the
intact animal following these acute measurements. Nephrotoxicity may
occur, however, when the radiocontrast agent is given in association with
experimental manoeuvres designed to reduce renal function. These include
repeated dehydration with furosemide injections, renal ischaemia (13),
associated HgCl glycerol-induced acute renal failure (14) or salt
depletion plus indomethacin (15). Other workers, however, could not
reproduce some of these results using comparable models (7-8).

ADMINISTRATION OF RADIOCONTRAST AGENTS TO DIABETIC RATS

Studies of nephrotoxicity in diabetic animals are very limited. We have
recently demonstrated that the rat with untreated streptozotocin-induced
diabetes is protected from the nephrotoxic effects of the aminoglycoside
gentamicin (16-18). This animal model also exhibits protection from low
dose cisplatin and reduced renal damage from low dose uranyl nitrate
(17). These studies prompted us to suggest that this model might be useful
for the evaluation of mechanisms of nephrotoxicity and its prevention
(17). Recent studies on the acute effects of intravenous radiocontrast
injection on renal function in anaesthetized diabetic rats have been
controversial. A protective effect was suggested by Reed et al (19),
whereas no changes were reported by Golman et al (20), and an impairment
of renal function was shown by Leeming et al (21). Data on renal effects
several hr or days after radiocontrast administration in diabetic rats
have not yet been reported.

Since the state of hydration and anaesthesia are known to influence the
effects of nephrotoxicans on renal function, we first designed an
experimental protocol in diabetic rats controlling for these variables. We
planned to assess the acute effects on renal function of the rapid
intravenous injection of radiocontrast in hydrated conscious and
anaesthetized diabetic and control rats.

Study 1. Acute renal effects of Renografin in anaesthetized and conscious diabetic and control rats.   Female Sprague-Dawley rats aged 4 to 9 months were used.   Diabetes was induced by injection of a single iv dose of 60 mg/kg body weight (bw) of streptozotocin.   Controls were age-matched rats. The duration of diabetes at the time of study ranged from 2 to 7 months. The radiocontrast agent injected in all studies was diatrizoate meglumine sodium in the form of Renografin 76% given intravenously as a bolus at a dose of 5 ml/kg bw, equivalent to 1.85 g of I/kg bw.   This dose is approximately 2 to 3 times the standard dose per kg bw used in humans. In preliminary studies, we demonstrated that the dose of radiocontrast used was sufficient to produce an adequate pyelogram at 15 and 30 min in both control and diabetic rats. The nephrographic effect and the radiographic density of the collecting system, however, were consistently less in the untreated diabetic rats, probably the consequence of the marked polyuria exhibited by these animals.

Animals used for studies in the conscious state were lightly anaesthetized with ether to allow for the placement of catheters. Rats were then placed in a plastic restrainer and allowed to recover from the light anaesthesia for 60 min. During the ensuing hr and subsequently throughout the experiment, ^{14}C-inulin in Ringer's solution was infused to measure GFR. Animals studied in the anaesthetized state were subjected to the same protocol except for the administration of Inactin to induce and maintain anaesthesia during the equilibration and experimental periods, There were 7 animals in each group. Eight urine collections were obtained after equilibration: two baseline periods of 20 min each and 6   post-radiocontrast periods, 2 each of 10, 20, and 30 min. Blood pressure (arterial caudal catheter) was measured during each time period and urine and blood samples were collected. Blood drawn was replaced with equal volumes of Ringer's solution.

The diabetic rats weighed less (238±11g vs controls, 292±11g P < 0.005) but had significantly higher kidney weights expressed as percent bw. Mean arterial pressure was slightly lower in diabetics, and as expected, diabetic rats had marked hyperglycaemia (509±27 mg/dl), polyuria (53±5 ul/min), glycosuria (4.6±0.5 mg/min), and higher sodium excretion (4.0±0.7 uEq/min) than control rats (201±33 mg/dl, P < 0.001 ; 12±2 ul/min, P < 0.001; 0.08±0.07 mg/min, P < 0.001; and 0.9±0.3 uEq/min, P < 0.005, respectively). At base-line, GFR was not significantly different between control and diabetic animals when expressed per g of kidney (1.6±0.7 and 1.5±0.1 ml/min/g kidney weight, respectively). However, when expressed per kg bw, or in ml/min, the diabetic animals had significantly higher clearance rates (15±0.8 vs controls, 11±0.5 ml/min/kg bw, P < 0.001). In both the conscious and anaesthetized groups, there were no differences in GFR between control and diabetic animals throughout the experiment, except for a slightly higher value for conscious controls at 60 min (Fig. 1). The peak increase in GFR observed in all groups immediately after the radiocontrast injection, though statistically significant from baseline, is partially due to a dilutional effect of the injection volume of radiocontrast on plasma inulin concentration, and to the marked increase in inulin excretion associated with the osmotic diuresis characteristic of this class of compounds. After this, GFR falls within 20 min and stabilizes at baseline levels in all animals throughout the 2 hr examined. It is clearly apparent that, although anaesthesia causes a significant lowering of GFR in both groups, there is no evidence of impairment of GFR after radiocontrast injection (Fig. 1).

Radiocontrast injection caused an immediate rise in urine flow that declined to baseline levels after approximately 60 min in conscious animals. In the anaesthetized animals, however, before the injection of radiocontrast, the diabetic rats had a significant reduction in their urine flow rate when compared to their conscious counterparts. In

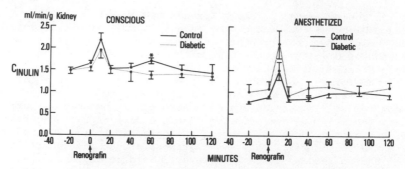

Fig. 1. Effect of Renografin on GFR in conscious and anaesthetized control and diabetic rats. Note that anaesthesia decreased GFR in diabetic and control rats, but did not modify the effect of the radiocontrast injection.

addition, the peak urine flow rates were attenuated during anaesthesia. A similar pattern was observed when urinary sodium excretion and fractional excretion of sodium were examined. As described earlier, the conscious diabetic rats have a baseline pressure slightly lower (122±2mm Hg) than control animals (130±2 mm Hg, P < 0.01). This difference was sustained throughout the experiment. During anaesthesia, however, the values of the control animals dropped to the level of diabetic rats. Although the diabetic animals showed a trend to have lower blood pressure under anaesthesia, the decrease did not achieve statistical significance.

In summary:

1. Both prior to and following radiocontrast administration, conscious diabetic rats had higher urine flow and sodium excretion rates but slightly lower mean arterial blood pressure than controls. GFRs per gram of kidney weight were not different.

2. Anaesthesia decreased GFR and urine flow in both groups, sodium excretion in diabetics, and mean arterial pressure in controls.

3. In both anesthetised and conscious rats, sodium excretion, and urine flow increased transiently after radiocontrast, returning to baseline within 40 to 60 min. These changes were attenuated by anaesthesia.

4. There was a transient measured increase in GFR at 10 min after radio-contrast, returning to baseline within 20 min. This most likely represents an artifact of the inulin clearance technique, as recently shown in the dog by Katzberg et al (12) utilizing an arterio-venous extraction method. Subsequently, in no case did GFR decrease after radiocontrast in either conscious or anaesthetized diabetic or control rats.

Study 2. Effects of radiocontrast on renal functions in conscious diabetic and control rats followed for 3 to 4 days. These studies are important for two reasons. First, two of the previously reported studies in diabetic animals examined renal function acutely, that is for only 40 (21) or 95 (9) min post-radiocontrast injection in anesthetized rats, and did not exclude or demonstrate the subsequent appearance of renal dysfunction or failure; a third study done in diabetic rabbits did not provide adequate data for evaluation (20). Secondly, in the present studies we tested the role of some of the risk factors thought to influence renal function in diabetes.

472

The animals were 6 months old and had had diabetes (induced by the injection of 65 mg/kg bw of streptozotocin) for four months at the time of the studies. Controls were age-matched rats. Animals were kept in individual metabolic cages for five days for adaptation, and were fed a normal rat chow and water ad libitum. The general experimental protocol consisted of a baseline day (day 0), immediately followed by the iv injection of Renografin at a dose of 5 ml/kg bw. After the radiocontrast administration, renal function was followed for 3 or 4 days with daily urine collections and blood samples.

The aims of these studies were three-fold: first, to evaluate if the untreated, normally hydrated diabetic rat exhibits enhanced sensitivity to radiocontrast (Study 2A); second, to assess if the risk factors dehydration and older age (Study 2B), or reduced renal function (Study 2C), enhance the sensitivity of untreated diabetic rats to radiocontrast; and third, to assess the effect of insulin therapy on the response of diabetic rats to radiocontrast (Study 2D), since we have shown that insulin treatment reverses the protection afforded by diabetes against gentamicin-induced acute renal failure (22). In these studies, impaired renal function was defined as a statistically significant decrease in endogenous creatinine clearance (Ccr) measured in 24-hr urine collections. The methods employed in these studies were previously described (16). Values are presented as means±SEM.

The baseline blood, urine and renal function values of the diabetic and control animals were similar to those in Study 1 and will not be described here.

Study 2A. Effect of Renografin on renal function in non-hydropenic diabetic and control rats. These animals were 6 months old at time of study and received 5 ml/kg bw of Renografin. Two animals in each group received a larger dose of Renografin, 12.5 ml/kg bw. The sequential changes in Ccr after Renografin are shown in Fig. 2. No changes occurred in the diabetic animals, while a tendency of the GFR to increase appeared in the control rats as the study progressed. Throughout the four days examined, the Ccr remained significantly higher in the diabetic rats. Similar results were observed in the animals that received the larger dose of radiocontrast agent. Thus, from this study we concluded that neither the young, normally hydrated, untreated diabetic nor the control animals developed impaired renal function following Renografin at the two dosages employed.

Study 2B. The role of dehydration, advanced age and prolonged duration of diabetes on the renal response to Renografin in untreated diabetic and control rats. These animals at the time of study were considerably older, 19 months of age and had had diabetes for a long time, 17 months. The protocol was essentially similar to that previously described, with the exception that an added 24-hr period of hydropenia (designated day OH) preceded the injection of Renografin. The baseline data with normal hydration was similar to that previously described. The only differences related to a higher proteinuria in the diabetic animals (54±9 mg/day vs 9±3 mg/day in controls; P < .005), and the absence in these older rats of differences in Ccr previously observed (16-18), see (Fig. 2) between diabetic (2.9±0.2 ml/min) and control groups (2.7±0.2 ml/min). Marked decreases in urine volume (diabetic 68%, P < 0.01; controls 61%, P < 0.001) and increases in urine concentration (diabetic 47% P < 0.001; controls 57%, P < 0.01) resulted from 24 hr of water deprivation in both groups. Most notable, was the 40% decrease in Ccr observed with hydropenia in the diabetic rats (baseline 2.9±0.2 ml/min; hydropenia 1.7±0.2 ml/min; P < 0.001), whereas in the controls, the changes in Ccr were not significant.

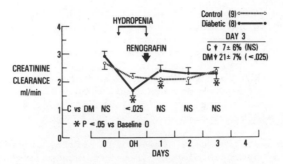

Fig. 2. Effect of Renografin on creatinine clearance in hydropenic old diabetic and control rats (Study 2A). The * indicates a significant difference from baseline. The P values shown are unpaired comparisons (Student's t-test) between control and diabetic rats.

The sequential changes in Ccr after Renografin are illustrated in Fig 3. Except during the hydropenic baseline day (Day OH), no differences in Ccr were apparent between groups. Following Renografin it should be noted, however, that in the diabetic animals, although Ccr recovered in part from dehydration, it still remained significantly below (20%) the non-hydropenic baseline value (Day 0). In addition, proteinuria increased in the diabetic rats after Renografin administration. This phase of our studies suggested that although 24 hr of dehydration immediately preceding the administration of Renografin to older diabetic rats might have had mild effects on renal function, as shown by a 20% decrease in Ccr and an increased proteinuria after three days, clearly acute renal failure did not develop in these animals during the period of observation.

Study 2C. Renal effects of Renografin in untreated diabetic and control rats with a remnant kidney. These animals (6 months of age, duration of diabetes 3-4 months) had half of the renal vasculature of the right kidney ligated first, and then the left kidney removed one week later. The animals were studied 4 days after nephrectomy with a protocol similar to that of Study 2A. As expected, serum creatinine concentration increased from 0.2±0.01 to 1.1±0.3 mg/dl in the diabetic (P < 0.025) and from 0.3±0.02 to 1.8±0.3 mg/dl in the control rats (P < 0.005). The latter values, were not different from each other at the time of Renografin administration. Other baseline values were similar to those previously described. Table 2 illustrates the sequential changes in Ccr. With two intact kidneys, the diabetic rats had a significantly higher clear ance, but with the ablation of renal mass the Ccr was reduced to about 25% of the baseline value in each group. It is quite apparent that the administration of Renografin did not induce any changes in Ccr in either remnant kidney group studied. Following Renografin there was a significant increase in proteinuria in the diabetic, but not the control animals.

Study 2D. Renal effects of Renogrifin in untreated and insulin-treated diabetic rats. These animals were 4 to 6 months old and had had diabetes induced 2 to 4 months prior to study. The untreated diabetic group used for comparison was that shown in Study 2A. In the insulin treated group, rats were implanted subcutaneously with mini-osmotic pumps (Alzet, Palo Alto, CA) which delivered 6 U of insulin per day at a constant rate as previously described (22). When animals had received insulin for 5 days, a baseline period was obtained. Subsequently, they were injected with Renografin and followed as before. The insulin-treated diabetic animals had a significantly lower baseline plasma glucose concentration, urine

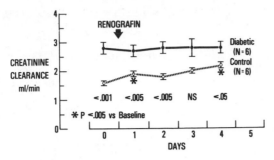

Fig. 3. Effect of Renogrifinon creatinine clearance in non-hydropenic young diabetic and control rats (Study 2B). Day 0 indicates the non-hydropenic baseline, day OH represents the hydropenic baseline, whereas days 1 to 3, the days after Renografin injection. The * indicates a significant difference from the non-hydropenic baseline (day 0) in both groups. Note that at baseline 0, the difference in Ccr between diabetic and control rats was no longer present in these older animals. Note also, that during dehydration (day OH) Ccr decreased 40% in the diabetic animals (P < 0.001).

Table 2.   EFFECT OF RENOGRAFIN ON CREATININE CLEARANCE IN DIABETIC   AND CONTROL RATS WITH REMNANT KIDNEYS (STUDY 2C)

	Diatetes (n = 7)		Controls (n = 8)
	creatinine clearance		(ml/min)
Baseline			
Two Kidneys	3.00±0.20	< 0.001	1.90±0.10
Remnant Kidney	0.74±0.24*	NS	0.41±0.08*
After Renografin			
Day 1	0.72±0.23 a	NS	0.37±0.07 a
Day 3	0.74±0.22 a	NS	0.44±0.08 a

* P < 0.001 from   two-kidney baseline.
a Not different (p > 0.1) from remnant kidney baseline or from day 1.

volume and Ccr than the untreated diabetic rats (Table 3).   Renografin did not cause changes in Ccr in either group.   Thus, the diabetic state per se (hyperglycaemia, glycosuria, polyuria, solute diuresis) appears not to influence the response of diabetic rats to the radiocontrast agent.

DISCUSSION

These studies demonstrated that normally hydrated, untreated young rats with streptozotocin-induced diabetes mellitus do not exhibit enhanced sensitivity to the renal effects of the intravenous administration of a relatively large dose of diatrizoate meglumine sodium (Renografin 76%). It may be argued that the marked polyuria and solute diuresis and elevated Ccr of these animals somehow protected them against the nephrotoxic effects of the radiocontrast used.   The fact that the non-diabetic control animals were also resistant to the nephrotoxic effects of Renografin makes this possibility unlikely.   Reed et al (19) reported a lesser decrease in renal haemodynamics of untreated diabetic rats after the injection of Renografin 60% into the renal artery. Unfortunately, in their study they

Table 3. EFFECT OF RENOGRAFIN ON Ccr IN UNTREATED AND INSULIN-TREATED DIABETIC RATS (STUDY SD)

	Diabetes Untreated a	P value c	Diabetes + Insulin b
	Creatinine	Clearance	(ml/min)
Baseline	2.8±0.2	< 0.025	2.0±0.1
After Renografin			
Day 1	2.7±0.2	NS	2.3±0.1
Day 3	2.8±0.3	NS	2.5±0.2

a n = 6, serum glucose 615±69 mg/dl; urine volume 134±10 ml/day.

b n = 4, serum glucose 197±89, p < 0.005 vs untreated diabetes; urine volume 55±7 ml/day, p < 0.001.

c Unpaired Student's t-test. NS = Non significant, p > 0.05.

did not establish the appearance (or protection from) acute renal failure beyond 60-90 min. On the other hand, a prolonged (40 min) decrease in GFR was reported by Leeming and co-workers (21) in diabetic rats.

When the selected assumed risk factors for radiocontrast nephrotoxicity (hydropenia, old age, and a 75% decrease in renal function and mass) were assessed in Studies 2B and 2C, the diabetic (and control) animals did not exhibit clear cut evidence of nephrotoxicity following Renografin. It may be argued that in Study 2B the association of hydropenia, old age and prolonged duration of diabetes was responsible for a Ccr that by day 3 was 20% lower than the non-hydropenic baseline value (Table 2). It should be noted, however, that the Ccr in the diabetic animals at that time already had increased above the lowest value obtained during hydropenia. Proteinuria increased following Renografin in Studies 2B and 2C. Holtas et al (23) have shown that proteinuria develops immediately (30 min) following the injection of radiocontrast agents into the renal artery of rats, suggesting that it may be an indication of injury.

Since it appears that pre-existing renal disease may be a definite risk factor in diabetic patients (4-6), it is possible that an animal model of renal disease (14), rather than the remnant model employed in Study 2C or a decrease in renal function greater than 75% of baseline may be necessary to predispose diabetic (and non-diabetic rats) to radiocontrast nephrotoxicity.

We have previously shown that insulin reverses the protection afforded by diabetes against gentamicin-induced acute renal failure (22). Administration of insulin to diabetic rats, however, did not influence Ccr after radiocontrast (Study 2D). Thus, it may be concluded that diabetes itself may not be a risk factor for radiocontrast-induced acute renal failure.

In conclusion, despite its successful use in other drug-induced nephrotoxicities (gentamicin, cisplatin, uranyl nitrate), the permutation of the diabetic, non-diabetic and the conscious or anaesthetized hydrated female Sprague-Dawley rat may not be an appropriate model to study the acute or chronic effects of radiocontrast-induced nephrotoxicity.

Studies of experimental radiocontrast nephrotoxicity in the rat may require the concomitant use of more than one of the known risk factors in order to mimic the clinical situation. These factors include: impaired renal function, hypovolaemia, ischaemia, severe dehydration, and prostaglandin synthesis inhibition. Furthermore, it appears reasonable that those studies in the rat that report transient or briefly documented changes in renal function after radiocontrast administration, should also document the appearance (or absence) of more persistent changes in the experimental animal to support the relevance of the observed changes to clinical radiocontrast nephrotoxicity.

ACKNOWLEDGEMENT

This work was supported by grants from the Veterans Administration and the Kidney Foundation of South Florida.

REFERENCES

1. C.A. Vaamonde, Risk factors in nephrotoxicity, _In_: "Homeostasis, nephrotoxicity, and renal abnormalities in the newborn", J. Strauss, ed., Martinus Nijhoff Publishing Co., Boston, (1986).

2. S.H. Hou, D.A. Bushinsky, J.B. Wish, J.J. Cohen and J.T. Harrington, Hospital-acquired renal insufficiency: a prospective study. _Am J Med_ 74:243 (1983).

3. S. Harkonen, and C. Kjellstrand, Contrast nephropathy, _Am J Nephrol_ 1:69 (1981).

4. J.L. Teruel, R. Marcen, J.M. Onaindia, A. Serrano, C. Quereda and J. Ortuno, Renal function impairment caused by intravenous urography, a prospective study. _Arch Intern Med_ 141:1271 (1981).

5. J.A. D'Elia, K.E. Gleason, M. Alday, C. Malarick, K. Godley, J. Warram, A. Kaldany and L.A. Weinrauch, Nephrotoxicity from angiographic contrast material. A prospective study. _Amer J Med_ 72:719 (1982).

6. C.P. Taliercio, R.E. Vlietstra, L.D. Fisher and J.C. Burnett, Risks for renal dysfunction with cardiac angiography. _Ann Intern Med_ 104:501 (1986).

7. C.S. McIntosh, I.F. Moseley, I.K. Fry and W.R. Cattell, Excretion urography. Toxicity studies in experimental acute renal failure. _Nephron_ 14:373 (1975).

8. T. Sherwood and D.J. Evans, Intravenous urography in experimental acute renal failure. Nephrograms and pyelograms in saline-loaded rats. _Nephron_ 14:373 (1975).

9. J-F. Moreau, D. Droz, L-H. Noel, J. Leibowitch, P. Jungers and J-R. Michel, Tubular nephrotoxicity of water-soluble iodinated contrast media. _Invest Radiol_ 15:S54 (1980).

10. L.H. Norby and G.F. DiBona, The renal vascular effects of meglumine diatrizoate. _J Pharmacol Exp Ther_ 193:932 (1975).

11. E.E. Cunningham, P. Barone, L. Nascimento and R.C. Venuto, Effect of a radiographic contrast agent on renal function in the rat. Comparison with equiosmolar mannitol. _Mineral Electrolyte Metab_ 12:157 (1986).

12. R.W. Katzberg, R.C. Pabico, T.W. Morris, K. Hayakawa, B.A. McKenna, B.J. Panner, J.A. Ventura and H.W. Fisher, Effects of contrast media on renal function and subcellular morphology in the dog. _Invest Radiol_ 21:64 (1986).

13. S.G. Schultz, K.J. Lavelle and R. Swain, Nephrotoxicity of radiocontrast media in ischemia renal failure in rabbits, Nephron 32:113 (1982).

14. M.S.F. McLachlan, S. Chick, E.E. Roberts and A.W. Asscher, Intravenous urography in experimental acute renal failure in the rat. Invest Radiol 7:466 (1972).

15. S.N. Heyman, C.A. Reubinoff, M. Brezis, F.H. Epstein and S. Rosen, Acute renal failure (ARF) from radiocontrast: selective injury to medullary thick ascending limbs (MTALs), a possible pathogenic mechanism. Clin Research 34:598A (1986).

16. R.B. Teixeira, F. Kelley, H. Alpert, V. Pardo and C.A. Vaamonde, Complete protection from gentamicin-induced acute renal failure in the untreated streptozotocin diabetes mellitus rat. Kidney Int 21:600 (1982).

17. C.A. Vaamonde, R.B. Teixeira, J. Morales, D. Roth, J. Kelly, H. Alpert, and V. Pardo, A new model for studying drug-induced acute renal failure: The rat with untreated diabetes mellitus, In: "Acute Renal Failure", H. E. Eliahou, ed., John Libbey & Co., London, (1982).

18. C.A. Vaamonde, R. Bier, W. Gouvea, H. Alpert, J. Kelly and V. Pardo, Effect of duration of diabetes on the protection observed in the diabetic rat against gentamicin-induced acute renal failure. Mineral Electrolyte Metab 10:209 (1984).

19. J.R. Reed, R.H. Williams and R.G. Luke, The renal hemodynamic response to diatrizoate in normal and diabetic rats. Invest Radiol 18:536 (1983).

20. K. Golman and T. Almen, Contrast media-induced nephrotoxicity. Survey and present state. Invest Radiol 20:592 (1985).

21. B.W.A. Leeming, K.C. Spokes and P. Silva, Effect of meglumine iothalamate on renal hemodynamics and function in the diabetic rat. Invest Radiol 20:971 (1985).

22. C.A. Vaamonde, D. Roth, J. Kelley, H. Alpert, V. Pardo and G.J. Kaloyanides, Insulin reverses the protection afforded by diabetes against gentamicin-induced acute renal failure. Clin Research 30:465A (1982).

23. S. Holtas, K. Golman and C. Tornquist, Proteinuria following nephroangiography. VIII. Comparison between diatrizoate and iohexol in the rat. Acta Radiol suppl 362:53 (1980).

RENAL MICROCIRCULATION DURING UROGRAPHIC CONTRAST MEDIA ADMINISTRATION

Sergio A. Ajzen, Mirian A. Boim, Horbcio Ajzen and Nestor Schor

Nephrology Division, Escola Paulista de Medicina, Rua Botucatu, 740 04023 S O Paulo, SP, Brazil

INTRODUCTION.

Around 10% of all acute renal failure (ARF) in hospitalised patients in 1983 was due to an intravascular contrast media (UCM) administration (1). There are various predisposition factors such as dose and age, multiple utilization of UCM, dehydration, diabetes, multiple myeloma, hypertension, atherosclerosis, prior kidney or liver diseases, the co-administration of nephrotoxic drugs and kidney transplantation. However, these factors have relative risk that can be identified.

Despite the utilization of new contrast media with lower nephrotoxicity, a progressive increase in the incidence of this ARF is suggested. This incidence is highly variable from 0-12% upto 100% in high risk patients (2,3). Among all contrast examinations, around 65% of ARF are seen after intravenous urography, 30% after arteriography and the rest, mainly by computerized tomography (4-6). This increase in the ARF observation could be due to a better monitoring and awareness of the patients given UCM. Moreover, with higher health standards, a prolonged survival of critical illness patients has been seen; thus patients are more prone to be submitted to a multiple X-ray contrast media examinations.

The pathophysiology of UCM-induced ARF is unclear, but many possible mechanisms are implicated. Tubular obstruction with an increase of tubular hydraulic pressure (P_T), and thus a decline of net transglomerular hydraulic pressure (ΔP) is one of the most commonly suggested mechanisms. A massive intratubular deposition of uric acid and/or calcium oxalate for instance, could account for the increases of P_T (7,8). Renal ischaemia leading to a decrease in one of the glomerular filtration determinant, such as the glomerular plasma flow rate (Q_A), has been suggested and, it is also possible that UCM caused effect on glomerular ultrafiltration coefficient, K_f (9-11). Haemodynamic effects of glomerular function and/or intrarenal flow distribution can contribute to this ARF. It is also well known that many hormonal systems were activated prior and/or during ARF (9-11). The present study was performed to define the role of renal haemodynamics in UCM-induced ARF.

MATERIALS AND METHODS.

Munich-Wistar rats (n = 8) were submitted to surgery for renal clearances and micropuncture studies as described in detail elsewhere (12). A control group (n = 5) was infused with saline and an additional group was treated with indomethacin (n = 7, 2mg/kg, iv), in bolus. The protocol was undertaken due to an increase use of the non-steroid anti-inflammatory drugs in many clinical situations. After an equilibration period of 40 min, a first study period was performed and, saline was given for time-control group or Conray (R)-400 (Mallinckrodt Diagnostics, USA) was infused as an UCM. After a new equilibration period a second study was undertaken. Since the osmolality of this contrast is around 2100 mOsm/kg it was also necessary to evaluate the effect of this high osmolality on renal function and, an additional vehicle-group was performed, osmolality-control group (n = 5).

RESULTS AND DISCUSSION

Table 1 shows a summary of whole kidney function before and after UCM administration.

Table 1 - Whole kidney function before and after urographic contrast media (UCM) administration.

	AP mmHg	GFR .... ml/min	RPF	TRVR mmHg.min/ml
BEFORE	109a +4	0.76 0.08	2.04 0.23	58.5 7.6
AFTER UCM	98* 3	0.31* 0.06	1.07* 0.18	87.6* 10.6

a X+SE, *p < 0.05 vs Before

After UCM the mean arterial pressure (AP) declined significantly (p < 0.05), but was within renal auto-regulatory levels. Also, mean glomerular filtration rate (GFR) and renal plasma flow (RPF) were reduced, but mean total renal vascular resistance (TRVR) increased. Figure 1 summarizes the glomerular haemodynamic data before and after UCM administration. Since mean tubular hydraulic pressure (P_T) is maintained in both study periods, 13±2 and 15±3 mmHg (X±SE) and glomerular capillary hydraulic pressure (PGC) increased from 40±1 to 48±3 mmHg (p < 0.05), the mean transglomerular hydraulic pressure difference (ΔP) increased, from 27±2 to 33±2mmHg (p < 0.05), as depicted in the top of the panel (Figure 1). There was a slight, but not significant decline in afferent arteriolar (R_A) and increase in efferent (R_E) arteriolar resistance. There was a significant (p < 0.05) reduction of the glomerular ultrafiltration coefficient (K_f) 0.059±0.004 vs 0.035±0.009 nl/(s.mmHg). Thus, despite the decline in K_f, a maintenance of the mean single nephron (SN) GFR was observed due to an increased ΔP.

A substantial difference in whole kidney function versus superficial nephron data (micropuncture data) was observed. GFR and RPF declined 60% and 47%, respectively, although mean SNGFR was unaffected and Q_A increased by 15%. Mean total renal vascular resistance (TRVR) increased by 50%, but total arteriolar resistance (R_T) was maintained. At least, two possibilities can explain the difference between whole renal and single nephron data. It is possible that UCM caused an important shift on the renal plasma flow from superficial to juxtamedullary nephrons. It is also possible a heterogeneous perfusion and/or filtration on superficial cortex and, without any our intention, we selected and punctured the

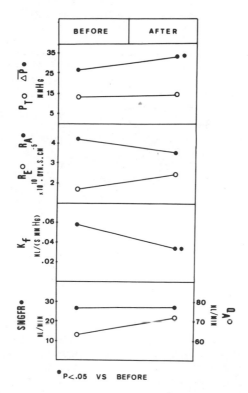

Figure 1 - Summary of glomerular haemodynamic data before and after
urographic contrast media (UCM) administration.

To test time-dependency on UCM studies, as well as the osmolality of better nephrons. Considering that the nephron rat population is around 60% to 80% of superficial and 20% to 40% of juxtamedullary nephrons it is not possible that only juxtamedullary nephron alteration occurred and thus, it is necessary to postulate that contrast media has heterogeneous effects on superficial nephrons.

Conray[R]-400, the respective control groups were performed. Table 2 shows that during both study periods, these rats, during time and osmolality-control (group/Conray vehicle) mean AP, HcT, GFR, RPF or TRVR were not affected.

Table 2. Whole kidney function during first (F) and second (S) study periods in time and osmolality control groups as well indomethacin group.

STUDY PERIODS	AP mmHg		HcT %		GFR	.. ml/min ..	RPF		TRVR mmHg.min/ml	
	F	S	F	S	F	S	F	S	F	S
TIME-CONTROL GROUP (n=5)	112a ±6	110 7	53 1	54 1	.85 .08	.80 .11	2.3 0.1	2.3 0.1	46 3	46 4
OSMOLALITY-CONTROL GROUP (n=5)	119 ±3	118 3	51 1	52 1	.82 .16	.91 .07	2.7 0.3	2.3 0.3	48 7	54 7
INDOMETHACIN +UCM TREATED GROUP (n=7)	127 ±5	117 5	52 1	55 1	.75 .04	.68 .03	1.9 0.2	1.8 0.3	71* 6	68* 9

a $\overline{X}$±SE, *p < .05 vs Groups

UCM caused a decline around 60% in GFR and 50% in RPF, with increases of 50% on total resistance (Figure 2). Indomethacin produced an unexpected protective effect on the mean GFR, RPF and total resistance, suggesting the participation of an important vasoconstrictor such as prostaglandin or thromboxane A2. It is also possible that UCM caused a direct and/or an indirect prostaglandin activation via the renin-angiotensin system or ADH release. These data have to be tested in a prospective clinical trial but, it is necessary to recall that many ARF can be provoked by non-steroid anti-inflammatory drugs as dehydration status, congestive heart failure, diabetes, nephrotic and hepato-renal syndromes, etc. In general, the mechanism of ARF induced by aspirin like-drugs in these clinical situations is due to a potentiation of vasoconstrictor effect of angiotensin II on renal function when a vasodilator prostaglandin was inhibited by this non-specific prostaglandin blocker. It may, therefore, be appropriate to start a prospective clinical trial with a new thromboxane synthesis inhibitor.

In conclusion, UCM Conray-400 in the present protocol study, caused an increase on total resistance, that is responsible for the decline in plasma flow and thus total renal glomerular filtration rate. The glomerular haemodynamic data suggest a decrease on K_f that was blunted by an increased PGC, which maintained superficial SNGFR. The mean Q_A and R_T were not substantialy altered by UCM. Comparative total renal and single

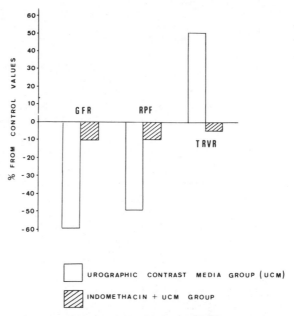

Figure 2. Summary of GFR, RPF and TRVR after UCM alone and after UCM plus Indomethacin administration from percentage control period.

nephron data suggest a higher juxtamedullary nephron susceptibility and/or a heterogeneous superficial nephron alteration in this ARF induced by UCM. Since no alteration on mean tubular hydraulic pressure was observed, no significant tubular obstructive mechanism is involved, at least on superficial nephron. Efferent (PAE) and peri-tubular capillary (PC) hydraulic pressures did not change (data not shown) thus, was possible to disclose an important backleak mechanism for this ARF. The use of a high osmolality-control-vehicle group excluded the possibility of an oncotic effect, per se, as an important factor in this pathophysiological mechanism. Indomethacin blunted the UCM-induced ARF due to a possible juxtamedullary nephron protection, by blocking a stimulated thromboxane and/or by modifying intrarenal haemodynamics.

ACKNOWLEDGEMENTS

These studies were supported largely by FAPESP, CNPq and IPEPENHI. We thank Ms. Marina Andre' da Silva for Secretarial Assistance.

REFERENCES

1. S.H. Hou, D.A. Bushinsky and J.B. Wish, Hospital-acquired renal insufficiency: A prospective study, Am. J. Med. 74:248 (1983).

2. R.L. Eisenberg, W.O. Bank and M.W. Hedgcock, Renal failure after major angiography, Am. J. Med. 68:43 (1980).

3. R.D. Swartz, J.E. Rubin, B.W. Leeming and P. Silva, Renal failure associated with administration of radiographic contrast material, JAMA 239:125 (1978).

4. J. Hanaway and J. Black, Renal failure following contrast injection for computerized tomography, JAMA 239:2056 (1977).

5. S. Harkonen and C.M. Kjellstrand, Intravenous pyelography in non-uremic diabetic patients, Nephron 24:268 (1979).

6. L.S. Fang, R.A. Sirota, T.H. Ebert and N.S. Lichtenstein, Low fractional excretion of sodium with contrast media-induced acute renal failure, Arch. Intern. Med. 140:53 (1980).

7. G.H. Mudge, Uricosuric action of cholecystographic agents: possible nephropoxicity, N. Engl. J. Med. 284:929 (1971).

8. R.H. Schwartz, W.E. Berdon and H.E. Wagner, Tamm-Horsfall urinary mucoprotein precipitation by urographic contrast agents, Am. J. Roehtgen 100:698 (1970).

9. W.J.H. Caldicott, N.K. Hollenberg and H.L. Abrams, Characteristics of response of renal vascular bed to contrast media. Evidence of vaso-constriction induced by renin-angiotensin system, Invest. Radiol. 5:539 (1970).

10. C.C. Chou, J.B. Hook and C.P. Hsieh, Effects of radiopaque dyes on renal vascular resistance, J. Lab. Clin. Med. 78:705 (1974).

11. R.W. Katzberg, T.W. Morris and F.A. Burgener, Renal renin and hemodynamic responses to selective renal artery catheterization and angiography, Invest. Radiol. 12:38 (1977).

12. N. Schor, I. Ichikwa and B.M. Brenner, Mechanism of action of various hormones and vasoactive substances on glomerular ultrafiltration in the rat, Kidney Int. 20:442 (1981).

HYPERTONIC RADIOCONTRAST MEDIUM AND THE KIDNEY: EFFECTS ON RENAL FUNCTIONS IN THE EUVOLAEMIC AND IN THE DEHYDRATED DOGS

Rufino C. Pabico, Richard W. Katzberg, Barbara A. McKenna, Thomas W. Morris, Janine A. Ventura, and Harry W. Fischer

The Departments of Medicine (Nephrology Unit) and Radiology, University of Rochester Medical Center, Rochester, NY 14642, U.S.A.

INTRODUCTION AND OBJECTIVES

There is an ever-increasing frequency in the use of radiocontrast media (RCM) in diagnostic radiology such as angiography, large-dose excretory urography, contrast-enhanced computerized automated tomography, digital subtraction arteriography, etc. This has raised the important issue which concerns most clinical nephrologists relating to the likelihood of a proportional rise in RCM-induced acute renal failure (ARF). Currently available data regarding the actual incidence of RCM-induced ARF are conflicting (1,2). Certain risk factors which may favour the development of RCM-induced ARF have been proposed, such as old age; renal parenchymal disease; diabetes mellitus; cardiac failure; dehydration; the dose, frequency and method of administration of RCM (3). In the presence of such risk factors, the development of ARF with the use of RCM could evolve from one or both of the following mechanisms:-

a) renal vasoconstriction with prolonged ischaemia leading to acute tubular necrosis (4), or

b) direct nephrotoxic effect (2,3).

In our study published recently, we showed that the intravenous (i.v.) administration of RCM to euvolaemic dogs led only to a transient change in renal haemodynamic functions and the rest of the functional changes were attributable to the effects of a brisk osmotic diuresis (5). However, in dehydrated dogs, marked changes in systemic and renal haemodynamic functions were observed following i.v. RCM (4). We extended our study using the same experimental animal model to determine if there would be any substantive difference between the euvolaemic and dehydrated animals with regard to the effect of RCM on the renal extraction of para-aminohippurate (E_{PAH}). A decline in E_{PAH} would mean a reduction in tubular transport (secretory) of the proximal tubules of the cortical nephrons and could indicate a toxic effect independent of the haemodynamic changes.

METHODS AND PROCEDURES

Mixed breed, healthy, euvolaemic dogs (n = 8) weighing 25-32 kg were anaesthetized with 30 mg/kg parenteral sodium pentobarbital and maintained by microdrip infusion of 50 ug/kg/min via a polyethylene catheter in the left femoral vein to maintain light anaesthesia. Twenty ml/kg of Dextrose 5% in 0.45% saline was given i.v. and maintained at 2-3 ml/min. The animals were intubated and ventilated via a Harvard respirator. They were kept warm with blankets and heating lamps. Systemic arterial pressure was monitored via a polyethylene catheter in the left femoral artery using a Statham p23dc pressure transducer. The right femoral artery was cannulated with a 7F Kifa heparinized catheter for blood sampling. The left renal artery was carefully isolated by blunt dissection following a left flank incision and either a 2.5 or 3.0 mm lumen diameter Statham electromagnetic flow probe placed around the mid to proximal aspect of the main renal artery. Selective catheterization of the left renal vein is achieved under fluoroscopic guide through a venotomy of the right external jugular vein. The proximal segment of the ipsilateral ureter was isolated and a small 5F silastic cannula inserted into the ureter via ureterotomy. Systemic arterial pressure and renal artery blood flow were continuously recorded on a Beckman Model 5525C type RM Dynograph Recorder.

Inulin (10%) and PAH (20%) in 0.9% saline were given i.v., with the priming doses calculated to provide plasma levels of 15-20 mg/dl and 2.0-3.0 mg/dl, respectively. Urinary losses of inulin and PAH were replaced with a maintenance dose delivered by a constant infusion pump. After an equilibration time of 60 min, 2-3 urine specimens were collected over 20 min each, and blood samples were obtained. Then RCM (Renografin-76 with osmolality of 1700 mOsm/kg), 2 ml/kg, was administered i.v. Urine specimens with paired blood specimens were collected at 5-min intervals for 15 min, then every 15 min for 45 min, and finally every 30 min for 60 min - a total of 2 hr from the time of i.v. RCM. Similar studies were done using 0.9% NaCl (n = 2) and hypertonic mannitol (n = 3) instead of RCM. Wedge sections were obtained from each kidney at the end of the experiment with the circulation intact. Then the hilus was clamped, both kidneys removed, and the animals sacrificed.

Blood specimens were allowed to clot and sera were collected. Urine specimen volumes were measured and aliquots were saved. Sera and urine specimens were frozen until the time of analyses. Inulin, PAH, osmolality, non-protein nitrogen, and electrolytes were measured and clearances and fractional excretions calculated described elsewhere (6). Values are expressed as mean±SEM, and when experimental values were compared with controls a $P < 0.05$ was considered significant. Similar studies were made on dehydrated dogs (n = 3).

RESULTS

The effects of i.v. RCM on glomerular filtration rate (GFR), as measured by inulin clearance, and effective renal plasma flow (ERPF), as measured by PAH clearance, are depicted in Figure 1. Both GFR and ERPF are significantly lower in the dehydrated dogs (closed circle) compared to the euvolaemic, hydrated animals (open circle) during the control period. During the first 5 min following i.v. RCM, there was a factitious increase in both GFR and ERPF brought about by the brisk osmotic diuresis and rapid urine flow. However, beyond the first period, both GFR and ERPF are not significantly different from the control values in the euvolaemic dogs. On the other hand, the renal haemodynamic functions, especially ERPF, declined significantly in the dehydrated dogs following i.v. RCM.

The effects on E_{PAH} by i.v. RCM are shown in Figure 2. The open symbols represent data from euvolaemic, hydrated dogs. Note that the i.v. administration of 0.9% NaCl and hypertonic mannitol (equiosmolal to the RCM) has no significant effect on E_{PAH} during the first hour; there is a slight increase in E_{PAH} during the second hour. There is a 14% decrease in E_{PAH} within the first 2-3 min following i.v. RCM in the euvolaemic dogs,

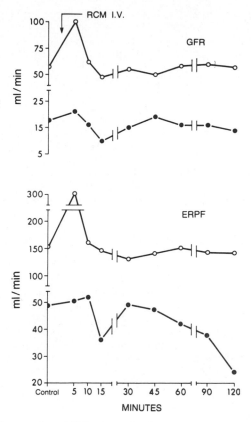

Figure 1. Effects of RCM on GFR and ERPF

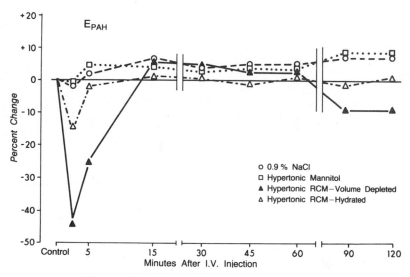

Figure 2. The effects of RCM on E_{PAH}

but E_{PAH} returns to control values during the rest of the experiment. In contrast, E_{PAH} decreased by 47% of control in dehydrated dogs within 2-3 min after i.v. RCM, and is still 25% depressed 5 min after i.v. RCM.

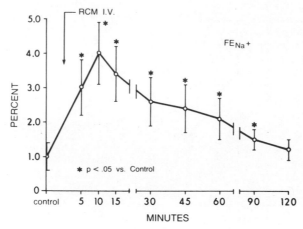

Figure 3.Tef effect of RCM on FE_{Na+}

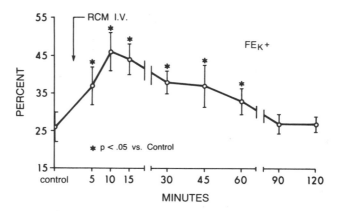

Figure 4.   The effect of RCM on FE_{K+}

E_{PAH} is back to control levels in 15 min, and remained stable for the remainder of the first hour. Note, however, that E_{PAH} is 10% lower than control during the second hour.

The changes in fractional excretion of sodium (FE_{Na}^{+}) and potassium (FE_{K}) following i.v. RCM are similar in both groups of animals. Figures 3 and 4 illustrate the significant natriuresis and kaliuresis, respectively, observed virtually throughout the duration of the study.

DISCUSSION

Hypertonic RCM, administered intravenously to dogs in doses similar to those given patients undergoing diagnostic radiocontrast studies, has been shown to affect renal haemodynamic and tubular functions. ˙In the euvolaemic, hydrated animals, the changes in GFR and ERPF are transient, and the changes in various renal functions are mainly the results of brisk osmotic diuresis (5). In the dehydrated animals, whose dehydration is sufficient to reduce GFR and ERPF, i.v. RCM further diminished the already compromised renal haemodynamic functions. In addition, renal tubular transport mechanism is impaired as evidenced by the marked reduction in

E_{PAH}.   Since both the competition for the same transport system   between RCM and PAH,   and the shift of blood flow from cortex to medulla have been ruled   out   as   the mechanism(s) for the depressed E_{PAH} (7),   the   likely explanation   for   the   reduction in E_{PAH} is   that   the   organic   iodinated portion   of RCM is toxic to the tubule (8).   The depressive effect on E_{PAH} by   RCM is not related to the osmotic properties of the organic   iodinated molecule of RCM (7).

REFERENCES

1.   R.D.   Swartz, V.E. Rubin, R.W. Leeming, et al, Renal failure following major angiography, Am. J. Med. 65:31-37 (1978).

2. B.E. VanZee, W.E. Noy, T.E. Talley, et al, Renal injury associated with intravenous   pyelography   in   non-diabetic   and   diabetic   patients,   Ann. Intern. Med. 89:51-54 (1978).

3.   G.E.   Mudge,   Nephrotoxicity of urographic radiocontrast drugs, Kidney Int. 18:540-552 (1980).

4.   R.W.   Katzberg,   T.W.   Morris,   E.C.   Lasser, et al, Acute systemic and renal   hemodynamic   effects   of   Meglumine/Sodium   Diatrizoate   76%   and Iopamidol in euvolemic and dehydrated   dogs,   Invest.   Radiol.   21:793-797 (1986).

5.   R.W.   Katzberg,   R.C.   Pabico, T.W. Morris, et al, Effects of contrast media   on   renal function and subcellular morphology in the   dog,   Invest. Radiol. 21:64-70 (1986).

6.   R.C.   Pabico,   B.A.   McKenna,   R.B. Freeman, Renal function before and after   unilateral   nephrectomy in   renal   donors,   Kidney   Int.   8:166-175 (1976).

7.   G.F.   DiBona, Effect of anionic and nonionic media on renal extraction of   para-aminohippurate in the dog,   Proc.   Exp.   Biol.   Med.   157:453-455 (1978).

8.   L.B.   Talner,   A.J.   Davidson,   Effect   of   contrast   media   on   renal extraction of PAH, Invest. Radiol. 3:301-309 (1968).

RENAL EFFECTS OF IONIC AND NONIONIC CONTRAST MEDIA: COMPARISON BETWEEN DIATRIZOATE MEGLUMINE AND IOPAMIDOL

Carlo Donadio, Gianfranco Tramonti, Roberto Giordani, Amalia Lucchetti, Andrea Calderazzi, Paola Sbragia, and Claudio Bianchi

Cattedra di Nefrologia Medica, Clinica Medica 2, Istituto di Radiologia, University of Pisa, I-56100 Pisa, Italy

INTRODUCTION.

Renal damage is a potential adverse side effect of the administration of iodinated contrast media (CM). Infact, CM represent one of the most frequent causes of renal failure (1,2). The renal damage determined by CM is sometimes irreversible (3). The mechanisms of this renal injury are not yet well understood. Hyperosmolality of the administered CM has been claimed to be an important factor of renal damage (4). No exhaustive data are available concerning the effects on renal function and nephrotoxicity of the different CM available. The aim of this study is the comparative evaluation of renal effects and nephrotoxicity of two different CM: diatrizoate meglumine (a high-osmolality ionic CM) and iopamidol (a new low-osmolality nonionic agent), after intravenous administration.

MATERIAL AND METHODS

Both diatrizoate (Angiografin 65% - Schering s.p.a) and iopamidol (Iopamiro 300 - Bracco s.p.a.) were administered by IV infusion.

Contrast media	Diatrizoate meglumine	Iopamidol
CM concentration (g/100ml)	65	61.2
Iodine concentration (g/100ml)	30.6	30.0
Osmolality (mOsm/kg)	1500	616
Volume infused (ml)	20-100	30-100
	mean 80.0	mean 76.9
Administerd dose	0.2-1.4	0.2-1.3
(CM g/kg bw)	mean 0.73	mean 0.71

Patients. Thirty-one adult patients (17 females and 14 males) participated in this study. Their main clinical data were as follows: - age 22-74 years, mean 50.7 - body weight 45.3-110.4 kg, mean 71.9 creatinine clearance 62-160 ml/min, mean 105.1. Intravenous urography was performed in 29 patients and computed body tomography in the remaining two. Fifteen patients were examined with diatrizoate and 16 patients with iopamidol in a randomized fashion. None of the patients had been examined with CM in the month preceeding this study, or was taking potentially nephrotoxic drugs. Two patients (one examined with diatrizoate and one with iopamidol) had type II diabetes.

Methods.   The following parameters of renal function were measured twice in the week preceeding the administration of CM and 1, 3 and 5 days after the examination: urine output (urine collected during the twelve night hours, 27 patients), urine protein concentration (27 patients), plasma creatinine and urea (27 patients), creatinine and urea clearances (25 patients). Glomerular filtration rate (GFR) (27 patients) and effective renal plasma flow (ERPF) (23 patients) were measured once in the basal period and after 3 to 5 days from CM administration. Their measurement was carried out by the noninvasive bladder cumulative method (5, 6), using diethylene-triamine-penta-acetic   acid labelled with 99mTc and 131I-hippuran as tracers. Urinary enzyme activities, indicators of tubular injury, were measured in the week preceeding the administration of CM and 1, 3 and 5 days after: alanine-aminopeptidase (AAP) (7) in 22 patients, gamma-glutamyltranspeptidase (GGT) (8) in 23 patients and N-acetyl-beta-D-glucosaminidase (NAG) (9) in 20 patients.

Statistical analysis of the difference between results obtained after administration of CM and the corresponding pre-treatment values was performed by the paired t-test.

RESULTS

A slight decrease of urine output was observed after one day from the administration of CM (from 906 to 754 ml/12 hrs with diatrizoate and from 801 to 688 with iopamidol, p < 0.05). Urinary concentration of proteins remained stable. Plasma creatinine and urea showed only minor changes. These variations were neither clinically nor statistically significant.

In Table I the effects on renal function of both CM are reported. Creatinine cl (as well as urea cl) remained almost unmodified. Similarly, mean values of GFR and ERPF did not change after administration of both CM. A decrease of GFR of more than 30 percent of the basal value was observed in one patient examined with diatrizoate (patient 9) and in two examined with iopamidol (patients 3 and 15). In patient 15 ERPF also decreased.

In Table II the effects on urinary enzyme activities are reported. Both CM produced a relevant increase of urinary enzymes (mainly brush border enzymes AAP and GGT). This increase was maximum after 1 day of examination with both CM and statistically significant. Urinary enzyme activities returned to basal values on the fith day after diatrizoate and on the third day after iopamidol. The increase of lysosomal enzyme NAG was slight. In particular, urinary AAP doubled in 9/11 patients examined with diatrizoate and in 6/11 with iopamidol; GGT doubled in 6/11 patients with diatrizoate and in 6/12 with iopamidol; NAG doubled in 4/8 patients with diatrizoate and in 3/12 with iopamidol.

DISCUSSION

The occurrence of acute renal failure after intravascular administration of iodinated CM is well recognized. Prospective studies seem to be necessary to evaluate the renal effects and nephrotoxicity of CM. In particular, it is necessary to evaluate:

1. effect on renal hemodynamics, mainly GFR (CM are mostly excreted by glomerular filtration);

2. effect on proximal tubule (main target of most nephrotoxins).

Table I. RENAL FUNCTION DATA SHOWN FOR INDIVIDUAL PATIENTS

A. Diatrizoate meglumide

Dosage g/kg	Cr cl ml/min before	after 1	3	5	GFR ml/min before	after	ERPF ml/min before	after
DAYS -->		1	3	5				
0.19	90.4	106.1	90.3	92.3				
0.27	106.3	94.4	101.6	99.1	79.9	64.8	460.7	414.1
0.34			74.6	58.2			419.5	284.6
0.41	160.4	119.3	159.8	170.6	77.6	65.1	375.6	396.4
0.51	138.7	109.2	142.5	148.1	109.0	113.4	279.0	389.5
0.59	101.1	91.7	114.7	91.3	74.5	85.2	662.1	540.0
0.72	111.0	163.8	134.1	115.2	66.8	55.0	349.3	346.3
0.77					54.2	52.6	296.1	271.1
0.87	116.7	102.8	93.2	94.2	68.4	44.8	333.3	251.7
0.88			72.9	75.3			272.9	264.2
0.98	106.8	105.5	70.0	96.9				
0.99	148.8	113.1	169.3	159.4	94.5	81.2		
1.01	87.1	90.5	116.6	98.8	69.6	75.2	258.3	512.9
1.08	86.8	61.7	87.7	88.5	74.0	54.7		
1.36	84.7	74.3	71.4	100.2	47.2	55.6		
mean	111.6	102.7	112.6	112.9	74.1	67.8	370.7	367.1
SD	25.4	25.2	33.0	29.2	15.6	18.3	121.8	102.8

B. Iopamidol

Dosage g/kg	Cr cl ml/min before	after 1	3	5	GFR ml/min before	after	ERPF ml/min before	after
DAYS -->		1	3	5				
0.21	77.0	67.2	78.5	92.2	47.0	62.1	189.3	274.8
0.24	119.9	120.5	102.2	116.2	105.8	108.1	345.7	351.9
0.27	94.1	104.4	93.3	90.8	73.1	50.8	397.7	363.1
0.28					100.9	98.6	269.3	299.9
0.31					66.7	68.4	227.9	217.9
0.58	137.6	157.7	113.4	95.6	68.3	56.1	345.6	277.5
0.77								
0.81	78.6	79.0	87.5	87.0	53.5	65.2	324.2	448.4
0.85	113.2	106.3	81.2	89.8	95.9	86.4	566.4	558.7
0.87	106.2	112.9	89.5	73.0	102.8	141.9		
0.88	74.4	72.7	81.3	101.7	48.4	58.5	241.5	287.3
0.89	72.2	64.7	40.3	50.8	31.8	30.4	149.1	134.0
0.94	109.4	125.1	113.8	114.3	76.0	71.2	485.5	418.2
0.94	160.2	146.1	195.6	108.3	57.5	68.0	318.9	298.8
1.22	97.2	132.7	97.1	97.2	88.6	45.5	391.4	250.0
1.25	93.1	134.3	73.8	118.1				
mean	102.5	109.5	96.0	95.0	72.6	72.2	327.1	321.4
SD	26.1	30.7	35.4	18.6	23.5	28.6	116.7	108.7

Cc-Cl creatinine clearance, GFR = glomerular filtration rate,
ERPF = effective renal plasma flow

Table II. URINARY ENZYME ACTIVITIES DATA SHOWN FOR INDIVIDUAL PATIENTS

A. Diatrizoate meglumine

Dosage g/kg	AAP U/g creatinine before	after			GGT U/g creatinine before	after			NAG uM/h/g creatinine before	after		
DAYS -->		1	3	5		1	3	5		1	3	5
0.19	1.8	1.7	2.5	3.2	24	30	17	28				
0.27	4.2	2.9	2.3	3.5	25	22	40	40	33	28	33	67
0.34												
0.41	1.4	1.7	3.3	1.5	34	55	43	38	8	10	18	10
0.51												
0.59												
0.72	1.5	6.3	1.9	1.1	31	301	74	62	36	33	29	56
0.77	2.3	7.9	4.4	1.1	47	185	51	42	27	35	62	27
0.87	2.7	8.7	3.3	2.9	39	85	31	27	18	19	24	23
0.88	6.7	6.9	15.2	12.1	111	98	97	67				
0.98	3.6	10.0	2.8	4.2	36	134	4	24	25	24	13	22
0.99												
1.01	14.4	33.3	20.0	8.8	45	195	61	38				
1.08	1.8	6.4	2.0	2.4	56	33	52	48	31	16	19	16
1.36	6.4	12.0	30.0	5.1	90	267	413	96	52	150	56	57
mean	4.3	8.9	8.0	4.2	48.9	127.7	80.3	46.4	38.8	39.4	31.8	34.8
SD	3.8	8.7	9.5	3.4	27.6	97.5	113.3	21.3	13.0	45.5	18.0	21.8
		*				*						

B. Iopamidol

Dosage g/kg	AAP U/g creatinine before	after			GGT U/g creatinine before	after			NAG uM/h/g creatinine before	after		
DAYS -->		1	3	5		1	3	5		1	3	5
0.21	9.8	10.1	8.1	3.8	55	65	61	64	143	76	87	133
0.24												
0.27	3.4	11.9	7.5	2.9	26	104	24	16	164	399	134	108
0.28												
0.31												
0.58					55	130	37	45	51	85	22	28
0.77	1.7	4.3	1.0	2.4	37	52	33	42	17	16	18	20
0.81	2.9	5.7	1.5	1.5	41	81	42	33	41	52	39	79
0.85	0.9	6.9	1.1	4.2	40	57	32	32	21	29	39	33
0.87	6.4	10.6	4.6	3.1								
0.88	6.5	5.8	7.5	5.2	42	58	22	19	147	160	131	203
0.89	2.7	5.8	3.0	2.8	43	214	51	3	37	29	40	41
0.94	1.7	1.6	2.1	1.8	30	18	35	19	21	20	10	12
0.94	3.2	3.2	1.0	1.7	51	65	34	36	16	17	14	14
1.22	4.5	12.9	6.9	2.3	61	171	60	48	68	67	144	61
1.25					40	107	50	58	26	108	11	18
mean	4.0	7.2	10.2	2.9	43.4	93.5	40.1	34.6	62.7	88.2	57.4	62.4
SD	2.6	3.7	21.7	1.1	10.4	55.6	12.9	18.1	55.8	107.0	52.0	59.0
		**				**						

* p < 0.025   ** p < 0.01

494

Conflicting results have been reported on both glomerular and tubular effects of CM (10-21). A lower nephrotoxicity for nonionic low-osmolal CM has been claimed by some authors, but not confirmed by others (14-16, 19, 21, 22). In our opinion it seems to be unlikely, in particular for urography, due to the dilution of contrast material in the blood-stream.

Up to now there has been no prospective study evaluating both glomerular and tubular effects of ionic and nonionic CM.

Our results demonstrate that both ionic and nonionic CM do not cause a marked impairment of renal hemodynamics. The moderate decrease of GFR observed in three patients (one with diatrizoate and two with iopamidol) was quite moderate. Both CM affect the proximal tubule, as demonstrated by the increased enzymuria observed in most patients. Infact, a marked increase of urinary enzyme activities (mostly brush border enzymes) occurred frequently, mainly after diatrizoate. The observed increase of urinary enzymes, which was completely reversible in a few days, suggests a tubular dysfunction, without indicating a clinically relevant renal damage. The mechanism of this tubular effect is not clear. Tke increase of AAP and GGT could be due to the contact of contrast material, contained in pre-urine, with the brush border of proximal tubular cells.

In conclusion, no significant differences have been observed between diatrizoate meglumine and iopamidol. Both CM do not cause clinically relevant renal effects. They can frequently induce a reversible tubular dysfunction and may occasionally cause a slight decrease of GFR.

Acknowledgements. This work has been supported in part by a research fund from the Ministero della Pubblica Istruzione. The help of Mr. Joseph Franceschina in preparing this manuscript was greatly appreciated.

REFERENCES

1. S.H. Hou, D.A. Bushinsky, 1.B. Wish, J.J. Cohen, and J.T. Harrington, Hospital-acquired renal insufficiency: a prospective study, Am. J. Med. 74:243 (1983).

2. D. Kleinknecht, P. Landais, and B. Goldfarb, Les insuffisances renales aigues associees h des medicaments ou A des produits de contraste iodes. Resultats d'une enquete cooperative multicentrique de la Societe de nephrologie, Nephrologie 7:41 (1986).

3. B.E. VanZee, W.E. Hoy, T.E. Talley, and J.R. Jaenike, Renal injury associated with intravenous pyelography in nondiabetic and diabetic patients, Ann. Intern. Med. 89:51 (1978).

4. J.B. Forrest, S.S. Howards, and 1.Y. Gillenwater, Osmotic effects of intravenous contrast agents on renal function, J. Urol. 125:147 (1981).

5. C. Bianchi, Noninvasive methods for the measurement of renal function, In: "Renal function tests. Clinical laboratory procedures and diagnosis", C.G. Duarte, ed., p. 65, Little, Brown, Boston (1980).

6. C. Bianchi, C. Donadio, and G. Tramonti, Noninvasive methods for the measurement of total renal function, Nephron 28:53 (1981).

7. J.E. Peters, I. Schneider, and R.J. Haschen, Bestimmung der 1-Alanyl: Peptidhydrolase (Alanil-Aminopeptidase, Aminosaure-Arylamidase) immenschlichen Harn, Clin. Chim. Acta 36:289 (1972).

8. G. Szasz, Gamma-Glutamyltranspeptidase-Aktivitat im Urin, Z. Klin. Chem. Klin. Biochem. 8:1 (1970).

9. L.J. Merle, M.M. Reindenberg, M.T. Camacho, B.R. Jones, and D.E. Drayer, Renal injury in patients with rheumatoid arthritis treated with gold, Clin. Pharmacol. Ther. 28:216 (1980).

10. N. Milman, and P. Gottlieb, Renal function after high-dose urography in patients with chronic renal insufficiency, Clin. Nephrol. 7:250 (1977).

11. T. Shafi, S.Y. Chou, J.G. Porush, and W.B. Shapiro, Infusion intravenous pyelography and renal function. Effects in patients with chronic renal insufficiency, Arch. Intern. Med. 138:1218 (1978).

12. A. Rahimi, R.P.S. Edmondson, and N.F. Jones, Effect of radiocontrast media on kidney of patients with renal disease, Br. Med. J. 282:1194 (1981).

13. J.L. Teruel, R. Marcen, J.M. Onaindia, A. Serreno, C. Quereda, and J. Ortuno, Renal function impairment caused by intravenous urography, Arch. Intern. Med. 141:1271 (1981).

14. G.A. Khoury, J.C. Hopper, Z. Varghese, K. Farrington, R. Dick, J.D. Irving, P. Sweny, O.N. Fernando, and J.F. Moorhead, Nephrotoxicity of ionic and non-ionic contrast material in digital vascular imaging and selective renal arteriography, Br. J. Radiol. 56:631 (1983).

15. M.E. Gale, A.H. Robbins, R.J. Hamburger, and W.C. Widrich, Renal toxicity of contrast agents: iopamidol, iothalamate, and diatrizoate, Am. J. Roentgenol. 142:333 (1984).

16. J.E. Scherberich, W. Mondorf, F.W. Falkenberg, D. Pierard, and W. Schoeppe, Monitoring drug nephrotoxicity. Quantitative estimation of human kidney brush border antigens in urine as a specific marker of tubular damage, Contrib. Nephrol. 42:81 (1984).

17. W.M. Thompson, W.L.Jr. Foster, R.A. Halvorsen, N.R. Dunnick, A.L. Rommel, and M. Bates, Iopamidol: new, nonionic contrast agent for excretory urography, Am. J. Roentgenol. 142:329 (1984).

18. H.J. Smith, K. Levorstad, K.J. Berg, K. Rootwelt, and K. Sveen, High dose urography in patients with renal failure. A double blind investigation of iohexol and metrizoate, Acta Radiol. Diagn. 26:213 (1985).

19. G. Cavaliere, G. Arrigo, G. D'Amico, P. Bernasconi, G. Schiavina, L. Dellafiore, and D. Vergnaghi, Tubular nephrotoxicity after intravenous urography with ionic high-osmolal and nonionic low-osmolal contrast media in patients with chronic renal insufficiency, Nephron 46:128 (1987).

20. R.F. Spataro, R.W. Katzberg, H.W. Fisher, and M.J. McMannis, High-dose clinical urography with the low-osmolality contrast agent hexabrix: comparison with a conventional contrast agent, Radiology 162:9 (1987).

21. C. Donadio, G. Tramonti, P. Lorusso, R. Giordani, A. Lucchetti, A. Calderazzi, C. Sbragia, P.L. Michelassi, and C. Bianchi, Effetti renali dei mezzi di contrasto: confronto tra diatrizoato di megluminae iopamidolo (risultati preliminari), G. Ital. Nefrol. in press.

22. S. Cedgard, H. Herlitz, K. Geterud, P. Attman, and M. Aurell, Acute renal insufficiency after administration of low-osmolar contrast media, Lancet 2:1281 (1986).

RENAL PROTON NUCLEAR MAGNETIC RESONANCE IN GENTAMICIN, CYCLOSPORIN A AND CISPLATINUM ACUTE RENAL FAILURE IN RATS

A. Iaina, S. Abrashkin*, J. Weininger*, and R.Azoury*

Department of Nephrology, Barzilai Medical Centre, Ashqelon 78306, and
*Soreq Nuclear Research Centre, Yavne, Israel

INTRODUCTION

Several studies suggest that it is possible to evaluate renal pathology by magnetic resonance imaging due to the sensitivity of the method in differentiating normal from pathological renal tissue (1-9). Proton magnetic resonance measurements are based on the properties of hydrogen nuclei that have spin. When placed in a magnetic field they orient themselves in the direction of the field. By application of a radio frequency pulse of suitable frequency, the direction of the spinning axis may be modified. After the pulse, the protons return to their original orientation emitting measurable signals. These signals grow and decay according to characteristic relaxation times; T_1 "spin-lattice" (longitudinal) and T_2 "spin-spin" (transverse) relaxation times. T_1 reflects the interaction of the hydrogen nucleus with its molecular environment, whereas T_2 reflects magnetic interactions between protons (10-12). In vitro magnetic resonance spectroscopy offers a direct measurement of different normal and abnormal tissues magnetic resonance properties (10-17). Using in vitro proton magnetic resonance measurements we demonstrated different profiles of relaxation times in different forms of experimental acute and chronic renal failure in rats (14,15).

Most of the protons in tissues and macromolecular solutions are bound in water molecules. Water in macromolecular solutions divides into free water and hydration water. Since proton magnetic resonance is essentially a measurement of water content, the future calculations of the bound and hydration water fractions would enhance sensitivity (18-25). According to a fast proton diffusion model (11,12), in which the free and hydration components result from fast proton diffusion from one compartment to another, it is assumed that the free and hydration water are two phases with distinguished relaxation times. The T_1 of a macromolecular solution is a result of the fast exchange of protons between the free and hydration compartments. The tissues T_1 are thus dominated by total tissue water content and the ability of the macromolecules to bind water in the hydration layer. Thus direct measurement of tissue T_1 and total tissue water content can be used to calculate both free water and the hydration water. In contrast to this, the T_2 parameter of tissues is strongly affected by the of crystalline water binding sites as well as the thickness of the hydration water multilayer, and may suggest structural changes.

The present study was performed to find the differences in the magnetic resonance properties and water distribution between normal and pathological renal tissue resulting from different kinds of nephrotoxic experimentally induced acute renal failure in rats.

MATERIALS AND METHODS

All experiments were performed on Charles River rats of both sexes weighing 250-300g (Yokneam, Israel). The rats were divided into three experimental groups. Gentamicin ARF was induced by one intraperitoneal injection per day for 8 days of 100mg gentamicin/kg body weight. The relaxation times and water content were measured on day 9. Cyclosporin A associated ARF was induced by intraperitoneal injections of 60 mg/kg body weight/day for 4 days, following right nephrectomy and 20 min left renal artery clamping (26). Cisplatinum ARF was induced by a single intraperitoneal injection of 5.5 mg Cisplatinum/kg body weight. Relaxation times and water content were measured 4 days thereafter. Normal rats were used as a control group. All rats were kept throughout the experiment in individual metabolic cages. The last 24-hr urine collection and blood sample taken at the end of the experiment were used for laboratory determinations. Creatinine clearance was calculated for each rat. MR parameters and water content determination: T_1 and T_2 relaxation times were measured in renal cortical and medullary slices weighing from 50 to 200 mg, within 5-10 min of excision, with a Bruker PC-20 Minispec spectrometer (Bruker, W. Germany Analytische Messtechnik GmbH, Rheinstetten) operating at 20 MHz at $37\pm1^\circ C$. T_1 was determined by the 180o r 90o method and a three-parameter fit, and T_2 by the Carr-Purcell-Meiboom-Gill (CPMG) spin echo sequence method. Water content (PW) of the samples was calculated as a percentage tissue weight - after 24 hr drying to constant weight. The fraction bound (FB = % water bound) and hydration fraction (HF = % water bound/g solid) were computed from the T_1 relaxation time, and the PW, according to a fast proton diffusion model (11-12). The theory and the derivation of the formulas used to convert T_1 relaxation time and PW in the various water compartments are beyond the scope of the present work. Statistical analysis: Mean$\pm$SD and one way analysis of variance were used to assess statistical significance, where $p < 0.05$ was considered significant.

RESULTS

In all three experimental groups the creatinine clearance decreased significantly ($p < 0.001$) and the blood urea increased ($p < 0.001$) compared to control rats (Table 1). The cortical relaxation times normal values were 473 ± 28 msec and 47 ± 4 msec for T_1 and T_2 respectively. In both gentamicin and cisplatinum groups both T_1 and T_2 were prolonged (Table 1). In the medulla the normal values were 691 ± 73 msec and 71 ± 8 msec for T_1 and T_2 respectively. The gentamicin and cyclosporin groups had prolonged T_2 values. The cisplatinum medullary T_1 is significantly prolonged compared with both normal and gentamicin groups. The cortical and medullary water compartments in the studied groups are given in Table 2. There were no significant changes in total water content in any group. In the cisplatinum group there was a significant decrease in cortical free and bound water compartments. In the cortex of the gentamicin group there was a small decrease in the fraction bound compared with the normal rats ($p < 0.05$) and both medullary FB and HF increased ($p < 0.05$) compared with the normal rats. In the medulla, the cisplatinum group had a small decrease in the fraction bound compared with the normal rats ($p < 0.05$).

DISCUSSION

Gentamicin, CyA and cisplatinum administration resulted in acute renal failure. In the present work, renal proton NMR spectroscopy was used to differentiate the renal effect of three important and widely studied nephrotoxic agents. This study demonstrates that significant changes occurred in renal cortex and medulla magnetic resonance properties in different types of experimental nephrotoxic ARF. Cisplatinum and gentamicin experimental ARF were found to have prolonged cortical T_1 and T_2 values. More prolonged medullary T_1 differentiate cisplatinum from gentamicin acute renal failure. CyA ARF differs from normal rats by a prolonged medullary T_2 and from gentamicin ARF by a prolonged medullary T_1 relaxation time. These

Table 1. Cortical and Medullary Proton Magnetic Resonance Relaxation Times and Renal Function in the Experimental Groups Studied

	CT_1	CT_2	MT_1	MT_2	Blood urea mg%	Ccr ul/min/100 g bw
N (n=22)	473 ± 28	47 ± 4	691 ± 73	71 ± 8	36 ± 4	408 ± 15
G (n=13)	$587\pm34*$	$74\pm7*$	670 ± 20	$81\pm4*$	$112\pm19*$	$280\pm21*$
CyA (n=6)	499 ± 8	51 ± 2	732 ± 11	$78\pm1*$	$92.8\pm7.6*$	$136\pm15*$
CP (n=8)	$523\pm22*$	$55\pm4*$	$758\pm79*\#$	78 ± 12	$124\pm9*$	$116\pm17*$

Mean$\pm$SD, N = normal, G = gentamicin, CyA = cyclosporin A, CP = cisplatinum acute renal failure and n = number of rats. * $p < 0.05$ (at least) vs N. # $p < 0.05$ vs G group.

Table 2. Water Distribution in the Different Experimental Groups Studied

	CORTEX			MEDULLA		
	PW	FB	HF	PW	FB	HF
N (n=22)	76 ± 0.8	11.0 ± 0.1	35.0 ± 0.2	79 ± 1.7	6.8 ± 0.1	26.3 ± 0.5
G (n=13)	77 ± 0.9	$9.9\pm0.2*$	32.8 ± 2.0	79 ± 0.4	$7.8\pm0.9*$	$29.0\pm2.5*$
CyA (n=6)	77 ± 0.8	11.0 ± 0.2	33.3 ± 3.0	80 ± 1.8	6.9 ± 0.2	27.0 ± 0.6
CP (n=8)	75 ± 2.6	$9.7\pm0.1*$	$28.7\pm0.6*$	80 ± 1.6	$6.0\pm0.3*$	24.8 ± 0.5

Mean$\pm$SD, n = number of rats, PW = % total tissue water, FB = fraction bound, HF = hydration fraction, N, G, CyA, CP as in table 1. * $p < 0.05$ (at least) vs N

results are in concordance with our previous work in which we found that in vitro proton NMR changes can differentiate several types of experimental acute and chronic renal failure (14,15).

The pathogenetic mechanisms of these models were extensively studied and focused on different cellular and molecular events (27-29). Using proton nuclear magnetic resonance in combination with the determination of tissue total water content measurement, we could determine renal water structure, ie. bound and free water distribution according to the fast proton diffusion model. Significant changes regarding the bound/free water ratio were found, whilst almost no changes were measured in the total water content. In the gentamicin acute renal failure, the cortical bound water fraction decreased compared with the normal rats. In the medulla, an increased bound water compartment was calculated. In the cisplatinum acute renal failure in both cortex and medulla, the bound water compartment decreased compared with the normal controls.

At the moment, we cannot indicate the biological importance of water structure changes found. The time sequences and relationship with the other intra-cellular functional changes in different types of experimental nephrotoxic acute renal failure remains to be determined.

In summary, using proton nuclear magnetic resonance technique, we demonstrated that significant changes occurred in the renal cortex and medulla magnetic resonance properties and tissue water distribution in rats with experimentally induced nephrotoxic acute renal failure. These findings may have clinical importance in magnetic resonance imaging and may have pathogenetic relevance, suggesting the importance of water structure changes in the development of renal failure.

REFERENCES

1. R.E. Steiner, The Hammersmith clinical experience with nuclear magnetic resonance, Clinical Radiology. 34:13 (1983).

2. H. Hricak, L. Crooks, P. Sheldon and L. Kaufman, Nuclear magnetic resonance imaging of the kidney, Radiology. 146:425 (1983).

3. H. Hricak and J.F. Newhouse, Magnetic resonance imaging of the kidney, Radiol. Clin. North Am. 22:287 (1984).

4. F.W. Smith, A. Reid, J.R. Mallard, J.M.S. Hutchinson, D.A. Pover, and G.R.D. Cato, Nuclear magnetic resonance tomographic imaging in renal disease, Diagnostic Imaging. 51:209 (1982).

5. L.J. Schultze, L. Te Strake, L.C. Paul, A.M. Tegzess, J.L. Bloem, J. Doornbos and R.G. Bluemm, Magnetic resonance imaging in renal transplants, In: "Proceedings EDTA-ERA" A.M. Davison and P.J. Guillou eds. Bailliere Tindal, London, pp 609-613 (1985).

6. I.R. Young, D.R. Bailes, M. Burl, A.G. Collins, D.T. Smith, M.J. MacDonald, J.S. Orr, L.M. Banks, G.M. Bydder, R.M. Greenspan and R.E. Steiner, Initial clinical evaluation of a whole body nuclear magnetic resonance (NMR) tomograph, J. Comput. Assist. Tomog. 6:1 (1982).

7. F. Terrier, H. Hricak, D.Revel, C. Alpers, P. Bretan and N.J. Feduska, Magnetic resonance imaging in the diagnosis of acute allograft rejection

and its differentiation from acute tubular necrosis necrosis; experimental study in the dog, Invest. Radiol. 20:617 (1985).

8. H. Hricak, F. Terrier and B. Demas, Renal allografts: evaluation by MR imaging, Radiology. 159:435 (1986).

9. H. Hricak, F. Terrier, M. Marotti, B.L. Engelstad, R.A. Filly, F. Vincenti, R.M. Duca, P.N. Bretan, C.B. Higgins and N. Feduska, Post-transplant renal rejection: comparison of quantitative scintigraphy, US and MR imaging, Radiology, 162:685 (1987).

10. P.T. Beall, D. Medina and C.F. Hazelwood, The "systemic effect" of elevated tissue and serum relaxation times for water in animals and humans with cancer, In: "NMR medicine", R. Damadian R, ed., Springer Verlag, New York, pp 39-57 (1981).

11. I.L. Cameron, V.A. Ord and G.D. Fullerton, Characterization of proton NMR relaxation times in normal and pathological tissues by correlation with other tissue parameters, Magnetic Resonance Imaging, 2:97 (1984).

12. G.D. Fullerton,J.L. Potter and N.C. Dornbluth, NMR relaxation of protons in tissues and other macromolecular water solutions, Magnetic Resonance Imaging, 1:209 (1982).

13. Z.H. Endre and P.W. Kuchel PW, Proton NMR spectroscopy of rabbit renal cortex, Kidney Int. 28:6 (1985).

14. A. Iaina, S. Abrashkin and J. Weininger, Proton MR study of different types of experimental acute renal failure in rats, Magnetic Resonance Imaging. 4:241 (1986).

15. S. Abrashkin, J. Weininger, L. Griffel, R. Schneider and A. Iaina, Proton magnetic resonance in experimental acute and chronic renal failure in rats, Renal Failure. 10:21 (1987).

16. D. London, P. Davis, R. Williams, L. Crooks, P. Sheldon P and C. Gooding, Nuclear magnetic resonance imaging of induced renal lesions, Radiology. 148;167 (1983).

17. Y. Yuasa and H.L. Kundel, Magnetic resonance imaging following unilateral occlusion of the renal circulation in rabbits, Radiology. 154:151 (1985).

18. G.N. Ling, Hydration of macromolecules, In:" Water and aqueous solutions: Structure, thermodynamics and transport processes", R. Horne, ed., pp 663-670, Wiley Interscience, New York (1972).

19. R.K. Outhred and E.P.George, A nuclear magnetic resonance study of hydrated systems using the frequency dependence of the relaxation process, Biophys. J. 13:83 (1973).

20. W.R. Inch, J.A. McCredie, C. Geiger and Y. Boctor, Spin-lattice relaxation times for mixtures of water and gelatin or cotton, compared with normal and malignant tissue, J. Nat. Canc. Inst. 53:689 (1974).

21. W.R. Inch, J.A. McCredie, R.R. Knispel, R.I. Thompson and M.M. Pintar, Water content and proton spin relaxation time for neoplastic and non-neoplastic tissues from mice and humans, J. Nat. Canc. Inst. 52:353 (1974).

22. H.J.C. Berendsen, Specific interactions of water with biopolymers, In: "Water a comprehensive treatise, Vol 5, Water in disperse systems", F. Franks, ed. Plenum Press, New York, pp 293-330 (1975).

23. C.F. Hazelwood, A view of the significance and understanding of the physical properties of cell-associated water, In: "Cell Associated Water", J. Clegg and W. Drost-Hanson, eds. Academic Press, New York, pp 165-259 (1979).

24. R. Mathur-De Vre, The NMR studies of water in biological systems, Prog. Biophys. Biol. 35:103 (1979).

25. K.R. Porter and J.B. Tucker, The ground substance of the living cell, Sci. Am. 244:56 (1981).

26. A. Iaina, D. Herzog, D. Cohen, S. Gavendo, S. Kapuler, I. Serban, G. Schiby and H.E. Eliahou, Calcium entry blockade with verapamil in cyclosporine A plus ischemia induced acute renal failure in rats, Clinical Nephrol. 25 (suppl 1):168 (1986).

27. B.D. Kaha, Cyclosporine nephrotoxicity: pathogenesis, prophylaxis, therapy and prognosis, Am. J. Kidney. Dis. 8:323 (1986).

28. J.M. Weinberg, The role of calcium overload in nephrotoxic renal tubular cell injury, Am. J. Kidney Dis. 8:284 (1986).

29. R. Safirstein, J. Winston, M. Goldstein, D. Moel, S. Dickman and J. Guttenplan, Cisplatin nephrotoxicity, Am. J. Kidney Dis. 8:356 (1986).

[31]PHOSPHORUS NMR STUDIES OF MERCURIC CHLORIDE NEPHROTOXICITY IN THE IN VITRO PERFUSED RAT KIDNEY

Z.H. Endre, P.J. Ratcliffe, L.G. Nicholls, J.G.G. Ledingham, J.D. Tange and G.K. Radda

Nuffield Department of clinical Medicine and Department of Biochemistry, University of Oxford, Oxford, UK

INTRODUCTION

[31]P Nuclear Magnetic Resonance (NMR) studies of the effect of hypoxia on ATP levels in the isolated perfused rat kidney have shown that a step-wise decrease in oxygen delivery is associated with a step-wise decrease in ATP to a new plateau level (1). The decrement in ATP was closely correlated with the volume extent of cellular necrosis determined from morphometric analysis of the same kidneys at the end of the perfusion period.

Renal injury caused by nephrotoxins may be modified or prevented by systemically acting vasoactive drugs, e.g. clonidine in experimental ARF induced by mercuric chloride in rats (2). The studies presented here address the general question of whether a directly-acting nephrotoxin can cause renal injury and ATP depletion in the absence of hypoxic or ischaemic injury.

The isolated perfused rat kidney (IPRK) provides a model system free of systemic hormonal or autonomic nervous regulation. The dose of mercury required to produce functional and morphological damage within the course of a three hour perfusion period was established in preliminary studies.

^{31}P NMR was then used to determine whether representative doses of mercuric chloride altered renal ATP levels since high doses of mercuric chloride produced marked changes in renal vascular resistance, the NMR studies were repeated in the non-filtering IPRK, since acute alterations of renal vascular resistance are abolished in this preparation (3).

METHODS

Right kidneys from Wistar rats 300-400g were perfused at a cannula tip pressure of 85-110 mm Hg with Krebs bicarbonate buffer supplemented with amino acids (4), 5 mmol/l glucose and 6.7 g/dl albumin (filtering kidneys, FK). Non-filtering kidneys (NFK) were perfused with the same medium except that 10 g/dl albumin was used and the perfusion pressure was 60-80 mm Hg. Mercuric chloride was added to the perfusate after 60 min of baseline perfusion. After a further 2 hours of perfusion, kidneys were perfusion-fixed with 2.5% glutaraldehyde and sectioned for routine morphological evaluation (5).

Renal function was estimated by ^{14}C-inulin clearance and urinary Na and K excretion. ^{31}P NMR measurements were obtained at 73.84 MHz (6) in a vertical bore 4.3T magnetic (Oxford Research Systems). Each spectrum averaged 452 scans collected via a solenoidal radiofrequency coil using a 35 us (67°) pulse at a 2 sec repetition rate. A line broadening of 20 Hz was applied prior to Fourier transformation of the data. Methylene diphosphonate (MDP) sealed in a glass capillary tube was used as an external chemical shift and intensity reference.

RESULTS

Mercuric chloride produced dose-dependent deterioration in parameters of renal function (Fig. 1) and in morphological damage. Doses of 2 and 8 mg/dl produced respectively mild and extensive histological damage, principally of proximal tubules. A typical ^{31}P NMR spectrum from normal in vitro perfused rat kidney is shown in Fig. 2. Both doses of mercuric chloride produced progressive dose-dependent decreases in total renal ATP (beta-ATP) levels and transient, dose-dependent increases in organic phosphate (Pi) levels. The effect of 8 mg/dl mercuric chloride is illustrated in Fig. 3, while the effect of both doses is summarized in Fig. 4.

Both doses of mercuric chloride also produced increases in renal vascular resistance with a profound biphasic decrease in perfusate flow rate at the 8 mg/dl dose (see also refs. 3 and 7), with the result that oxygen delivery was reduced from 30 umol/min to 60 umol/min at the higher dose. Consequently, the ^{31}P NMR studies were repeated in the NFK since changes in renal vascular resistance do not occur in this preparation, even at the 8 mg/dl dose of mercuric chloride (3). ß-ATP levels decreased in NFK following 8 mg/dl mercuric chloride, however the extent of ATP depletion was reduced from 80-100% in FK to 40-60% in NFK (Fig. 4).

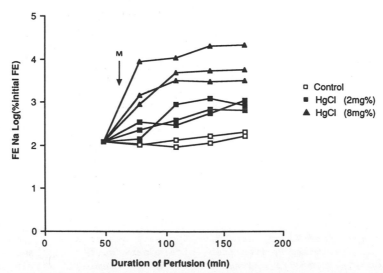

Fig. 1. Effect of mercuric chloride on fractional sodium excretion (FE$_{Na}$) in the isolated perfused rat kidney. Mercuric chloride was added after 60 min of baseline perfusion to the concentration indicated. FE$_{Na}$ is shown as percentage of the value prior to addition of mercuric chloride; a log scale has been used to compress the scale of the ordinate.

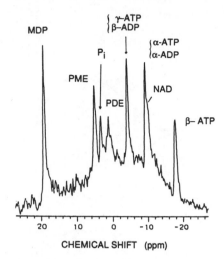

Fig. 2. Typical ^{31}P NMR spectrum of isolated perfused rat kidney. Key: MDP methylene diphosphonate (external reference), PME phosphomonoester, Pi inorganic phosphate, PDE phosphodiester, alpha-, beta-. and gamma-phosphate resonances of ATP or ADP, NAD oxidised or reduced nicotinamide adenine dinucleotide.

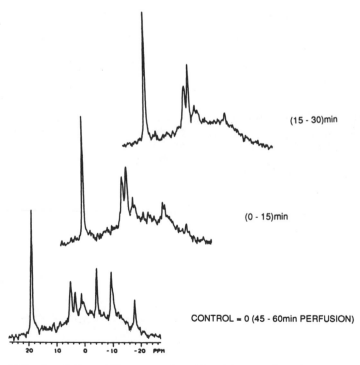

Fig. 3. Effect of 8 mg/dl mercuric chloride on phosphorus metabolites in perfused kidney. ^{31}P NMR spectra were acquired as described in the text.

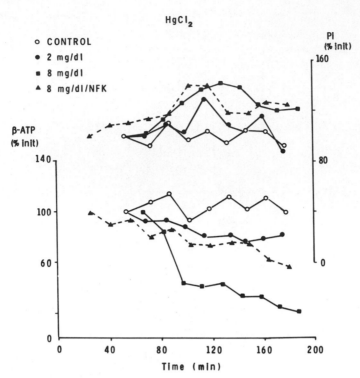

Fig. 4. Dose dependence of changes in total renal ATP (ß-ATP) and inorganic phosphate (Pi) levels following addition of mercuric chloride to the isolated perfused rat kidney. ß-ATP and Pi levels are given as percentage of the value prior to addition of mercuric chloride. Unbroken lines refer to experiments in filtering kidneys, broken lines show an experiment in the non-filtering kidney (hyperoncotic albumin).

DISCUSSION

These studies in IPRK illustrate that even in the absence of systemic effects, the nephrotoxic actions of mercuric chloride include direct cellular toxicity at both luminal and peritubular cell surfaces and indirect toxicity through a reduction in oxygen delivery as a result of profound increases in renal vascular resistance.

At a dose of 8 mg/dl, the renal hypoxia induced by reductions in perfusate flow contribute substantially to the observed decrease in ATP. However, even in the absence of changes in oxygen delivery in the NFK, mercuric chloride significantly reduced total renal ATP. The corollary of these findings is that detection of reduced renal ATP levels by NMR does not distinguish between ischaemic and direct nephrotoxic injury.

REFERENCES

1. Z.H. Endre, J.G.G. Ledingham, G.K. Radda, P.J. Ratcliffe and J.D. Tange, J. Physiol., 384:41 (1987)

2. G. Eknoyan, R.E. Bulger and D.C. Dobyan, Lab. Invest., 46: 613 (1982)

3. P.J. Ratcliffe, Z.H. Endre, L.G. Nicholls, J.D. Tange and J.G.G. Ledingham, The isolated perfused rat kidney: filtering and non-filtering models in the assessment of altered renal vascular resistance in nephrotoxicity, (this Symposium).

4. B.D. Ross, F.H. Epstein and A. Leaf, Amer. J. Physiol., 225: 1165 (1973)

5. H.J. Schureck and W. Kriz, Lab. Invest., 53:145 (1985)

6. P.J. Ratcliffe, Z.H. Endre, S.J. Scheinmann, J.D. Tange, J.G.G. Ledingham and G.K. Radda, Phosphorus nuclear magnetic resonance study of steady state ATP levels during graded hypoxia in the isolated perfused rat kidney, submitted for publication

7. Z.H. Endre, L.G. Nicholls, P.J. Ratcliffe and J.G.G. Ledingham, Prevention and reversal of mercuric chloride-induced increases in renal vascular resistance (RVR) by captopril, (this Symposium).

APPLICATION OF ^{1}H NMR URINALYSIS TO THE EXAMINATION OF NEPHROTOXIC LESIONS INDUCED BY MERCURIC CHLORIDE, HEXACHLORO-1,3-BUTADIENE, AND PROPYLENEIMINE

Kevin P. R. Gartland (1), F. W. Bonner (2), and J. K. Nicholson (1)

(1) Department of Chemistry, Birkbeck College, University of London, Malet Street, London WC1E 7HX and (2) Department of Toxicology, Sterling-Winthrop Research Centre, Alnwick, Northumberland NE66 2JH, U.K.

INTRODUCTION

In recent years proton nuclear magnetic resonance (^{1}H NMR) spectroscopic analysis of urine has been shown to provide sensitive indications of renal damage induced in rats by mercuric chloride (1) and p-aminophenol (2,3). Notable among these is the excretion of considerable quantities of glucose and lactic acid following p-aminophenol (2,3). Both of these parameters were later quantified employing conventional UV methods and found to be dose-related. Mercuric chloride has also been reported to produce a considerable lacticaciduria in fasted Sprague-Dawley rats (1). Prior to these studies, the appearance of lacticaciduria following nephrotoxic insult had not been reported.

We therefore propose that lactic acid may be a novel marker of proximal tubular injury in the rat and chose to employ two proximal tubular toxins, mercuric chloride and hexachloro-1,3-butadiene (HCBD), and one medullary toxin propyleneimine, (PI) to test this hypothesis. In addition, we considered it appropriate to apply ^{1}H NMR urinalysis to these nephrotoxins in an effort to provide profiles or fingerprints of site-specific damage within the kidney.

EXPERIMENTAL

Animals and Treatments.   Male Fischer 344 rats employed in this study were allocated to 5 groups of 5 rats each and were housed individually in metabowls for 5 days prior to treatment to permit acclimatization. Animals received a single i.p. injection of saline or corn oil control, a 100 mg/ml HCBD in corn oil, a 1 mg/ml solution of $HgCl_2$ or a 1% PI in saline, equivalent to doses of 200 mg/kg HCBD, 2 mg/kg $HgCl_2$, and 20 ul/kg PI respectively.

Urine was collected over ice for 24 hr prior to and at 8, 24, and 48 hr after dosing. Animals were killed 48 hr after dosing and blood removed for measurement of plasma urea (Beckman kit).

Conventional Urinalysis.   N-acetyl-ß-D-Glucosaminidase (NAG) was measured in desalted urine (Sephadex G25M) by the method of Maruhn (4). Perchloric acid extracts of urine were tested for acetic and lactic acids employing commercially available diagnostic kits, urinary glucose was measured by the hexokinase method employing a Sigma diagnostic kit, and urine osmolality was determined by freezing point depression on an Advanced Instruments 3W2 Osmometer.

^{1}H NMR Urinalysis.   For NMR, 0.45 ml urine was diluted with 0.05 ml ^2H_2O (field frequency lock) containing sodium 3-(trimethylsilyl)-[2,2,3,3-^2H]-1-propionate (0 ppm) as an internal shift reference. Single pulse experiments were employed with the following conditions: 64 free induction decays (FIDs) were collected into 16,384 computer points using 380 pulses, acquisition time 1.3 seconds. A further delay of 2.0 seconds between pulses was added to ensure that the spectra were fully T_1 relaxed. A continuous secondary irradiation field was applied at the resonance frequency of water to suppress the intense water signal.

Samples were examined either non-lyophilized or after a lyophilization step (to correct for any increase in urine flow rate) by high resolution ^{1}H NMR spectroscopy at a field strength of 9.4 Tesla (400 MHz ^{1}H).

RESULTS

Mercuric Chloride.   Damage to the pars recta of the proximal tubule by $HgCl_2$ is manifest as transient but considerable enzymuria (Fig. 1), glycosuria (Fig. 2) together with a reduction in urine osmolality (Fig. 3) and a later increase in urine flow rate (Fig. 4). Mercuric chloride caused the greatest elevation in blood urea nitrogen (BUN) at 48 hr after dosing Table 1.

Proton NMR urinalysis (Fig. 5) reveals glycosuria and lacticaciduria (Table 2) 8-24 hr and 24-48 hr after dosing combined with a reduction in urinary citrate. Other changes seen at 8-24 hr include the appearance of the amino acids alanine and valine, a reduction in citrate excretion, and in addition, increased amounts of acetic acid and ethanol.

Hexachlorobutadiene.   Enzymuria (Fig. 1), sustained glycosuria (Fig. 2), with reduced osmolality (Fig. 3) and a great increase in urine flow rate (Fig. 4) can be seen following HCBD.

Proton NMR urinalysis (Fig. 6) highlights changes confirmed by conventional methods (glycosuria) and also changes, principally lacticaciduria (Table 2), aminoaciduria (alanine, valine and glutamine) and also the appearance of increased amounts of acetic acid.

Table 1.   Blood Urea Nitrogen

BUN (mg/100ml)

Control	(saline)	18.04 ± 0.54	(5) [a]
Control	(corn oil)	16.01 ± 0.68	(5) $p < 0.05$
$HgCl_2$		170.80 ± 13.62	(4) $p < 0.001$
HCBD		34.98 ± 2.61	(5) $p < 0.001$
Propyleneimine		23.83 ± 2.10	(5) $p < 0.05$

[a] Data presented as x ± SE(n)

The NMR profile of urine from a rat after HCBD resembles very closely that seen after p-aminophenol, a nephrotoxin producing damage in the pars convoluta of the proximal tubule (Fig. 7).

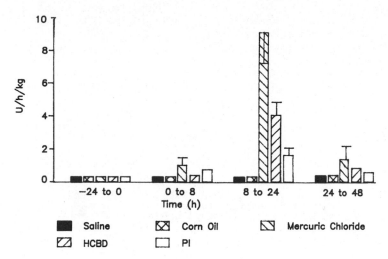

Figure 1. The effect of nephrotoxins on urinary N-acetyl-ß-D-glucosaminidase

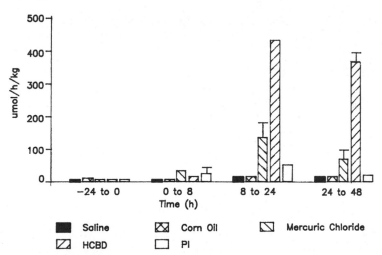

Figure 2. The effect of nephrotoxins on urinary urine glucose excretion.

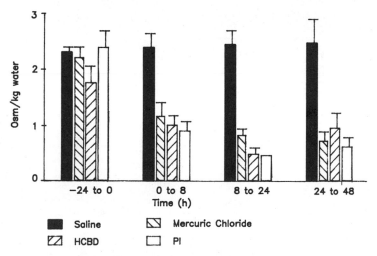

Figure 3. The effect of nephrotoxins on urine osmolality.

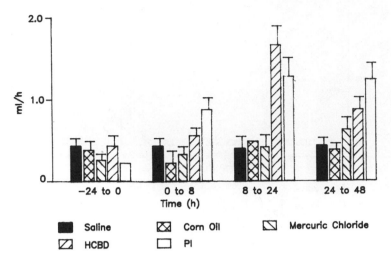

Figure 4.   The effect of nephrotoxins on urine flow rate.

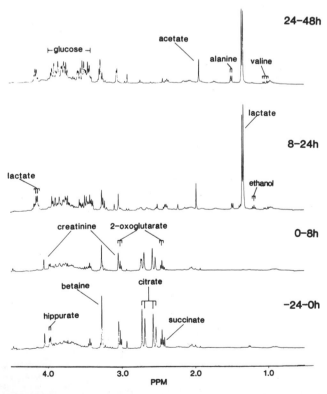

Figure 5.   400 MHz Proton NMR spectra of urine collected from rats receiving 2 mg/kg $HgCl_2$.

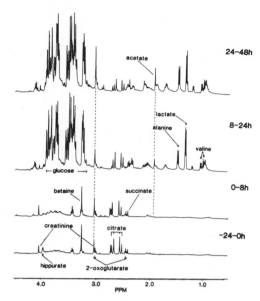

Figure 6. 400 MHz Proton NMR spectra of urine collected from rats receiving 200 mg/kg HCBD.

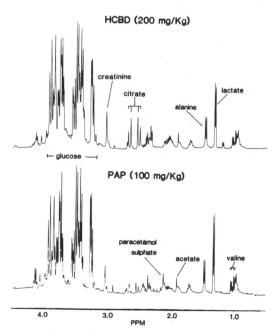

Figure 7. 400 MHz Proton NMR spectra of 16 urines collected between 8-24 hr after rats were given 100 mg/kg p-aminophenol; 200 mg/kg HCBD.

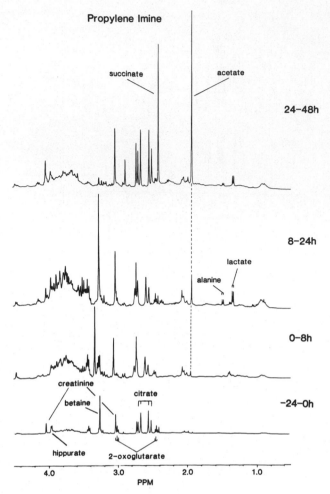

Figure 8. 400 MHz Proton NMR spectra of urine collected from rats receiving propyleneimine.

Table 2.   Urinary lactic acid

umol/h/kg	TIME OF URINE COLLECTION			
	-24 - 0	0 - 8	8 - 24	24 - 48 h [a]
HCBD (n = 5)	5.60± 0.76	6.51±* 0.56	66.67±** 2.28	44.35±** 4.19
HgCl$_2$ (n = 4)	4.39± 0.44	5.17±* 0.60	39.24±*+ 13.74	48.64±++ 21.43

[a] Data presented as x ± SE(n)

* = NS; ** = p < 0.001;   *+ = p < 0.05; ++ = p < 0.1

<u>Propyleneimine</u>.   Treatment with the papillary toxin produces the earliest increase in urine flow rate (Fig.   4) and the greatest reduction in urine osmolality (Fig.   3).   Minor elevations in urine glucose (Fig. 2) together with significant enzymuria (Fig. 1) can also be seen.

Changes   in   the NMR profile of urine are seen as early as 8 hr   after   PI (Fig.   8).   At   8-24 hr the appearance of lactate and alanine can be   seen (perhaps heralding secondary cortical damage) together with elevations   in urinary acetate and betaine.   Succinate and   acetate   are   considerably elevated 24-48   hr   after PI.   This elevation   in   urinary   acetate   was confirmed by the conventional UV method for acetate (Table 3).

Table 3.   Urinary   acetic acid

umol/h/kg	TIME OF URINE COLLECTION			
	-24 - 0	0 -- 8	8 - 24	24 - 48 h [a]
Propylene-	1.65±	3.12±	5.49±	30.23±
imine	0 17	1.05	1.43	4.99
		NS	p < 0.05	p < 0.001

[a] Data presented as x ± SE (n = 5)

DISCUSSION

The   present   study demonstrates the usefulness of high resolution   proton NMR in the detection of nephrotoxicity by studying the changing pattern of low molecular weight urine components.   A high   resolution   proton   NMR spectrum of urine can be obtained in a matter of minutes.   Thus   the   NMR method is rapid requiring no preselection of metabolites for detection and only minimum sample pretreatment.   All those molecules with suitable NMR-detectable protons and present in urine at near millimolar   concentrations are likely to give resonances, allowing a large number of important inter-mediary metabolites and excretion products present in urine to be studied simultaneously.

Although not as sensitive as more conventional biochemical assay   methods, NMR   can   provide   an excretion profile or 'fingerprint'   of the   changes occurring in the excretion of low molecular weight metabolites in urine.

In those rats receiving mercuric chloride and HCBD, NMR urinalysis uncovered elevations in the excretion of glucose,   and also certain   amino acids   (alanine,   glutamine   and   valine).   Failure to reabsorb   such   low molecular   weight   components   as glucose and amino   acids   is   a   typical manifestation   of proximal tubular damage reflecting functional defects in this segment and reduced solute reabsorption efficiency.

In addition to glycosuria and aminoaciduria,   NMR urinalysis also revealed lacticaciduria   following mercuric chloride and HCBD,   again confirmed   by conventional method. Lacticaciduria has previously been reported following nephrotoxic   insult   by   mercuric chloride and p-aminophenol (2,3)   both proximal tubular toxins.   However,   such a finding has not previously been reported   for   HCBD.   Nicholson   et al (1)   suggested   the   lacticaciduria observed   following mercuric chloride resulted from increased   utilization of   anaerobic   pathways   within the kidney.   While this   may   in   fact   be occurring in this case, we feel that a more probable explanation is linked to the site of nephrotoxic injury. All of the nephrotoxins which have been demonstrated to produce lacticaciduria all cause damage to the proximal tubule. We therefore suggest that the lacticaciduria seen with all of the proximal tubular nephrotoxins arises from decreased reabsorption since lactic acid is known to be reabsorbed throughout this segment (5,6). The mercuric chloride-induced hypocitraturia has been described previously and has been attributed to toxin-induced alterations in acid-base status (1).

A number of changes can be seen in the NMR profile of urine following challenge with PI. Urinary betaine (N,N,N-trimethylglycine), elevated after PI, may prove to be a novel site-specific marker of papillary damage. Betaine is confined almost exclusively to the inner medulla of the kidney in rats and rabbits and has been suggested to play a role in the maintenance of intracellular osmotic balance in this region (7). Modest elevations in urine lactate and alanine were observed following PI, probably reflecting secondary cortical involvement.

Other changes highlighted by NMR were increases in the excretion of acetic and succinic acids. Elevations in urinary acetate and succinate were reported in rats following a 24-hr fasting period, and were further increased following nephrotoxic doses of mercuric chloride (1). Propylene-imine may bring about the elevations witnessed in urinary acetate and succinate in one of, or a combination of three ways:

i) decreased reabsorption,
ii) overflow of elevated plasma levels and
iii) Kreb's Cycle block at the condensing enzyme and succinic dehydrogenase.
Studies in which these substances are quantitated in blood-free cortical and medullary tissue, and also plasma, in addition to assay of the above two enzymes may shed light on the mechanism of this organic aciduria.

Employing high resolution proton NMR, we have succeeded in uncovering a reproducible pattern, or 'fingerprint' of toxin-induced damage to the proximal tubule, and have further noted that this is distinct from the pattern of low molecular weight urine components seen following medullary insult.

Proton NMR urinalysis, in combination with conventional biochemical methodology, is a very powerful tool with which to examine the effects of nephrotoxic chemicals, and also therapeutic compounds (eg diuretics), on renal function.

REFERENCES

1. J.K. Nicholson, J.A. Timbrell and P.J. Sadler, Proton NMR Spectra of urine as indicators of renal damage. Mercury-induced nephrotoxicity in rats, Mol. Pharamacol., 27:644-651 (1985).

2. K.P.R. Gartland, J.K. Nicholson, J.A. Timbrell and F.W. Bonner, Detection and assessment of p-aminophenol-induced nephrotoxic lesions by Proton NMR spectroscopy, Human Tox. 5:122-123 (1986).

3. J.K. Nicholson and K.P.R. Gartland, In: Cells, Membranes and Disease, including Renal, ed. E. Reid, G.M.W. Cook and J.P. Luzio, Methodological Surveys in Biochemistry and Analysis Vol. 17, pp. 397-408, Plenum Press, New York, (1987).

4. D. Maruhn, Rapid colorimetric assay for ß-galactosidase and N-acetyl-ß-D-glucosaminidase in human urine, Clin. Chim. Acta, 73:453-461 (1976).

5. F. Dies, G. Ramos, E. Avelar and M. Lennhoff, Renal excretion of lactic acid in the dog, Am. J. Physiol., 216:106-111 (1969).

6. B. Hohmann, P.P. Frohnert, R. Kinne and K. Baumann, Proximal tubular lactate transport in rat kidney: a micropuncture study, Kidney Int., 5:261-270 (1974).

7. S. Bagnasco, R. Balaban, H.M. Fales, Y.M. Yang and M. Burg, Predominant osmotically active organic solutes in rat and rabbit renal medullas, J. Biol. Chem., 261:5872-5877 (1986).

PATHOGENESIS OF PROTEIN DROPLET NEPHROPATHY AND ITS RELATIONSHIP TO RENAL CARCINOGENESIS IN THE MALE RAT

Brian G. Short, Vicki L. Burnett, and James A. Swenberg

Chemical Industry Institute of Toxicology, Research Triangle Park, North Carolina, 27709

INTRODUCTION

Male rats chronically exposed to inhaled unleaded gasoline (UG) or other petroleum hydrocarbon fuels developed a low but dose-related increase in the incidence of renal adenomas and carcinomas (3,10). Elucidation of the mechanism of this sex and species-specific carcinogenic response to UG is essential for determining the potential human health risk from exposure to UG. Genotoxic assays of UG, including a recently developed in vivo/in vitro unscheduled DNA synthesis assay for the kidney, have been predominately negative (5,13,14,18).

Male rats are also uniquely susceptible to renal toxicity following acute or subchronic exposure to a variety of volatile hydrocarbon compounds, including UG, or isoparaffinic fractions of UG, such as 2,2,4-trimethylpentane (TMP) (1,9,15). Although these chemicals cause minimal renal functional impairment, a protein droplet nephrosis develops, progressing to mild tubular degeneration, necrosis, and regeneration after several weeks of treatment (4,8,15,21). A chronic regenerative response subsequent to moderate proximal tubular damage in the kidney of petroleum hydrocarbon-exposed male rats may be an important stimulus in renal tumour formation caused by this group of chemicals (19,22). Loury et al. (14) have shown a 5 to 8-fold increase in S phase of renal cells induced by UG using an in vitro-in vivo approach. We have recently localized the renal proliferative effects of gavaged TMP to the P2 segment of the proximal tubule of the male rat via pulse-dose [^{3}H-TdR] autoradiography studies (19). To further characterize possible dose-response relationships between UG or TMP-induced protein droplet nephrosis, localized cell proliferation, and renal tumourigenesis, we have conducted continuous [^{3}H-TdR] administration studies during the last week of a three week exposure regimen to UG or TMP. This report provides initial evidence of the role of protein droplet nephrosis in UG-induced renal cancer of this sex and species.

MATERIALS AND METHODS

Male F-344 rats were gavaged five consecutive days per week for three weeks with 0, 0.2, 0.5, 2, 5, 20 or 50 mg/kg of 2,2,4-trimethylpentane (TMP) or exposed to vapourised unleaded gasoline (PS-6, American Petroleum Institute) at concentrations approximating 0, 2, 20, 200, and

2000 ppm for six hours per day, five days per week, for three weeks. Each dose group contained three animals. Since the proximal tubule has been found to be the primary site of damage in response to UG and TMP, quantitative autoradiography was conducted on this region following continuous (7 day) administration of [^{3}H-TdR] (1 mCi/ml, 40-60 Ci/mmol) during the last week of exposure via subcutaneous osmotic pumps (Alzet 2ML, Alza Corp., Palo Alto, Ca). Following the three week exposure period, rats were killed, and 2% paraformaldehyde/1% glutaraldehyde perfusion-fixed kidneys were collected for protein droplet assessment and histoautoradiography.

Histological examination of kidneys for protein droplets was performed on glycol methacrylate (GMA) embedded sections cut at 2 and stained with Lee's methylene blue-basic fuchsin (LMBBF) (2). Slides were graded according to extent and severity of crystalloid protein droplet accumulation (0 = minimal; 1+ = mild; 2+ = moderate; 3+ = severe; 4+ = markedly severe), without knowledge of treatment group. Slides for autoradiography were dipped in Kodak NTB2 emulsion, exposed for three weeks at -20°F, and developed in Kodak D-19 developer. Slides were examined by dark field microscopy but quantitative autoradiography was conducted by light microscopic examination of LMBBF stained autoradiographic sections to identify cell type as well as labelling status. A minimum of 3000 proximal tubule cells were counted per slide for each animal. Each proximal tubule cell counted was classified as P1, P2, or P3 and labelling status recorded. The labelling index (LI) for each cell type was calculated as the percent of labelled cells among total labelled and unlabelled cells of that cell type for each animal analysed. Mean dose group LIs of each proximal tubule segment and the total proximal tubule LI were calculated in each experiment (mean+sem) and analysed for treatment effect within each segment by one-way analysis of variance (ANOVA). Significant ($P < 0.05$) differences among LIs of dose groups from both experiments were further analysed by a Newman-Keuls multicomparison test to detect which dose groups were significantly different from each other.

RESULTS

Histology. Kidneys from animals exposed to either TMP or UG were characterized by protein droplet-filled cells that occupied a slightly larger portion of the cortical labyrinth and medullary rays compared to controls, including adjacent P1 and P3 segments. The majority of renal tubular protein droplets from TMP- or UG-treated rats were increased in size and angularity compared to controls, similar to that demonstrated previously (19). Grading of protein droplet accumulation in kidneys from TMP treated animals demonstrated a significant ($P < 0.05$) dose-responsive increase in protein droplet score from animals dosed with 2-50 mg/kg TMP (Fig 4A). Protein droplet-laden P2 cells were sometimes swollen, with varying degrees of degeneration and necrosis characterized by cytoplasmic basophilia or vacuolation and karyorrhexis. Protein droplet score was a dose-responsive parameter of protein droplet nephrosis induced by 2-50 mg/kg TMP.

Dark Field Autoradiography. Autoradiography by this method revealed clear treatment-related effects of increased cell proliferation compared to controls (Fig. 1). Although detailed segment identification could not be determined with this technique, linear arrays of intense cell labelling were present within the cortex of treated animals from both experiments, corresponding to the location and extent of protein droplet accumulation. The outer stripe of the outer medulla of kidneys from animals exposed to 50 mg/kg TMP or 2000 ppm UG had more labelled cells than controls or lower dose groups. The junction of the outer stripe of outer medulla and inner

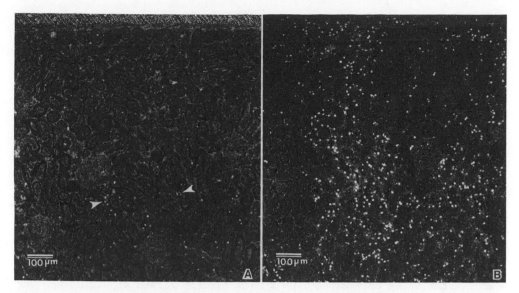

Fig 1. Dark-field illumination of kidney autoradiograph from control (A) and 2000 ppm UG-exposed (B) male rat after continuous (7 day) administration of [^{3}H]TdR. A few tubular epithelial cell nuclei are labelled (arrowheads). B, An increased number of labelled nuclei are present in the cortex compared to control slide.

stripe of the outer medulla contained localized intense cell labelling, especially within the epithelium surrounding granular casts. The inner stripe of outer medulla and inner medulla of the 2000 ppm UG kidneys had an evenly dispersed mild increase in labelled cells.

Quantitative Autoradiography. A consistent finding in kidneys from control groups of both experiments was an elevation of the P2 LI which were 2.8 to 4.0 times higher than adjacent P1 and P3 LI (P < 0.05) (Fig 2). P2 tubules containing the greatest extent of protein droplets also appeared to have the highest number of labelled cells (Fig. 3A). The occurrence of protein droplet formation and occasional necrotic, desquamated cells appeared to be associated with increased cell proliferation within the P2 segment of control male rats.

The LI of the proximal tubule (PT) from animals treated with 20 or 50 mg/kg TMP were significantly (P < 0.05) elevated above PT LI of controls and the two lowest dose groups (Fig. 2A). Analyses of LI from individual proximal tubule segments demonstrated that the P2 cells were primarily responsible for the increased cell proliferation within the PT (Fig. 2A). The LI of P2 cells from the 2-50 mg/kg dose groups were increased in a dose-responsive manner 1.9 to 4.8 times higher than the P2 LI of control and lower dose groups (0.2 and 0.5 mg/kg TMP) (P < 0.05). Kidneys with the highest proportions of labelled cells usually had the greatest severity of crystalloid protein droplet accumulation (Fig. 3B). A strong correlation (r=0.82, p 0.05) between the dose-responsive increases in P2 LI and protein droplet score was present in the TMP-treated rats (Fig. 4A).

The LI of the PT from animals exposed to 200 or 2000 ppm UG were 2.4 to 6.4 times higher (P < 0.05) than the PT LI from control, 2, or 20 ppm UG dose groups (Fig. 2B). Again, as in TMP treated animals, these increases were due to the increased LI of the P2 cells which were 3.3 to 5.8 times

521

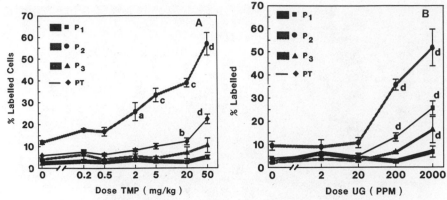

Fig. 2. Effect of 21 days of 0-50 mg/kg TMP(A) or 0-2000 ppm UG (B) on continuous uptake of [^{3}H]TdR by P1, P2 and P3 segments of the proximal tubule epithelium. Labeling index (LI) is percentage of labelled cells within each segment. Proximal tubule (PT) LI represents mean cell turnover rate for the entire (P1+P2+P3) proximal tubule. Each test point is the mean (+sem) value determined from 3 rats (except 2 rats at 0.2 mg/kg TMP test point). Dosage is presented on log scale.
a = significantly greater than control (P < 0.05), Newman-Keuls multi-comparison test
b = significantly greater than control and 0.5 mg/kg TMP dose groups (P < 0.05), Newman-Keuls multicomparison test
c = significantly greater than control, 0.2, and 0.5 mg/kg TMP dose groups (P < 0.05), Newman-Keuls multicomparison test
d = significantly greater than all lower dose groups (P < 0.01), Newman-Keuls multicomparison test

higher (P < 0.05) than mean P2 LI of controls and lower exposures. However, increased cell turnover was not limited to the P2 segment of the high dose (2000 ppm) animals, as the LI of the P3 segment was 2.5 to 6.8 times higher than the mean P3 LI of controls and all other UG dose levels (P < 0.05). Increased P3 cell labelling from these animals was prominent in the tubular epithelium surrounding granular casts at the junction of the outer stripe of outer medulla and inner stripe of outer medulla (Fig. 3C) or near regions of P2 cell labelling.

DISCUSSION

The use of continuous labelling techniques in this report has revealed a dose-related increase in cell proliferation of the P2 segment from male rats exposed to gavaged TMP or inhaled UG. This increase represented a local, compensatory regenerative response of the adjacent, viable tubular epithelium, as suggested in our earlier [^{3}H-TdR] pulse dose autoradiography studies (19). This compensatory, rather than mitogenic stimulus is similar although probably milder than regenerative responses seen with other nephrotoxins such as $HgCl_2$ (7) or cis-platinum (11). Protein droplet composition in control and treated rat kidneys has been shown to consist primarily of alpha-2u-globulin, a sex-specific protein (MW 18,000) synthesised in large quantities by the sexually mature male rat, excreted, and reabsorbed by the P2 segment of the proximal tubule (1) (Burnett, et al., 1987, unpublished data). Recent reports described elsewhere at this symposium have detected reversible binding of a metabolite of TMP to alpha-2u-globulin in the male rat kidney (12). Perhaps altered endocytosis or lysosomal handling of this reversibly bound

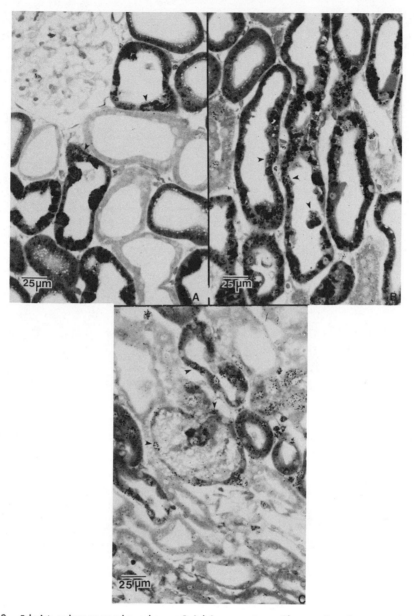

Fig. 3. Light microscopic view of kidney autoradiographs from control(A), 50 mg/kg TMP-treated(B) and 2000 ppm UG-exposed(C) male rats following continuous [^{3}H]TdR labelling procedure. A, The few labelled cells present are located primarily within the protein droplet filled P2 segments (arrowheads). Note the paucity of labelled nuclei in adjacent P1 segments and other surrounding cells. B, A striking increase in the number of labelled cells occurring within P2 segments lined by protein droplet-filled cells. Note occasional exfoliated cells. C, Increased labelling is present in terminal P3 segments and adjacent epithelium lining granular casts (arrows).

alpha-2u-globulin-TMP metabolite complex may play a significant role in triggering increased cell turnover of the P2 cells via lysosomal enlarge-

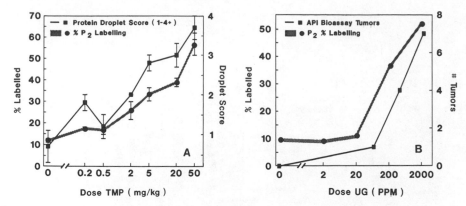

Fig. 4. A) Graph summarizing the dose-responsive relationship between protein droplet score and P2 cell proliferation in TMP-treated male rats. B) This graph shows the dose-dependent similarity of P2 cell LI observed in male rats during three weeks of UG inhalation exposure in this study and the number of renal epithelial tumours (adenomas and carcinomas) found in male rats exposed to inhaled UG in a 2-yr bioassay (Kitchen, 1984). Chronic bioassay contained 60 rats/dose group at 26 month sacrifice time.

ment and/or instability, leading to cell death.

Elevated cell replication rates as demonstrated in this report may represent a potentially increased risk of cancer within the kidney, similar to that suggested in other organs such as liver (6,17). A remarkable similarity in dose-response to UG exists between P2 cell replication rates found in this report and the number of renal adenomas and carcinomas found in the 2 year bioassay of UG (10) (Fig 4B). Fixation of spontaneous mutations to create "initiated" cells and promotion of spontaneously initiated cells may explain the low, but significantly increased incidence of tumours resulting from nongenotoxic chemicals, such as UG. If sex and species specific increases in protein droplet accumulation and cell replication continue during chronic exposure to TMP or UG, it is likely that the male rat represents an inappropriate model for meaningful risk estimates of human renal cancer from UG exposure.

REFERENCES

1. C.L. Alden, R.L. Kanerva, G. Ridder, and L.C. Stone, The pathogenesis of the nephrotoxicity of volatile hydrocarbons in the male rat, p. 107, In: "Renal Effects of Petroleum Hydrocarbons," M.A. Mehlman, ed., Princeton Scientific Publishers, Inc., New Jersey (1984).

2. H.S. Bennet, A.D. Wyrick, S.W. Lee, and J.H. McNeel, Science and art in preparing tissues embedded in plastic for light microscopy with special reference to glycol methacrylate, glass knives, and simple stains, Stain Technol 51:71-97 (1976).

3. R.H. Bruner, Pathologic findings in laboratory animals exposed to hydrocarbon fuels of military interest, p. 133, In: "Renal Effects of Petroleum Hydrocarbons," Vol. VII, M.A. Mehlman, ed., Princeton Scientific Publishers, Inc., New Jersey (1984).

4. W.M. Busey and B.Y. Cockrell, Non-neoplastic exposure-related renal

lesions in rats following inhalation of unleaded gasoline vapors, p. 57, In: "Renal Effects of Petroleum Hydrocarbons," Vol. VII, M.A. Mehlman, ed., Princeton Scientific Publishers, Inc., New Jersey (1984).

5. C.C. Conaway, C.A. Schreiner, and S.T. Cragg, Mutagenicity evaluation in petroleum hydrocarbons, p. 89, In "Applied Toxicology of Petroleum Hydrocarbons," M.A. Mehlman, ed., Princeton Scientific Publishers, Inc., New Jersey (1984).

6. V.M. Craddock, Cell proliferation and experimental liver cancer, pp. 153-201, In: "Liver Cell Cancer," A.M. Cameron, C.A. Linsell, and G.P. Warwick, eds., Elsevier Publishing Corp., Amsterdam (1976).

7. F.E. Cuppage and A. Tate, Repair of the nephron following injury with mercuric chloride, Am J Pathol 51:405 (1967).

8. C.L. Gaworski, J.D. MacEwen, E.H. Vernot, R.H. Bruner, M.J. Cowan, Jr., Comparison of the subchronic inhalation toxicity of petroleum and oil shale JP-5 jet fuels, p. 33, In: "Applied Toxicology of Petroleum Hydrocarbons," H.N. MacFarland, C.E. Holdsworth, J.A. MacGregor, R.W. Call, and M.L. Lane, eds., Princeton Scientific Publishers, Inc., New Jersey (1984).

9. C.A. Halder, C.E. Holdsworth, B.Y. Cockrell, and V.J. Piccirillo, Hydrocarbon nephropathy in male rats: Identification of the nephrotoxic components of unleaded gasoline, Toxicol Ind Health 1:67-87 (1985).

10. D.N. Kitchen, Neoplastic renal effects of unleaded gasoline in Fischer F344 rats, p. 65, In: "Renal Effects of Petroleum Hydrocarbons," M.A. Mehlman, ed., Princeton Scientific Publishers, Inc., New Jersey (1984).

11. C.J. Kovacs, P.G. Braunschwerger, L.L. Schenken, and D.R. Burholt, Proliferative defects in renal intestinal epithelium after Cis-archlorodiamine platinum (II), Br J Cancer 45:286 (1982).

12. E.A. Lock, M. Charbonneau, J. Strasser, J.A. Swenberg, and J.S. Bus, The reversible binding of a metabolite of 2,2,4-trimethylpentane to a renal protein fraction, Toxicol Appl Pharmacol 91:182-192 (1987).

13. D.J. Loury, T. Smith-Oliver, S. Strom, R. Jirtle, G. Michalopoulos, and B.E. Butterworth, Assessment of unscheduled and replicative DNA synthesis in hepatocytes treated in vivo and in vitro with unleaded gasoline or 2,2,4-trimethylpentane, Toxicol Appl Pharmacol 85:11-23 (1986).

14. D.J. Loury, T. Smith-Oliver, and B.E. Butterworth, Assessment of unscheduled DNA synthesis and cell replication in rat kidney cells exposed in vitro or in vivo to unleaded gasoline, Toxicol Appl Pharmacol 87:127-140 (1987).

15. R.D. Phillips and B.Y. Cockrell, Kidney structural changes in rats following inhalation exposure to C10-C11 isoparaffinic solvent, Toxicology 33:261 (1984).

16. R.D. Phillips and B.Y. Cockrell, Effects of certain light hydrocarbons on kidney function and structure in male rats, p. 89, In: "Renal Hydrocarbons," M. A. Mehlman, ed., Princeton Scientific Publishers, Inc., New Jersey (1984).

17. M.F. Rajewsky, Tumorigenesis by exogenous carcinogens: Role of

target cell proliferation and state of differentiation, pp. 215-223, In: "Age Related Factors in Carcinogenesis," IARC Scientific Publ. 58, A. Likhachev, ed., IARC, Lyon (1985).

18. K.A. Richardson, J.L. Wilmer, D. Smith-Simpson, and T.R. Skopek, Assessment of the genotoxic potential of unleaded gasoline and 2,2,4-trimethylpentane in human lymphoblasts in vitro, Toxicol Appl Pharmacol 82:316 (1986).

19. B.G. Short, V.L. Burnett, and J.A. Swenberg, Histopathology and cell proliferation induced by 2,2,4-trimethylpentane in the male rat kidney, Toxicol Pathol 14:194 (1986).

20. M.D. Stonard, P.G.N. Phillips, J.R. Foster, M.G. Simpson, and E.A. Lock, alpha-2u-Globulin: measurement in rat kidney following administration of 2,2,4-trimethylpentane, Toxicol 41:161-168 (1986).

21. F.B. Thomas, C.A. Halder, C.E. Holdsworth, and B.Y. Cockrell, Hydrocarbon nephropathy in male rats. Temporal and morphologic characterization of the renal lesions, pp. 477-480, In: "Renal Heterogeneity and Target Cell Toxicity," P.H. Bach, and E.A. Lock, eds., John Wiley & Sons, Chichister (1985).

22. B.F. Trump, T.W. Jones, and M.M. Lipsky, Light hydrocarbon nephropathy, p. 493, In: "Renal Heterogeneity and Target Cell Toxicity," P.H. Bach and E.A. Lock, ed., John Wiley & Sons, New York (1985).

23. C. Viau, A. Bernard, F. Gueret, P. Maldague, P. Gengoux, and R. Lauwerys, Isoparaffinic solvent-induced nephrotoxicity in the rat, Toxicology 38:227 (1986).

LIGHT HYDROCARBON-INDUCED NEPHROTOXICITY: THE INTERACTION OF 2,2,4-TRIMETHYLPENTANE WITH ALPHA-2U-GLOBULIN IN THE MALE RAT KIDNEY

E.A. Lock, M. Charbonneau (1), J. Strasser (1), J.A. Swenberg (1) and J.S. Bus (1)

Imperial Chemical Industries PLC, Central Toxicology Laboratory, Alderley Park, Cheshire. SK10 4TJ, UK and (1) Chemical Industries Institute of Toxicology, Research Triangle Park, North Carolina 27709, USA

INTRODUCTION

Inhalation exposure to unleaded gasoline for 2 years has been shown to produce a small increase in the incidence of renal tumours (adenomas and adenocarcinomas) in male Fischer 344 rats, but not in female rats or mice of either sex (MacFarland, 1984; Kitchen, 1984). Following subchronic inhalation exposure of unleaded gasoline to male rats, nephrotoxicity occurred and was characterised by an increase in protein (hyaline) droplets in proximal convoluted tubules (Halder et al, 1984), the accumulation of casts at the cortico-medullary junction and single cell necrosis and regeneration of the nephron (Short et al, 1987). Autoradiographic analyses of various segments of the nephron, following continuous administration of [^{3}H]-thymidine via osmotic pumps, showed a dose-related increase in cell turnover in the P2 segment (Short et al, 1987). Thus unleaded gasoline produces nephrotoxicity in the male rat following subchronic exposure. Various light hydrocarbon mixtures and individual branched-chain saturated hydrocarbon components of these mixtures, such as 2,2,4-trimethylpentane (TMP), have been shown to produce similar nephrotoxic effects (Halder et al, 1985; Stonard et al, 1986; Short et al, 1986; Phillips and Egan, 1984 and, Viau et al, 1986). In addition, other chemicals such as decalin (Alden et al, 1984) and 1,4-dichlorobenzene (Charbonneau, 1987b) also produce the nephropathy.

The basis for the marked sex difference in nephrotoxicity is not fully understood, but two important components have been identified:-

i) the protein droplets seen after TMP or unleaded gasoline administration appear to contain the male rat-specific protein alpha-2u-globulin (Stonard et al, 1986; Loury et al, 1987; Lock et al, 1987; Olson et al, 1987), and

ii) there are small but important differences in the sex dependent disposition of TMP. Female rats rapidly metabolise TMP and excrete it in urine, while in male rats the compound is eliminated more slowly and is retained in the kidneys (Kloss et al, 1985). Recent studies have also shown that TMP is metabolised in male and female rats to trimethyl-pentanols, pentanoic acids and hydroxypentanoic acids (Olson et al, 1985; Charbonneau et al, 1987a).

This paper summarises some of our recent findings aimed at relating the metabolism of TMP to the accumulation of alpha-2u-globulin in the kidneys of male rats.

METABOLISM AND DISPOSITION OF 2,2,4-TRIMETHYLPENTANE IN THE RAT

Following oral administration to male or female rats, TMP is mainly eliminated from the body by exhalation as unchanged TMP and in urine as water soluble metabolites (Kloss et al, 1985); there is however some retention of radioactivity in the kidneys of male rats. Following a single oral dose of $[^{14}C]$-TMP at 0.5g/kg (equivalent to 4.4mmol/kg) to male or female rats, peak tissue concentrations of radioactivity occurred after 12hr in the males and 8hr in the females. The peak concentration in the kidney of males was twice that observed in females, 1252 versus 577 nmol equivalents/g wet weight respectively (Charbonneau et al, 1987a), whereas the peak liver and plasma concentrations found in males were no different from those found in females. There thus appeared to be a marked difference in the disposition of TMP in the male versus the female rat, the female rat eliminating the TMP-derived radiolabel more rapidly in urine over the first 24hr (Charbonneau et al, 1987a, Table 1). This dose of TMP produces a four-fold increase in the renal concentration of alpha-2u-globulin in the male but not female rat (Table 1, Stonard et al, 1986; Charbonneau et al, 1987a).

Identification and quantitation of the metabolites of TMP in the urine of male and female dosed rats, showed that metabolism occurred via the same pathways and at a similar rate (Figure 1). Oxidation of TMP occurred at carbon-5 to give 2,4,4,-trimethyl-1-pentanol, 2,4,4,-trimethylpentanoic acid and 2,4,4,-trimethyl-5-hydroxypentanoic acid (Olson et al, 1985). This was the major metabolic pathway for both sexes; the percentage of the dose excreted in the urine over 24hr being 4.4% and 4.6% for females and males respectively (Charbonneau et al, 1987a). TMP oxidation at carbon-1 to form 2,2,4-trimethyl-1-pentanol, 2,2,4-trimethylpentanoic acid and 2,2,4-trimethyl-5-hydroxypentanoic acid was a minor pathway leading to 1.9% and 1.6% in the urine over 24hr in females and males respectively (Charbonneau et al, 1987a). TMP oxidation to form 2,4,4-trimethyl-2-pentanol was also a minor pathway, although female rats appeared to excrete more in the urine (Figure 1, Charbonneau et al, 1987a). Two metabolites, 2,4,4-trimethyl-2-pentanol and 2,4,4,-trimethylpentanoic acid were detected in liver, kidney and plasma (Charbonneau et al, 1987a). 2,4,4-Trimethyl-2-pentanol was the predominant metabolite detected, being present in the male rat kidney at 8, 12 and 24hr after dosing. In contrast it was absent from the female kidney at these times. This observation supports the hypothesis of a kidney-specific accumulation of a TMP metabolite leading to the male rat-specific nephrotoxicity.

REVERSIBLE BINDING OF 2,4,4-TRIMETHYL-2-PENTANOL TO ALPHA-2U-GLOBULIN

Administration of TMP to male rats produced a dose-related increase in the concentration of TMP-derived radiolabel in the kidney which appeared to parallel the dose-related accumulation of alpha-2u-globulin (Stonard et al, 1986; Charbonneau et al, 1987a). Studies were therefore undertaken to examine the nature of the radiolabel retained in the male rat kidney following TMP administration and to determine the nature of the association, if any, of 2,4,4-trimethyl-2-pentanol with alpha-2u-globulin. Gibson and Bus (1987) postulated that the male rat-specific nephrotoxicity produced by TMP may be the result of a stable Schiff-base product formed in the liver between an aldehyde metabolite of TMP and the epsilon-amino residue of lysine in the protein, alpha-2u-globulin. No evidence for a marked covalent interaction between radioactivity from TMP and renal proteins has been found (Loury et al, 1987; Lock et al, 1987), in fact more covalent binding was found in protein from female kidneys than in

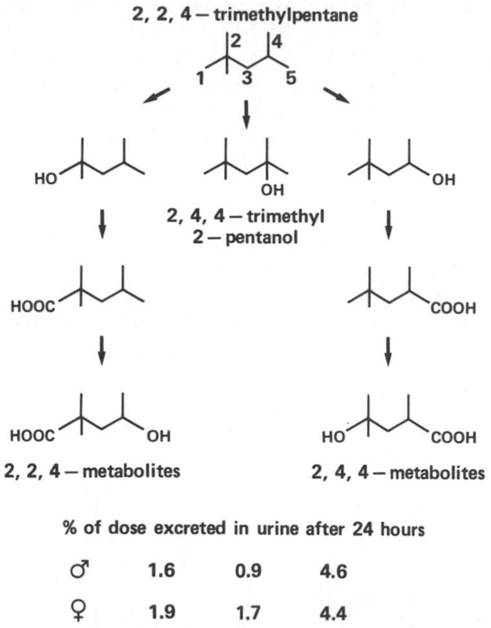

2, 2, 4 – trimethylpentane

2   4
1   3   5

HO⌐⌐⌐   ⌐⌐⌐ OH (center, OH)   ⌐⌐⌐ OH

**2, 4, 4 – trimethyl
2 – pentanol**

HOOC⌐⌐⌐   ⌐⌐⌐ COOH

HOOC⌐⌐⌐ OH   HO⌐⌐⌐ COOH

2, 2, 4 – metabolites   **2, 4, 4 – metabolites**

% of dose excreted in urine after 24 hours

♂	1.6	0.9	4.6
♀	1.9	1.7	4.4

Figure 1. Pathways of metabolism of 2,2,4-trimethylpentane in male and female Fischer-344 rats. Modified from Charbonneau et al 1987a.

protein from male kidneys. Schiff-base interactions between aldehyde metabolites of TMP and protein would be labile under acidic conditions, but can be stabilised by the addition of sodium cyanoborohydride (Dottavio-Martin and Ravel, 1978; Jentoft and Dearborn, 1979). The addition of sodium cyanoborohydride did not alter the retention or chromatographic profile of radioactivity in the male kidney (Loury et al, 1987; Lock et al, 1987), indicating that a Schiff base may not be formed.

Subcellular fractionation of the kidney of male rats 24hr after a dose of [^{3}H]-TMP showed that the bulk of the radioactivity was found in the cytosol fraction (116,000g supernatant); the fraction which contained the highest concentration of alpha-2u-globulin (Table 2, Lock et al, 1987). Little radiolabel was present in the lysosomal fraction, the presumed site of alpha-2u-globulin processing, after its renal reabsorption and it is possible that homogenization of the kidney led to lysosomal disruption and the release of this protein. A more detailed study using specific enzyme markers for each fraction in the renal cortex would be of value to establish the specific localisation of the radiolabel, although any homogenization procedure, however gentle, is likely to disrupt the lysosomes.

Fractionation of male renal cytosol, from rats treated 24hr previously with [^{3}H]-TMP, on Sephadex G-75 resolved the low molecular weight proteins from the larger molecular weight proteins (Figure 2), and showed that about 26% of the radiolabelled material co-eluted with the fractions which contained alpha-2u-globulin the remainder of the radiolabel eluting in the low molecular weight region (Lock et al, 1987). Dialysis of the cytosol fraction from male rat kidney against phosphate buffer led to selective loss of the small molecular weight material, assumed to be water soluble mainly acidic, metabolites of TMP (Olson et al, 1985; Charbonneau et al,

1987). The radiolabelled material remaining after dialysis of male rat cytosol from TMP-treated rats could be separated from the protein by the addition of sodium dodecylsulphate which destroys the tertiary structure of proteins (Lock et al, 1987). This finding indicates a reversible binding of TMP or a metabolite to a fraction enriched in alpha-2u-globulin, and explains why equilibrium dialysis in the presence of strong acidic conditions and/or sodium dodecylsulphate (Loury et al, 1987) failed to detect the association.

The finding that protein denaturation liberated the radioactivity, enabled it to be extracted into solvent and identified by gas chromatography and mass spectral analysis as 2,4,4-trimethyl-2-pentanol. This finding is consistent with the finding of 2,4,4-trimethyl-2-pentanol in the male but

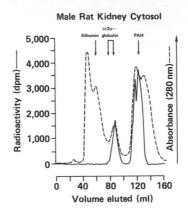

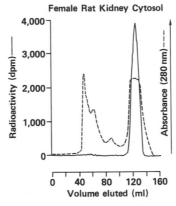

Figure 2.Elution patterns of protein and radiolabelled material on Sephadex G-75 of male or female rat kidney cytosol from animals given [^{3}H]-TMP, 0.5g/kg and 230uCi/kg, 24hr previously. For experimental details see Lock et al (1987).

not female rat kidney (Charbonneau et al, 1987a), and provides the first evidence for an interaction in vivo between a metabolite of TMP and a protein fraction enriched in a male rat-specific low molecular weight protein (Lock et al, 1987). Studies using female rat renal cytosol (Figure 2), male rat hepatic cytosol (Figure 3) and male rat plasma (Figure 3) showed no evidence for an interaction of radiolabelled material from TMP with low molecular weight protein fractions. These findings suggest that the interaction does not occur in the liver or plasma of male rats, although the protein is present in these tissues, albeit at a low concentration. However we cannot exclude the possibility that the technique is not sensitive enough to detect the interaction. Chromatography of male rat urine from [^{3}H]-TMP-treated rats showed evidence of an interaction between an alpha-2u-globulin enriched fraction and radiolabel (Lock et al, 1987). Chromatography of male rat kidney cytosol from rats exposed to 300ppm unleaded gasoline (which contains TMP) showed evidence of an interaction between 2,4,4-trimethyl-2-pentanol and an alpha-2u-globulin enriched fraction (Charbonneau et al, 1988).

In summary, these studies provide evidence to support the hypothesis that a metabolite of TMP interacts with a protein fraction enriched in alpha-2u-globulin in the kidney of male, but not female, rats. The precise nature of this interaction and its relevance to the male rat-specific nephrotoxicity produced by TMP and other volatile hydrocarbons remains to be elucidated. It is possible that the renal accumulation of this protein-metabolite-complex may reduce the ability of cells in the P2 segment of the proximal tubule to catabolise the protein. Excessive accumulation of the protein-chemical-complex could lead to lysosomal fragility, the release of proteolytic enzymes and the metabolite into renal cells and their ultimate demise. This could also explain the selective increase in cell turnover in the P2 segment of the proximal tubule of the male rat following TMP administration (Short et al, 1986).

This finding of an interaction of a metabolite of a component in unleaded gasoline with a protein fraction enriched in alpha-2u-globulin may well be of relevance to nephrotoxicity produced by other chemicals. For example, 2,5-dichlorophenol, a metabolite of 1,4-dichlorobenzene, has been shown to be associated with this protein fraction (Charbonneau et al, 1987b). Similarly the selective retention of the 2-decalone metabolites of decalin in the male rat kidney (Olson et al, 1986) may be due to a chemical-protein-complex.

Table 1. Tissue concentration of radioactivity from [^{14}C]-TMP (0.5g/kg, equivalent to 4.4mmol/kg) and renal alpha-2u-globulin content: comparison between male and female Fischer-344 rats 24hr after dosing.

Tissue	Male	Female
Kidney (nmol eq/g wet wt)	1180 (0.1%)[a]	300 (0.03%)[a]
Liver (nmol eq/g wet wt)	950	250
Plasma (nmol/ml)	405	165
Urine (% dose)	12.2	19.5
Renal alpha-2u-globulin (mg/g wet wt)	28.1	<2

Data from Charbonneau et al 1987a.

[a] Data expressed as percentage of administered dose.

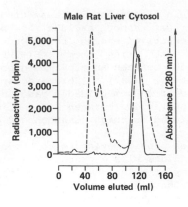

Male Rat Liver Cytosol

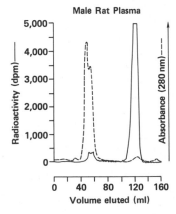

Male Rat Plasma

Figure 3. Elution patterns of protein and radiolabelled material on Sephadex G-75 of male rat hepatic cytosol or plasma from animals given [^{3}H]-TMP, 0.5g/kg and 230uCi/kg, 24hr previously. For experimental details see Lock et al (1987).

Table 2. Intrarenal distribution of radioactivity from [^{3}H]-TMP, 24hr after a single oral dose of 0.5g/kg to male rats.

Subcellular Fraction	Total Radiolabelled Material (nmol equiv)	% In fraction	2u-globulin
Whole homogenate	830	100	++
Cell debris and nuclei	187	22	+
Mitochondria	31	4	-
Lysosomal	27	3	++
Microsomal	18	2	+
Cytosol	497	60	++++

Data from Lock et al (1987), the alpha-2u-globulin content was determined on an arbitrary basis of +, present to a very small extent to 4+, present in a high concentration in the various tissue fractions.

REFERENCES

ALDEN, C.L., KANERVA, R.L., RIDDER, G., AND STONE, L.C. (1984). The pathogenesis of the nephrotoxicity of volatile hydrocarbons in the male rat. In: Renal Effects of Petroleum Hydrocarbons. Advances in Modern Environmental Toxicology (M.A. Mehlman, C.P. Hemstreet, J.J. Thorpe, and N.K. Weaver, Eds.), Vol. VII, pp. 107-120. Princeton Sci. Pub., Princeton, NJ.

CHARBONNEAU, M., LOCK, E.A., STRASSER, J., COX, M.G., TURNER, M.J., AND BUS, J.S. (1987a). 2,2,4-Trimethylpentane-Induced Nephrotoxicity. I. Metabolic disposition of TMP in male and female Fischer-344 rats. Toxicol. Appl. Pharmacol. 91, 171-181.

CHARBONNEAU, M., STRASSER, J., LOCK, E.A. AND SWENBERG, J.A. (1987b). 1,4-Dichlorobenzene (1,4-DCB)-induced nephrotoxicity : similarity with unleaded gasoline (UG)-induced renal effects. Proceedings 3rd. Int. Symp. on Nephrotoxicity. 3-7 August. Guildford, Surrey, UK.

CHARBONNEAU, M., SHORT, B.G., LOCK, E.A. AND SWENBERG, J.A. Mechanisms of petroleum-induced sex-specific protein droplet nephropathy and renal cell proliferation in Fischer-344 rats : relevance to humans. In: Trace Substances in Environmental Health (1988). In press.

DOTTAVIO-MARTIN, D., AND RAVEL, J.M. (1978). Radiolabeling of proteins by reductive alkylation with [^{14}C]formaldehyde and sodium cyanoborohydride. Anal. Biochem. 87, 562-565.

GIBSON, J.E., AND BUS, J.S. (1987). Current perspectives on gasoline (light hydrocarbon) induced male rat nephropathy. N. Y. Acad. Sci., in press.

HALDER, C.A., WARNE, T.M., AND HATOUM, N.S. (1984). Renal toxicity of gasoline and related petroleum naphthas in male rats. In: Renal Effects of Petroleum Hydrocarbons. Advances in Modern Environmental Toxicology (M.A. Mehlman, C.P. Hemstreet, J.J. Thorpe, and N.K. Weaver, Eds.), Vol. VII, pp. 73-88. Princeton Sci. Pub., Princeton, NJ.

HALDER, C.A., HOLDSWORTH, C.E., COCKRELL, B.Y., AND PICCIRILLO, V.J. (1985). Hydrocarbon nephropathy in male rats. Identification of the nephrotoxic components of unleaded gasoline. Toxicol. Ind. Health 1, 67-87.

JENTOFT, N., AND DEARBORN, D.G. (1979). Labeling of proteins by reductive methylation using sodium cyanoborohydride. J. Biol. Chem. 254, 4359-4365.

KITCHEN, D.N. (1984). Neoplastic renal effects of unleaded gasoline in Fischer 344 rats. In: Renal Effects of Petroleum Hydrocarbons. Advances in Modern Environmental Toxicology (M.A. Mehlman, C.P. Hemstreet, J.J. Thorpe, and N.K. Weaver, Eds.), Vol. VII, pp. 65-71. Princeton Sci. Pub., Princeton, NJ.

KLOSS, M.W., COX, M.G., NORTON, R.M., SWENBERG, J.A., AND BUS, J.S. (1985). Sex-dependent differences in the disposition of ^{14}C-5-2,2,4-trimethylpentane in Fischer 344 rats. In: Renal Heterogeneity and Target Cell Toxicity (P.H. Bach and E.A. Lock, Eds.), pp. 489-492. Wiley, Chichester.

LOCK, E.A., CHARBONNEAU, M., STRASSER, J., SWENBERG, J.A., AND BUS, J.S. (1987). 2,2,4-Trimethylpentane-induced nephrotoxicity. II. The reversible binding of a metabolite of 2,2,4-trimethylpentane to a renal protein fraction containing alpha-2u-globulin. Toxicol. Appl. Pharmacol. 91, 182-192.

LOURY, D., SMITH-OLIVER, T., AND BUTTERWORTH, B.E. (1987). Assessment of the binding potential of 2,2,4-trimethylpentane to the rat alpha-2u-globulin. Toxicol. Appl. Pharmacol. 88, 44-56.

MacFARLAND, H.N. (1984). Xenobiotic induced kidney lesions: Hydrocarbons. The 90-day and 2-year gasoline studies. In: Renal Effects of Petroleum Hydrocarbons. Advances in Modern Environmental Toxicology (M.A. Mehlman, C.P. Hemstreet, J.J. Thorpe, and N.K. Weaver, Eds.), Vol. VII, pp. 51-56. Princeton Sci. Pub., Princeton, NJ.

OLSON, C.T., YU, K.O., AND SERVE, M.P. (1985). Identification of urinary metabolites of the nephrotoxic hydrocarbon 2,2,4-trimethylpentane in male rats. Biochem. Biophys. Res. Commun. 130, 313-316.

OLSON, C.T., YU, K.O., AND SERVE, M.P. (1986). Metabolism of nephrotoxic cis- and trans-decalin in Fischer-344 rats. J. Toxicol. Environ. Health 18, 285-292.

OLSON, M.J., GARG, B.D., MURTY, C.V.R. AND ROY, A.K. (1987). Accumulation of alpha-2u-globulin in the renal proximal tubules of male rats exposed to unleaded gasoline. Toxicol. Appl. Pharmacol. 90, 43-51.

PHILLIPS, R.D., AND EGAN, G.F. (1984a). Effect of C10-C11 isoparaffinic solvent on kidney function in Fischer 344 rats during eight weeks of inhalation. Toxicol. Appl. Pharmacol. 73, 500-510.

PHILLIPS, R.D., AND EGAN, G.F. (1984b). Subchronic inhalation exposure of dearomatized white spirit and C10-C11 isoparaffinic hydrocarbon in Sprague-Dawley rats. Fundam. Appl. Toxicol. 4, 808-818.

SHORT, B.G., BURNETT, V.L., AND SWENBERG, J.A. (1986). Histopathology and cell proliferation induced by 2,2,4-trimethylpentane in the male rat kidney. Toxicol. Pathol. 14, 194-203.

SHORT, B.G., BURNETT, V.L., COX, M.G., BUS, J.S. AND SWENBERG, J.A. (1987). Site specific renal cytotoxicity and cell proliferation in male rats exposed to petroleum hydrocarbons. Lab. Invest. In press.

STONARD, M.D., PHILLIPS, P.G.N., FOSTER, J.R., SIMPSON, M.G., AND LOCK, E.A. (1986). Alpha-2u-Globulin: Measurement in rat kidney following administration of 2,2,4-trimethylpentane. Toxicology 41, 161-168.

VIAU, C., BERNARD, A., GUERET, F., MALDAGUE, P., GENGOUX, P., AND LAUWERYS, R. (1986). Isoparaffinic solvent-induced nephrotoxicity in the rat. Toxicology 38, 227-240.

MALE RAT SPECIFIC ALPHA$_{2u}$GLOBULIN NEPHROPATHY AND RENAL TUMOURIGENESIS

C. L. Alden, Miami Valley Laboratories, The Procter and Gamble Company, Cincinnati, OH 45247, USA

INTRODUCTION

Male Rat Unique Proximal Convoluted Tubule (PCT) Protein Reabsorption Droplets

Weinbren [see 1] characterised spontaneously occurring hyaline droplets in the otherwise normal mature male rat kidney. The ultrastructural characteristics of the spontaneous PCT hyaline body was characterised by Maunsbach as a phagolysosomal protein reabsorption droplet and defined as a male rat specific increased size and propensity for crystalloid change in comparison to the female rat or higher species, including humans [1].

In the 1970's Neuhaus and Roy [1] described a unique primary male rat urinary protein occurring from 50 to 150 days of age. This protein migrated as an alpha$_{2u}$globulin and was thus designated alpha$_{2u}$globulin, with the "u" signifying urogenous. In the 1980's we [1] linked these observations demonstrating that the spontaneous hyaline droplet in the otherwise normal male rat kidney consists exclusively of alpha$_{2u}$globulin [1]. Two-dimensional protein electrophoretic separation of renal cortex protein, including cellular fractionation and immunocytochemistry techniques were utilized. The female rat does not contain mRNA for alpha$_{2u}$globulin in the liver, but this protein can be induced by ovariectomy and testosterone therapy.

Alpha$_{2u}$globulin

Approximately 50mg of alpha$_{2u}$globulin is synthesised per day in the young mature male. Since alpha$_{2u}$globulin is a low molecular weight protein of 18,600 Daltons it is rapidly filtered and poorly reabsorbed (approximately 60% is reabsorbed, with 40% lost in the urine) and represents only 3mg% of the serum protein. That which is reabsorbed is poorly hydrolyzed, thus accumulating in the PCT epithelium as morphologically visible hyaline droplets (Figure 1). Renal parenchyma thus consists of 3%, by weight, of alpha$_{2u}$globulin. Geerstzen has demonstrated a t-1/2 of 8 hours for alpha$_{2u}$globulin under physiological conditions [1].

The glomerular filtrate of the mature male rat contains a full complement of low molecular weight proteins as does the female and higher species, including humans. Neuhaus has demonstrated that the rat glomerular

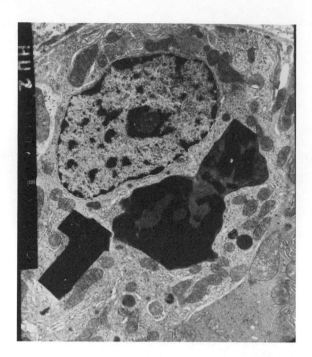

Figure 1.   Crystalloid alpha$_{2u}$globulin inclusion in perinuclear location in a proximal convoluted tubular cell cytoplasm.

filtrate contains approximately 50mg of albumen over a 24-hour period, an amount comparable to alpha$_{2u}$globulin filtrate loads. Albumen, however, is efficiently reabsorbed (>90%) and rapidly catabolized and thus does not accumulate in the kidney [see 1].   Alpha$_{2u}$globulin is believed to function as a pheromone carrier.   Exposure of female rats via aerosol results in localization of this protein in the pituitary and reflex increase in follicle stimulating hormone release. Alpha$_{2u}$globulin injected in the male protects the testicle against the effects of injected oestrogen [see 1].

Male mice also excrete a sex-related protein resulting in urinary protein levels 2.5 to 3 times that of female mice. Mature male mice and rats are thus physiological proteinuric compared to female counterparts or to higher species of either sex.   The male mouse sex-associated urinary protein, is not poorly hydrolyzable and thus does not accumulate in PCT epithelium. Higher species, including humans, are not reported to excrete sex-association urinary proteins.   Furthermore, Pesce and Anderson [2] in independent reviews of urinary protein profiles in normal and abnormal humans do not report presence of proteins migrating as alpha$_2$globulin.

XENOBIOTIC EXACERBATION OF ALPHA$_{2u}$GLOBULIN ACCUMULATION

Several chemicals specifically significantly increase alpha$_{2u}$globulin accumulation in PCT epithelium of the male rat as the primary acute toxicological effect, including d-limonene, unleaded gas, trimethylpentane (TMP), and decalin.   d-Limonene comprises over 90% of the oil of the orange.   d-Limonene is widespread in natural foodstuffs.   The average daily consumption of d-limonene has been estimated as 2mg/kg.   This dose is very near an effect level, supporting to the exquisite sensitivity of the male rat. The primary effect of $\underline{d}$-limonene has been established utilizing light microscopy, ultrastructural morphology, and two-dimensional electrophoretic protein separation analyses and immunocyto-chemistry.

In time sequence studies, $\underline{d}$-limonene and unleaded gasoline induce exacerbated hyaline droplet formation and accelerated apoptosis, leading to granular cast formulation with entrapment in the pars recta, nephron obstruction and then exacerbated chronic nephrosis. This triad, hyaline droplets, granular casts, and exaggerated chronic nephrosis, comprises a very specific spectrum of injury common to a growing list of diverse chemicals, but distinct from primary acute effects and subchronic sequelae of a variety of well-characterised comparative nephrotoxins such as heavy metals, aminoglycoside antibiotics, mycotoxins and nonsteroidal anti-inflammatory drugs (3-8).

CHRONIC CONSEQUENCE OF ALPHA$_{2u}$GLOBULIN NEPHROPATHY

Chemicals that have been demonstrated to induce the specific triad described above also induce a very specific spectrum of chronic injury characterised by linear mineralisation of the renal papilla, pelvic urothelial hyperplasia, exacerbated chronic timepoints. The linear papilla mineralisation is thought to represent mineralised remnants of the necrotic debris in the cast that migrate with time from the pars recta to the prebend segment of Henle's Loop [1].

ALPHA$_{2u}$GLOBULIN ASSOCIATED TUMORIGENESIS

Inducers of alpha$_{2u}$globulin nephropathy consistently induce renal tubular tumours. Currently 13 chemicals have been identified as inducers of this phenomenon (Table 1 and 2). No chemical inducing this nephropathy has been recognised that does not lead to tubular tumour formation. Several of these chemicals affect male rat kidneys only and are nongenotoxic.

Table 1. NTP REPORT OF MALE RAT RENAL CARCINOGENS ASSOCIATED WITH ALPHA$_{2U}$GLOBULIN NEPHROPATHY

ASSOCIATIONS:	Male Rat Renal Tumours	Mouse Liver Tumours	Other Tumours	Genotoxicity
XENOBIOTIC:				
Hexachloroethane	Yes	?	?	?
Paradichlorobenzene	Yes	Yes	No	No
Dimethylmethylphosphonate	Yes	No	No	Yes
Isophorone	Yes	No	No	Yes
Pentachloroethane	Yes	Yes	No	Yes
$\underline{d}$-Limonene	Yes	No	No	No

Table 2. XENOBIOTICS WHICH PRODUCE ALPHA$_{2U}$GLOBULIN NEPHROPATHY/TUMOURS IN MALE RATS.

JP-4, JP-TS, JP-7,	C_{10}-C_{12} Isoparaffins
RJ-5, JP-10, Diesel Fuel (Marine)	Unleaded Gasoline

Currently elucidated mechanistic concepts include the following potential associations:

1.   Non-specific linkage between male rat renal toxicity and renal tumourigenicity

2.   Non-specific linkage between male rat renal replicative rate increase and renal tumourigenicity

3.   Specific linkage between male rat renal tubular cell phagolysosomal $alpha_{2u}$globulin overload and renal tumourigenesis

Support for the concept that toxicity always precedes renal oncogenicity includes a survey of NTP bioassays and the published literature in which rat renal tumourigens consistently induce morphological alterations in subchronic studies. However, agents causing renal toxicity (e.g., Mirex and N-phenyl-2-napthylamine; S. Eustis, Personal Communication, 1987) do not always lead to tubular tumour formation, mitigating against constancy of this association.

Support for the concept that replicative rate increase non-specifically represents a male rat renal tumour risk exists. Decalin, a model chemical for this specific nephropathy, causes increased proximal convoluted tubular cell replication and increased apoptosis (Table 3 and 4). Increased apoptosis presumably reflects the cell injury of $alpha_{2u}$globulin overload. However, renal toxins such as Netilmicin presumably increase apoptosis and replicative rate but do not lead to tubular tumour formation (Black, H. - Personal Communication; Schulte-Hermann, R. - Personal Communication, 1987). Lysosomal overload does not appear non-specifically to represent a tumour risk since mannitol and aminoglycoside antibiotics cause lysosomal overload but not tumourigenesis [9]. Nitrilotriacetate does cause lysosomal overload, zinc loading and renal tubular tumour formation, but probably does not cause increased apoptosis, thus probably reflecting a different mechanism of tumourigenesis [10].

Table 3.   PERCENT OF LABELLED RENAL CORTICAL TUBULAR CELLS

Group* (Males - 11 weeks old)	N	Average
Untreated	3	1.2
Decalin 50 mg/kg	2	8.8**
Decalin 250 mg/kg	3	9.5*

* Twenty-eight day gavage study   ** Statistically significant

It is important to note that in $alpha_{2u}$globulin nephropathy replicative rate increase occurs in the cell affected by toxicity, and thus probably represents the target cell for tumourigenicity. This is in contrast to the genotoxic carcinogen that typically is injurious. Replicative response, and presumably tumour response, occurs in a subpopulation of cells resistant to the toxicity. This is also in contrast to the classical promoter, phenobarbital, that is not toxic and causes replicative rate increase but decreased apoptosis.

Table 4.   MEAN URINARY RENAL EPITHELIAL CELL COUNTS/HOUR
(d-Limonene Influence on Apoptosis)

Treatment	Renal Epithelial Cells		Renal Epithelial Cell Clumps/Casts	
	Day 7	Day 14	Day 7	Day 14
Corn Oil	0	69	0	0
d-Limonene 75 mg/kg bid	5,346	38,794	15	5,341

Finally, this leads us then to consider that a specific association exists between male rat renal tubular cell alpha$_{2u}$globulin phagolysosomal overload and renal tumourigensis. We hypothesised that alpha$_{2u}$globulin might have a mitogenic influence in the kidney cortex. By neutering the female, followed by testosterone therapy, we can force hepatic synthesis of alpha$_{2u}$globulin and its renal accumulation with hyaline droplet formation. This regimen, however, has no influence on replicative rate (Table 4). However, the alpha$_{2u}$ load in this model is substantially less than in the normal mature control male and orders of magnitude less than the treated mature control male.   Thus, we infused the female rat with 50mg intraperitoneally with a crude alpha$_{2u}$globulin protein preparation twice per day for two weeks. During the second week we implanted osmotic pumps for slow release of tritiated thymidine with subsequent autoradiography. This regimen significantly increased replicative rate (Table 5).   These data suggest that alpha$_{2u}$globulin overload is the toxic and mitogenic stimulus linked with the tumourigenic response. The xenobiotics may simply mediate the overload.

Conceptually, three possibilities emerge as testable hypotheses for a specific mechanism in alpha$_{2u}$globulin nephropathy-associated tubular tumourigenesis.

Table 5.   INFLUENCE OF ALPHA$_{2U}$GLOBULIN SYNTHESIS ON REPLICATIVE RATE

	INTACT FEMALE	NEUTERED 11 WEEK OLD FEMALE TREATED WITH TESTOSTERONE
MEAN (N = 5)	1.2%	1.2%
RANGE	0.9-1.4%	0.9-1.7%

1.   The crystalloid inclusion of perinuclear location (Table 6) is reminiscent of the phenomenon in which phagocytosed asbestos assumes a perinuclear position and injures chromosomes during cell mitosis.

2.   Phagolysosomal protein overload has been reported to result in leakage of lysosomal enzymes such as RNA and DNAases into cytosol. During mitoses these enzymes might cause chromosomal injury [11].

3.   Finally, a third conceptual specific link with oncogenesis can be found if the phagolysosomal alpha$_{2u}$ overload correlates with proportional increase in proton pump activity.   Increased activity could lead to cytoplasmic alkalinisation and cytosol sodium elevation.   Increased cytoplasmic sodium and increased proton pump activity have recently considered been mitogenic, if not oncogenic, stimuli [12].

Table 6.   INFLUENCE OF ALPHA$_{2u}$GLOBULIN INFUSION IN FEMALE RATS (N=3).

Treatment 2 Week Duration	Mean Replicative Rate
Control	3.3%
Alpha$_{2u}$globulin at 50 mg b.i.d. (crude preparation)	7.8% statistically significant

EXTRAPOLATION TO HUMANS

Kidneys of species that do not synthesise alpha$_{2u}$globulin are not affected by treatment with d-limonene, including female rats and mice, and dogs of both sexes. Because of the prerequisite role of alpha$_{2u}$globulin in the toxicological response, the male rat should not be considered predictive of a human response. In addition, since the toxicological response seems inexorably linked to the tumourigenic response the male rat again probably is not predictive for humans.

REFERENCES

1.   Mehlman, M.A., Hemstreet, C.P., Thorpe, J.J. and Weaver, N.K. (1984) [Editors] Renal Effects of Petroleum Hydrocarbon, Princeton Scientific Publishers, Princeton.

2.   Anderson, N.L., Nance, S.L., Pearson, T.W and Anderson, N.G. 1982. Specific antigerum staining of 2 dimensional electrophoretic patterns of human plasma proteins embolished on nitrocellulose. Electrophoresis. 3, 135.

3.   Pesce, A.J., Clyne, D.H., Pollak, V.E., Kant, S.F., Foulkes, E.C. and Selenke W.M. 1980. Renal tubular interactions of proteins. Clin. Biochem. 13, 209.

4.   Stone, L.C., Kanerva, R.L., Burns, J.L., and Alden, C.L.: Decalin-induced nephrotoxicity: light and electron microscopic examination of the effects of oral dosing on the development of kidney lesions in the rat. Fd. Chem. Toxic. 25:43-52, 1987.

5.   Kanerva, R.L., McCracken, M.S., Alden, C.L., and Stone, L.C.: Characterization of spontaneous and decalin-induced hyaline droplets in kidneys of adult male rats. Fd. Chem. Toxic. 25:63-82, 1987.

6.   Kanerva, R.L., McCracken, M.S., Alden, C.L., and Stone, L.C.: Morphogenesis of decalin-induced renal alterations in the male rat. Fd. Chem. Toxic. 25:52-61, 1987.

7.   Stone, L.C., McCracken, M.S., Kanerva, R.L., and Alden, C.L.: Development of a short-term model of decalin inhalation nephrotoxicity in the male rat. Fd. Chem. Toxic. 25:35-41, 1987.

8. Kanerva, R.L., Ridder, G.M., Lefever, F.R., and Alden, C.L.: Comparison of short-term renal effects due to oral administration of decalin or d-limonene in young adult male Fischer-344 rats. Fd. Chem. Toxic. 1987.

9. Kanerva, R.L., and Alden, C.L.: Review of kidney sections from a subchronic d-limonene oral dosing study conducted by the National Cancer Institute. Fd. Chem. Toxic., 1987.

10. Abdo, K.M., Huff, J.E., Haseman, K.J. and Alden, C.L.: No evidence of carcinogenicity and D-mannitol and propylgallate in F-344 rats or B6C3F1 mice. Fd. Chem. Toxic. 24:1091-1097, 1986.

11. Anderson, R.L., Alden, C.L. and Merski, J.A.: The effects of nitrilotriacetate on cation disposition and urinary tract toxicity. Fd. Chem. Toxic. 20:105-122, 1988.

12. Maack, T., Johnson, V., Kau, S.T., Figueirido, J. and Sigulem, D.: Renal filtration, transport, and metabolism of low molecular weight proteins: a review. Kidney Int. 16:251, 1986.

13. Cameron, I.L., Smith, N.K., Pool, T.B., and Sparks, R.L.: Intra-cellular concentration of sodium and other elements as related to mitogenesis and oncogensis in vivo. Cancer Research, 40:1493-1500, 1980.

NEPHROTOXICITY AND STUDIES ON THE REABSORPTION AND DISPOSAL OF ALPHA 2U-GLOBULIN

Otto W. Neuhaus

Department of Biochemistry, University of South Dakota, Vermillion, South Dakota

INTRODUCTION

Alpha-2u-globulin, a low-molecular weight (LMW) protein of 19,000 dalton, is synthesised by the male rat liver as a family of isoforms; pI = 4.6-5.2. This protein is an important constituent of the physiological proteinuria in adult male rats. At maturity the total urinary protein is 20-30% alpha-2u and 10% albumin. At 160 days of age the excretion of albumin and total urinary proteins are markedly increased. By one year, albumin represents nearly 60% of the total protein while alpha-2u is less than 10%. This reversal in relative content may be the consequence of a progressive glomerulonephrosis, associated with an apparent spontaneous accumulation of hyaline droplets. The nephrotic condition may be the consequence of the burden of excreting alpha-2u. Its early onset is sex-dependent; female rats do not exhibit the proteinuria until a later age.

Recent publications concerning nephrosis in rats dosed with certain hydrocarbons showed an accumulation of hyaline droplets which were seen only in the male rat. These intracellular droplets consist of alpha-2u-globulin.

In both ageing and the response to hydrocarbons, the common pathological factor may be the accumulation of alpha-2u, It is conceivable that this sex-dependent protein is handled by the kidney cells via a susceptible pathway not shared with other proteins. This sex-dependent process could occur either at the endocytotic level whereby proteins are absorbed or during the intracellular handling of the invaginated protein. These options are the subject of the following study.

A SPECIFIC VERSUS A COMMON ABSORPTIVE PROCESS

Recently, it was reported that the renal absorption of alpha-2u is probably via a general endocytotic mechanism acting on LMW proteins such as lysozyme (1). These studies have been expanded to demonstrate that the characteristics of this process are similar to those reported for other marker proteins. Earlier studies indicated that a positively charged protein or a positively charged region of the protein is bound to negative binding sites located on or in the membranes of the microvilli (2,3). Binding is followed by invagination and insertion into the cytosol either as endosomes or possibly in the free state.

The current studies were performed using the continuously infused, anaesthetized adult male rat (1). Infusion was performed through the femoral vein using a mildly diuretic, modified Krebs-Ringer medium. The urinary bladder was cannulated and urine samples were collected at 20 min intervals. Urinary alpha-2u and albumin were measured using an immunological technique. Typical results are presented in Figure 1. Data for both alpha-2u and albumin are described as the excretion rates in ug/min. Control values are given by the excretion rate at zero-time (t_o). To determine if a given protein would successfully compete with alpha-2u absorption, a bolus of a test LMW protein was infused at t_o. As seen in Figure 1, when cytochrome c was injected, the excretion rate for alpha-2u was increased but not that for albumin. These results are similar to those published for lysozyme and support the concept that proteins are absorbed by two general systems, one for LMW and the other for HMW proteins. Figure 2 shows that this inhibitory process is dose-dependent. To establish whether net protein charge plays a role in this absorptive process, five LMW proteins of varying isoelectric points were tested. As seen in Figure 3 each increased the excretion rate for alpha-2u regardless of isoelectric point. Cytochrome c and beta-lactoglobulin, for example, were equally effective despite divergent pIs of 10.6 and 5.2. It is especially interesting that both possess 13-19 lysyl residues comparable with alpha-2u. Perhaps the lysyl residues or specifically its epsilon ammonium groups are of greater significance than the net charge of the protein molecule. This is further indicated by the fact that gentamicin, an aminoglycoside, also inhibits the absorption of alpha-2U (1). Similarly the polyamine, spermine, increased the alpha-2u excretion from a control value of 4.4 ± 2.3 to an experimental of 12.5 ± 2.3 ug/min. Certain amino acids were used to confirm the importance of the ammonium groups. Figure 4 illustrates the structures of two model amino acids used, namely, epsilon aminocaproic acid (EACA) and tranexamic acid. Both have amino groups equidistant from the carboxyl as in L-lysine. As seen in Figure 5, the injection of a bolus of L-lysine caused an immediate increase in alpha-2u excretion with little effect on albumin. Since large doses of lysine may damage renal tubule cells, the reversibility of its effect was demonstrated by a sequential administration of 3 doses of lysine, as seen in Part B of Figure 5. Figure 6 shows that the model amino acids EACA and tranexamic acid each increased the excretion rate for alpha-2u. The osmotic effect caused by the large amount of solute was considered by comparing the results with the effect of an equimolar quantity of sodium chloride. EACA and tranexamic acid exerted equally significant increases in excretion rate for alpha-2u. These data support the conclusions reached by others (2-4), indicating that the presence of basic amino acids and their configuration are of greater importance than the net charge of the protein itself. It is concluded that alpha-2u globulin is transported into the cell by a process having properties comparable to those for other LMW proteins and, therefore, does a not utilize a unique mechanism.

AN INTRACELLULAR FATE UNIQUE TO ALPHA 2U-GLOBULIN

Once internalized the proteins may be degraded by proteolysis within the phagolysosomes or may be degraded in the cytosol by an ATP-dependent, ubiquitin-requiring system. It is also conceivable that some proteins may be restored to the blood stream by translocation through the basolateral membrane.

Recent studies using the hydrocarbon, 2,2,4-trimethylpentane, demonstrated a renal accumulation of alpha-2u globulin in adult male rats (5). This accumulation may be the consequence of the blockage of a unique disposal pathway for alpha-2u. To test this possibility, trimethylpentane was administered by gavage of a single dose of 12 mmole/kg. Urine, blood serum

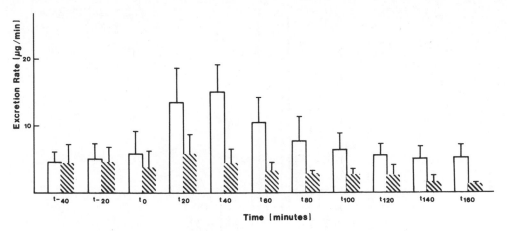

Fig. 1. Response of excretion rates to the iv injection at to of cytochrome C (20 mg/kg).

Open bars = alpha-2u; closed = albumin. Data = means±SD.

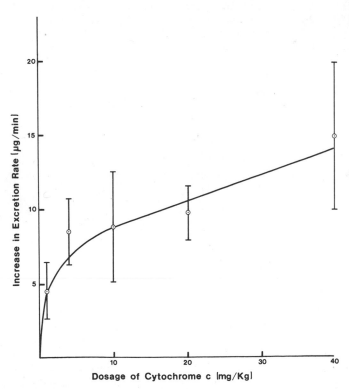

Fig. 2. Dose-dependency of the effect of cytochrome c excretion of alpha-2u in the adult male rat.

Each point represents the maximal increase in excretion rate above the control (t$_o$); means±SD.

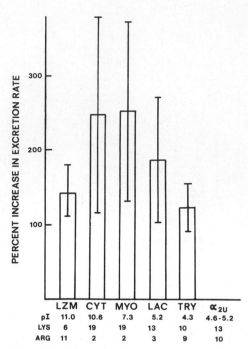

	LZM	CYT	MYO	LAC	TRY	α_{2U}
pI	11.0	10.6	7.3	5.2	4.3	4.6-5.2
LYS	6	19	19	13	10	13
ARG	11	2	2	3	9	10

Fig. 3. Effect of isoelectric point of various proteins on the excretion rates of alpha-2u. CYT = cytochrome c; MYO = myoglobin; LAC = beta-lactoglobulin; TRY = soybean trypsin inhibitor; LZM = lysozyme. Data are maximal percent increases above to using 40 mg/kg; mean±SD.

L-LYSINE   EACA   TRANEXAMIC ACID
                                (CYCLOCAPRONE)

Fig. 4. Comparison of the structural formulas for the model amino acids, epsilon aminocaproic acid (EACA) and tranexamic acid with the basic amino acid, L-lysine.

and kidney samples were collected. The kidney tissues were homogenised and solubilized with Triton X-100. Immunoassays were performed for alpha-2u and albumin. TMP treatment resulted in a striking increase in renal alpha-2u concentration 24, 48 and 72 hr after treatment (Figure 7), but albumin concentration was not affected. The alpha-2u in the blood serum and urine also were unaffected by TMP. These data indicate that alpha-2u and albumin are handled in the kidneys by separate processes, one affected by TMP and the other not. It is suggested that the alpha-2u may be disposed by a specific, perhaps sex-dependent, process in the male rat kidney whereas the disposal of albumin may represent a more general process.

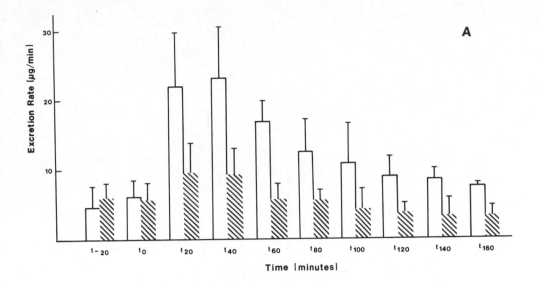

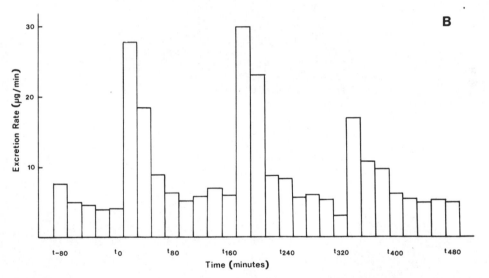

Fig. 5. A. Response of alpha-2u excretion to the iv injection of L-lysine (4.5 mmole/kg) at t_o = Open bars are alpha-2u; closed are albumin; each represents the mean$\pm$SD. B. Sequential injection of 3 equal doses of L-lysine.

In conclusion, it has been shown that the endogenous sex-dependent protein of the adult male rat, alpha-2u globulin, is absorbed by the renal tubule cells via a general process for LMW proteins. These studies support the suggestion that the presence of the epsilon ammonium group of lysine is of greater importance than the net molecular charge of the protein. Studies with the nephrotoxic agent TMP indicate that the disposal of alpha-2u, but not that of albumin is inhibited. It is suggested that the anionic, LMW protein alpha-2u is internalized into the renal tubule cells by a common process, shared with LMW proteins in general, but is handled within the cell by a process unique to this protein.

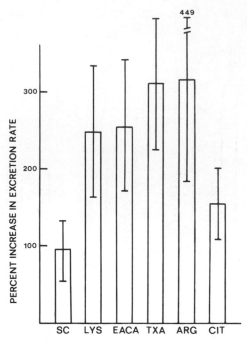

Fig. 6. Comparison of effects on alpha-2u excretion of equimolar amounts of amino acids with sodium chloride (SC). LYS = L-lysine; EACA = epsilon aminocaproic acid; TXA = tranexamic acid; ARG = L-arginine; CIT = L-citrulline. Data = mean±SD.

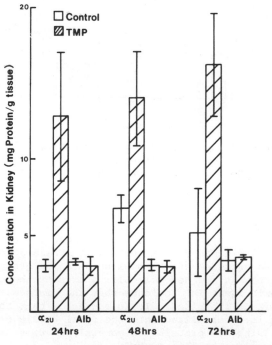

Fig. 7. Effect of a single dose (gavage) of 2,2,4-trimethylpentane on the concentration of alpha-2u and albumin in the kidneys of the adult male rat. Open bars = corn oil control; Closed = TMP (12 mmole/kg).

REFERENCES

1. O.W. Neuhaus, Renal reabsorption of low-molecular weight proteins in adult male rats: alpha-2u globulin, <u>Proc. Soc. Expt. Biol. Med</u>. 182:531 (1986).

2. B.E. Sumpio and T. Maack, Kinetics, competition and selectivity of tubular absorption of proteins, <u>Am. J. Physiol</u>. 243:F379 (1982).

3. K. Baumann, C. Cojocel and W. Pape, Effect of molecular charge of protein on its reabsorption in microperfused proximal renal tubules, <u>In</u>: "The Pathogenicity of Cationic Proteins", P.P. Lambert, P. Bergmann and R. Beauwens, eds., Raven Press, New York (1983).

4. C.E. Mogensen, K. Solling and E. Vittinghus, Studies on mechanisms of proteinuria using amino acid-induced inhibition of tubular reabsorption in normal and diabetic man, <u>In</u>: "Contributions to Nephrology", G.M. Berlyne, S. Giovannetti and S. Thomas, eds., S. Karger, Basel (1981).

5. M.D. Stonard, P.G.N. Phillips, J.R. Foster, M.G. Simpson and E.A. Lock, Alpha-2u globulin: measurement in rat kidney following administration of 2,2,4-trimethylpentane, <u>Toxicol</u>. 41:161 (1986).

INDUCTION OF HYALINE DROPLET ACCUMULATION IN RENAL CORTEX OF MALE RATS BY AROMATIC COMPOUNDS

Ernst Bomhard[1], Georg Luckhaus[1], Manfred Marsmann[2] and Andreas Zywietz

[1]Fachbereich Toxicology, Bayer AG, Wuppertal, F.R.G.
[2]Institute of Pharmacokinetics, Bayer AG, Wuppertal, F.R.G.
[3]Laboratory of Molecular Design, Bayer AG, Pflanzenschutzzentrum Monheim, F.R.G.

INTRODUCTION

Repeated oral and inhalation exposure of male rats to unleaded gasoline and a variety of petroleum-derived naphthas, solvents, and distillates has been reported to induce a characteristic spectrum of changes in the kidney which has been referred to as "light hydrocarbon nephropathy" (Mehlmann et al., 1984; Craig, 1986). Most of the identified compounds belong to the class of branched-chain alkanes. A select few of the investigated aromatics were inactive (Halder et al., 1984; Halder et al., 1985). Recently, corresponding effects were seen in short- and long-term studies with p-dichlorobenzene (NTP, 1986; Bomhard et al., 1987). Accumulation of hyaline droplets in the tubular epithelium occurs within a few days after treatment with these compounds and precedes the subsequent tubular lesions (Thomas et al., 1985). This study evaluated "light hydrocarbon nephropathy" inducing potential of several aromatic hydrocarbons by histological judgement of hyaline droplet accumulation (HDA).

Little is known about common molecular properties of compounds inducing nephropathies other than that a certain degree of branching and an egg-like shape have been postulated as prerequisites for activity (Halder et al., 1985; Craig, 1986). Molecular modelling (Fruehbeis et al., 1987) has emerged as a tool for the rigorous examination of structure based properties and is used to derive an interaction model between nephropathy inducing hydrocarbons and a putative binding site on a male rat specific protein in the present study.

MATERIAL AND METHODS

5 male Wistar rats (age 10 to 12 weeks) each were administered the test substances in peanut oil once daily for 7 days. Dose level initially was 500 mg/kg/d for all groups but had to be reduced to 250 mg/kg/d on day 3 in the case of 1,2,4-trichlorobenzene and chlorobenzene due to frank toxicity. Sections of both kidneys were stained with azan according to Heidenhain.

Computer graphics modelling of a putative binding site common to HDA inducing compounds was based on published data of aliphatic hydrocarbons. Lowest energy molecular structures were obtained from molecular mechanics calculation (MM2)* volumes were calculated from standard von der Waals radii and further operated on utilizing features of the molecular modelling software SYBYL*. Octanol-water partition coefficients were either calculated with the CLOGP* programme or taken as experimental values from associated database.

*)   Programmes used:
    MM2:   Quantum Chemistry Programme Exchange, Bloomington, Indiana,
              No. 395.
    SYBYL: Tripos Ass., St. Louis, MO 63117
    CLOGP: A. Leo, Ponoma Medical College, Claremont CA 91711.

RESULTS

Presence or absence of hyaline droplet accumulation is presented for each of the compounds in the Table.

Test substance	HDA
Chlorobenzene	−
o-Dichlorobenzene	−
m-Dichlorobenzene	−
p-Dichlorobenzene	+
1,2,3-Trichlorobenzene	−
1,3,4-Trichlorobenzene	−
1,3,5-Trichlorobenzene	+
o-Xylene	+
m-Xylene	−?
1,2,3-Trimethylbenzene	−
1,2,4-Trimethylbenzene	−
1,3,5-Trimethylbenzene	−
N,N-Diethyl-m-toluamide	+

In accordance with published data 1,2,4-trimethylbenzene and o-dichlorobenzene were negative (Craig, 1986; Halder et al., 1985). m-xylene has been reported to be negative (Craig, 1986; Halder et al., 1985) and the score in any of the 5 rats did not exceed that found in controls. Based on the incidence, 3 of 5 animals, it was classified questionable. N,N-diethyl-m-toluamide showed strongest activity, followed by 1,3,5-trichlorobenzene, o-xylene and p-dichlorobenzene.

Structure-activity considerations have identified a Log Kow>3.5, the presence of an isopentyl unit and a certain size and shape of their spatial structures as main factors discriminating active and inactive aliphatic hydrocarbons. A 3D-model of a putative binding site has then been derived by superimposing the most potent branched chain alkanes and calculating their cumulative molecular volume (Fig. 1a). The boundaries of this model are gradually established, as inactive analogues show a common excess volume on docking them into the binding site (Fig. 1b). Although the model has solely been derived from acyclic compounds it also accommodates cycloaliphatics like decalin and tricyclodecane that have been reported as inducers of "light hydrocarbon nephropathy" (Fig. 2). In the case of aromatics the mere steric fit into the binding site model is not sufficient to explain the observed differences in activity.

DISCUSSION AND CONCLUSIONS

The potential of inducing light hydrocarbon nephropathy in male rats via hyaline droplet accumulation is also a feature of several aromatic

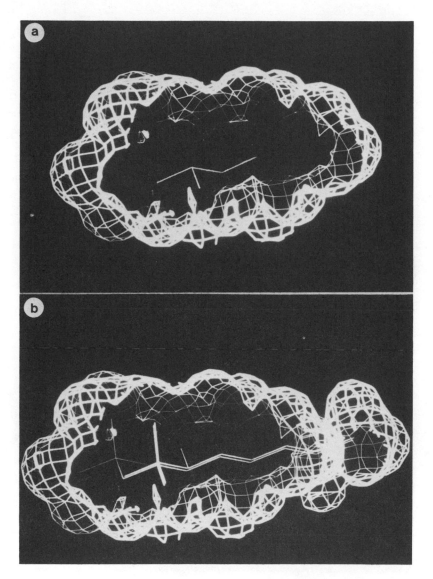

Fig. 1. Cumulative volume obtained from van der Waals spheres centred on atoms of superimposed structures.
a) most potent branch-chain hydrocarbons with essential isopentyl unit.
b) less potent compounds with small excess volume.

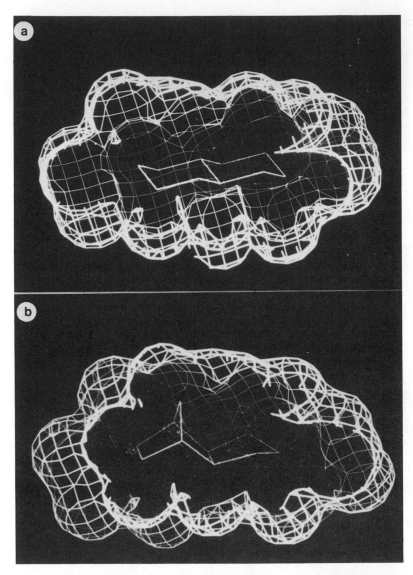

Fig. 2. Docking of a) trans-decalin and b) tricyclodecane into the putative binding site model, probably at the alpha $_{2u}$-globulin molecule.

hydrocarbons. This potential can be evaluated by a short-term screening test using 5 animals per test compound. Long-term treatment of male rats with hydrocarbons inducing the typical nephropathy is regularly followed by subsequent cytolysis and compensatory cell proliferation. This sustained increase in cell proliferation is believed to lead to increased "fixation" of spontaneous DNA damage, resulting in mutations and subsequent carcinogenesis. All light hydrocarbon nephropathy inducing compounds tested so far in adequate long-term experiments have indeed let to an increase in cortical kidney tumour (Craig, 1986; NTP 1983, 1986). Therefore it is speculated that long-term administration of the investigated aromatic hydrocarbons results in increased incidences of renal cortical tumours in male rats. This nephrocarcinogenicity seems to have no relevance for man.

There is evidence that HDA inducing light hydrocarbons or derivatives thereof interact with a male rat specific protein, most probably alpha-globulin, at a common putative binding site. A first 3D-model of this binding site has been derived from computer graphics analyses of the molecular shape of active and inactive acyclic hydrocarbons. It has been shown that this model also explains the observed cycloaliphatics. Further research is in progress to identify the physical-chemical properties other than steric fitting that are responsible for the binding of aromatics to the male rat specific protein. To our present knowledge these are most probably related to the polarity of the compounds since HDA activity only occurs with those chlorobenzenes that carry no dipole moment. A refinement of the current model to yield a quantitative correlation between structural properties and HDA activity is also worked on.

REFERENCES

Bomhard, E., Luckhaus, G. Voigt, W.-H. and Loeser, E. Induction of Light Hydrocarbons Nephropathy by p-Dichlorobenzene. Arch Toxicol., in press.

Craig, P. Paper presented at the Toxicology Forum, 1986. Annual Summer Meeting, Aspen, Colorado.

Fruehbeis, H., Klein, R. and Wallmeier, H. Computergestuetztes Molekueldesign (CAMD) - ein Ueberblick, Angew. Chem., 99 (1987) 413-428.

Halder, C.A., Holdsworth, C.E. and Cookrell, B.Y. Hydrocarbon Nephropathy in Male Rats. Identification of the Nephrotoxic Components of Gasoline. In: Monographs in Applied Toxicology. No. 2. Renal Heterogeneity and Target Cell Toxicity. P.H. Bach and E.A. Lock (eds.). John Wiley & Sons, Chichester, (1985) pp. 481-484.

Halder, C.A., Warne, T.M. and Hatoum, N.S. Renal Toxicity of Gasoline and Related Petroleum Naphthas in Male Rats. In: Advances in Modern Environmental Toxicology. Vol. VII. Renal Effects of Petroleum Hydrocarbons. M.A. Mehlmann et al., (eds.) Princeton Scientific Publishers, Inc., Princeton, NY (1984) pp. 73-87.

Mehlmann, M.A., Hemstreet, C.P., Thorpe, J.J. and Weaver, N.K. (eds.) Renal Effects of Petroleum Hydrocarbons. Advances In: Modern Environmental Toxicology, Vol. VII., Princeton Scientific Publishers, Inc., Princeton, NY (1984).

NTP Technical Report on the Toxicology and Carcinogenesis Studies of 1,4-Dichlorobenzene (CAS No. 106-46-7) in F 344/N Rats and B6C3F1 Mice (Gavage Studies). NIH Publication No. 86-2575, Department of Health and Human Services, Research Triangle Park, NC, 1986.

NTP Technical Report on the Carcinogenesis Bioassay of Pentachloroethane (CAS No. 76-01-7) in F 344/N Rats and B6C3F1 Mice (Gavage Studies) <u>NIH Publication No., 83-1788</u>, Department of Health and Human Services, Research Triangle Park, NC, 1983.

Thomas, F.B., Halder, C.A., Holdsworth, C.E. and Cockrell, B.Y. Hydrocarbon Nephropathy in Male Rats. Temporal and Morphological Characterization of the Renal Lesions. <u>In</u>: Monographs in Applied Toxicology. Renal Heterogeneity and Target Cell Toxicity. P.H. Bach and E.A. Lock (eds.). John Wiley & Sons, Chichester, (1985).

1,4-DICHLOROBENZENE-INDUCED NEPHROTOXICITY: SIMILARITY WITH UNLEADED GASOLINE (UG)-INDUCED RENAL EFFECTS

Michel Charbonneau, Josef Strasser, Edward A. Lock, Max J. Turner, and James A. Swenberg

Chemical Industry Institute of Toxicology, Department of Biochemical Toxicology and Pathobiology, P.O. Box 12137, Research Triangle Park, NC, U.S.A. 27709

INTRODUCTION

1,4-Dichlorobenzene (1,4-DCB) administered (150 or 300 mg/kg/day, po) 5 days per week for 104 weeks caused a dose-related increase in the incidence of renal adenomas and/or carcinomas in male rats, but not female F-344 rats or either sex of B6C3F1 mice (NTP, 1987). 1,2-Dichlorobenzene (1,2-DCB), an isomer of 1,4-DCB, caused no increase in the incidence of male rat renal tumours (NTP, 1985); the doses used were, however, 2.5 times lower than those employed for the 1,4-DCB study. Exposure to vapours of unleaded gasoline (UG) for 114 weeks also produced a dose-related increase in the incidence of renal adenomas and carcinomas in male, but not female F-344 rats or either sex of mice (Kitchen, 1984). The incidence of male rat renal tumours was dose-dependent but relatively low for both compounds. Assessment of the genotoxic properties of 1,4-DCB and UG by a battery of tests has shown that the chemicals are non-genotoxic. Our hypothesis to explain renal tumour formation is based on a multi-stage carcinogenesis model: Cells, in which spontaneous DNA alterations naturally occur, replicate following chemically-induced cell proliferation causing a mutated cell. Mutated cells undergo clonal expansion due to increased cell proliferation. This greatly increases the likelihood of additional spontaneous mutations occurring, leading to an increased incidence of renal cancer.

Acute or subchronic gavage or inhalation of UG or 2,2,4-trimethylpentane (TMP) increased cell proliferation and protein droplet formation in male but not female rats (Short et al., 1986, 1987). The increased renal cell proliferation is mainly localized to the P2 segment, the site where increased protein droplet formation is also primarily localized. Short et al. (1987) also reported that over a range of doses, increases in the mean score for droplets paralleled increases in cell proliferation. Immuno-histochemistry studies showed that protein droplets contain alpha-2u-globulin (alpha-2u), a low molecular weight protein produced by male but not female rats that is filtered at the glomerulus and partly reabsorbed and hydrolyzed by the P2 segment cells. 2,4,4-Trimethyl-2-pentanol has been shown to be reversibly bound to alpha-2u after TMP or UG administration to male rats (Lock et al., 1987). Our current hypothesis to explain the relationship between the renal accumulation of the metabolite-alpha-2u complex, protein droplet formation and cell proliferation proposes that the renal accumulation of this metabolite-protein complex disrupts lysosomes, and the release of lysosomal enzymes into the cells alters essential cell functions leading to cell death and compensatory cell proliferation. The present studies were undertaken to determine if acute exposure of 1,4-DCB causes a male rat-specific increase DCB or a metabolite reversibly binds to alpha-2u. 1,2-DCB was used as a negative control.

MATERIALS AND METHODS

Treatment of Animals. Sexually mature male (200-250 g) and female (175-200 g) F-344 rats were used after two weeks of quarantine. The animals were housed (21°C, 12-hour light/dark cycle) in polystyrene cages with stainless steel tops and runners. Rats were allowed access to food and water ad libitum.

1,4-DCB (99+%), 1,2-DCB (99.0%), [^{14}C]-1,4-DCB (>98%, 11 mCi/mmol) and [^{14}C]-1,2-DCB (>98%, 11 mCi/mmol) were obtained commercially. Animals were dosed by gavage (5 ml/kg) with a single dose of [^{14}C]-1,4 or 1,2-DCB in corn oil at 300 or 500 mg/kg (170 mCi/kg) or with 7 daily doses of 1,4-DCB or 1,2-DCB. Animals were killed 24 hr after dosing and 33% kidney and liver homogenates (67 mM phosphate buffer, pH 7.2) were prepared. Samples were fixed in 10% buffered formalin, embedded in glycol methacrylate, and 2mm sections were stained with Lee's methylene blue-basic fuchsin.

Protein Droplet Evaluation. Stained sections for 6 animals per group were examined by light microscopy without knowing from which group the tissues were derived; values represent the mean scores calculated from 3 analysts. The presence of protein droplets was assessed using a 0 to 4+ scoring scale; 1+: occasional droplets in some proximal tubules, 2+: a mild response with droplets in a large number of tubules; 3+: a moderate response with a more widespread cortical distribution and; 4+: an extensive response with widespread distribution in the cortex.

Cell Proliferation Evaluation. Alzet pumps [10 ml/hr, 7 days] filled with [^{3}H]-TdR (0.5 mCi/ml) were implanted s.c. on the back of 6 animals per group. Rats were dosed 1 hr after pump implantation and daily for the next 6 days, and were killed 24 hr after the last dose. Renal DNA was extracted (Schulte-Herman, 1977) and assayed (Burton, 1956 as modified by Richards, 1974).

Column Chromatography of Kidney and Liver Cytosol and Plasma. Samples of male rat kidney or liver cytosol were applied to a Sephadex G-75 column and eluted with 67 mM phosphate buffer, pH 7.2. The column was calibrated using bovine serum albumin (66,000 d), alpha-2u (19,000 d) and [^{3}H]-p-aminohippuric acid (194 g). The column eluate was monitored at 260 nm using a U.V. monitor and radioactivity measured in each fraction.

Isolation and Identification of Chemicals Bound to alpha-2u-Globulin. Kidney cytosol from 1,4- or 1,2-DCB-treated male rats was eluted on the Sephadex column, fractions 80 to 95 were pooled and lyophilised, and resuspended in distilled water. Chemicals in the reconsistuted fraction were extracted into ethyl acetate (pH < 1) and identified by electron-ionization mass spectra of the organic phase on a model 4500 gas chromatograph-mass spectrometer (Finnigan Corp., CA) fitted with a DB-5 fused silica capillary column (J and W Scientific, CA) inserted directly into the source.

Equilibrium Dialysis. Kidney or liver cytosol from male rats treated with [^{14}C]-1,4 or [^{14}C]-1,2-DCB was dialyzed (Sun and Dent, 1980) against 10 mM phosphate buffer [with or without 0.1% sodium dodecyl sulphate (SDS)] for 36 hr, using cellulose dialysis tubing (M.W. cutoff = 1000).

Aliquots of the dialyzed samples and dialysate were taken for determination of radioactivity.

Statistics. [^{3}H]-TdR incorporation into renal DNA was compared using a Newman-Keuls multiple range test. Scores for protein droplets were compared using a Kruskal-Wallis multiple comparison test. Percentages of radiolabel bound to male rat kidney or liver proteins were tested using Student's t-test. In all cases, the level of significance used was 0.05.

RESULTS AND DISCUSSION

The 7 daily doses of DCB administered to male rats for the protein droplet and cell proliferation studies corresponded to the high dose used in the 1,2-DCB (120 mg/kg) and 1,4-DCB (300 mg/kg) 2-year studies. Mean scores for droplets and [^{3}H]-Tdr incorporation into renal DNA, a biochemical measurement of cell proliferation, were significantly increased compared to control values for the 1,4-DCB- but not 1,2-DCB-treated rats (Table 1). TMP administered to male rats at a dose one-half the low dose of 1,4-DCB produced a mroe severe increase in protein droplet formation and cell proliferation. After a single oral dose (500 mg/kg), the mean scores for droplets were 1.2$\pm$0.1, 3.2$\pm$0.3, 1.6$\pm$0.2 and 3.4$\pm$0.1 for controls, 1,4-DCB-, 1,2-DCB- and TMP-treated rats, respectively. Female rats treated with 500 mg/kg 1,4-DCB, 1,2-DCB or TMP showed a mean score for droplets lower than 1.

Table 1 Protein droplets formation and [^{3}H]-TdR incorporation into male rat renal DNA following multiple doses of 1,4-DCB, 1,2-DCB or TMP.

Treatment	Mean Score for Droplets (1+ to 4+)	^{3}H-Tdr Incorporation (dpm/μg DNA)
Corn oil	1.0 ± 0.0[b]	94.3 ± 3.4[b]
1,4-DCB 120 mg/kg	2.2 ± 0.3[c]	138.5 ± 6.5[c]
1,4-DCB 300 mg/kg	3.5 ± 0.3[c]	159.2 ± 5.6[c]
1,2-DCB 120 mg/kg	1.6 ± 0.3	97.8 ± 8.2
1,2-DCB 300 mg/kg	1.8 ± 0.3	90.6 ± 4.3
TMP 50 mg/kg[d]	3.1 ± 0.2[c]	192.5 ± 0.2[c]

[a] Rats were dosed with one of the chemicals (5 ml in corn oil) every morning for 7 days, and were killed 24 hr after the last dose.

[b] Results are mean ± SEM for 6 rats.

[c] Significantly different from control (p<0.05).

[d] 50 mg/kg TMP is equal to 0.44 mmol/kg, whereas 120 and 300 mg/kg 1,4- or 1,2-DCB are equal to 0.82 and 2.04 mmol/kg, respectively.

The precentage of kidney DCB equivalent in cytosol was similar for both isomers (3.4 mmol/kg; 49.8 and 55.9% for 1,4- and 1,2-DCB, respectively) and was similar to that observed for TMP-treated rats (4.4 mmol/kg; 60%). The cytosolic fraction prepared from male rat kidney had a high content of alpha-2u. Thus, a reversible association between a 1,4- or 1,2-DCB derived chemical and alpha-2u similar to that reported for TMP was investigated. Gel filtration of male rat kidney cytosol showed that radiolabel derived from [^{14}C]-1,4-DCB or [^{14}C]-1,2-DCB co-eluted with alpha-2u. The following ranking order was observed for the percentage of radiolabel co-eluting with alpha-2u-globulin: TMP > 1,4-DCB > 1,2-DCB (Table 2).

Equilibrium dialysis of male rat kidney cytolsol against buffer containing

0.1% SDS led to an additional loss of a substantial amount of chemical compared with dialysis against buffer without SDS (Table 3). SDS is a detergent which destroys the secondary and tertiary structures of proteins; chemicals bound to the protein via weak forces (e.g. hydrogen bonds) will be dissociated from it and released into the dialysis buffer upon addition of SDS. Thus, as was the case for TMP, our findings indicated a reversible association between 1,4-DCB- or 1,2-DCB-derived radiolabel and alpha-2u. Co-elution of radiolabel with alpha-2u remained after dialysis against buffer without SDS. 1,2-DCB has been shown to bind covalently to kidney proteins (NTP, 1985); our results are in agreement with this observation since after dialysis against buffer containing SDS a relatively high percentage of 1,2-DCB equivalent remained bound (Table 3). In addition, radiolabel from 1,2-DCB, but not 1,4-DCB, co-eluted with high molecular weight liver proteins, and dialysis in the presence or absence of SDS showed that the radiolabel was covalently bound to the liver macromolecules [(-SDS): 39,5$\pm$5.1%, (+SDS): 40.8$\pm$5.9%, p > 0.05].

Analysis of extracts from kidney cytosol prepared from rats treated with 0.5 or 1.0 g/kg 1,4-DCB showed that 2,5-dichlorophenol and 1,4-DCB were bound to alpha-2u, whereas analysis of an extract from kidney cytosol prepared from 2.0 g/kg 1,2-DCB-treated rats showed that only 1,2-DCB was present. Space-filling models for 2,5-dichlorophenol, 2,4,4-trimethyl-2-pentanol and 1,2-DCB showed that although the DCBs and the TMP metabolite are not structurally related, their 3-dimensional arrangement has similarity. Three common features were observed:-

1) A bulky and similarly oriented lipophilic group (bulkier in the TMP metabolite which forms a stronger association with alpha-2u than 1,4-DCB metabolite);

2) A hydrogen available to form a hydrogen bond with an acceptor on the protein;

3) In 2,5-dichlorophenol, 2,4,4-trimethyl-2-pentanol an oxygen available to form a hydrogen bond with a donor on the protein. 1,2-DCB possesses only two of these components and is only loosely associated with alpha-2u-globulin; the same is probable for 1,4-DCB.

Table 2   Radiolabel in renal cytosol prepared from male rats treated with [^{14}C]-1,4-DCB, [^{14}C]-1,2-DCB or [^{3}H]-TMP.

Isomer	Radiolabel co-eluting with α_{2u}-globulin (nmol equiv.)	Total Radiolabel recovered from elution of 1 ml of kidney cytosol (nmol equiv.)	% Radiolabel co-eluting with α_{2u}-globulin
1,4-DCB 300mg/kg	10.2 ± 0.8 [b]	76.1 ± 8.6	13.6 ± 0.6
1,4-DCB 500 mg/kg	33.5 ± 9.4	244.5 ± 46.8	14.5 ± 4.6
1,2-DCB 300mg/kg	10.5 ± 2.7	119.3 ± 13.0	8.7 ± 1.6
1,2-DCB 500mg/kg	21.4 ± 2.6	252.1 ± 34.0	8.7 ± 0.9
TMP 500 mg/kg [c]	134.9 ± 8.5	575.3 ± 48.6	24.8 ± 1.6

[a] Rats were treated orally (5 ml/kg in corn oil) with the radiolabel chemicals and were killed 24 hr later.

[b] Results are mean ± SEM for 3 animals/group.

[c] 500 mg/kg TMP is equal to 4.4 mmol/kg, whereas 500 mg/kg 1,4-DCB or 1,2-DCB is equal to 3.4 mmol/kg.

Table 3 The effect of dialysis in the presence and absence of SDS on the binding of radiolabel from $[^{14}C]$-1,4-DCB, $[^{14}C]$-1,2-DCB or $[^3H]$-TMP to male rat kidney cytosol.

Treatment	Dialysis Buffer[b]	Radiolabeled material associated with kidney cytosol (nmol equiv.)		% Bound
		Before dialysis	After dialysis	
1,4-DCB	- SDS	147.9 ± 45.1[c]	26.2 ± 4.3	19.4 ± 3.3
1,4-DCB	+ SDS	147.9 ± 45.1	4.7 ± 0.8	3.4 ± 0.6[d]
1,2-DCB	- SDS	241.0 ± 22.7	40.2 ± 3.1	16.7 ± 0.3
1,2-DCB	+ SDS	241.0 ± 22.7	18.7 ± 4.2	7.6 ± 2.2[d]
TMP[e]	- SDS	400.8 ± 78.2	69.6 ± 11.6	19.3 ± 2.4
TMP[e]	+ SDS	400.8 ± 78.2	6.8 ± 2.4	1.6 ± 0.4

[a] Male rats were dosed orally (5 ml/kg) with $[^{14}C]$-1,4-DCB, $[^{14}C]$-1,2-DCB [500 mg/kg (3.4 mmol/kg); 170 μCi/kg in corn oil, or $[^3H]$-TMP [500 mg/kg (4.4 mmol/kg); 230 μCi/kg in corn oil. The animals were killed 24 hr after dosing, their kidneys removed and homogenized, and the cytosol prepared as described in Methods.

[b] Samples (1 ml) were dialyzed for 18 hr against 10 mM phosphate buffer (pH 7.2) in the presence or absence of 0.1% SDS and the amount of radiolabeled material remaining determined as described in Methods.

[c] Results are the mean ± SEM of cytosols from 3 separate animals.

[d] Significantly different from data for the sample dialyzed in buffer without SDS.

[e] Results are reprinted from Lock et al. (1987).

In summary, similarities between 1,4-DCB- and UG-induced nephrotoxicity consist of a male rat-specific increase in the incidence of renal tumours following chronic exposure, a male rat-specific increased protein droplet formation, cell proliferation and reversible binding of the chemical or a metabolite to alpha-2u following acute exposure (using TMP as a model comound for UG). However, 1,2-DCB did not produce male rat-specific renal tumours, increased protein droplet formation, or cell proliferation, but did bind to alpha-2u. The extent of binding was less than that for 1,4-DCB and was not totally reversible. 1,2-DCB also showed a greater potential for covalent binding to macromolecules. Thus, at equimolar doses 1,4-DCB- and 1,2-DCB-induced renal effects are dissimilar.

REFERENCES

BURTON, K. (1956). A study of the conditions and mechanism of the diphenylamine reaction for the colorimetric estimation of deoxyibonucleic acid. Biochemistry 62, 315-322.

KITCHEN, D.N. (1984). Neoplastic renal effects of unleaded gasoline in Fischer 344 rats. In: Renal effects of petroleum hydrocarbons (M.A. Mehlman, C.P. Hemstreet, J.J. Thorpe, N.K. Weaver, eds.), Advances in modern environmental toxicology, Vol. VII, pp. 65-71, Princeton Scientific Publishers, Inc., Princeton, New Jersey.

LOCK, E.A., CHARBONNEAU, M., STRASSER, J., SWENBERG, J.A., AND BUS, J.S. (1987). 2,2,4-Trimethylpentane (TMP)-induced nephrotoxicity. II- The reversible binding of a TMP metabolite to a renal protein fraction containg alpha-2u-globulin. Toxicol. Appl. Pharmacol 91, 182-192.

NATIONAL TOXICOLOGY PROGRAM (NTP) (1985). Toxicology and carcinogenesis studies of 1,2-dichlorobenzene in F344/N rats and B6C3F1 mice. NTP TR 255. U.S. Department of Health and Human Services, Public Health Service, National Institutes of Health.

NATIONAL TOXICOLOGY PROGRAM (NTP) (1987). Toxicology and carcinogenesis studies of 1,4-dichlorobenzene in F344/N rats and B6C3F1 mice. NTP TR 319. U.S. Department of Health and Human Services, Public Health Service, National Institutes of Health.

RICHARDS, G.M. (1974). Modifications of the diphenylamine reaction giving increased sensitivity in the estimation of DNA. Anal. Biochem. 57, 369-376.

SCHULTE-HERMANN, R. (1977). Two-stage control of cell proliferation induced in rat liver by alpha-hexachlorocyclohexane. Cancer. Res. 37. 166-171.

SHORT, B.G., BURNETT, V.L., AND SWENBERG, J.A. (1986). Histopathology and cell proliferation induced by 2,2,4-trimethylpentane in the male rat kidney. Toxicol. Pathol. 14, 194-203.

SHORT, B.G., BURNETT, V.L., COX, M.G. BUS, J.S., AND SWENBERG, J.A. (1987). Site specific renal cytotoxicity and cell proliferation in male rats exposed to petroleum hydrocarbons. Lab. Invest. 57, 564-577.

SUN, J.D. AND DENT, J.G. (1980). A new method for measuring covalent binding of chemicals to cellular macromolecules. Chem.-Biol. Interac. 32, 41-61.

COMPARISON OF THE SUBACUTE NEPHROTOXICITY OF INDUSTRIAL SOLVENTS IN THE RAT

Alfred Bernard, Raphaella de Russis, Jean-Claude Normand and Robert Lauwerys

Unite de Toxicologie Industrielle et Medecine du Travail Universite Catholique de Louvain Clos Chapelle-aux-Champs 30.54 B-1200 Brussels, Belgium

INTRODUCTION

The question whether chronic exposure of low or moderate intensity to nonsubstituted organic solvents can lead to some types of renal diseases is still open. Most of the experimental work carried out so far to address this problem (1-7) report effects occurring only in male rats, which presumably are irrelevant for the human situation. None of these studies have compared the nephrotoxicity of the solvents commonly used in industry using quantitative indicators of renal damage to help identify the potentially most nephrotoxic solvents. To fill this gap, we have compared the effects on the urinary excretion of albumin, ß2-microglobulin (ß2-m) and ß-N-acetylglucosaminidase of the most widely used industrial solvents when subacutely administered to female Sprague-Dawley rats.

MATERIALS AND METHODS

Female Sprague-Dawley rats, 2 to 4 months old, weighing 150-250 g were used for all experiments. Rats were injected intraperitoneally, 5 times per week, for two weeks with the solvents dispersed in olive oil or water. Control rats were injected with olive oil only (2.5 ml/kg). The urinary concentration of albumin and, ß2-m was determined by an automated immunoassay based on latex particle agglutination (8). The activity in urine of ß-N-acetylglucosaminidase was assayed by the method of Tucker et al (9). The glomerular filtration rate (GFR) and the renal plasma flow (RPF) were estimated simultaneously from the clearance of ^{51}Cr-EDTA and ^{121}I-iodohippurate respectively (10). The kidney concentrating ability was determined by measuring the osmolality of urine (Wescor vapour pressure osmometer, Logan UT) collected during 8 hours following a 24-hour water deprivation period (food ad libitum). The concentrations of cyclohexanol and cyclohexanone in rat urine were determined by gas chromatography according to the method of Perbellini and Brugnone (11). The difference between the groups were assessed by one-way analysis of variance followed by Dunett's multiple comparison test with $p < 0.05$ considered as statistically significant. For the urinary excretion of albumin and ß2-m, the statistical analysis was performed on log transformed data.

RESULTS AND DISCUSSION

In a first series of experiments we compared the subacute nephrotoxicity of 17 industrial solvents administered to rats at doses approximately equitoxic in terms of the LD50. The only significant effect observed under these conditions is an increased urinary excretion of ß2-m in rats challenged with cyclohexane (Table 1). None of the solvents affected the urinary excretion of albumin or ß-N-acetylglucosaminidase (results not shown).

Table I. Urinary excretion of ß-N-acetylglucosaminidase, ß2-microglobulin and albumin in female rats given repeated intraperitoneal injections of several industrial solvents.

Solvent [a]	Dose [b]		ß2-microglobulin
		% of	
	g/Kg	oral LD	(ug/24 h)
Controls (oil)			2.29±0.42 [c]
Ethylene glycol monomethyl ether (EGME)	0.4	25	4.81±0.51
Ethylene glycol mono-n-butyl ether (EGBE)	0.055	10 [d]	1.87±0.33
Dipropylene glycol mono-methyl ether (DPGME)	1	20	2.22±0.29
Controls (oil)			3.57±0.86
n-Hexane	1	10 [d]	3.32±0.20
Ethylbenzene	0.35	10	3.51±1
Trichloroethylene	0.5	10	2.12±0.54
Tetrachloroethylene	1	9	3.02±0.64
Cyclohexane	1.5	5	24.8±10 *
Methanol	1	7.7	2.19±0.17
Styrene	0.5	10 [d]	5.09±1.39
1,1,1-Trichloroethane	0.5	10	4.3 ±1.7
Controls (oil)			2.19±0.30
m-xylene	0.5	10	1.95±0.15
2-nitropropane	0.01	10	1.97±0.46
2-butanone	0.34	10	2.13±0.40
Isophorone	0.23	10	2.35±0.46
Furfural	0.013	10	2.66±0.31
1,2-dibromoethane	0.011	10	2.24±0.27

a   5 animals per group
b   five i.p. injections per week for 2 weeks
c   mean ± SE
d   i.p. LD50
*   significantly different from control value

Since in this experiment the dose of cyclohexane administered to rats was higher than that of other solvents, another experiment was performed to compare the subacute nephrotoxicity of cyclohexane with that of other solvents administered at the same dose. Rats were repeatedly injected i.p. With 1 g/kg of cyclohexane, toluene, styrene or trichloroethylene. Xylene and ethylbenzene were also administered, but at the dose of 0.75 g/kg which was the highest dose the animals could tolerate. As shown in Table II, under these conditions styrene was the most tubulotoxic producing on the average a 7-fold increase of ß2-globulinuria against a 3.2-fold increase for cyclohexane. Because of the great scatter of the results, the latter effect was not statistically significant. The other solvents tested at the 1 g/kg dose (i.e. toluene, trichloroethylene, tetrachloroethylene, dipropylene glycol monomethylether, n-hexane and methanol) did not affect the ß2-m excretion (Tables I and II).

Table II. Subacute nephrotoxicity of selected industrial solvents in female rats

	Dose[a] % of the oral (g/Kg)	LD50	ß2-microglobulinuria (ug/24 h)
Controls			1.71 (0.55 - 2.92)[b]
Cyclohexane	1	3.33	5.50 (1 - 40)
Toluene	1	20	3.31 (1.3 - 7.1)
Styrene	1	20	11.9 (2.44 - 134)*
Trichoroethylene	1	20	2.47 (0.94 - 6.71)
Xylene	0.75[c]	15	2.10 (1.23 - 5.60)
Ethylbenzene	0.75[c]	20	3.04 (1.48 - 3.5)

a five i.p. injections per week for 2 weeks
b geometric mean (range) of 5 animals
c the highest dose the animals could tolerate in this experiment
* significantly different from control value.

As cyclohexane is a widely used industrial solvent with a threshold limit value higher than that of styrene (300 vs 50 ppm), we have carried out several experiments in order to characterize its subacute tubulotoxicity. Fig. 1 shows the time course of the urinary excretion of ß2-m in female rats repeatedly injected i.p. with cyclohexane (0.375, 0.75 or 1.5 g/kg) or cyclohexanol (0.4 g/kg), the main urinary metabolite of cyclohexane. The increase of ß2-microglobulinuria caused by cyclohexane is both dose- and time-dependent. It is of interest to note that cyclohexanol causes a ß2-microglobulinuria pattern very similar to that of cyclohexane, which suggests that cyclohexanol is the metabolite responsible for the nephro- toxicity of cyclohexane. The examination of the renal function of these animals at the end of the treatment disclosed no change in the GFR, the RPF or in the relative kidney weight. The renal concentrating ability (urinary osmolality, mmoles/kg), however, was significantly depressed in rats treated with 1.5 g/kg of cyclohexane (mean $\pm$ SE: 1283 $\pm$ 180) or with 0.4 g/kg (1120 $\pm$ 141) of cyclohexanol compared to controls 1870 $\pm$ 112) (n = 5 in each group).

We have also examined the effect on ß2-m excretion of three other metabolites which may be formed during exposure to cyclohexane: cyclohexanone, 1,4-cyclohexanediol and 1,4-cyclohexanedione. Administered i.p. at the dose of 0.5 g/kg daily, these compounds caused no change in ß2-m excretion, which thus reinforces our hypothesis that the nephrotoxicity of cyclohexane is due to cyclohexanol. The cyclic character of cyclohexane seems to be an important determinant in the nephrotoxicity of this solvent. No sign of tubulotoxicity was found when saturated unsubstituted C_6 hydrocarbons such n-hexane, 2- or 3-methylpentane were subacutely administered to female rat.

The finding that the subacute nephrotoxicity of cyclohexane is greater than that of most industrial solvents, was rather unexpected. It remains to assess whether these observations are relevant for human populations chronically exposed to this solvent. To our knowledge, the only epidemiological study which has been carried out on workers exposed to cyclohexane is that of Mutti et al (13). These authors have examined shoe factory workers exposed to C_5-C_7 hydrocarbon mixtures, mainly to n-hexane and cyclohexane. The TLV for the mixture was exceeded in most workplaces. Total protein excretion was significantly increased in exposed workers. The albuminuria of these workers was not increased but several of them presented with elevated values of lysozyme and ß-glucuronidase in urine.

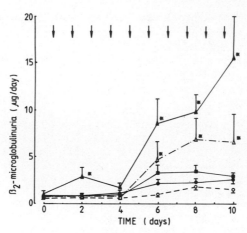

Fig. 1. Time course of urinary ß2-microglobulin in rats given repeated i.p. injections of cyclohexane (●, 0.375; ■, 0.75 and ,▲ 1.5 g/kg) or cyclohexanol (△, 0.4 g/kg) and in controls (○). The arrows represent the time of injection. mean ± SE of 5 animals. * p < 0.05.

The authors concluded that exposure to C_5-C_7 hydrocarbon mixtures may lead to a mild tubular damage. These observations are consistent with the present experimental data.

ACKNOWLEDGEMENTS

We gratefully acknowledge X. Dumont and M. Dasnoy for their technical assistance. At the time of the study R. de Russis was research fellow of the University of Bari, ltaly while J.C. Normand was research fellow of the University Claude Bernard Lyon 1, France. A. Bernard is Research Associate of the Belgian Fund for Scientific Research.

REFERENCES

1. R.D. Phillips, B.Y. Cockrell, Kidney structural changes in rats following inhalation exposure to C^{10}-C^{11} isoparaffinic solvent, Toxicology, 33:261 (1984)

2. C. Viau, A. Bernard, F. Gueret, P. Maidague, P. Gengoux, and R. Lauwerys, isoparaffinic solvent-induced nephrotoxicity in the rat, Toxicology 38:227 (1986).

3. M. D. Stonard, J. R. Foster, M. G. Simpson, and E. A. Lock, Alpha-2u-globulin: measurement in rat kidney following administration of 2,2,4-trimethylpentane, Toxicology 4:161 (1986).

4. C.L. Alden, R.L. Kanerva, G. Ridder, and L.C. Stone, The pathogenesis of the nephrotoxicity of volatile hydrocarbons in the male rat, In: "Advances in Modern Environmental Toxicology", vol. VII, M.A. Mehlman, ed., Princeton Scientific Publishers, Princeton (1984).

5. C.A. Halder, C.E. Holdsworth, and B.Y. Cockrell, Hydrocarbon nephropathy in male rats. Identification of the nephrotoxic component of gasoline, In: "Renal heterogeneity and target cell toxicity", P.H. Bach and E.A. Lock, ed., John Wiley & Sons, Chichester (1985).

6. M.D. Stonard, P.G. Phillips, J.R. Foster, M.G. Simpson and E.A. Lock, alpha-2u-globulin: measurement in rat kidney following administration of 2,2,4-trimethylpentane, Toxicology 41:161 (1986).

7. S.K. Chakrabarti, L. Labelle, and B. Tuchweber, Studies on the subchronic nephrotoxic potential of styrene in Sprague-Dawley rats, Toxicology 44:355 (1987).

8. A. Bernard, and R. Lauwerys, Continuous flow system for automation of latex immunoassay, Clin. Chem. 29:1007 (1983).

9. S.M. Tucker, P.J. Boyd, A.E. Thompson, and R.G. Price, Automated assay of N-acetyl-ß-glucosaminidase in normal and pathological urine, Clin. Chim. Acta 62:333 (1973).

10. A.P. Provoost, M.H. de Keijzer, E.D. Wolff and J.C. Molenaar, Development of renal function in the rat. The measurement of GFR and ERPF and correlation to body and kidney weight, Renal Physiol. 6:1 (1971).

NEPHROTOXIC RESPONSES TO MULTIPLE CHEMICAL EXPOSURE

William O. Berndt

University of Nebraska Medical Center, Department of Pharmacology, Omaha, Nebraska 68105, USA

INTRODUCTION

Contemporaneous exposure to more than one chemical represents a practical toxicological problem. The scientific community has long examined the effects of various single toxic agents on renal function in well-controlled laboratory experiments. These studies have given us insights into tubular sites of action of specific chemicals, mechanisms of actions (at least in some instances) and an understanding of the breadth of chemical substances which can produce damage to the kidney. Taken together, these investigations have been extremely valuable in describing, and provided part of the basis for an understanding of the chemically-induced nephrotoxic response resulting in acute renal failure. Perhaps most noteworthy are studies on the heavy metals, but a variety of organic compounds have also been studied almost as thoroughly. None of these studies, however, no matter how carefully conceived and conducted help the toxicologist address the "real world" problem. In fact, human exposure to toxic chemicals rarely occurs with a single substance, but rather to multiple substances. This is true with environmental exposures as well as those encountered in the industrial setting. Although these circumstances are obvious and well recognized, relatively few studies have been under-taken in the laboratory setting to examine the possibility that interactive effects may occur with multiple exposure to chemicals and that such interactions might lead to results which would not be predicted from the effects of the individual chemical substances.

The studies summarized below were not designed to mimic the "real life" situation for exposure to these or any other combination of chemical substances. Rather, the experiments were designed to test the hypothesis that exposure of animals in the laboratory setting to two nephrotoxicants simultaneously might lead to effects on renal function that could not be predicted from the individual actions of the test compounds. The substances· studied in these experiments all have nephrotoxic potential: mercuric chloride, potassium dichromate, citrinin, and hexachloro-1,3-butadiene (HCBD). The dose of dichromate selected for these studies was one which showed only minimal effects in these experimental protocols. The other compounds were tested with multiple doses, at least some of which were significantly nephrotoxic. Some of the results of these experiments have been published in detail, and the interested reader is referred to those articles (Baggett and Berndt 1984a,b, 1985, 1986; Haberman et al., 1987; Jensen and Berndt 1986).

METHODS

Standard procedures for the assessment of the actions of xenobiotics on renal function were used in all of these studies and are described briefly below. Details are presented in the published literature (see above). Male, Sprague-Dawley rats (200-250g) were housed individually in stainless steel metabolism cages. Urine samples were collected at 24-hr intervals and analysed for various chemicals useful for the assessment of renal function. At the termination of the experiments, rats were killed and blood and tissue samples removed for various chemical and biochemical analyses. In some experiments, kidneys were removed after appropriate periods of pre-treatment, renal slices prepared free hand from the cortices and were used to determine the accumulation of an organic anion, p-aminohippurate (PAH), and an organic cation, tetraethylammonium (TEA). In each instance, the ^{14}C-labelled compound was used to monitor uptake during an incubation of 90-120 min in a Dubnoff shaker under an oxygen atmosphere. The accumulation data are expressed as the slice-to-medium ratio (S/M ratio), i.e., the radio-activity per gram of tissue divided by the radioactivity per ml of bathing solution. For the preparation of isolated membrane vesicles, the method of Boumendil-Podevin and Podevin (1983) was used after modifications to make the technique more suitable for rat tissue. This permitted the preparation of both basolateral and brush border membranes from a single Percoll centrifugation of a crude membrane preparation. The extent of membrane separation was established by appropriate enzyme analyses. The isolated membranes were used either immediately or frozen for no longer than 72 hr before use. PAH transport by the basolateral membrane vesicles was accomplished by the rapid filtration technique after exposure of the membranes to mercuric chloride, potassium dichromate, or both metals for 15-30 min. For all pretreatment experiments, mercuric chloride was administered subcutaneously (sc) as was potassium dichromate. Citrinin and HCBD were administered intraperitoneally. Appropriate statistical tests were applied, usually the Analysis of Variance with the difference between the means assessed by the Student-Newman-Keuls. Differences were taken as significant if $P < 0.05$.

RESULTS AND DISCUSSION

The first part of the data relates to experiments designed to examine potential interaction of mercuric chloride and potassium dichromate on renal function in the rat. The data in Table 1 were obtained from animals treated with the test compounds either individually or together. The animals were treated on day 0 and the average control value for all groups before treatment was 11.0 ml/24 hr $\pm$ 3.5. Except for the group treated with the combination of agents, the urine volumes on day one were similar to those of the control day. The data for the combination group was significantly different on day 1 and on day 2 from all other groups. No data are presented for the combination group for day 4 since all animals succumbed. The data in Table 2 are from the same experiments as in Table 1 and highlight effects of the individual nephrotoxicants and their combination on potassium concentration in the urine. As with urine volume changes, the effects produced on potassium excretion by the combination of mercuric chloride and potassium dichromate were significantly different from all other groups on at least 2 of the 4 experimental days. In each instance, these results represent a potentiation of the mercuric chloride effect in that the effects produced by the combination of metals was always greater than the sum of the individual effects.

TABLE 1. Effect of $HgCl_2$, $K_2Cr_2O_7$ and the Combination on Urine Flow in the Rat

Values as ml/24 hr $\pm$ SE for N=4

Days after treatment	1	2	3	4
Control	12.2	9.5	9.9	10.1
	±20	±2.5	±1.5	±1.0
$HgCl_2$ (4mg/kg)	14.5	11.8	15.0	17.0
	±2.0	±2.5	±4.0	±4.0
(10mg/kg)	±1.5	±2.0	±1.3	±2.0
Combination	18.5*	2.1*	9.5	--
	±2.0	±1.0	±3.5	

*Values significantly different from all other values on the same day.

TABLE 2. Effect of $HgCl_2$, $K_2Cr_2O_7$ and the Combination on Potassium Concentration in the Urine of Rats

	Values are mEq/l $\pm$ SE for N=4			
Days after treatment	1	2	3	4
Control	98.5	120	125	155
	±10	±11.5	±13	±16.5
$HgCl_2$ (4mg/kg)	120	91	58	56
	±13.5	±12	±9.5	±10
$K_2Cr_2O_7$ (10mg/kg)	130	96	105	140
	±12	±10	±9.5	±18
Combination	50*	45*	35	--
	±4.5	±6.0	±6.0	

*Values significantly different from all other values on the same day.

Not all renal function parameters responded with a potentiation. For example, blood urea nitrogen (BUN) increased about 7-fold 24 hr after a single 4 mg/kg dose of mercuric chloride. Potassium dichromate (10 mg/kg) produced no increase in BUN at 24 hr. The combination of metals produced a response identical to that of mercuric chloride alone. That is, the response to the combination was additive.

The ability of dichromate to potentiate mercuric chloride was seen more readily in the renal slice studies. For these experiments, rats were pre-treated 24 hr before the slice study was conducted. The data in Table 3 are from some of those experiments. Although in these experiments no statistically significant effects were observed on the accumulation of PAH (with or without lactate) after pretreatment with mercuric chloride or significantly reduced the accumulation of PAH in the presence of lactate. As with the accumulation of TEA by the renal cortical slices, the effect on PAH in the presence of lactate was significantly different than all other groups. Hence, these data represent a potentiation of potassium dichromate on mercuric chloride effects on organic ion transport, effects similar to that seen on whole animal renal function given above.

TABLE 3. Effect of HgCl$_2$, K$_2$Cr$_2$O$_7$ and the Combination on Organic Ion Accumulation by Renal Cortical Slices

Values are S/M ratios ±SE for N=4

	Control	K$_2$Cr$_2$O$_7$ mg/kg	HgCl$_2$ mg/kg		Hg+Cr mg/kg	
	0	10	3	5	3/10	5/10
PAH	3.0 ±0.2	3.7 ±0.5	4.1 ±0.5	3.3 ±0.8	3.2 ±0.8	2.7 ±0.6
PAH (+ lactate)	6.8 ±0.3	6.0 ±0.4	8.1 ±0.7	5.1 ±0.6	3.0* ±0.2	2.4* ±0.3
TEA	11.5 ±0.3	12.1 ±0.4	11.9 ±0.3	10.2 ±0.6	5.7* ±0.3	5.4* ±0.5

*Indicates values statistically different from control, chromate alone, and mercuric chloride alone. Experiments were performed 24 hr after pretreatment.

It was of interest to know whether or not the effect of mercuric ion and dichromate on organic ion transport could be observed under strictly in vitro conditions. To study this possibility, renal cortical slices were prepared from healthy, non-pretreated rats, and the metal ions were added directly to the incubation media, either alone or in combination. As can be seen in Table 4, at the concentrations used in this study, the metal ions alone had little or no effect on PAH uptake by the slices. However, when mercuric chloride and potassium dichromate were added together a statistically significant reduction in PAH accumulation was observed. The magnitude of this response was far less than that observed in slices from pretreated rats. Nonetheless, a significant effect was observed and this may be important in helping understand the underlying mechanisms of the enhanced nephrotoxicity.

TABLE 4. Effect of HgCl$_2$, K$_2$Cr$_2$O$_7$ and the combination on PAH accumulation by renal cortical slices

Values are S/M ratios ± SE for N=3

Control	17.1 ± 0.8
K$_2$Cr$_2$O$_7$, 10^{-5}M	16.0 ± 1.0
HgCl$_2$, 5×10^{-6}M	15.9 ± 1.8
10^{-5}M	15.4 ± 1.1
K$_2$Cr$_2$O$_7$, 10^{-5}M plus HgCl$_2$ 5×10^{-6}M	11.6 ± 1.0*
K$_2$Cr$_2$O$_7$, 10^{-5}M plus HgCl$_2$ 10^{-5}M	12.1 ± 0.8*

*Indicates values significantly different from control, chromate alone and mercuric chloride alone.

Several studies have been undertaken to examine possible mechanisms by which chromate might enhance mercuric chloride-induced nephrotoxicity. Various experimental protocols designed to examine kinetic factors which might alter the effect of mercuric chloride have proven negative. For example, there was no effect of chromate to alter mercuric ion delivery to the kidney (i.e., no change in renal blood flow), and there was no alteration in the accumulation of mercuric ion by renal tissue as assessed by ^{203}Hg accumulation, after chromate administration. Similarly, distribution of ^{203}Hg to other organs was unaffected. ^{203}Hg-Mercuric chloride excretion after the administration of potassium dichromate was the same as in the absence of chromate over the first 36 hr after treatment. Further, the subcellular distribution of mercuric ion and its binding to metallothionein were unaltered by chromate whether added to fresh renal cortex slices in vitro or administered to rats in a pretreatment protocol. These data suggest that simple kinetic factors do not underlie the dichromate-enhancement of the nephrotoxic response observed with mercuric chloride, at least with respect to target organ distribution or relocation within the target organ.

Since the renal plasma membrane of the tubular cells may contact mercuric chloride and/or potassium dichromate earlier than other cellular organelles, experiments were undertaken to examine the possible interaction of these metal ions on cell membrane function. Furthermore, data in the literature indicate that membrane disruption may be involved both with mercuric chloride and dichromate (Gritzka and Trump, 1968; Evan and Dial, 1974; Ganote et al., 1975; Kempson et al., 1977; Carmichael and Fowler, 1980). These studies suggested that the renal tubular membrane may be a primary site of action, and demonstrated the sensitivity of membrane response to these metals. For the cell membrane experiments, basolateral membranes were separated from those of the brush border in a crude membrane preparation of renal cortex by Percoll gradient centrifugation. The separation was undertaken with an appropriate modification of the Percoll concentration to adapt this procedure for use with rat tissue. The basolateral membrane vesicles were used to assess the transport of PAH in the presence and absence of mercuric chloride, potassium dichromate, or the combination of the two metals. The data in Table 5 are from those experiments wherein the metals were added directly to the freshly prepared vesicles. Low concentrations of the metal ions added individually for 15-30 min to the vesicles before the conduct of a rapid filtration experiment showed no effect on PAH uptake. Indeed, the individual metal ions had no effect on PAH transport in concentrations up to 10^{-5}M. However, when the two metal ions were added together at the same concentrations (10^{-9}M each) a marked reduction in the accumulation of PAH was observed at the two earlier time points. PAH transport reached equilibrium at the same time in the treated as in control vesicles despite the inhibition of transport at the earlier time points. These data suggest that the plasma membrane may be a site for the interaction of these metal ions and might be the preliminary step which leads to overall renal dysfunction and an ultimately enhanced acute renal failure.

TABLE 5. Effects of $Cr_2O_7{}^{2-}$ and Hg^{2+} on basolateral PAH transport

Concentration (moles/litre)		% of Equilibrium Value		
$Cr_2O_7{}^{2-}$	Hg^{2+}	15 sec.	30 sec.	60 sec.
0	0	55 ± 1.5	65 ± 0	78 ± 1.7
10^{-9}	0	50.3 ± 2.0	66.7 ± 6.8	79 ± 6.1
0	10^{-9}	59 ± 5.1	70.2 ± 5.3	77 ± 3.5
10^{-9}	10^{-9}	36.6 ± 0.9*	51.3 ± 0.9*	64 ± 3.7

*Significantly different from other values at same time.

It has also been possible to demonstrate interesting interactions of potassium dichromate with various organic compounds. In Table 6 are data which demonstrate an interaction of citrinin and dichromate on the renal slice accumulation of tetraethylammonium. For these experiments, rats were pretreated 24 hr before the experiment with the doses indicated. Only minimal effects of citrinin or dichromate alone were observed on TEA accumulation by the slices. However, when the combination of citrinin and dichromate were used in the pretreatment protocol, a significant reduction in the accumulation of TEA was observed. In each instance, the response seen with the combination was significantly greater than the sum of the individual effects again suggesting that a potentiation has occurred. A similar potentiated response of citrinin was observed on overall renal function, specifically with respect to urine flow and glucose excretion. HCBD is a well-known nephrotoxicant.

TABLE 6. Effect of Citrinin $K_2Cr_2O_7$ and the Combination on TEA Accumulation by Renal Cortical Slices

Values are S/M ratios $\pm$ SE for N=4

	S/M Ratio $\pm$ SE
Control	14.0 $\pm$ 1.0
$K_2Cr_2O_7$ (10 mg/kg)	13.7 $\pm$ 0.6
Citrinin 35 mg/kg	11.8 $\pm$ 3.4
55 mg/kg	11.0 $\pm$ 3.0
Citrinin (35) + $K_2Cr_2O_7$	5.1 $\pm$ 0.4*
Citrinin (55) + $K_2Cr_2O_7$	3.0 $\pm$ 0.1*

*Values significantly different from respective individual values.

The data presented in Figure 1 demonstrate that potassium dichromate may interact with HCBD to produce an effect which is greater than that anticipated from the sum of the individual actions. The data are for urine glucose concentration on a enhancement of glucose excretion was observed. Again, these data suggest that a potentiated response is observed in the presence of both compounds, a response not seen with either agent alone.

The ability of agents to interact to produce an enhanced response are not confined simply to interactions with metals. The data presented in Table 7 are from experiments where the effects of HCBD were examined on renal slice accumulation of TEA both in the presence and absence of the sulphydryl depletor, diethylmaleate (DEM). Neither DEM nor HCBD alone significantly reduced TEA transport. Indeed, the lack of an effect on TEA accumulation by slices has been uniformly reported by several laboratories. When the combination of DEM and HCBD were studied, however, a dramatic reduction in TEA accumulation was observed. This effect is most noteworthy since, as indicated above, the general consensus has been that HCBD fails to affect TEA movement by renal slices at any dose.

The data presented here are given as an example of interactive effects of nephrotoxicants which can be studied in the laboratory setting. The experiments were designed to test the hypothesis that the combinations of chemicals might produce responses which could not be predicted from the actions of the individual chemicals. The interactions appear to be wide

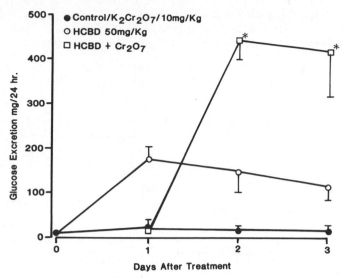

Figure 1.   The effects of potassium dichromate, HCBD and both compounds on glucose excretion by rats.

TABLE 7.   Effect of HCBD, DEM and the Combination on TEA Accumulation by Renal Cortical Slices

Values are S/M Ratios $\pm$ SE for N=4

	TEA S/M Ratio
Control	16.0 ± 0.7
HCBD, 300 mg/kg	15.4 ± 1.2
DEM 0.7 ml/kg	15.7 ± 0.8
0.35 ml/kg	15.3 ± 1.0
DEM (0.35 ml/kg) + HCBD	$4.8 \pm 0.7*$
DEM (0.7 ml/kg) + HCBD	$5.3 \pm 0.8*$

*Indicates values significantly different from Control, DEM alone and HCBD alone.

spread involving not only metals with metals, but metals with organic compounds and some organic compounds with other organic compounds.   The mechanisms which underlie these interactions are not entirely clear, although with the mercuric ion-dichromate interaction there is a suggestion that membrane effects may be very important.   In any event, these data emphasize the necessity for studies on the interactions of chemicals since this approach tends to better mimic the "real world" situation than studies on individual agents and because these interaction studies may give insights into mechanisms of actions not only of the interactive responses, but of the individual compounds as well.

REFERENCES

Baggett, J. McC. and Berndt, W.O., 1984, Interaction of potassium dichromate with the nephrotoxins, mercuric chloride and citrinin, Toxicology, 33:157.

Baggett, J. McC. and Berndt, W.O., 1984, Renal and hepatic glutathione concentrations and renal transport in rats after treatment with hexachloro-1,3-butadiene and citrinin, Arch. Toxicol., 56:46.

Baggett, J. McC. and Berndt, W.O., 1985, The effect of potassium dichromate on the urinary excretion, organ and subcellular distribution of [203]Hg-mercuric chloride, Toxicol. Lett., 29:115.

Baggett, J. McC. and Berndt, W.O., 1986, Renal function in the rat after pre-treatment with mercuric chloride and potassium dichromate, Fund. Appl. Toxicol., 6:98.

Carmichael, N.G. and Fowler, B.A., 1980, Effects of separate and combined chronic mercuric chloride and sodium selenate administration in rats: histological, ultrastructural, and X-ray microanalytical studies of liver and kidney, J. Envir. Path. Toxicol., 3:399.

Dial, W.G., Jr. and Evan, A.P., 1974, The effects of sodium chromate on the proximal tubules of the rat kidney, Lab. Invest., 6:704.

Ganote, C.E., Reimer, K.A. and Jennings, R.B., 1974, Acute mercuric chloride nephrotoxicity, Lab. Invest., 6:633.

Gritzka, T.L. and Trump, B.F., 1968, Renal tubular lesions caused by mercuric chloride, Am. J. Pathol., 6:1225.

Haberman, P., Baggett, J. McC. and Berndt, W.O., 1987, The effect of chromate on citrinin-induced renal dysfunction, Toxicol. Lett., 38:88.

Jensen, R. and Berndt, W.O., 1987, Mercuric and chromate effects on renal vesicle membrane transport, Toxicologist, 7:28.

Kempson, S.A., Ellis, B.G. and Price, R.G., 1977, Changes in rat renal cortex, isolated plasma membranes and urinary enzymes following the injection of mercuric chloride, Chem. Biol. Interact., 18:217.

DICHLOROVINYL CYSTEINE ACCUMULATION AND ß-LYASE ACTIVITY IN THE DEVELOPING MOUSE KIDNEY

P.O. Darnerud, A.-L. Gustafson and V.J. Feil*

Dept. of Toxicology, Uppsala University, BMC, Box 594, S-751 24, Uppsala, Sweden and *MRRL, US Dept. of Agriculture, Fargo, ND 58105, USA

INTRODUCTION

The nephrotoxin S-(1,2-dichlorovinyl)-L-cysteine (DCVC) is formed by trichloroethylene extraction of proteinaceous substances. This compound was first identified in extracted animal food in the late 50's (McKinney et al., 1957), and has been widely used as a model compound in nephrotoxicity studies. DCVC is accumulated in the proximal tubules, where it is bioactivated by cysteine conjugate ß-lyase (Bhattacharya and Schultze, 1967) and causes tubular damage (Terracini and Parker, 1965). It has also been shown that the DCVC accumulation in the kidney is dependent on an active carrier system for organic anions (Elfarra et al.,1986).

While many papers have been devoted to the study of DCVC bioactivation and toxicity in adult animals, the situation in the newborn/young has been sparsely studied. This study will present data on the ^{14}C-DCVC accumulation in the mouse kidney and liver at different developmental stages. Also, the ß-lyase activity has been measured in these organs at the same points. The age-related changes in DCVC accumulation and ß-lyase activity are compared and the correlation between these discussed.

METHODS

^{14}C-Labelled DCVC was synthesised according to Schultze et al. (1959) and used for whole-body autoradiography on new-born mice (day 1-3 from birth). The mice were given 0.125 uCi (40 ug)/g body weight i.p. or orally and were killed 6h later. Some sections were washed with various solvents to extract non-covalently bound radioactivity.

The accumulation of ^{14}C-DCVC was measured quantitatively: ^{14}C-DCVC was given orally (0.025 uCi (8 ug)/g body wt.) to mice at different developmental stages (day of birth - adult). Twenty-four hours after the administration the animals were killed and the radioactivity in the kidney and liver measured by liquid scintillation counting.

The ß-lyase activity was determined by measuring the formation of 2-mercaptobenzothiazole spectrophotometrically (321 nm) in the kidney and liver homogenates from untreated mice at different developmental stages (two days before birth - adult), using S-(2-benzothiazolyl)-cysteine (BTC)

as the substrate (Dohn and Anders, 1982). In short, 10% (w/v) organ homogenates were incubated with BTC (2 mM) and pyridoxal phosphate for 5 min at 37°C and pH 8.6, trichloroacetic acid was added and the supernatant was used for spectrophotometrical determination.

RESULTS AND DISCUSSION

Whole-body autoradiography of a new-born mouse given ^{14}C-DCVC is shown in Fig. 1. A strong accumulation of firmly bound radioactivity was present in the kidney cortex and, to a lesser extent, in the liver, in accordance with earlier results on adult mice (to be published). In addition, labelling was also seen in the intestinal contents, and in the mucosa of the mouth and oesophagus in the newborn. In conclusion, the autoradiographical data suggests that the kidney may also be the target organ for toxicity at an early developmental stage.

Quantitative measurements of the kidney and liver radioactivity accumulation at different developmental stages is given in Fig. 2. The kidney accumulation of radioactivity increased steeply from about day 10 of age. This is in contrast to the permanently low levels seen in the liver during this developmental period. These data suggest an increased sensitivity for DCVC-induced kidney damages in the adult mouse compared to the newborn. Similar findings have been reported using cephaloridine where the newborn animal is more resistant to nephrotoxicity than the adult rabbit (Tune, 1975). These finding for DCVC differ from those for hexachlorobutadiene (Kuo and Hook, 1983; Lock et al., 1984), where nephrotoxicity increased in the young rat and mouse, compared to the adult one.

Development of ß-lyase activity in mouse kidney and liver is shown in Fig. 3. Both kidney and liver enzyme activity increased over the time period. The liver values showed the largest increase, and the adult values were about 4 times that of the kidney (3.3 and 0.8 nmol product/min/mg protein, respectively). In the study of Dohn and Anders (1982), the corresponding ß-lyase activity in adult male rats was 5.5 and 6.2 nmol in the liver and

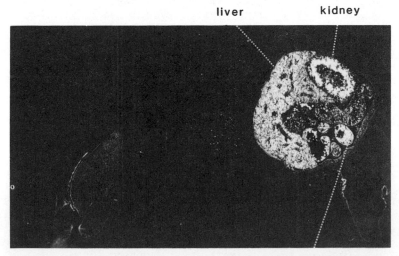

liver   kidney

intestinal contents

Fig. 1. Whole-body autoradiogram of a new-born mouse (day 2), 6h after oral administration of ^{14}C-DCVC. Note the uptake of radioactivity in the kidney cortex, liver and intestinal contents.

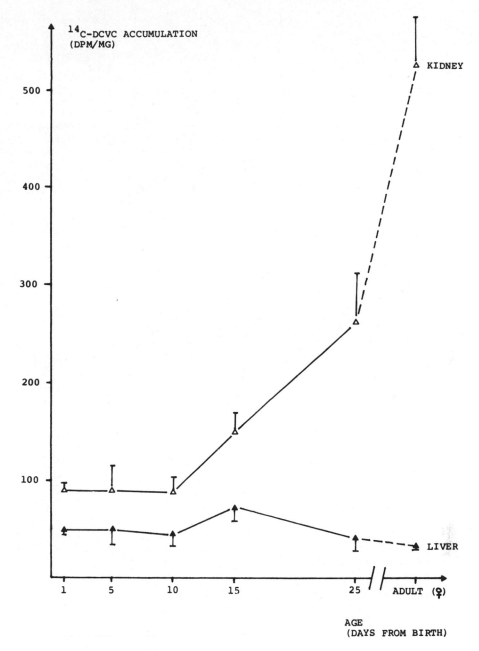

Fig. 2. Quantitative ^{14}C-measurements of kidney and liver tissue after oral administration of ^{14}C-DCVC (0.025 uCi/g body wt.). Mean of 4-6±SD.

kidney, respectively. The reason for the discrepancy between our values and those presented by Dohn and Anders could include differences in enzyme specificity for the substrate, BTC, could be due to species- or sex-related differences in the specificity for the BTC substrate.

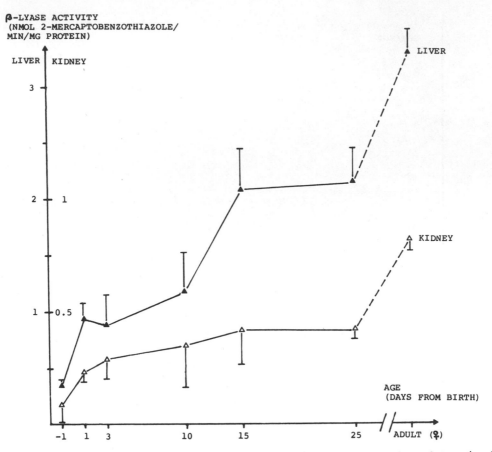

Fig. 3. ß-Lyase activity in kidney and liver homogenates, determined with S-(2-benzothiazolyl)cysteine (2mM) as substrate. Incubation conditions: 37°C, pH 8.6, 5 min, +pyridoxal phosphate. Mean of 4-6±SD.

Both the radioactivity accumulation and the ß-lyase activity in the kidney increased during the studied developmental period. However, the ^{14}C accumulation and ß-lyase activity curves showed no good correlation, and therefore the increase in kidney ^{14}C-DCVC accumulation does not seem to be primarily dependent on the increase in enzyme activity. This suggestion is strengthened by the results of the liver ß-lyase values, which are constantly higher than the kidney values, whereas the ^{14}C-DCVC accumulation values for the liver are permanently low. Other factors more important than the ß-lyase activity for DCVC accumulation in the kidney may relate to transport mechanisms for DCVC into the tubule cells. Consequently, future studies are needed to reveal the role of this uptake mechanism for the decreased DCVC accumulation in the newborn and juvenile animal.

CONCLUSIONS

1. Whole-body autoradiography with ^{14}C-DCVC resulted in a firm binding of radioactivity in the inner cortex of the kidney and in the liver of the newborn mouse, in accordance with earlier results on adult mice.

2. Quantitative measurements on the ^{14}C-DCVC accumulation showed a marked increase of the kidney values with age, whereas the liver values were constantly low during the developmental period. The kidney values suggests an increased sensitivity for DCVC induced kidney damages in the adult mouse, compared to the newborn.

3. The kidney ß-lyase activity increased to about 10 times the initial activity during the studied period. However, the liver values were always considerably higher.

4. The results show that the ^{14}C-DCVC accumulation does not directly mirror the ß-lyase activity in the developing mouse kidney. Other factors, such as uptake and transport mechanisms, may play a more important role for the ^{14}C-DCVC accumulation in vivo.

REFERENCES

Bhattacharya, R.K., and Schultze, M.O., 1967, Enzymes from bovine and turkey kidneys which cleave S-(1,2- dichlorovinyl)-L-cysteine, Comp. Biochem. Physiol., 22:723.

Dohn, G.G., and Anders, M.W., 1982, Assay of cysteine conjugate ß-lyase activity with S-(2-benzothiazolyl)cysteine as the substrate, Anal. Biochem., 120:379.

Elfarra, A.A., Lash, L.H., and Anders, M.W., 1986, Metabolic activation and detoxication of nephrotoxic cysteine and homocysteine S-conjugates, Proc. Natl. Acad. Sci., 83:2667.

Kuo, C.-H., and Hook, J.B., 1983, Effects of age and sex on hexachloro-1,3-butadiene toxicity in the Fisher 344 rat, Life Sci., 33:517

Lock, E.A., Ishmael, J., and Hook, J.B., 1984, Nephrotoxicity of hexachloro-1,3-butadiene in the mouse: The effect of age, sex, strain, monooxygenase modifiers, and the role of glutathione, Toxicol. Appl. Pharmacol., 72:484.

McKinney, L.L., Weahly, F.B., Eldridge, A.C., Campbell, R.E., Cowan, J.C., Picken Jr, J.C., and Biester, H.E., 1957, S- (Dichlorovinyl)-L-cysteine: An agent causing total aplastic anemia in calves, J. Am. Chem. Soc., 79:3932.

Schultze, M.O., Klubes, P., Perman, V., Mizuno, N.S., Bates, F.W., and Sautter, J.H., 1959, Blood dyscrasia in calves induced by S-(dichloro-vinyl)-L-cysteine, Blood, 14:519.

Terracini, B., and Parker, V.H., 1965, A pathological study on the toxicity of S-(dichlorovinyl)-L-cysteine, Food Cosmet. Toxicol., 3:67.

Tune, B.M., 1975, Relationship between the transport and toxicity of cephalosporine in the kidney, J. Infect. Dis., 132:189.

REGIOSELECTIVE TOXICITY BY DICHLOROVINYLCYSTEINE IN RABBIT RENAL CORTICAL SLICES

G.H.I. Wolfgang, A.J. Gandolfi and K. Brendel

Department of Pharmacology and Toxicology, University of Arizona, Tucson, AZ 85724, USA

INTRODUCTION

S-(1,2-dichlorovinyl)-L-cysteine (DCVC) is a potent specific nephrotoxin which produces proximal tubular damage in vivo and in vitro (Elfarra, 1986 a,b; Lash, 1986b). In vivo DCVC causes its primary lesion in the straight segment (S-3) of the proximal tubule. Previous in vitro systems (proximal tubule suspensions and cells) have not allowed for the expression of a specific lesion. Cultured precision-cut renal cortical slices retain their architecture thus allowing the expression of specific lesions in addition to changes in biochemical indices.

Cysteine conjugates such as DCVC are metabolized to their ultimate toxic species by cysteine conjugate ß-lyase. DCVC is metabolized by this enzyme to yield pyruvate, ammonia and a reactive thiol (Anderson, 1965). This reaction has been shown by several investigators to play a role in the nephrotoxicity of DCVC (Lash, 1986a, 1986b). ß-lyase has been found to predominate in cytosolic and mitochondrial fractions (Lash, 1986a) and be pyridoxal phosphate dependent. The enzyme activity can be inhibited by pyridoxal phosphate inhibitors such as aminooxyacetic acid (AOAA) and propargylglycine (Elfarra, 1986a). In addition to monitoring enzyme activity, renal cortical slices can be utilized to assess modulation of enzyme activity and the resultant effects on toxicity.

METHODS

Chemicals were obtained from commercial sources; DCVC was synthesised (McKinney, 1959), as was S-(2-benzothiazolyl)-cysteine (Dohn 1982).

Kidneys from male NZW rabbits (1.5-2.0kg) were excised, decapsulated and cored along their cortical-papillary axis. Cortical slices were prepared using a Krumdieck tissue slicer (Ruegg, 1987). Slices were incubated in an open slice support system (Ruegg, 1987) with serum-free D4E/F12 media for up to 12 hr (95/5, O_2/CO_2, room temperature). DCVC was added to the media in given concentrations. Slices were removed at designated time points for measurement of intracellular potassium (K^+), intracellular lactate dehydrogenase (LDH), organic anion and cation accumulation, histopathology or ß-lyase activity. To identify whether DCVC was gaining access to the cell via the organic acid transport system, slices were incubated in the presence of increasing concentrations of DCVC and a fixed concentration of

^{14}C para-aminohippurate (PAH). The kinetic uptake of PAH was then measured. For inhibition studies, slices were preincubated for 30 min with AOAA, then incubated with DCVC and AOAA in the medium. K^+ was measured by flame photometry (Stacey, 1978) and LDH by a kinetic assay (Sigma 228-10). Organic anion (PAH) and cation (tetraethylammonium, TEA) accumulation were assessed by 40 min incubations with ^{14}C-labelled substrates and ^3H_2O as a volume marker. The organic ion accumulation is expressed as the slice ($^{14}C/^3H$) to medium ratio as determined by liquid scintillation counting. ß-Lyase activity was measured using S-(2-benzothiazolyl)-cysteine (Dohn, 1982). Samples for histology were fixed and embedded in methacrylate plastic, 2 um sections were stained with Toluidine blue.

The results were analysed by ANOVA and treatment differences were identified by Newman Keuls multiple comparison tests. A 0.05 level of probability or less was used as a criteria of significance.

RESULTS AND DISCUSSION

DCVC produced time and concentration dependent decreases in biochemical indices (Figure 1). Whereas 10^{-6}M DCVC produed no changes from control slices 10^{-5}M, $5x10^{-5}$M and 10^{-4}M DCVC showed increasing toxicity (Figure 2). PAH and TEA were earlier indicators of toxicity than K^+, alterations in LDH occurred last and concurrently with histopathological changes. 10^{-5}M DCVC caused a straight proximal tubular (S3) lesion between 8 and 12 hr. $5x10^{-5}$M DCVC caused a similar lesion between 4 and 8 hr, and a distinct S3 pattern was observed at 8 and 12 hr. The highest dose (10^{-4}M) causes an S3 lesion between 2 and 4 hr, however by 8 hr all the proximal tubules were damaged.

Although DCVC decreases PAH accumulation, it does not appear to use the same transport process. In a kinetic study, varying concentrations of DCVC were incubated with PAH to assess competition for transport. No inhibition was observed with 10^{-6}-10^{-4}M DCVC, however probenecid completely inhibited PAH transport (Figure 3). PAH accumulation is most likely affected by a disruption of mitochondrial metabolism and thus energy status, (Reimer, 1971) not by a competitive inhibition of transport activity.

Table 1. Effect of AOAA on DCVC Toxicity$_a$

	Intracellular K^+_b	Intracellular LDH$_c$
Control	35.08±1.13	10.12±1.00
$5x10^{-5}$M DCVC	17.36±0.62*,**	7.43±0.51*
$5x10^{-5}$M DCVC + 10^{-3}M AOAA	29.96±1.70*	8.97±0.54

a All slices incubated for 8 hr, those with AOAA were preincubated for 30 min. Data is expressed as mean±SE of 12 observations.

b nmoles K^+/ug DNA

c Units LDH/mg DNA

* Significantly different from control (p < 0.05)
** Significantly different from AOAA treated (p < 0.05)

Slices maintained ß-lyase activity throughout the 12 hr incubation period, although decreases were observed at later time points (Figure 4). Aminooxyacetic acid (10^{-4}M and 10^{-3}M), inhibited ß-lyase activity almost completely (> 90%) by 1 hr and continued to inhibit enzyme activity

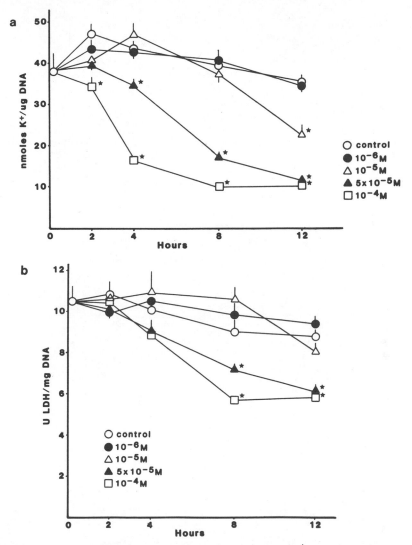

Figure 1. Effects of DCVC on (a) intracellular K^+ and (b) intracellular LDH measured in rabbit cortical slices exposed in vitro. Each point represents mean±SE of 8 observations. Stars indicate a significant difference from controls at the same time point.

throughout the 12 hr period. 5×10^{-5}M DCVC also inhibited ß-lyase activity, but to a lesser extent than AOAA. Inhibition of enzyme activity by DCVC may be due to structural damage to the proximal tubules rather than interference with the enzyme itself, since inhibition of the enzyme has a similar time course as the toxicity of DCVC.

Preincubation of slices with 10^{-3}M AOAA inhibited DCVC toxicity (Table 1) although the inhibition was incomplete. This incomplete inhibition may be explained by the relatively rapid non-enzymatic degradation of DCVC (Lash, 1986b) or the multiplicity (cytosolic, mitochondrial) of the ß-lyase itself (Lash, 1986a). Histopathology (Figure 5a) shows a distinct S3 lesion produced by 5×10^{-5}M DCVC. AOAA (Figure 5b) provided protection to

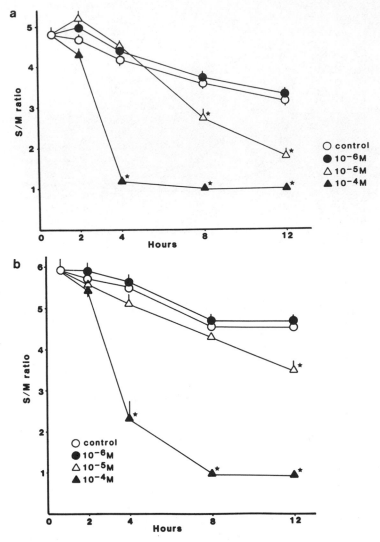

Figure 2. Effects of DCVC on a) PAH accumulation and b) TEA accumulation measured in rabbit cortical slices exposed in vitro. Each point represents mean±SE of 8 observations.

Stars indicate a significant difference from controls at the same time point.

the slices, no pattern of damage was observed although minor damage was evident.

Slices are shown to be viable throughout a 12 hr incubation by structural indices (K^+, LDH), functional indices (PAH, TEA, ß-lyase activity) and histological assessment. This in vitro model allows for the correlation between biochemical and pathological effects of DCVC. A distinct S3 lesion can be visualized before toxicity extends to all proximal tubules; this chronology also being observed in vivo (Hassall, 1983).

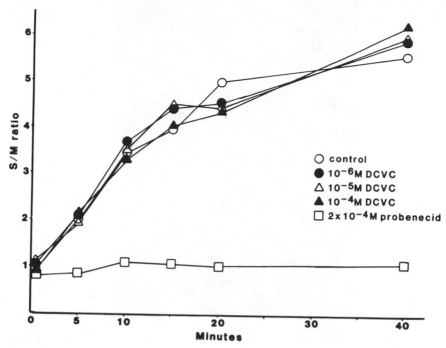

Figure 3. Effect of DCVC on the kinetic accumulation of PAH. Values represent the mean of 2 slices.

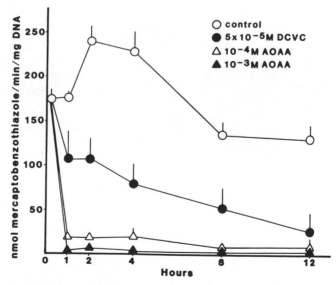

Figure 4. Inhibition of slice ß-lyase activity by DCVC and AOAA. Each point represents mean±SE of > 3 observations.

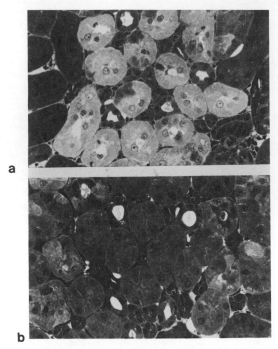

Figure 5. (a) Histopathology of rabbit cortical slices exposed to 5×10^{-5} M DCVC (8 hr, 100x). (b) Histopathology slices exposed to 5×10^{-5} M DCVC and AOAA. (30 min preincubation with AOAA, 8 hr, 100x).

ACKNOWLEDGEMENTS

Supported by Johns Hopkins CAAT and NIH GM 328290.

REFERENCES

Anderson P.M., Schultze M.O. (1965). Cleavage of S-(1,2-dichlorovinyl)-L-Cysteine by an enzyme of bovine origin. <u>Arch. Biochem. Biophys</u>. 111, 593-602.

Dohn D.R., Anders M.W. (1982). Assay of cysteine conjugate ß-lyase activity with S-(2-benzothiozolyl)-cysteine as the substrate. <u>Anal</u>. <u>Biochem</u>. 120, 379-386.

Elfarra A.A., Jacobson I., Anders M.W. (1986a). Mechanism of S-(1,2-dichlorovinyl) glutathione-induced nephrotoxicity. <u>Biochem. Pharm</u>., 35, 283-288.

Elfarra A.A., Lash L.H., Anders M.W. (1986b). Metabolic activation and detoxification of nephrotoxic cysteine and homocysteine S-conjugates. <u>Proc. Natl. Acad. Sci</u>., 83, 2667-2671.

Hassall C.D., Gandolfi A.J., Brendel K. (1983). Correlation of the in vivo and in vitro renal toxicity of S-(1,2-dichlorovinyl)-L-cysteine. <u>Drug Chem. Tox</u>. 6, 507-520.

Lash L.H., Elfarra A.A., Anders M.W. (1986a). Renal cysteine conjugate ß-lyase. Bioactivation of nephrotoxic cysteine S-conjugates in mitochondrial outer membrane. J. Biol. Chem. 261, 5930-5935.

Lash L.H., Anders M.W. (1986b). Cytotoxicity of S-(1,2-dichlorovinyl)-glutathione and S-(1,2-dichlorovinyl)-L-cysteine in isolated rat kidney cells. J Biol. Chem., 261, 13076-13081.

McKinney L.L., Picken J.C., Jr., Weakley F.B., Eldridge A.C., Campbell R.E., Cowan J.C., and Biester H.E. (1959). Possible toxic factor of trichloroethylene-extracted soybean oil meal. J. Am. Chem. Soc., 81, 909-915.

Reimer K.A., Jennings R.B. (1971). Alterations in renal cortex following ischemic injury. PAH uptake by slices of cortex after ischemia or autolysis. Lab. Invest., 25, 176-184.

Ruegg C.E., Gandolfi A.J., Nagle R.B., Krumdieck C.L., Brendel K. (1987). Preparation of positional renal slices for study of cell-specific toxicity. J. Pharm. Methods, 17, 111-123.

Stacey N.H. (1978). Toxicity of halogenated volatile anesthetics in isolated rat hepatocytes. Anesthesiology 48, 17-22.

USE OF LLC-PK[1] MONOLAYERS AS AN IN VITRO MODEL FOR NEPHROTOXICITY

Jos J.W.M. Mertens, John G.J. Weijnen, Wim J. van Doorn, Bert Spenkelink, Johan H.M. Ternink, and Peter J.van Bladeren

Department of Toxicology, Agricultural University Wageningen, De Dreyen 12, 6703 BC Wageningen, The Netherlands

INTRODUCTION

When cell cultures are used for in vitro nephrotoxicity studies, the cells are usually grown on a solid surface, which allows only apical treatment with xenobiotics. However, in vivo, xenobiotics can gain access to the proximal tubule cell from the apical as well as from the basolateral side. Functional differences exist between the apical and basolateral membranes, especially with regard to transport phenomena, and thus different mechanisms may underlie a possible nephrotoxicity. To study these mechanisms in vitro, the cells should have the same functional differences between apical and basolateral membranes and should be grown as a confluent monolayer on a porous support, to allow both apical and basolateral exposure.

The LLC-PK[1] cell line is such a cell line with a typical epithelial polarity. It possesses several features typical of the proximal tubular epithelium. A number of transport systems (1), and enzymes, like gamma-glutamyltranspeptidase (GGT)(2), that play a role in the mercapturic acid pathway are present.

The present paper summarizes our investigations on the usefulness of LLC-PK1 cells grown on a porous membrane as an in vitro nephrotoxicity model. The confluency of the monolayer on the support was checked by scanning electron microscopy, and the hexachlorobutadiene metabolites, S-(1,2,3,4,4-pentachlorobutadienyl)glutathione (PCBD-GSH) and N-acetyl-S-(1,2,3,4,4-pentachlorobutadienyl)-L-cysteine (PCBD-NAC) were used as test compounds. In the nephrotoxicity of these compounds transport systems seem to play a decisive role (3,4). We therefore also investigated the existence of transcellular organic anion and cation transport.

METHODS

LLC-PK1 cells were cultured in William's Medium E, supplemented with 10 % foetal calf serum, 100 IU of penicillin, and 100 mg/l of streptomycin. Cells were seeded at 0.8×10^6 cells/membrane on porous membranes of transwell cell culture chambers (Costar). Medium was renewed on day 3-4, and experiments were performed on day 6. For scanning electron microscopy standard procedures were followed. Cytotoxicity was determined after overnight incubation with varying concentrations of test compounds by

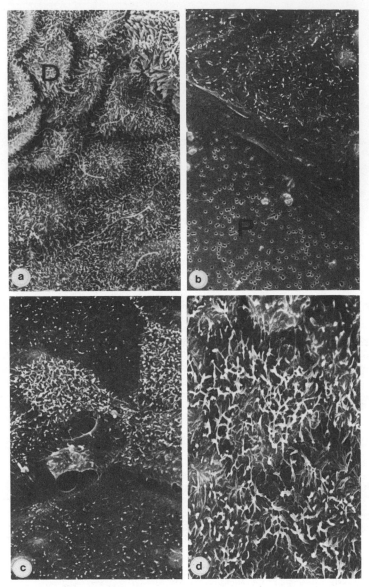

Fig. 1. Scanning electron micrograph of LLC-PK[1] cells cultured on a solid (a) or a porous surface during 1 (b), 3(c) or 6(d) days, 3000 x.   (D: dome and P: pores of the membrane)

Table 1. Toxicity as a result of apical or basolateral exposure

| | Concentration | | |
Compound	Apical	Basolateral	% LDH
CONTROL			3 ± 3
PCBD-GSH	150		48 ± 11
		150	13 ± 4
PCBD-NAC	500		4 ± 2
		500	3 ± 3

(Data from ref. 5)

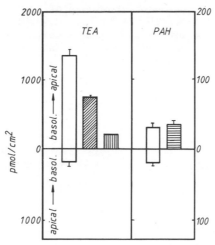

Fig. 2. Transcellular organic ion transport. LLC-PK[1] monolayers were incubated with (^{14}C)-PAH (42.7 mCi/mmol) in Earle's Balanced Salt Solution without phenol red and supplemented with 2.4 mM HEPES (pH 7.5), in the absence (☐) or presence of inhibitors: ouabain (0.1 mM) (▨), quinine (0.1 mM) (▥) or probenecid (1 .0 mM) (☰). Data from (5)

measuring LDH leakage and expressed as percentage of maximal release, from control cells treated with 0.5% Triton X-100. Transcellular organic ion transport was studied using the radio-labelled anion para-aminohippurate (PAH) and the cation tetraethylammonium (TEA) (for details see legend to Fig. 2).

RESULTS AND DISCUSSION

LLC-PK[1] cells cultured on a solid support form characteristic domes when they reach confluency indicating that transcellular transport occurs in these cells (Fig. 1a). When monolayers are grown on a porous membrane the cells maintain their polarity as evidenced by a well developed brushborder (Fig. 1d), but domes are no longer present suggesting that solutes can pass through the membrane. In order to allow separate treatment of the cells, either from the apical or from the basolateral side, confluency is a pre-requisite. As can be seen in figure 1 (compare a, b and c), six days of cell growth resulted in a confluent monolayer.

When confluent LLC-PK[1] monolayers were exposed from the apical side to PCBD-GSH, toxicity was considerable higher than after basolateral exposure (Table 1), indicating that GGT, which catalyses the first step of the break-down of the conjugate to the ultimate reactive intermediate, is predominantly present at the apical membrane. Apical or basolateral treatment with PCBD-NAC, however, elicited no toxicity even at rather high concentrations, since PCBD-NAC can only enter cells by way of basolaterally located anion transporters (4), the absence of an organic anion transporter could be an explanation for this finding. This was investigated with specific radio-labelled substrates (Fig. 2). No probenecid sensitive transcellular PAH transport could indeed be measured, whereas a TEA transport was clearly present. Quinine as well as ouabain could inhibit this organic cation transport.

The absence of an organic anion transporter limits the usefulness of the

LLC-PK1 cell for studying the nephrotoxicity of compounds, like PCBD-NAC, needing this transport to enter the cells. However, the finding of an active basolateral organic cation transporter, together with GGT and dipeptidase, makes this system especially interesting for testing all compounds that use these transport systems.

REFERENCES

1. J.S. Handler, Use of cultured epithelia to study transport and its regulation, J. Exp. Biol. 106,55 (1983).

2. A. Perantoni and J.J. Berman, Properties of Wilms' tumor line (TuWi) and pig kidney line (LLC-PK1) typical of normal kidney tubular epithelium, In Vitro, 15,446 (1979).

3. E.A. Lock and J. Ishmael, Effect of the organic acid transport inhibitor probenecid or renal cortical uptake and proximal tubular toxicity of hexachloro-1,3-butadiene and its conjugates, Toxicol. Appl. Pharmacol., 81,32 (1985).

4. E.A. Lock, J. Odum and P. Ormond, Transport of N-acetyl-S-pentachloro-1,3-butadienylcysteine by rat renal cortex, Arch. Toxicol., 59,12 (1986).

5. J.J.W.M. Mertens, J.G.J. Weijnen, W.J. van Doorn, A. Spenkelink, J.H.M. Tenmink and P.J. van Bladeren, Differential toxicity as a result of apical and basolateral treatment of LLC-PK1 monolayers with S-(1,2,3,4,4-penta-chlorobutadienyl)glutathione and N-acetyl- S-(1,2,3,4,4-pentachlorobutadi-enyl)-L-cysteine, submitted.

BIOACTIVATION MECHANISM AND CYTOTOXICITY OF S(2-CHLORO-1,1,2-TRIFLUORO-ETHYL)-L-CYSTEINE

Lawrence H. Lash, Wolfgang Dekant* and M.W. Anders

Department of Pharmacology, University of Rochester, Rochester, NY 14642, U.S.A. * Present address: Institut fur Toxickologie, Universitat Wurzburg, D-8700 Wurzburg, Federal Republic of Germany

INTRODUCTION

Glutathione conjugation of electrophilic xenobiotics is an important cellular detoxication mechanism. The nephrotoxicity and nephrocarcino-genicity of certain halogenated alkenes, however, may be attributed to glutathione S-conjugate formation followed by metabolism of the glutathione S-conjugates to the corresponding cysteine S-conjugates, which are metabolised by renal cysteine conjugate ß-lyase (ß-lyase) to ammonia, pyruvate and a thiol (Dekant et al., 1986a,b; Elfarra and Anders, 1984). The thiols thus formed are thought to lose hydrogen halide or tautomerise to yield reactive, electrophilic species (Anders et al., 1987; Dekant et al., 1986c) that may be the ultimate toxic metabolites. The chemical nature of these metabolites formed from cysteine S-conjugates has, however, not been characterized.

Chlorotrifluoroethylene is a potent nephrotoxin (Potter et al., 1981) and is metabolised by hepatic cytosolic and microsomal glutathione S-transferases to S-(2-chloro-1,1,2-trifluoroethyl)glutathione (Dohn et al., 1985a), which is nephrotoxic in rats and cytotoxic in isolated, rat kidney proximal tubular cells (Dohn et al., 1985b). The corresponding cysteine S-conjugate S-(2-chloro-1,1,2-trifluoroethyl)-L-cysteine (CTFC) is also nephrotoxic in rats and cytotoxic in isolated kidney cells, and its bio-activation is dependent on metabolism by renal ß-lyase (Dohn et al., 1985b). Pyruvate and hydrogen sulphide have been identified as metabolites of CTFC (Banki et al., 1986; Lash et al., 1986).

The objective of the present study was to investigate the bioactivation mechanism of CTFC. Purified ß-lyase from bovine kidney cytosol and a pyridoxal model, which catalyzes ß-elimination reaction from S-substituted cysteines (Kondo et al., 1985), were used to study CTFC metabolism, and the metabolites formed were identified by ^{19}F-NMR and mass spectrometry. Isolated, renal proximal tubular cells were employed to assess the cytotoxicity of CTFC and its metabolites.

METHODS

Instrumental analyses. ^{1}H and ^{19}F NMR spectra were recorded with a Bruker WP-270-SY FT-NMR spectrometer operating at 270.13 MHz (^{1}H) or 254.17 MHz (^{19}F). [1]H Chemical shifts are expressed in ppm upfield from 1%

trifluoroacetic acid in deuterium oxide (76.55). High resolution mass spectra were recorded with a Finnigan-MAT Model 8500 mass spectrometer operating at 70 eV. Gas chromatography/mass spectrometry was performed with a Hewlett-Packard 5790 gas chromatograph (12 m x 0.2 mm, 0.33 um film thickness, HP-1 crosslinked methyl silicone column, splitless injection) coupled to a Hewlett-Packard 5970B Mass Selective Detector.

Syntheses. N-Dodecylpyridoxal bromide, chlorofluoracetic acid, methyl chlorofluoroacetate, N,N-diethyl chlorofluorothioacetamide, and benzyl-2-chloro-1,1,2-trifluoroethyl sulphide were synthesised by previously published procedure (Kondo et al., 1985; Scheeren et al., 1973; Young and Tarrant, 1949) or as described by Dekant et al. (1987).

Purification of renal cytosolic cysteine conjugate ß-lyase. ß-Lyase was purified from bovine kidneys by a modification of the procedure of Ricci et al. (1986) for glutamine transaminase K (EC 2.6.1.64); glutamine transaminase K is identical to ß-lyase (Stevens et al., 1986). Glutamine transaminase K activity was assayed as described by Cooper (1978), and ß-lyase activity was measured as described by Dohn and Anders (1982) in the presence of 5 mM 4-methylthio-2-oxobutanoic acid. The specific activity of the purified enzyme was 126 nmol 2-mercaptobenzothiazole formed/min per mg protein.

Isolation of renal proximal tubular cells. Isolated, renal proximal tubular cells were prepared by the collagenase perfusion method of Jones et al. (1979) from male Fischer 344 rats (200-300 g). Cell viability was estimated by determining the percentage of cells that excluded trypan blue was typically 85-95%.

Incubation conditions. Incubations of CFTC with N-dodecylpyrridoxal bromide were performed at $37^{\circ}C$ in 5 mm NMR tubes containing 10 mM phosphate buffer (pH 8.0), 0.25 mM N-dodecylpyridoxal bromide, 5 mM CTFC, 3mM cetyl-trimethylammonium chloride, and 1 mM tetrasodium EDTA in a final volume of 0.5 ml. For trapping experiments, diethylamine or benzyl bromide was added 1 min after the start of the reaction to a final concentration of 2 mM. At the end of the incubation period, the incubation mixtures were extracted twice with 2 ml of ether, the ether phases were concentrated, and the residue was analyzed by GC/MS. ß-Lyase (0.14 mg) was incubated with CFTC (0.1 mM) in 1.5 ml of 0.1 M phosphate buffer (pH 7.4) containing 4-methyl-thio-2-oxobutanoic acid (5 mM). Samples (0.5 ml) were taken at 0 and 60 min, and protein was precipitated by the addition of 50 ul of 30% (w/v) trichloroacetic acid. After centrifugation, the samples were analyzed by ^{19}F NMR. Isolated, renal proximal tubular cells ($1x10^6$/ml) were incubated at $37^{\circ}C$ in Krebs-Henseleit buffer, pH 7.4, supplemented with 25 mM HEPES, 2.5 mM $CaCl_2$, 25 mM $NaHCO_3$, and 2% (w/v) bovine serum albumin. All buffers used in experiments with isolated cells were equilibrated with 95% O_2:5% CO_2.

Measurement of cellular oxygen consumption. Cellular oxygen consumption was measured polarographically at $37^{\circ}C$. Measurements were begun by the addition of 3.3 mM succinate to $1x10^6$ cells in a final volume of 1.5 ml.

RESULTS AND DISCUSSION

^{19}F NMR analysis of reaction mixtures containing CTFC and either the pyridoxal model of bovine kidney ß-lyase showed a time-dependent loss of the multiplets of CFTC and the appearance of a singlet and a doublet in a 2:1 ratio (Fig. 1). The singlet exhibited a chemical shift identical to that of inorganic fluoride; the doublet was identical in chemical shift and coupling constants to synthetic chlorofluoroacetic acid (CFAA). A multiplet (δ approx 10 ppm) was also observed in the spectrum, but has

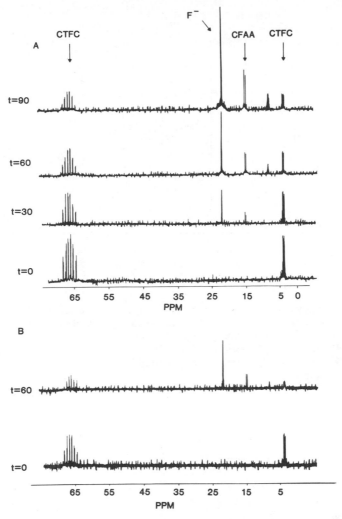

Fig. 1 ^{19}F NMR spectra of incubation mixtures containing S-(2-chloro-1,1,2-trifluoroethyl)-L-cysteine and N-dodecylpyrodoxal bromide (A) or cysteine conjugate ß-lyase (B). (Data are from Dekant et al., 1987, reprinted with permission.)

not been identified.

To identify potential reaction intermediates formed from CTFC, trapping experiments were conducted. The expected product of a B_6-dependent ß-elimination reaction from CTFC would be 2-chloro-1,1,2-trifluoroethane-thiol. Benzyl bromide was used to trap this putative thiol as a stable thioether. GC/MS analysis of the ether extracts of incubation mixtures containing CTFC, N-dodecylpyridoxal bromide, and benzyl bromide revealed a peak (5.4 min) whose mass spectrum (m/z 91, $C_7H_7^+$; 65, $C_5H_5^+$; 240; 242) and gas chromatographic retention times were identical with those of benzyl 2-chloro-1,1,2-trifluoroethyl sulphide.

Because of its chemical instability, 2-chloro-1,1,2-trifluoroethanethiol should eliminate hydrogen fluoride to yield chlorofluorothionoacetyl

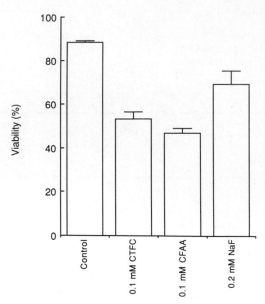

Fig. 2   Cytotoxicity of S-(2-chloro-1,1,2-trifluoroethyl)-L- cysteine (CFTC) and metabolites in isolated rat kidney cells.   Isolated kidney cells (1x10^6/ml) were incubated with 0.1 mM CTFC, 0.1 mM chlorofluoroacetic acid (CFAA), or 0.2 mM NaF at 37°C.   After 1 h, cell viability was determined by the exclusion of trypan blue.   Results are the means±S.E. of 3 cell preparations.

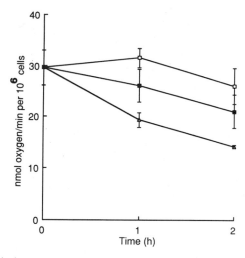

Fig. 3.   Inhibition of cellular oxygen consumption by CFAA.   Isolated kidney cells (1x10^6/ml) were incubated with buffer (□), 0.02 mM CFAA (■), or 0.1 mM CFAA (△) at 37°C.   Oxygen consumption was measured with 3.3 mM succinate.   Results are the means±S.E. of 3 cell preparation.

fluoride, which is a strong acylating agent.   GC/MS analysis of ether extracts from incubation containing CFTC and N-dodecylpyridoxal bromide in the presence of diethylamine revealed the presence of a single volatile compound whose retention time (3.8 min) and mass spectrum (m/z 44, 60, 88, 114, 148, 183) were identical to those of synthetic N,N-diethyl chloro-

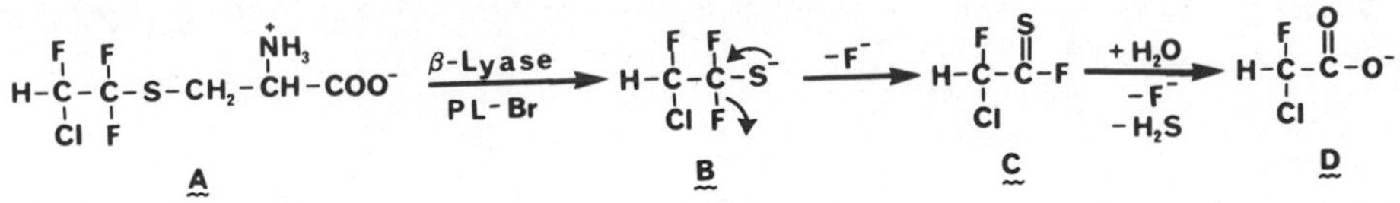

Fig. 4. Bioconversion of **1**, S-(2-chloro,1,1,2,-trifluoroethyl)-L-cysteine to **2** 2-chloro-1,1,2-trifluoroethanethiol, **3** chloro-fluorothiono-acetyl fluoride and **4** chlorofluoroacetic acid.

fluorothioacetamide; the thioamide apparently arose by acylation of diethylamine by chlorofluorothionoacetyl fluoride. Hydrolysis of the thionoacyl fluoride gives the terminal metabolites CFAA, inorganic fluoride and hydrogen sulphide.

The relative roles of reactive intermediates and terminal metabolites in the toxicity of CFTC are unresolved. Acylation of cellular nucelophiles by chlorofluorothionoacetyl fluoride may be important in CTFC and both CFTC and hydrogen sulphide are mitochondrial poisons, the mitochondrial toxicity of CTFC is not attributable to hydrogen sulphide formation (Banki et al., 1986). Inorganic fluoride is nephrotoxic (Whitford and Taves, 1973) and thus may pay a role in CTFC-induced cytotoxicity. To assess whether CFAA and inorganic fluoride contribute to CTFC-induced cytotoxicity, isolated, renal proximal tubular cells were incubated with CFAA andinorganic fluoride and effects on cell viability were measured. Previous studies (Dohn et al., 1985b) showed that CTFC markedly reduced cell viability in isolated kidney cells. Incubation of isolated kidney cells with either 0.1 mM CTFC or 0.1 mM CFAA for 1 h reduced cell viability by similar amounts (Fig. 2). Incubation of isolated cells with 0.2 mM NaF produced a small decrease in cell viability. CFAA also produced time- and concentration-dependent inhibition of cellular oxygen consumption with succinate as the respiratory substrate (Fig. 3). These results indicate, therefore, that both CFAA and inorganic fluoride may play a role in CTFC-induced cytotoxicity.

In conclusion, the present study defines a bioactivation mechanism for CTFC (Fig. 4). The first product formed is the unstable thiol 2-chloro-1,1,2-trifluoroethanethiol, which loses hydrogen fluoride to form the acylating agent chlorofluorothionoacetyl fluoride; the hydrolysis of which yields the stable, terminal metabolites CFAA, inorganic fluoride, and hydrogen sulphide. In addition to the intermediate acylating agent, CFAA and inorganic fluoride may contribute to CTFC-induced cytotoxicity.

ACKNOWLEDGEMENTS

The authors thank Dr. George A. Maylin, Mr. Thomas Lomangino, Prof. Otto Hutzinger, and Dr. Joy U. Daggett for their generous assistance, and Ms Sandra Morgan for preparing the manuscript. This work was supported by N.I.E.H.S. Grant ES03127 to M.W.A. and National Research Service Award ES05357 to L.H.L.; W.D. was supported by the Deutsche Forschungsgemeinschaft.

REFERENCES

Anders, M.W., Elfarra, A.A., and Lash, L.H., 1987, Arch. Toxicol., 60:103.

Banki, K., Elfarra, A.A., Lash, L.H. and Anders, M.W., 1986, <u>Biochem.</u>
<u>Biophys. Res. Commun.</u>, 138:707.

Cooper, A.J.L., 1978, <u>Anal. Biochem.</u>, 89:451.

Dekant, W., Metzler, M., and Henschler, D., 1986a, <u>Biochem. Pharmacol.</u>,
35:2455.

Dekant, W., Metzler, M., and Henschler, D., 1986b, <u>J. Biochem. Toxicol.</u>,
1:57.

Dekant, W., Vamvakas, S., Berthold, K., Schmidt, S., Wild, D., and
Henschler, D., 1986c, <u>Chem.-Biol. Interact.</u>, 60:31.

Dekant, W., Lash, L.H., and Anders, M.W., 1987, <u>Proc. Natl. Acad. Sci.</u>
U.S.A., in press.

Dohn, D.R., and Anders, M.W., 1982, <u>Anal. Biochem.</u>, 120:379.

Dohn, D.R., Quebbemann, A.J., Borch, R.F., and Anders, M.W., 1985a,
<u>Biochemistry</u>, 24:5137.

Dohn, D.R., Leininger, J.R., Lash, L.H., Quebbemann, A.J., and Anders,
M.W., 1985b, <u>J. Pharmacol. Exp. Ther.</u>, 235:851.

Elfarra, A.A., and Anders, M.W., 1984, <u>Biochem. Pharmacol.</u>, 33:3729.

Jones, D.P., Sundby, G.-B., Ormstad, K., and Orrenius, S., 1979, <u>Biochem.</u>
<u>Pharmacol.</u>, 28:929.

Kondo, H., Kikuchi, J., Uchida, S., Kitamikado, T., Koyanagi, E., and
Sunamoto, J., 1985, <u>Bull. Chem. Soc. Japan</u>, 58:675.

Lash, L.H., Elfarra, A.A., and Anders, M.W., 1986, <u>J. Biol. Chem.</u>,
261:5930.

Potter, C.L., Gandolfi, A.J., Nable, R.B., and Clayton, J.W., 1981,
<u>Toxicol. Appl. Pharmacol.</u>, 59:431.

Ricci, R., Nardini, M., Federici, G., and Cavallini, D., 1986, <u>Eur. J.</u>
<u>Biochem.</u>, 157:57.

Scheeren, J.W., Ooms, P.H.J., and Nivard, R.J.F., 1973, <u>Synthesis</u>,
1973:149.

Stevens, J.L., Robbins, J.D., and Byrd, R.A., 1986, <u>J. Biol. Chem.</u>,
261:15529.

Whitford, G.M., and Taves, D.R., 1973, <u>Anesthesiology</u>, 39:416.

Young, J.A., and Tarrant, P., 1949, <u>J. Am. Chem. Soc.</u>, 71:2432.

ROLE OF BIOTRANSFORMATION IN ACUTE N-(3,5-DICHLOROPHENYL)SUCCINIMIDE-INDUCED NEPHROTOXICITY

G.O. Rankin, D.J. Yang, V.J. Teets, H.C. Shih and P.I. Brown

Departments of Pharmacology and Anatomy, Marshall University School of Medicine, Huntington, West Virginia 25704-2901, U.S.A.

INTRODUCTION

N-(3,5-Dichlorophenyl)succimide (NDPS) was developed as an agricultural fungicide during the early 1970s (Fujinami et al, 1972). Although preliminary field testing of NDPS was promising, the usefulness of NDPS as an agricultural fungicide has been limited because of potential toxicity. NDPS has been shown to produce tubular necrosis following acute exposure which is characterized by diuresis, proteinuria, glucosuria, haematuria, increased blood urea nitrogen (BUN) concentration and kidney weight, and decreased organic ion accumulation by renal cortical slices (Rankin, 1982; Rankin et al., 1985). Chronic exposure to NDPS produces interstitial nephritis (Sugihara et al., 1975). In addition, NDPS has been shown to promote the activity of several renal carcinogens including the nitrosamines (Ito et al, 1974) and citrinin (Shinohara et al., 1976).

The ultimate nephrotoxic species following acute NDPS administration is unknown. However, recent studies from our laboratory have demonstrated that NDPS nephrotoxicity is produced at least in part via one or more metabolites (Rankin et al., 1986; Rankin et al., 1987 a,b). Of the known NDPS metabolites only N-(3,5-dichlorophenyl)succinamic acid (NDPSA) has been evaluated (Yang et al., 1985), and found to be only weakly nephrotoxic. Since the nephrotoxic potential of the known metabolites resulting from oxidation of the succinimide ring have not been examined, we examined the role of these metabolites in NDPS-induced nephrotoxicity. This biotransformation pathway has been described by Ohkawa et al. (1974) and begins with oxidation of NDPS at the methylene bridge of the succinimide ring to form N-(3,5-dichlorophenyl)-2-hydroxysuccinamic acid (NDHSA) which is subsequently decarboxylated to form N-(3,5-dichlorphenyl)malonamic acid (DMA). In this study, we report the nephrotoxic potential of NDHS, NDHSA and DMA in male Fischer 344 rats.

METHODS

Male Fischer 344 rats (200-300g) were housed singly in metabolism cages. Following 2 control days, rats (4 per group) were administered a single intraperitoneal injection of NDPS or a NDPS metabolite (0.2, 0.4 or 1.0 mmol/kg) or sesame oil (2.5 ml/kg), and renal function was monitored at 24 and 48 hr as previously described (Yang et al., 1985). Urine contents were monitored using Multistix strips (Ames Division, Miles Laboratories,

Inc.). Tail blood samples were obtained prior to housing the rats in metabolism cages and at 48 hr for determination of the BUN concentration. Kidney weights and accumulation of [^{14}C]-p-aminohippurate (PAH) and [^{14}C]-tetraethylammonium (TEA) by renal cortical slices were determined at 48 hr. In all experiments, pair-fed control rats were used to assure that renal effects were chemically induced and not due to decreased food intake.

RESULTS

Urine volume was increased on both post-treatment days by NDPS (0.4 or 1.0 mmol/kg), NDHS (0.2 or 0.4 mmol/kg) or NDHSA (0.2 to 0.4 mmol/kg) administration (Table 1). DMA was only weakly diuretic. Proteinuria was increased by NDPS (0.4 or 1.0 mmol/kg) from +1 to +3 at 24 and 48 hr post-treatment. Similar increases in proteinuria were observed following NDHS (0.2 or 0.4 mmol/kg) and NDHSA (0.2 mmol/kg). Proteinuria increased only to +2 at 24 hr following NDHSA (0.4 mmol/kg), while DMA administration did not alter proteinuria. Glucosuria (trace to +1) and haematuria were observed when increased proteinuria was present.

TABLE 1. Effect of NDPS Metabolites on Urine Volume (ml)

Dose (mmol/kg)	Day 0 Control	Treated	Day 1 Control	Treated	Day 2 Control	Treated
NDPS						
0.2	9±1	8±1	9±1	14±3	8±1	12±3
0.4	12±1	13±1	13±1	27±3*#	5±1*	18±3#
1.0	13±3	12±1	10±3	31±2*#	7±1	21±1*#
NDHS						
0.2	14±1	12±1	15±1	21±3*#	8±1*	25±2*#
0.4	13±1	13±1	14±1	22±2*#	8±1	23±4*#
NDHSA						
0.2	9±1	10±1	8±1	22±3*#	7±1*	33±6*#
0.4	9±1	12±1	11±1	17±2*#	6±1	34±2*#
DMA						
0.4	11±1	8±1	8±1*	8±1	8±1*	6±1*
1.0	12±2	9±1	5±1*	17±1*#	6±1*	6±1*

Values are means±S.E. for n=4.

*Significantly different (P < 0.05) from day 0 value within the group.

#Significantly different (P < 0.05) from appropriate pair-fed control group.

BUN concentration and kidney weight also were increased following NDPS (0.4 or 1.0 mmol/kg), NDHS (0.2 or 0.4 mmol/kg) or NDHSA (0.2 or 0.4 mmol/kg) administration (Table 2). DMA treatment did not result in altered BUN concentration or kidney weight.

Basal and lactate-stimulated PAH uptake were decreased by NDPS (0.4 or 1.0 mmol/kg), NDHS (0.4 mmol/kg) or NDHSA (0.2 or 0.4 mmol/kg) treatment, while NDHS (0.2 mmol/kg) decreased only basal PAH uptake (Table 3). However, TEA accumulation was decreased by NDPS (0.4 or 1.0 mmol/kg), NDHS (0.2 or 0.4 mmol/kg) and NDHSA (0.2 or 0.4 mmol/kg) administration. NDPS (0.2 mmol/kg) or DMA administration did not decrease PAH or TEA accumulation.

TABLE 2.   Effect   of   NDPS Metabolites on BUN Concentration   and   Kidney
weight at 48 h Post-treatment

Dose	Concentration (mg%)		Kidney Weight (g/100g B.W.)	
(mmol/kg)	Control	Treated	Control	Treated
NDPS				
0.2	19±1	18±1	0.42±0.02	0.38±0.02
0.4	14±1	142±7*	0.43±0.01	0.62±0.04*
1.0	14±1	168±12*	0.36±0.01	0.62±0.05*
NDHS				
0.2	17±1	153±16*	0.38±0.01	0.62±0.03*
0.4	17±1	173±30*	0.39±0.01	0.62±0.02*
NDHSA				
0.2	30±1	119±21*	0.39±0.01	0.58±0.04*
0.4	19±2	92±23*	0.41±0.01	0.56±0.02*
DMA				
0.4	20±1	19±1	0.36±0.01	0.36±0.02
1.0	19±1	19±1	0.35±0.01	0.35±0.01

Values are means ± S.E. for n = 4.

*Significantly different (P < 0.05) from the control group values.

TABLE 3.   Effect of NDPS Metabolites on Organic Ion Accumulation

			S/M Ratio			
Dose	PAH		PAH + Lactate		TEA	
(mmol/kg)	Control	Treated	Control	Treated	Control	Treated
NDPS						
0.2	3.0±0.2	3.3±0.2	9.4±0.9	9.5±1.1	18.0±0.4	17.3±1.3
0.4	3.1±0.1	2.1±0.1*	6.9±0.4	4.8±0.3*	16.2±0.3	14.8±0.8*
1.0	2.8±0.1	1.9±0.1*	5.6±0.1	3.0±0.1	14.8±1.0	13.9±1.1
NDHS						
0.2	3.7±0.2	2.9±0.4*	5.9±0.3	5.4±0.8	18.3±0.8	13.0±0.8*
0.4	4.2±0.2	2.1±0.1*	9.4±0.6	4.3±0.7*	17.5±0.4	10.5±0.7*
NDHSA						
0.2	4.2±0.3	2.5±0.1*	11.6±0.8	6.1±0.4*	20.0±0.7	14.1±0.7*
0.4	4.8±0.3	2.5±0.3*	10.8±0.4	6.5±0.7*	17.6±0.3	12.2±1.2*
DMA						
0.4	4.3±0.3	4.7±0.4	8.8±0.6	10.9±0.4*	17.4±0.8	16.3±1.1
1.0	3.9±0.1	4.2±0.1*	9.8±0.4	10.4±0.6	18.8±0.7	19.6±1.4

Values are means±S.E. for n = 4.   The slice-to-medium (S/M)   ratio is
determined by dividing S, the radioactivity (dpm) per g tissue, by M, the
radioactivity (dpm) per ml incubation medium.

*Significantly different (P < 0.05) from appropriate control group.

Morphological changes produced by NDHS or NDHSA were indistinguishable from those produced by NDPS (0.4 or 1.0 mmol/kg) (Rankin et al., 1985). These changes were characterized as extensive proximal tubular necrosis with atrophy of proximal tubules and alteration in lumina size.

DISCUSSION

Results from previous studies in our laboratory have suggested that the nephrotoxic metabolite(s) of NDPS result from oxidation of the succinimide ring (Rankin et al., 1986) and may originate from extrarenal tissue (Rankin et al., 1987 a,b). The results of the present study support these earlier observations.

The finding that NDHS and NDHSA, metabolites originating from succinimide ring oxidation, are nephrotoxic metabolites supports the conclusion that oxidation at the methylene bridge of NDPS produced nephrotoxic metabolites. In addition, the observation that NDPSA was weakly nephrotoxic (Yang et al., 1985), while its 2-hydroxy derivative NDHSA is markedly nephrotoxic when administered to rats, also supports the conclusion that hydroxylation of the succinimide ring is an important bioactivation step.

We also previously noted that probenecid attentuated NDPS nephrotoxicity (Rankin et al., 1987b) while phenobarbital markedly enhanced NDPS-induced renal effects (Rankin et al., 1987a). These results suggested that an organic acid of extrarenal origin contributed to NDPS nephrotoxicity. The finding that NDHSA is more nephrotoxic than NDPS suggests that NDHSA could be the organic acid contributing to NDPS-induced nephropathy with probenecid blocking entry of NDHSA into proximal tubular cells. The inability of probenecid to completely block NDPS-induced renal effects could be the result of passive diffusion of NDPS and/or NDHS, both neutral molecules, into renal issue. However, it is not known if NDPS exerts a direct toxic effect on renal tissue or must first be bioactivated to the ultimate nephrotoxic species.

Previously we had suggested that the succinimide ring must be cyclic and nonalkyl substituted for optimal nephrotoxic potential (Yang et al., 1985). However, the finding that the acylic metabolite NDHSA is nephrotoxic indicates that a cyclic succinimide ring is not essential for maximal nephrotoxic potential.

The ultimate nephrotoxic species following NDPS administration remains unclear, but the results of the present study show that metabolites arising from succinimide ring oxidation may be, or at least lead to, the ultimate nephrotoxicant. Therefore, it appears that NDHS and/or NDHSA might be the ultimate nephrotoxic species or that they are converted to an as of yet unidentified metabolite. It also is not known whether NDHS is a direct nephrotoxicant or must first be hydrolyzed to NDHSA before the nephrotoxic response is observed. The observation that NDHS (0.4 mmol/kg) administration tends to produce slightly greater nephrotoxicity (more proteinuria, glucosuria, increased BUN concentration and kidney weight) than NDHSA (0.4 mmol/kg) suggests that NDHS is a nephrotoxicant independent of biotransformation to NDHSA. However, further studies are necessary to clearly delineate the direct contributions of NDHS and NDHSA or the role of further biotransformation of these metabolites to NDPS-induced nephropathy.

ACKNOWLEDGEMENTS

The authors would like to thank Darla Kennedy for her assistance in preparing this manuscript. This work was supported by NIH Grant DK 31210.

REFERENCES

Fujinami, A., Ozaki, T., Nodera, K., and Tanaka, K., 1972, Studies on biological activity of cyclic imide compounds. Part II. Antimicrobial activity of 1-phenylpyrrolidine-2,5- diones and relates compounds, _Agric. Biol. Chem._, 36:318.

Ito, N., Sugihara, S., Makiura, S., Arai, M., Hirao, K., Denda, S., and Nishio, O., 1974, Effect of N-(3,5-dichlorophenyl)succinimide on the histological pattern and incidence of kidney tumors in rats induced by dimenthylnitrosamine, _Gann_, 65:131.

Ohkawa, H., Hisada, Y., Fujiwara, N., and Miyamoto, J., 1974, Metabolism of N-(3,5-dichlorophenyl)succinimide in rats and dogs, _Agric. Biol. Chem._, 7:1359.

Rankin, G.O., 1982, Nephrotoxicity following acute administration of N-(3,5-dichlorophenyl)succinimide in Sprague-Dawley rats, _Toxicology_, 23:21.

Rankin, G.O., Yang, D.J., Cressey-Veneziano, K., and Brown, P.I., 1985, N-(3,5-Dichlorophenyl)succinimide nephrotoxicity in the Fischer 344 rat, _Toxicol. Lett._, 24:99

Rankin, G.O., Yang, D.J., Richmond, C.D., Teets, V.J., Wang, R.I. and Brown, P.I., 1987a, Effect of microsomal enzyme activity modulation on N-(3,5-dichlorophenyl)succinimide-induced nephrotoxicity, _Toxicology_ (in press).

Rankin, G.O., Yang, D.J., Teets, V.J., and Brown, P.I., 1986, Deuterium isotope effect in acute N-(3,5-dichlorophenyl)succinimide-induced nephrotoxicity, _Life Sci._, 39:1291.

Rankin, G.O., Yang, D.J., Teets, V.J., Lo, H.H., and Brown, P.I., 1987b, The effect of probenecid on acute N-(3,5- dichlorophenyl)succinimide-induced nephrotoxicity in the Fischer 344 rat, _Toxicology_, 44:181.

Shinohara, Y., Arai, M., Hira, K., Sugihara, S., Nakanishi, K., Tsunoda, H., and Ito, N., 1976, Combination effect of citrinin and other chemicals on rat kidney tumorigenesis, _Gann_, 67:147.

Sugihara, S., Shinohara, Y., Miyata, Y., Inoue, K., and Ito, N., 1975, Pathology analysis of chemical nephritis in rats induced by N-(3,5-dichlorophenyl)succinimide. _Lab. Invest._, 33:219.

Yang, D.J., Richmond, C.D., Teets, V.J., Brown, P.I., and Rankin, G.O., 1985, Effect of succinimide ring modification on N-(3,5-dichlorophenyl)-succinimide-induced nephrotoxicity in Sprague-Dawley and Fischer 344 rats, _Toxicology_, 37:65.

CHLOROFORM NEPHROTOXICITY AND RENAL UPTAKE OF CALCIUM

B.A.S. Skeer and W.E. Lindup

Department of Pharmacology and Therapeutics, University of Liverpool, P.O.
Box 147, Liverpool L69 3BX

INTRODUCTION

The pathology of necrosed cells from various causes such as ischaemia,
chemicals, viruses and radiation is often similar and it has been
suggested that intracellular accumulation of calcium is involved (Farber,
1981). Nephrotoxicity, hepatotoxicity and myocardial necrosis, for
example, are all associated with increased concentrations of intracellular
calcium (Mallov, 1983; Berndt et al., 1984; Schanne et al., 1979). A
major point of controversy however is whether the entry of untoward
amounts of calcium through the damaged cell membrane is a cause or
consequence of cell death (Fariss and Read, 1985).

Chloroform is a popular experimental nephrotoxin and it increases kidney
calcium as measured by a titration method (Masuda and Nakayama, 1983).
The aim of this work was to confirm with radiolabelled [^{45}Ca] calcium that
a nephrotoxic dose of chloroform does increase renal calcium and to see
whether chlorpromazine, a membrane stabilizer, could reduce any such
increase in calcium and either ameliorate or prevent the nephrotoxicity.

MATERIALS AND METHODS

Inbred CBA male mice (20 - 30g) were used. Mice were dosed with
chloroform (0.2ml/kg) dissolved in corn-oil (1ml/25ml corn-oil) and
administered ip, 0.05ml/10g body weight. Control mice received the same
dose of corn-oil alone. Each mouse also received an ip dose of [^{45}Ca]
calcium chloride (1 to 8uCi) in aqueous solution not more that 90 seconds
after the first injection. The effect of chlorpromazine (20mg/kg; ip)
administration 1 hr prior to the injection of ^{45}Ca and chloroform was also
investigated.

Blood was collected by cardiac puncture under diethylether anaesthesia
with heparin as the anticoagulant at either 4 or 24 hr after injection.
Plasma creatinine was measured by the alkaline picrate method and the mice
were then killed by decapitation. The injections of chloroform and
^{45}CaCl$_2$ were given between 0930 and 1000 hours.

Measurement of Renal Calcium. The kidneys were excised, weighted and
homogenised in 10ml of cold 0.9% NaCl with an Ultra-Turrax homogenizer. An
aliquot (0.5ml) of the kidney homogenate was digested in 2M-NaOH (2ml) for

1 hr at $50^{\circ}C$. The solution was neutralised with 2M-NaOH (2ml) and then the radioactivity measured by liquid scintillation counting.

RESULTS

Plasma creatinine concentrations were not significantly raised 4 hr after injection of chloroform, but had increased significantly ($p < 0.05$) by 24 hr from 0.36 ± 0.25 (controls) to 2.81 ± 0.30 mg/100 ml (treated). The kidneys removed from the chloroform-treated mice were, without exception, considerably paler in colour than those from the controls.

Table 1. Effect of chloroform on renal ^{45}Ca in male mice

Time (hr)	Renal ^{45}Ca (dpm/g wet wt.)	
	Control	Chloroform
4	$6,612 \pm 1,984$ (6)	$17,115 \pm 7,047$[a] (6)
24	$1,500 \pm 119$ (4)	$37,930 \pm 30,258$[a] (4)

Dose of $^{45}CaCl_2$ was 4uCi
Mean values ($\pm$ s.d.) with number of mice in parentheses.
[a] = $p < 0.05$ relative to control.

Table 2. Effect of chloroform on renal ^{45}Ca in male mice

Time (hr)	Renal 45Ca (dpm/g wet wt.)	
	Control	Chloroform
4	$8,416 \pm 2,073$ (4)	$13,062 \pm 4,560$ (4)
24	$2,768 \pm 1,716$ (14)	$119,657 \pm 53,658$[a] (16)

Dose of $^{45}CaCl_2$ was 8uCi.
Mean values ($\pm$ s.d.) with number of mice in parentheses.
[a] = $p < 0.01$ relative to control.

Table 3. Effect of chlorpromazine pretreatment (20mg/kg; ip) on renal concentration of ^{45}Ca in male mice 24 hours after administration of chloroform.

Pretreatment Group	Renal ^{45}Ca (dpm/g wet wt.)	
	Control	Chloroform
Saline	$2,768 \pm 1,716$ (14)	$119,657 \pm 53,658$[a] (16)
Chlor-promazine	$8,094 \pm 2,416$ (14)	$18,349 \pm 5,215$[b] (14)

Dose of $^{45}CaCl_2$ was 8uCi
[a,b] Plasma creatinine concentrations were 2.81 ± 0.30 and 0.88 ± 0.79 mg/100ml respectively.

Tables 1 and 2 show that in control mice the concentration of ^{45}Ca in the kidney declined between 4 and 24 hr after a dose of either 4 or 8uCi. The concentrations of ^{45}Ca in the kidneys of chloroform treated mice were significantly higher however and increased, rather than decreased, between 4 and 24 hr. This increase coincided with the increase in plasma creatinine concentration.

Table 3 shows that pretreatment with chlorpromazine prior to administration of chloroform depressed the chloroform-induced increase of both renal calcium concentration and plasma creatinine. All the kidneys removed from mice (both control and chloroform-treated) pretreated with chlorpromazine appeared normal and had none of the paleness encountered with chloroform-treated mice.

DISCUSSION

The increase in renal calcium concentration produced by a nephrotoxic dose of chloroform has been confirmed with the use of [^{45}Ca] calcium chloride. The extent of the increase was similar to that reported by Masuda and Nakayama (1983) who used the EDTA titration method to measure kidney calcium. More work is required however to optimize the dose, timing and route of administration of the radiotracer, but it offers a convenient way to monitor toxin-induced changes in the calcium uptake of major organs. Thus injury to several organs can be monitored simultaneously and even if a toxin-induced increase in tissue concentration of calcium does not prove that calcium caused the injury, there is nevertheless evidence (Hulmes, 1986) that tissue calcium levels are a good measure of the amount of injury.

Pretreatment with chlorpromazine had a protective effect on the mouse kidney, perhaps by virtue of its membrane stabilizing properties although other mechanisms such as inhibition of the formation of chemically reactive metabolites of chloroform are also possible.

REFERENCES

Berndt, W.O., Hayes, A.W. and Baggett, J. McC., 1984, Effects of fungal toxins on renal slice calcium balance, Toxicol. Appl. Pharmacol., 74: 78.

Farber, J.L., 1981, The role of calcium in cell death, Life Sci., 29: 1289.

Fariss, M.W. and Reed, D.J., 1985, Mechanism of chemical-induced toxicity II. Role of extracellular calcium, Toxicol. Appl. Pharmacol., 79:296.

Humes, H.D., 1986, Role of calcium in pathogenesis of acute renal failure, Am. J. Physiol., 250:F579.

Mallov, S., 1983, Role of calcium and free fatty acids in epinephrine-induced myocardial necrosis, Toxicol. Appl. Pharmacol., 71:280.

Masuda, Y. and Nakayama, N., 1983, Protective action of diethyldithio-carbamate and carbon disulfide against renal injury induced by chloroform in mice, Biochem. Pharmacol., 32:3127.

Schanne, F.A.X., Kane, A.B., Young, E.E. and Farber, J.L., 1979, Calcium dependence of toxic cell death: A final common pathway, Science, 206:700.

RENAL PATHOLOGY OF ORALLY ADMINISTERED L-TRIIODOTHYRONINE (T3) IN THE RAT

Sandra J. Kennedy and Huw B. Jones

Department of Pathology, Smith Kline and French Research Limited, The Frythe, Welwyn, Herts., AL6 9AR

INTRODUCTION

In addition to the endocrinological uses in hormone replacement therapy L-triiodothyronine (L-T_3) has been of both pharmacological and clinical interest in its potential value as an adjunct to tricyclic anti-depressant therapy due to its CNS effects (1) and in the treatment of hyper-cholesterolaemia (2). The documentation of any toxicity is of some importance, but there is an absence of published information concerning the effects repeated doses of L-T_3.

The adverse effects on the heart due to L-T_3 are well known since one of the limiting features of T3 administration for lowering plasma lipids is the cardiac side effects (The Coronary Drug Project Research Group, 1972). Therefore the dosages administered to rats must be a carefully modulated to prevent death due to cardiac damage. We have established in our laboratory that a dose of 1 mg/kg/day L-T_3 causes a high incidence of mortality in rats resulting from myocardia degeneration and necrosis. Therefore dose levels of 0.1 and 0.25 mg/kg/day L-T_3 were used in this investigation for periods of up to 75 days in rats and effects of this compound in the kidney are reported.

MATERIALS AND METHODS

L-T_3 was administered orally by gavage to 6 week old rats of the SK&F Wistar strain in 2 studies. The first investigation was of 14 days duration at a dose level of 0.25 mg/kg/day to 5 male and 5 female rats with comparable control groups. The second study involved treating a total of 70 rats with 0.1 mg/kg/day L-T_3 and sacrificing 5 males and 5 females at 2, 5, 10, 15, 31, 75 days and one group which was treated for 31 days and allowed to recover for 44 days. Matching controls were killed after the same time periods. Analysis of the urinary protein levels and the urinary enzyme markers: N-acetyl-ß-D-glucosaminidase (NAG), alkaline phosphatase (AKP) and total lactate dehydrogenase (LDH) were performed on urine samples taken on the day prior to each necropsy in the time course study only. At the end of both investigations all the animals were killed by exposure to CO_2 gas and exsanguinated. A detailed post-mortem examination was carried out. The kidneys were removed and fixed in neutral buffered formalin prior to embedding in paraffin wax and 5um sections stained with haematoxylin and eosin. Kidney samples from the time course study were taken and fixed in glutaraldehyde prior to routine processing into resin blocks for electron microscopy.

RESULTS/DISCUSSION

Oral administration of L-T_3 to rats revealed two novel lesions in the kidney which have not been hitherto reported in the literature. The first of these findings was necrosis of the tip of the papilla (Fig. 1), and the other was the occurrence of multinucleated epithelial cells in the distal tubules (Fig. 2). The incidence of these changes for the 2 investigations are shown in Tables 1 and 2.

Papillary necrosis was only evident in the 14 day study at the higher dose level of L-T_3, namely 0.25 mg/kg/day. It occurred, unilaterally, in 3/10 rats and consisted of necrosis of the papillary tip with a mild neutrophilic infiltration, focal haemorrhage and marked hyperplasia of the adjacent viable collecting duct epithelium and also of the epithelium overlying the papillary tip. Mitotic figures were frequent in the epithelium.

Table 1. T_3-Induced Lesions in the Rat Kidney - 14-Day Oral Study

	Control	0.25 mg/kg/day
Papillary necrosis	-	3
Multinucleate epithelial cells - distal tubules	-	10

n = 10

Table 2. Multinucleate Epithelial Cells in Distal Tubules Time Course Study

Duration of exposure (days)		2	5	10	15	31	75	31+44R
Control	M	-	-	-	-	-	-	-
	F	-	-	-	-	-	-	-
0.1 mg/kg/day T_3	M	-	-	2	3	2	5	5
	F	-	-	1	-	4	4	4

n = 5

31+44R = 31 days exposure + 44 days recovery

There is an extensive literature concerning the induction of papillary necrosis due to a wide variety of xenobiotic compounds, the most widely reported of which are the non-steroidal anti-inflammatory drugs (3). It is considered that the lesions starting at the papillary tip may be largely due to a result of the local concentration of the drugs and their metabolites in the inner medulla and of structural factors unique to the vasculature of the region. Associated hyperplasia of the overlying papillary epithelium, as seen in the present study, has been recorded in such instances (4). The pathogenesis of such a finding remains to be elucidated.

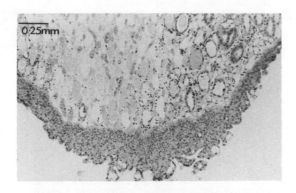

Figure 1. Rat kidney following 14 days dosing with 0.25mg/kg/day L-T$_3$. Tip of renal papilla showing necrosis and associated hyperplasia of overlying epithelium and adjacent collecting duct epithelium.

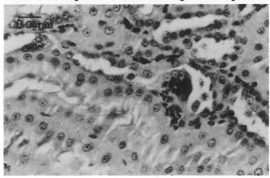

Figure 2. Rat kidney following dosing with 0.1mg/kg/day L-T$_3$. Multinucleated epithelial cells in the distal tubule.

The second histological finding in the kidneys attributable to L-T$_3$ administration was the presence of multinucleated epithelial cells in the distal tubules. These cells occurred sporadically in the distal nephron and contained up to 20 nuclei. There was no histological or ultrastructural evidence of any associated tubular changes or any increase in mitotic figures at any of the time points or doses examined. Electron microscopical examination of these cells confirmed their distal tubular location and revealed no nuclear/nucleolar abnormalities and the cells were obviously multinuclear. The only nuclear variations were a difference in chromatin pattern with some nuclei having a more open appearance with little heterochromatin indicating a nucleus active in DNA/RNA synthesis and some nuclei with more electron-dense heterochromatin suggesting a more inactive state (Fig. 3). The cytoplasm of these cells did not exhibit any overt abnormalities.

The affected distal tubular epithelial cells were present in the kidneys all rats which had received 0.25 mg/kg/day L-T$_3$ for 14 days. They were also apparent in the time course study where they were first seen in a few animals after 10 days administration of 0.1 mg/kg/day T$_3$. There was a slight tendency for these cells to be more evident in the males rather than the females, but their overall appearance and incidence within an affected kidney did not vary with time. However, there was some increase in the number of rats affected from 10 to 75 days, and the animals which were treated for 31 days and allowed to recover for 44 days did not show any evidence of a diminution in overall incidence or change in appearance. Indeed, the number of rats affected in the 75 day and 31 day + 44 day

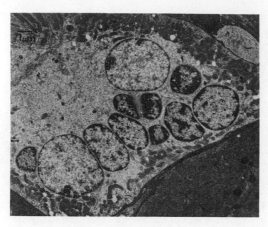

Figure 3. Electron Micrograph. 0.1mg/kg/day L-T$_3$, Multinucleate epithelial cell in distal tubule.

recovery groups were identical. Therefore there was no indication of progression of this lesion over this time period but equally there was no sign of a regression.

The urinalysis results from the time course investigation showed a trend towards an increase in urinary protein, more especially in the females from as early as day 10. In the absence of structural abnormalities this may be linked to an increase in food intake and protein turnover due to the increased metabolic activation attributable to L-T$_3$. There were also minimal to moderate increases in the activity of various urinary enzymes at all time points from 2-75 days; these parameters were AKP, NAG and LDH. All these parameters had returned to within the normal range of values in the recovery rats. There were no histological abnormalities seen to support these changes.

The multinucleated epithelial cells in the distal nephron may represent karyokinesis without cell division. Such a finding has been reported in the rat kidney in the proximal tubule but has invariably been associated with degenerative changes and an increase in mitotic rate, for example with lysinoalanine (5) and with heavy metals (6) and the subsequent development of renal adenomas. Multinucleated epithelial cells have also been seen in rats treated with the fungus Penicillium verrucosum which mimic Balkan nephropathy (7). Once again the lesions occur in the proximal tubule and are associated with degenerative changes, an increased mitotic rate and abnormal nuclei including micronuclei and nucleolar segregation. There is no evidence apparent in the literature of multinucleated epithelial cells occurring in the distal as opposed to the proximal nephron in the absence of degenerative changes and nuclear abnormalities.

CONCLUSION

These data have shown the renal effects of oral administration of toxicological doses of an endogenous hormone, L-T$_3$, to the rat. The findings included the occurrence of renal papillary necrosis with hyperplasia of the overlying epithelium and adjacent collecting duct epithelium after exposure to 0.25 mg/kg/day L-T$_3$ for 14 days. In addition, multinucleated epithelial cells were noted in the distal tubules in all rats, in this study and in a subsequent time course study at a lower dose of 0.1 mg/kg/day. This lower dose did not elicit papillary necrosis, but the multinucleateal cells developed after 10 days dosing and their presence was consistent up to 75 days. There was no evidence of progression of this lesion over time or regression in a recovery group. The pathogenesis of both these L-T$_3$-induced changes is unknown at present and further investigation is in progress.

REFERENCES

1. A.J. Prange, P.J. Lossen, I.C. Wilson and M.A. Lipton, The therapeutic uses of hormones of the thyroid axis in depression, In: Neurobiology of Mood Disorders, R.M. Post, and J.C. Ballenger (ed) Williams and Wilkins, Baltimore (1984).

2. A.H. Underwood, J.C. Emmett, D. Ellis, S.B. Flynn, P.D. Lesion, G.M. Benson, R. Novelli, N.J. Pearce and V.P. Shah, A thyromimetic that decreases plasma cholesterol without increasing cardiac activity, Nature, 324, 425-429 (1986).

3. H.E. Black, Renal toxicity of non-steroidal anti-inflammatory drugs, Tox. Path. 14, 83-90 (1986).

4. E.A. Molland, Experimental renal papillary necrosis, Kidney Intern., 13, 5-14 (1978).

5. J.C. Woodard and D.D. Short, Renal toxicity of N-(DL-2-amino-2-carboxyethyl)-L-lysine (lysinoalanine) in rats. J. Cosmet. Toxicol, 15, 117-119 (1977).

6. B.J. Payne, L.Z. Saunders, Heavy metal nephropathy of rodents, Vet. Pathol, 15 (Suppl 5), 51-87 (1978).

7. G.C. Peristianis, P.K.C. Austwick and R.L. Carter, An ultrastructural investigation of nephrotoxicity in rats induced by feeding cultures of Penicillium verrucosum var, Cyclopium. Virchows Arch B Cell Path., 28, 321-337 (1978).

LIPID PEROXIDATION AS A POSSIBLE CAUSE OF OCHRATOXIN A TOXICITY

A.D. Rahimtula, M. Castegnaro, J.C. Bereziat, V. Bussachini-Griot, L. Broussole, J. Michelon and H. Bartsch

International Agency for Research on Cancer, 150 Cours Albert Thomas, 69372 Lyon Cedex 08, France

INTRODUCTION

Ochratoxin A (OA), a dihydroisocoumarin containing mycotoxin, is a widespread natural contaminant of a variety of food and feedstuffs at levels ranging from 9-27500 ug/kg (1). Ingestion of OA has been shown to induce nephropathy in several species (1) while dietary feeding induced renal adenomas and hepatocellular carcinomas in mice (2). OA did not produce genetic or related effects in a variety of in vitro short term-tests, but it has been shown to induce single strand breaks in DNA of liver, kidney and spleen (3). OA is suspected of being the main aetiologic agent responsible for Balkan endemic nephropathy (BEN) and associated urinary tract tumours, diseases which affect multiple members of families residing in restricted areas of Bulgaria, Yugoslavia and Romania (1).

Lewis (extensive metabolizers) and DA (poor metabolizers) rat strains show genetic polymorphism for the gene regulating debrisoquine-4-hydroxylase in a manner analogous to human metabolism. In previous in vitro studies (4,5) we have demonstrated that liver and kidney microsomal OA-hydroxylase activity was much lower in DA rats than in Lewis rats. This may be relevant to OA toxicity since it has been shown that individuals who are more susceptible to BEN are predominantly phenotyped as extensive metabolizers of debrisoquine (6,7).

Despite the carcinogenic and toxic properties of OA, the mechanism of its action is not known. Our results suggest that induction of lipid peroxidation by OA may be a possible cause of its toxicity. Furthermore, differences in metabolism and excretion of OA in DA and Lewis rats may help to explain the increased susceptibility of humans who are extensive metabolizers of debrisoquine to OA, and the development of BEN.

MATERIALS AND METHODS

Chemicals. OA, Sigma Chemical Co.; [^{3}H]OA, Amersham.

Animals. Male Wistar rats (150-250 g), IFFA-CREDO, Lyon; Female DA rats (160-180 g), Zentral Institut fur Verchstiere, Hannover; Female Lewis rats (225-250 g); C.S.E.A.L.-CNRS, Orleans. DA and Lewis rats were phenotyped using debrisoquine (8).

Lipid peroxidation. In vitro lipid peroxidation was carried out in 0.1M phosphate buffer (pH 7.4) and contained per ml: 2 mg liver microsomal protein and 125 nmol OA. Lipid peroxidation was initiated by the addition of either NADPH (1 umol) or ascorbate/$FeSO_4$ (1umol/5 nmol). Malondialdehyde (MDA) formed was estimated by the thiobarbituric acid method (9). In vivo lipid peroxidation was assessed by measuring the levels of ethane exhaled (9) by Wistar rats following administration of OA (6.0 mg/kg).

Ochratoxin A metabolism. In vitro metabolism of OA was carried out in 0.1 M phosphate buffer and contained per ml: 2 mg microsomal protein, 125 nmol OA and 1 umol NADPH. After 1 hr, 0.1ml of HCl was added and OA and its metabolites were extracted into chloroform and subjected to HPLC separation (4). For protein binding, 125 nmol of [^{3}H]OA (80 dpm/pmole) was used and the work up was carried out as described earlier (10).

In vivo metabolic studies were carried out in DA and Lewis rats after administration of either a single dose of OA or during long-term dosing. For single dose studies, rats were orally intubated with OA (0.5 mg or 5.0 mg/kg) in sodium bicarbonate solution (n = 3 rats for 0.5 mg OA and n = 4 for 5.0 mg OA) and immediately placed in individual metabolic cages.

Urine was collected every 24 hours for up to 96 hr. For long-term dosing studies, rats (n = 9 for DA rats; n = 10 for Lewis rats) were orally intubated with OA (1.5 mg/kg) 5 times a week (Monday-Friday) for 8 weeks. Urine samples were collected on the following days: week 1, day 4; week 3, days 5; week 5, day 5; week 7, day 5; week 8, day 4. Aliquots (10 ml) of each urine sample were adjusted to pH 2.4 and successively extracted with 5 ml of chloroform:methanol (2:1) and twice with 5 ml of chloroform. The pooled organic extracts were dried (anhydrous Na_2SO_4), evaporated to dryness and the residue redissolved in 5 ml of chloroform. The mixture was passed through a Sep-Pack cartridge and eluted with 20 ml of chloroform:acetic acid (100:0.2) followed by 50 ml of chloroform:methanol:acetic acid (95:5:0.2). Each fraction was evaporated to dryness and the residues subjected to HPLC separation for determination of OA and 4-OH-OA levels as described earlier (4).

RESULTS AND DISCUSSION

Addition of OA to liver microsomes stimulated both the enzymatic (NADPH-dependent) and the chemically induced (ascorbate/$FeSO_4$-dependent) lipid peroxidation (Fig. 1). Free active oxygen species such as superoxide anions, hydrogen peroxide or hydroxyl radicals, appear not to be involved since superoxide dismutase (SOD), catalase and mannitol were without effect (Table 1). As expected, the antioxidant BHT and the iron chelator desferal abolished lipid peroxidation. The cytochrome P-450 inhibitor metyrapone was without effect, but alpha-naphthoflavone (0.1 mM) inhibited lipid peroxidation by 35% presumably due to its antioxidant properties (11). It is thus possible that OA enhances lipid peroxidation by facilitating the NADPH (or ascorbate) dependent reduction of Fe^{3+} to Fe^{2+} and/or by facilitating the initiation step of lipid peroxidation. In vivo administration of OA to Wistar rats resulted in about a 7-fold increase in the level of ethane exhaled (Fig. 2) thus confirming the in vitro results.

In the presence of NADPH, OA is metabolized to two epimeric hydroxyl derivatives (4S)-4-OH-OA and (4R)-4-OH-OA (12), as well as to a reactive species that binds irreversibly to proteins (Table 1). In the absence of NADPH, there was no significant metabolism of OA; however, extensive binding to protein occurred. This is not unexpected, since it has been shown (13) that OA binds tightly to serum albumin. BHT and desferal drastically reduced (>80%) the level of (4S)-4-OH-OA, but not of (4R)-4-

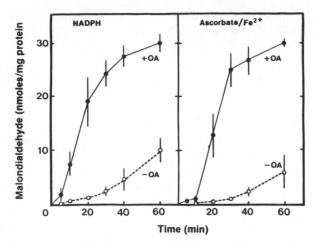

Figure 1. Enhancement of microsomal lipid peroxidation in the presence of ochratoxin A. Incubations were carried out as described in the Methods section. Each point represents the mean±S.D. of duplicate incubations from 5 different experiments.

OH-OA, suggesting that the (4S) epimer is formed in a lipid peroxidation dependent pathway and possibly requires the presence of free radicals. Desferal and BHT also inhibited protein binding of OA by 46-58%, suggesting that about half the binding of OA to protein is lipid peroxidation dependent. That the other half of protein binding is due to the cytochrome P-450 dependent activation pathway is suggested by the fact that metyrapone, which inhibits the formation of (4R)4-OH-OA by 40%, also inhibits protein binding by 20%. However, lipid peroxidation and formation of (4S)-4-OH-OA are not affected (Table 1). Similar results are obtained through the use of alpha-naphthoflavone.

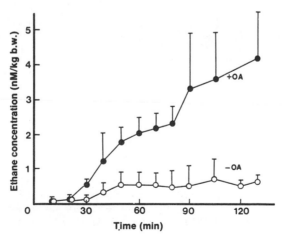

Figure 2. Effect of ochratoxin A administration on exhalation of endogenous ethane. Details are as described in the Methods section. Data are expressed as nM ethane/kg and each point represents the mean±S.D. of 6 rats.

Table 1. Effect of Various Agents on Ochratoxin A-dependent Lipid Peroxidation, Metabolism and Protein Binding.

Addition to system	MDA formed	Metabolism (4S)	(4R)	Protein binding
-NADPH (Blank)	<3	<3	6	111
No addition	100	100	100	100 *
SOD (20 ug)	98	104	101	102
Catalase (20 ug)	99	106	104	104
Mannitol (100 mM)	96	98	102	101
BHT (20 uM)	0	20	85	42
Desferal (0.1 mM)	1	17	151	54
Metyrapone (0.1 mM)	105	109	60	80
alpha-Naphtho-flavone (0.1 mM)	65	47	38	56

Incubations were carried out in duplicate for 60 min at $37^{\circ}C$ in 1 ml of 0.1 M phosphate buffer and contained 2 mg liver microsomal protein, 125 uM OA or [^{3}H]OA and 1mM NADPH. Values are expressed relative to "No addition" as 100 which corresponded to 30.1 nmol/mg protein of MDA, 335 pmol/mg protein of (4S)-4-OH-DA, 755 pmol/mg protein of (4R)-4-OH-OA and 276 pmol/mg protein of OA bound (net value).

*Net value after subtraction of blank (-NADPH).

Formation of reactive oxygen species possibly resulting in enhancement of lipid peroxidation and/or binding of reactive metabolites to critical cellular macromolecules are considered likely mechanisms for the enhancement of xenobiotic toxicity. It is thus possible that OA exerts its toxic effects via such pathways.

In vivo studies revealed that, in all cases, the OA metabolic ratios were higher in DA rats than in Lewis rats (Fig. 3 and 4). In the single dose experiment (Fig. 3), excretion of the 4-OH metabolite was complete by 96 hr while OA was still being excreted. In fact, at the high OA dose (5.0 mg/kg), excretion of OA tended to rise after 4 days. This may indicate greater initial binding to serum albumin and its subsequent release. At the end of 96 hr, the OA metabolic ratio for DA rats was 21.8 (0.5 mg/kg) and 22.5 (5.0 mg/kg) while, for Lewis rats, the corresponding values were 7.4 and 7.8 (Fig. 3) indicating that OA metabolic ratios were 2.9-fold higher in DA rats. This status was maintained in DA and Lewis rats fed OA on a long-term basis (Fig. 4). These results confirm our earlier in vitro studies (4,5) that OA-4-hydroxylase activity is lower in hepatic and renal microsomes preparations from DA rats than from Lewis rats. It has yet to be demonstrated that DA rats are less susceptible than Lewis rats to the nephrotoxic and/or carcinogenic effects of OA. However, in preliminary experiments, we have shown that administration of DA results in an increase in ethane exhalation in Lewis but not in OA rats. This lack of effect in DA rats may possibly be due to the more rapid elimination of OA in DA rats (Fig. 3).

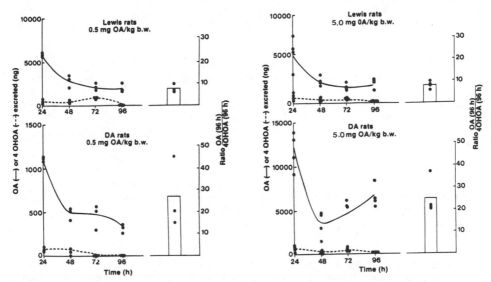

Figure 3. Levels of urinary ochratoxin A and 4-hydroxyochratoxin A in Lewis and DA rats following administration of ochratoxin A. Details are as described in the Methods section. Each point represents the level of OA or 4-OH-OA excreted by individual rats at the various time points. In each panel, the graph to the right represents the cumulative OA metabolic ratio at the end of 96 hr.

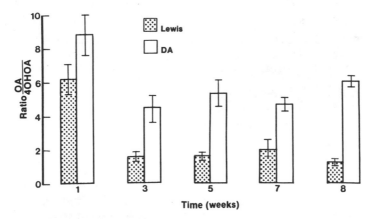

Figure 4. Urinary ochratoxin A metabolic ratios in Lewis and DA rats following chronic administration of ochratoxin A. Details are described in the Methods section.

REFERENCES

1.   P. Krogh & S. Nesheim. Ochratoxin A, In "Environmental Carcinogens - Selected Methods of Analysis, Vol. 5: Some Mycotoxins. Stoloff, L., Castegnaro, M., Scott, P., O'Neill, I.K. & Bartsch, H., eds, IARC Scientific Publications No. 44, International Agency for Research on Cancer, Lyon (1982).

2.   A.M. Bendele, W.W. Carlton, P. Krogh and E.B. Lillehoj. Ochratoxin A Carcinogenesis in B6C3F1 Mouse. J. Natl. Cancer Inst., 375:733 (1985).

3.   E.E. Creppy, A. Kane, G. Dirheimer, C. Lafarge-Frayssinet, S Mousset and C. Frayssinet. Genotoxicity of Ochratoxin A in Mice: DNA single-strand break evaluation in spleen, liver and kidney. Toxicol. Lett., 28:29 (1985)

4.   E. Hietanen, C. Malaveille, A.-M. Camus, J.-C. Bereziat, G. Brun, M. Castegnaro, J. Michelon, J.R. Idle and H. Bartsch. Interstrain comparison of hepatic and renal microsomal carcinogen metabolism and liver S9-mediated mutagenicity in OA and Lewis rats phenotyped as poor and extensive metabolizers of debrisoquine. Drug Metab. Dispos., 14:118 (1986).

5.   E. Hietanen, H. Bartsch, M. Castegnaro, C. Malaveille, J. Michelon and L. Broussolle. Use of antibodies (Ab) against cytochrome P-450 isozymes to study genetic polymorphism in drug oxidations. J. Pharm. Clin., 4:71 (1985).

6.   J.C. Ritchie, M.J. Crothers, L.R. Idle, J.B. Crieg, T.A. Connors, I.G. Nikolov and I.N. Chernozemsky. Evidence for an inherited metabolic susceptibility to endemic (Balkan) nephropathy. In: "Proceedings of the 5th Symposium on Endemic Balkan Nephropathy", S. Strahinie and V. Stefanovic, eds. p. 23 (1983).

7.   M. Castegnaro, I.N. Chernozemsky and H. Bartsch. Meeting Report: Endemic Nephropathy and Urinary Tract Tumors in the Balkans. Cancer Res., (1987) (in press).

8.   S.G. Dabbagh, J.R. Idle and R.L. Smith. Animal modelling of human polymorphic drug oxidation, the metabolism of debrisoquine and phenacetin in rat inbread strains. J. Pharmacol., 33:161 (1981).

9.   A.D. Rahimtula, J.-C. Bereziat, V. Bussachini-Griot and H. Bartsch. Lipid peroxidation as a possible cause of ochratoxin A toxicity. Biochem. Pharmacol., (submitted for publication).

10.   Z.A. Shamsuddin and A.D. Rahimtula. Metabolic activation of 2,6-dimethyl-naphthalene by liver microsomes and effect on tissue glutathione levels in vivo. Drug Metab. Dispos., 14:724 (1986).

11.   P.R. Miles, J.R. Wright, L. Bowman and H.D. Colby. Inhibition of hepatic microsomal lipid peroxidation by drug substrate without drug metabolism. Biochem. Pharmacol., 29:565 (1980).

12.   F.C. Stormer, C.E. Hansen, J.I. Pedersen, G. Hvistendahl and A.J. Aasen. Formation of (4R) and (4S)-4-hydroxyochratoxin A from ochratoxin A by liver microsomes from various species. Appl. Environ. Microbiol., 42:1051 (1981).

13.   F.S. Chu. Interaction of ochratoxin A with bovine serum albumin. Biochem. Biophys., 147:359 (1971).

SILICON IN URAEMIC RATS

Shinichi Hosokawa, Mayiml Morinaga, Hiroshi Nishitani, Osamu Yoshida*

Utano National Hospital, Kyoto University Hospital*, 8 Ondoyama-cho, Ukyo-ku, Kyoto-city, 616, Japan

INTRODUCTION

Silicon is one of essential trace elements for normal growth, bone formation and development in rats (1) and also plays an important role in other vital processes in animals (2). Silicon is found in brain, liver, lung, kidney (especially in mitochondria), and in bone, blood and urine.

Silicon may also be toxic and causes lung fibrosis (3), liver disease (4), nephropathy (5) and neuropathy (6) in man. Serum silicon has been found to be very high in uraemic patients (7,8), but there is no information regarding the role of these increased levels on the development or progression of renal changes. In this paper, the relationship between renal function and anaemia, and silicon levels of uraemic rats were examined.

MATERIALS AND METHODS

Normal male Wistar rats (n = 5; 250g) and matched rats (n = 5) were made uraemic by performing a 5/6 nephrectomy. Serum, corpuscular and renal tissue silicon levels were measured. When collecting blood, plastic cannuli and containers that had been acid-leached and screened to ensure that they were silicon free, were used. Serum, corpuscular and renal tissue samples were all handled in the same manner. Silicon concentration were determined by a standard dilution method. Silicon levels were measured with flameless atomic absorption spectrophotometry (Hitachi, Japan), equipped with a silicon hollow-cathode tube, using a 251.6 nm wavelength and nitrogen gas system (gas flow: 1 l/min) designed to gradually increase the temperature. The low-threshold silicon levels were 0.1 ug/dl. The variation coefficient for replicate measurement was 1%, and the recovery of added silicon by this method 100 $\pm$ 1.1 %. Blood urea nitrogen (BUN) and serum creatinine were assessed by standard methods, and red blood cell count (RBC) and haemoglobin (Hb) values were measured with Coulter counter. Student's t-tests were used.

RESULTS

The relationship between BUN and serum, corpuscular and renal tissue silicon levels. The relationship between BUN levels and serum silicon levels was statistically significant (r = 0.79, p < 0.01). There was significant negative relationship between BUN levels and corpuscular silicon levels ($r = -0.78$, $p < 0.01$). There was no significant relationship between BUN levels and renal tissue silicon levels.

The relationship between serum creatinine levels and serum, corpuscular and renal tissue silicon levels. The relationship between serum creatinine levels and corpuscular silicon levels was negative significant ($r = -0.82$, $p < 0.05$). We did not find any significant relationship between serum creatinine levels and renal tissue levels.

The relationship between silicon levels in RBC and serum, corpuscular and renal tissue levels. There was significant ($r = -0.90$, $p < 0.01$) relationship between serum silicon levels and RBC. The relationship between RBC and corpuscular silicon levels was significant ($r = 0.81$, $p < 0.01$). We found significant ($r = -0.67$, $p < 0.05$) relationship between RBC and renal tissue silicon levels.

The relationship between Hb values and serum corpuscular and renal tissue levels. There was significant ($r = -0.93$, $p < 0.01$) relationship between serum silicon levels and Hb levels and corpuscular silicon levels ($r = 0.82$, $p < 0.01$). We also found a significant relationship between Hb values and renal tissue silicon levels ($r = -0.80$, $p < 0.01$).

The relationship between haematocrit (Hct) levels and serum, corpuscular and renal tissue silicon levels. A significant correlation between serum silicon levels and Hct values was found ($r = -0.93$, $p < 0.01$). There was also a significant relationship between Hct levels and corpuscular silicon levels ($r = 0.83$, $p < 0.01$). The relationship between Hct values and renal tissue silicon levels was also significant ($r = -0.61$, $p < 0.05$).

DISCUSSION

Silicon is an essential trace element for growth in rats (1) and bone formation (2). Recently, Mauras et al. (9) reported that silicon is a good indication of renal failure because serum silicon levels showed a good correlation with creatinine. While Berlyne et al. (10) reported that urine silicon excretion is significantly related to creatinine clearance. Silicon is partly eliminated by the kidneys and excessive amounts accumulate in these organs in some patients heavily exposed to inhalation and cause nephropathy (11). Our data showed that BUN levels have good correlation with serum and corpuscular silicon levels. Also, our results showed that there were, significant relationship between serum creatinine levels and serum corpuscular silicon levels. However, we did not find any correlation with renal tissue silicon levels and BUN values and serum creatinine levels.

These results suggest that serum and corpuscular silicon levels are good indicators of renal function, and that silicon is a nephrotoxic substance. Serum silicon levels show a good negative correlation with RBC, Hb and Hct values. There were positive relationship between corpuscular silicon levels and RBC, Hb and Hct levels. We found negative relationship between renal tissue silicon levels and RBC, Hb and Hct values. These results suggest that silicon is a haematotoxic substance, and that serum silicon levels are good indicator of anaemia.

CONCLUSION

In rats with a surgically induced uraemia:-

1) Serum silicon levels were high.

2) Corpuscular silicon levels were low.
3) Renal tissue silicon levels were high.
4) Serum and corpuscular silicon levels are good indicators of renal function.
5) Serum, corpuscular and renal tissue silicon levels are indicators of anaemia.
6) Silicon may exert its effects by being a direct nephrotoxic and haematotoxic substance.

REFERENCES

(1) Schwarz K, Milne DB. Growth-promoting effects of silicon in rats. Nature, 239: 339, 1972.

(2) Carlisle DM. Silicon: An essential element for the chick. Science, 178: 619, 1972.

(3) Leong ASY. Pathologic findings in silicone spallation: Autopsy and biopsy studies. Annals Academy Med, 12: 304-310, 1983.

(4) Laohapand T, Osman EM, Morley AR, Word MK, Kerr DNS. Accumulation of silicon elaster in regular dialysis. Proc. EDTA. 19:143, 1982.

(5) Hauglustaine D, Van Damme B, Daeness P, Michielsen P. Silicon nephropathy: a possible occupational hazard. Nephron. 26: 219, 1980.

(6) Hershey CO, Ricantai ES, Hershey LA, Varnes AW, Lavin PJM, Strain WH. Silicon as a potential uremic neurotoxin: trace element analysis in patients with renal failure. Neurology, 33: 786, 1986.

(7) Hosokawa S, Morinaga M, Nishitani H, Maeda T, Yoshida O. Silicon in chronic hemodialysis patients. ASAIO transaction, 33: 1987 (in press).

(8) Berlyne GM, Adler AJ, Ferran N, Bennett S, Holt J. Silicon metabolism. Nephron. 44:36, 1986.

(9) Mauras Y, Riberi P, Cartier F, Allain P. Increase in blood silicon concentration in patients with renal failure. Biomedicine, 33:228, 1980.

(10) Berlyne GM, Dudek E, Adler A3, Rubin JE, Seidman M. Silicon metabolism: the basic facts in renal failure. Kidney Int. 28 suppl 17:175, 1985.

(11) Goligorsdy MS, Chaimovilz Cidio, Nir Y, Rapopert J, Kol R, Yehuda J. X-ray microanalysis of uremic nephrocalcinosis: Cellular distribution of calcium, aluminium and silicon in uremic nephrocalcinosis. Mineral Electrolyte Metab. 11:301, 1985.

NEPHROTOXICITY OF EXPERIMENTAL ENDOTOXAEMIA IN RATS

Jocemir R. Lugon, Mirian A. Boim, Oswaldo L. Ramos and Nestor Schor

Nephrology Division, Escola Paulista de Medicina, Rua Botucatu, 740 0423 S O Paulo, SP, Brazil

INTRODUCTION

Endotoxaemia is frequently associated with acute renal failure (ARF) and continues to offer a very poor prognosis despite the recent progress in antibiotic therapy (1). During endotoxaemia an important release of vasoconstrictor and/or dilator hormones have been measured suggesting a that there is a hormonal role in this type of ARF (2). However, the understanding of this pathophysiology is very complex since the renal function is compromised by multifactorial effects such as pre-existing diseases (eg. diabetes, multiple myeloma, etc.) the frequent administration of potential nephrotoxins (eg. aminoglycoside therapy) and/or prostaglandin inhibitors which all serve to complicate the assessment of renal function. Furthermore, systemic haemodynamic alterations can, per se, affect renal microcirculation.

This study was undertaken to evaluate the glomerular haemodynamics in the absence of any important systemic haemodynamic effects during the endo-toxaemia status. For this purpose euvolaemic adult Munich-Wistar rats were studied during two time periods and after a first study period received a single intravenous dose of lypopolysaccharide (LPS) from E.Coli 0111:B4 (Difco, USA) at a maximal dosage of 100ug/kg, which had no substantial effect on the mean arterial pressure, so as to maintain the animals within renal auto-regulatory levels and avoiding any of thee systemic haemodynamic alterations seen in patients with endotoxaemia.

These animals were submitted to a micropuncture measurements for glomerular haemodynamic studies, using the techniques detailed elsewhere (3).

RESULTS AND DISCUSSION

Figure 1 summarizes whole renal function after LPS administration. As shown, glomerular filtration rate (GFR), renal plasma flow (RPF) and total filtration fraction (FF) declined significantly by 57, 31 and 40% respectively ($p < 0.05$). However, total renal vascular resistance (RVR), increased by 74% ($p < 0.05$).

Figure 2 shows glomerular haemodynamic data before and after LPS administration. Single nephron glomerular filtration rate (SNGFR) and

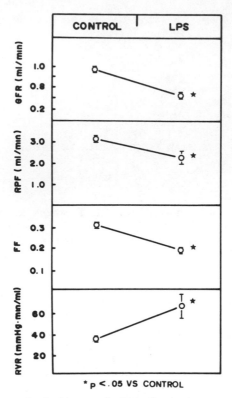

Figure 1 - Summary of whole renal function after LPS administration.

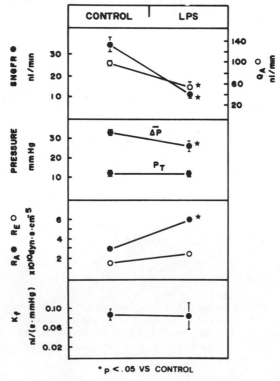

Figure 2 - Summary of glomerular haemodynamic data after LPS administration.

glomerular plasma flow (Q_A) declined significantly after LPS. Since mean SNGFR was predominantly affected, single nephron filtration fraction also declined from 0.35±0.01 to 0.22±0.03 (X±SE, p < 0.05).

Mean tubular hydraulic pressure (P_T) was not affected by LPS, thus the decline on mean transglomerular hydraulic pressure, $\triangle P$, was due to a decrease on mean glomerular capillary hydraulic pressure, PGC. The decline of mean PGC and Q_A were due to an increase on total arteriolar resistance, R_T, mainly by the afferent one, R_A (p < 0.05). No difference was observed on glomerular ultrafiltration coefficient, K_f.

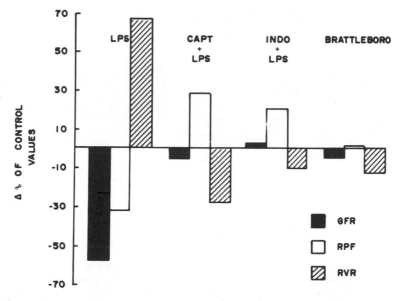

Figure 3 - Summary of mean glomerular filtration rate (GFR), renal plasma flow (RPF), and total renal vascular resistance (RVR) in the groups.

In addition, the possible role of the renin-angiotensin and prostaglandin systems were assessed by treating rats with a continuous iv inhibition of captopril (CAPT, n = 6, 2 mg/kg/h, iv) or a bolus of indomethacin, (INDO, n = 6, 2 mg/kg, iv). LPS was administered in the study second study period as described above. The effects of the absence of endogenous vasopressin was assessed in Brattleboro rats (n =6), a genetic diabetes insipidus strain, using the same protocol of LPS administration after a control study period. Figure 3 summarizes mean GFR, RPF and RVR in the groups LPS, CAPT + LPS, INDO + LPS and in the Brattleboro rats group, compared with baseline control period, percentage of variation.

Acute LPS administration at the dose level used in this study caused a decline in GFR and RPF and an increase on RVR. The administration of

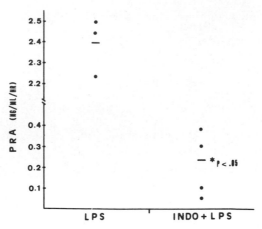

Figure 4 – Plasma renin-activity (PRA) in LPS alone and after simultaneous indomethacin (INDO) treatment.

captopril and indomethacin or the use of Brattleboro rats decreased the LPS related effects on total renal function. It is of interesting that the increase on mean plasma renin activity (Figure 4) after LPS, was also blunted by a simultaneous treatment with indomethacin, suggesting therefore that renin-angiotensin system is secondarily activated by prostaglandin stimulation. Thus LPS caused a decline on total and super-ficial nephron glomerular filtration rate, on flows and filtration fractions, with increases on the resistances. However, superficial nephrons appear to be more affected, suggesting a preferential cortical ischaemia as also observed by Conger et al (4) in female Munich-Wistar rats (MW). Furthermore, it was in someway expected, as it is known that higher doses of LPS are able to induce selective necrosis of renal cortex (4) a lesion also described in human sepsis (5).

The present glomerular haemodynamic data indicated that LPS infusion caused a marked increase in R_A which leads to a reduction in mean PGC and thereby determining a significant decrease in ΔP. No change was found in K_f, which is an an unexpected finding, considering that blood levels of many hormones (eg. prostaglandins, angiotensin II) which are able to reduce the ultrafiltration coefficient and AVP are markedly elevated in endotoxaemia (2). An attractive hypothesis to explain the maintenance of the K_f as a direct action of LPS on mesangial cells, impairing its contraction ability, but this needs to be tested. Another alternative is that higher levels of atrial natriuretic factor (ANF) could account for the unmodifyed K_f since it prevents mesangial contraction in some experimental situations (6). ANF levels have apparently not been measured in sepsis.

Pretreatment with captopril or indomethacin and the absence of AVP all minimize LPS-induce whole renal function alterations. It is expected that the absence of one vasopressor, might prevent a vasoconstriction mediated alterations. Using saralasin, for instance, Conger et al (4) prevented the LPS-induced reduction in GFR by 50% in female MW rats. Prostaglandins inhibition is known to impair kidney function under vasoconstrictor stimulus, thus the prevention of LPS-induced renal function reduction by indomethacin is surprising. However, there are several demonstrations of increase survival rate in septic or endotoxaemic animals which received indomethacin (7,8). Unfortunately, informations about renal function are missing in these studies.

Our preliminary results with indomethacin led us to speculate that its protective effects had been mediated, at least partially, by direct inhibition of thromboxane A2 synthesis and/or indirectly, by inhibition of prostaglandins-dependent angiotensin release pathway. We did not selectively investigate thromboxane A2 role, but, in a similar protocol study, Badr et al (9) observed that the synthesis inhibition of this hormone prevented LPS-induced reduction in GFR by 70%. The measurement of plasma renin activity at the end of our experiments showed that animals treated with indomethacin had mean levels 10 times lower than those of LPS treated animals, indicating that prostaglandins-dependent renin pathway is very active in the present experimental model.

Taken together these data, clearly suggest that the renal protective effect of indomethacin in endotoxaemia can be partially accounted for the eventual synthesis impairment of two vasoconstrictors, thromboxane A2 and angiotensin II. Additional interactions involving different vasoactive systems that are known to be activated in endotoxaemia like leukotrienes, AVP, histamine, kinins, endorphins and others have to be studied.

In summary, by using an experimental model in which low doses of LPS were administered to rats in order to minimize its systemic effects, we were able to investigate mainly the direct action of LPS on renal haemodynamics. The main finding was SNGFR reduction that resulted from declines in both Q_A and ΔP caused by an outstanding elevation in R_A. Mean K_f, in the present protocol, remained unaltered. Moreover, the data suggest that inhibition of some hormonal pathways can significantly reduce the impact of LPS over the renal function. Of special clinical relevance is the finding that prior non-steroid anti-inflammatory drugs administration, in opposition to what was thought, actually improved renal function during endotoxaemia opening the perspective of its utilization in clinical trials.

ACKNOWLEDGEMENTS

This work was supported by grants from FAPESP, CNPq, CAPES and IPEPENHI. The authors thank Ms. Clara Versolato for technical assistance and Marina Andre' da Silva for secretarial assistance.

REFERENCES

1. W.R. McCabe, T.L. Treadwel and A. de Maria Jr, Pathophysiology of bacteremia, Am. J. Med. 75:7 (1983).

2. M.F. Wilson and D.J. Brackett, Release of vasoactive hormones and circulatory changes in shock, Circ. Shock 11:225 (1983).

3. N. Schor, I. Ichikawa and B.M. Brenner, Mechanisms of action of various hormones and vasoactive substances on glomerular ultrafiltration in the rat, Kidney Int. 20:442 (1981).

4. J.D. Conger, S.A. Falk and S.J. Euggenheim, Glomerular dynamics and morphologic changes in the generalized schwartzman reaction in postpartum rats, J. Clin. Invest. 67:1334 (1981).

5. N.K. Holenberg, M. Epstein, S.M. Rosen, R.I. Basch, D.E. Oken and J.P. Merril, Acute oliguric renal failure in man: evidence for preferential renal cortical ischemia, Medicine 47:455 (1968).

6. J.M. Lopez-Novoa, G. Arriba, A.F. Cruz, L. Hernando and D.R. Puyol, Atrial natriuretic peptide modulates isolated rat glomeruli contraction, The First Annual Meeting on ANF: 99A (1986).

7. R.R. Butler Jr, W.C. Wise, P.V. Haluska and J.A. Cook, Gentamicin and indomethacin in the treatment of septic shock: Effects on prostacyclin and thromboxane A2 production, J. Pharmacol. Exp. Ther. 225:94 (1983).

8. J.R. Fletcher, The role of prostaglandins in sepsis, Scand. J. Invest. Dis. 31 (Suppl):55 (1982).

9. K.F. Badr, V.E. Kelley and B.M. Brenner, Selective antagonism of thromboxane A2 and sulfidopeptide leukotrienes ameliorates endoxotin-induced renal ischemia, Kidney Int. 27:227 (A) (1985).

STUDIES ON A PHYSIOLOGICAL MODEL FOR THE HUNMAN RENAL FANCONI SYNDROME

Karl S. Roth

Virginia Commonwealth University, Medical College of Virginia, Box 239, MCV Station Richmond, Virginia 23298, USA.

INTRODUCTION

The human renal Fanconi syndrome (FS) is unique among the many nephrotoxic disorders because of its association with a wide variety of inherited metabolic disorders as well as with numerous exogenous substances (1,2). This broad spectrum of known aetiologies lends credence to the concept that the renal tubular dysfunction of the FS represents the result of a common, underlying effect of a number of different agents on the kidney. Accordingly, investigators have utilized several animal models for the FS in efforts to elucidate the biochemical mechanism(s) implicit in this disorder. The most thoroughly-studied of these models is that generated by treatment of the rat with maleic acid, both in vivo (3,4) and in vitro (5-8). To date, the specific biochemical action by which maleate affects transport of sugars, amino acids and various other endogenous materials remains elusive, although many intracellular and membrane transport phenomena have been demonstrated (5-10). However, the most significant disadvantage inherent in all studies using this compound is the fact that maleate is not an endogenously produced substance in mammals. Therefore, until very recently, no model system was available with which to study the FS associated with genetic disease in man.

Succinylacetone (SA) is a compound formed and excreted in abnormal quantities in urine of humans affected by the autosomal recessive genetic disorder, hereditary tyrosinemia (11). Such individuals also suffer from a secondary and reversible renal FS which includes glucosuria and generalized aminoaciduria (1,2). Accordingly, we have undertaken an investigation into the use of SA in creation of an animal model for the study of the biochemical basis of the FS. Such a model would have a very distinct advantage over the maleic acid-treated animal, in which the inciting substance is non-physiologic and may, therefore, bear little or no relevance to the human disorder.

METHODS AND MATERIALS

Adult male Sprague-Dawley rats weighing 150-175g were purchased from Charles River Breeding Laboratories (Wilmington, MA). Animals were weighed and housed individually in metabolic cages: each rat was given free access to Purina chow and water ad libitum. Following an overnight period of acclimatization, urine was collected for a 24-h period and frozen at -20°C. The animals were then injected intraperitoneally with neutralized (pH 7.0) SA. Controls were given equal volume of normal saline intraperitoneally. Urines were collected over the subsequent 24-h period and frozen at -20°C until analysed. Amino acid quantitation was performed using a JEOL JLC-5AH automated amino acid analyser.

Isolated renal tubules were prepared by collagenase digestion of minced cortical slices, as previously described (5). The experimental method for determining substrate uptake by tubules has been described by us and others in detail (7-9). "Trapped medium" space and total water were 15.2% and 80% respectively (5). Tissue substrate concentrations and distribution ratios (cpm/ml intracellular fluid to cpm/ml medium) were determined as previously described (12). All data were analysed for significance by Student's t-test. The suspensions were either untreated or treated with 4 mM SA. Oxygen consumption was measured polarographically at 30°C with a Clark fixed-voltage electrode.

Brushborder membrane vesicles were then prepared using the method of Booth and Kenny (13) modified as described by Weiss et al (14). The final membrane pellet was suspended to a protein concentration of 0.3-0.4 mg/ml as determined by the method of Lowry, et al. (15). All measurements of uptake were performed using Millipore filtration on HAWP filters (0.45 um) according to the technique described by McNamara et al. (16). The vesicles demonstrated osmotic activity and did not metabolise substrate. Results are expressed as nmoles (or pmols) of substrate uptake/mg protein.

RESULTS

Although 24-h urinary volume did not differ significantly during pre- and post-injection periods, administration of SA intraperitoneally resulted in proteinuria (> 300 mg/dl) and glucosuria (> 250 mg/dl). Quantitative measurement of urinary amino acids revealed increases in several following SA injection.

Studies in Isolated Tubule Fragments. The steady-state distribution ratio achieved by the tubules for alpha-methyl-D-glucoside (AMG) and alpha-aminoisobutyric acid (AIB) were significantly depressed (P < 0.001) in the presence of 4 mM SA, compared to controls. Any further increase in concentration of the inhibitor to 8 mM did not produce a proportionately greater effect on the steady-state concentration gradient achieved. The inhibitory effect of SA was exerted fully by 30 min of incubation, by which time both control and experimental tissue achieved and maintained steady-states. Preincubation with 4 mM SA for 30 min did not further increase the difference in steady-state levels achieved. Initial rates of uptake in the presence of SA appeared to differ from controls.

Tubules were incubated for 30 minutes in three separate flasks, two of which contained 4 mM SA. At the end of this incubation, the tissue was separated from the original buffer and resuspended in buffer alone or buffer + 4 mM SA. Substrate was then added and an uptake experiment was carried out. No significant difference (P > 0.05) in uptake of AMG or AIB was observed between control tubules and those exposed to 4 mM SA and resuspended in buffer alone. On the other hand, continued exposure to SA resulted in inhibition of AMG and AIB, uptake, thus demonstrating the reversibility of the transport effects of SA. Finally, oxygen consumption by the tubules was examined with and without 4 mM SA after a 30-min preincubation. SA treatment reduced oxygen consumption compared to controls by 50% in the presence of endogenous substrate alone (controls = 82.8 nmol O_2/min per ml versus 40.0 nmol O_2/min per ml) on five separate determinations. A similar relationship between SA-treated tubules pertained with fortilied respiration (115.4 versus 76.1 nmol O_2/min per ml) on four separate determinations. A 30-min preincubation of tubules with 4 mM SA in the presence of various metabolic substrates, alone or in combination, did not result in any increase in distribution ratio of AIB over that observed with SA alone. Uptake of AMG was noncompetitively inhibited by 4 mM SA. Determination of 15-min velocity of uptake at 0.045-30 mM AIB without added 4 mM SA needed a two-limbed plot using the Hofstee transformation. Addition of 4 mM SA under otherwise identical conditions also resulted in a two-limbed plot showing non-competitive inhibition.

Studies in Renal Brushborder Membrane Vesicles. Uptake of 0.06 mM glycine by membrane vesicles incubated in 100 mM NaCl gradient reached the peak overshoot at 3 minutes, as compared to vesicles allowed to equilibrate in 100 mM NaCl prior to the start of incubation with glycine. Addition of 4 mM SA to gradient-incubated vesicles significantly (P < 0.0001) reduced the overshoot peak achieved at 3 minutes (Fig. 1). At the earliest time of incubation (30 sec) the uptake by SA-treated vesicles was significantly reduced compared to the controls (P < 0.0001). A similar phenomenon was observed with other substrates, SA in each case causing a reduction in the amount of material taken up with time compared to controls when the vesicles were incubated in a 100 mM NaCl gradient (Table 1). Further, in the cases of glycine and lysine, where uptake is known to occur simultaneously on heterogeneous transport systems, SA exerted an inhibitory effect on uptake at both low and high substrate concentrations.

TABLE 1. Effect of 4.0 mM Succinylacetone on Membrane Uptake of Sugars and Amino Acids

		UPTAKE (nmol/mg)		
SUBSTRATE	(mM)	CONTROL	4 mM SA	P
Glycine	0.06	0.729$\pm$0.045	0.398$\pm$0.54	0.0002
	1.1	5.83$\pm$0.361	3.84$\pm$0.413	0.001
L-Lysine	0.06	0.434$\pm$0.021	0.24$\pm$0.027	0.02
	2.1	13.2$\pm$1.002	6.80$\pm$0.931	0.001
alpha-CH$_3$-Glucoside	0.06	0.780$\pm$0.069	0.571$\pm$0.072	0,02
D-Glucose	0.06	0.623$\pm$0.043	0.212$\pm$0.061	0.001

Vesicles were incubated for 3 minutes at 25° in 100 mM NaCl gradient, with or without added 4 mM SA. Uptake values are given as the means of at least 9 separate determinations $\pm$ standard error. P values were determined as described under "Methods".

In view of the fact that transport inhibition caused by 4 mM SA in the isolated tubule is reversible, we were concerned that our observations might indicate the presence of physical damage to the membrane integrity. Thus, we further examined the basis for our observations by testing for reversibility in the membrane vesicles. Vesicles were pre-incubated in either THM or THM + 4 mM SA for 30 seconds at 25°C. The vesicles were then recentrifuged, the supernatant discarded and the vesicles in each tube resuspended in fresh THM with no SA added. Uptake of 0.06 mM glycine was examined. Results clearly demonstrated no differences in glycine uptake between control and SA-treated vesicles.

In order to better assess the nature of the inhibition by SA on glycine and AMG uptake, we examined changes occurring in concentration-dependent uptake by membrane vesicles. The membranes were incubated for 30 seconds at 25°C in 100 mM NaCl with or without 4 mM SA. Glycine concentration varied from 0.021 mM to 7.6 mM, while AMG varied from 10 ÌM to 0.51 mM. Glycine concentration-dependent uptake over the entire substrate range

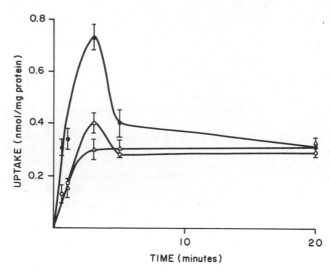

Figure 1. Glycine uptake by brushborder membrane vesicles. Control (●),
control + 4 mM SA (○), and sodium-equilibrated (△) are shown as S.E. of 12
separate determinations.

appeared to be competitively-inhibited by 4 mM SA, while inhibition of AMG
uptake was also non-competitive in nature.

DISCUSSION

Unavailabiltiy of appropriate naturally-occurring animal models has
significantly hampered investigations into the biochemical basis for
various human disorders, especially those with genetic aetiologies. This
is particularly true of diseases in which it is not clear that the
phenotypic   manifestations   are   secondary   to   identifiable   endogenous
metabolic products rather than to the primary genetic defect, as in
cystinosis. In cystine storage the renal FS is not reversible and does not
occur naturally in animals; thus one cannot distinguish between cystine
nephrotoxicity and mutant gene expression aetiologically.

The potential for a physiologic animal model for study of the human FS was
created by the description of succinylacetoacetate and SA excretion in
urine of patients with hereditary tyrosinemia associated with renal
tubular dysfunction (11). Subsequent work demonstrating a relationship
between increased flux through the tyrosine catabolic pathway and
reversible tubular dysfunction in affected individuals (17) provided
further support for embarking on the present investigations.

Our in vivo data provide evidence for a relationship between endogenous SA
produced as a consequence of a genetic defect in humans and a secondary
renal FS. The nephrotoxicity caused by SA could be enhanced by succinylacetoacetate, but we did not attempt to examine this possibility in our
studies. Appearance of glucosuria and aminoaciduria subsequent to
injection of healthy male rats excited our curiosity about renal tubular
cellular events underlying this finding.

Based on our earlier observations in the isolated tubule that SA
reversibly reduces O_2 consumption while affecting membrane transport of

sugars and amino acids in a non-competitive fashion, we anticipated finding little, if any effect of SA on uptake by the brushborder vesicle. However, the present data leave little room for doubt that, in the presence of 4 mM SA the vesicle uptake of several physiologic substrates is significantly reduced. On the other hand, our data are equally definitive in demonstrating the reversible nature of this reduction. Such findings point to an important difference between the SA- and maleic acid-induced models: in the latter, maleate-treated isolated tubules show transport inhibition of sugars (5) and amino acids (6) without demonstrable effects on membrane vesicle uptake (18). Thus, the transport-related actions of SA on the intact tubule cell appear to be more complex than those of maleate. Since our studies were carried out over hexose and amino acid concentration ranges corresponding to normal blood levels in the rat, we believe that our observations may reflect actual physiologic events attributable to SA.

We have now demonstrated that SA, unlike maleate, holds inhibitory properties for rat renal proximal tubular epithelium at both the membrane and mitochondrial levels, and that this inhibition affects the transport of sugars and amino acids, as well as O_2 consumption. These factors are highly significant to the study of a model system for the human renal FS, inasmuch as SA is endogenously produced in humans while maleate is not. Thus, further characterization of the SA model would be of great value to an understanding of the biochemical basis for the renal tubular dysfunction seen in the Fanconi syndrome.

ACKNOWLEDGEMENTS

This work was supported by Grant #RO 1 AM35319-02 from the National Institutes of Health, Bethesda, MD.

REFERENCES

1. Roth, K.S. and Segal, S. In: Nephrology, J. Hamburger, J. Crosner and J.-P. Grunfeld, eds., pp. 945-975. Wiley, NY 1979

2. Roth, K.S., Foreman, J.W. and Segal, S. Kidney Int. 20:705, 1981

3. Rosenberg, L.E. and Segal, S. Biochem. J. 92:345, 1964

4. Hergeron, M. and Vadeboncoeur, M. Nephron 8:367, 1971

5. Roth, K.S., Hwang, S.M. and Segal, S. Biochim Biophys Acta 426:675, 1976

6. Roth, K.S., Goldmann, D.R. and Segal, S. Pediat Res 12:1121, 1978

7. Scharer, K., Yoshida, T., Voyer, L., Berlow, S., Pietra, G. and Metcoff, J. Res. Exp. Med. 157:136, 1972

8. Rogulski, J., Pacanis, A., Adamowicz, W. and Angielski, S. Acta Biochim Polon 21:403, 1974

9. Pacanis, A. and Rogulski, J. Acta Biochim Polon 24:3, 1977

10. Szczepanska, M. and Angielski, S. Amer. J. Physiol. 239, F50, 1980

11. Lindblad, B., Lindstedt, S. and Steen, A. Proc. Natl. Acad. Sci. USA 74:4641, 1977

12. Rosenberg, L.E., Blair, A. and Segal, S. *Biochim. Biophys. Acta* 54:479, 1961

13. Booth, A.G. and Kenny, A.J. *Biochem. J*. 142:575, 1974

14. Weiss, S.D., McNamara, P.D., Pepe, L.M. and Segal, S. *J. Membr. Biol*. 43:91, 1978

15. Lowry, O.H., Rosebrough, N.J., Fan, A.L. and Randall, R.J., *J. Biol. Chem*. 193:265, 1951.

16. McNamara, P.D., Ozegovic, B., Pepe, L.M. and Segal, S. *Proc. Natl. Acad. Sci. USA* 73:4521, 1976

17. Fallstrom, S.P., Lindblad, B. and Steen, A. *Acta Paediatr. Scand*. 70:315, 1981

18. Reynolds, R., McNamara, P.D. and Segal, S. *Life Sci* 22:39, 1978.

CHRONIC URETER CANNULA IN PIG

Ei-ichi Kokue, Minoru Shimoda, Nobue Tanaka and Toyoaki Hayama

Tokyo University Agriculture and Technology, Department of Veterinary Medicine, Fuchu, Tokyo, Japan 183

INTRODUCTION

The renal clearance is an important parameter of the drug disposition. It is calculated from the amount of urinary drug per unit time and plasma concentration. Using experimental animals the exact value of renal clearance cannot be determined, because urine is voided spontaneously (Shimoda et al, 1986). It may be preferable to collect urine and blood at the same time under the continuous urinary flow, but we report here experience based on the chronic ureter cannulation of pigs.

MATERIALS AND METHODS

Animals.   Twenty-four pigs from commercial breed, weighing 28-45 kg and 1 Goettingen minipig, 30kg, were used. They were given commercial mashed feed (2% of body weight) without any antibacterial agent, and water ad libitum. They were housed in individual metabolic cage after surgery.

Surgical Operation.   Two kinds of silicon tubes were used as the cannula. One was thin, (1.0 mm id and 2.5 mm od), the other was thick, (2.5 mm id and 4.0 mm od).   Ketamine was injected (im, 10 mg/kg) as a pre-anesthetics, and animals were anaesthetized using halothane. After the midline incision, the ureters were exposed at the upper level of the urinary bladder. The cannula was inserted into the ureter and advanced cranially up to the beginning of ureter, and fixed on the Muscle psoas minor. The distal ends were advanced subcutaneously and fixed on Muscles transversus abdominis. They were brought out from body on a flank (F-zone), on a hypogastric zone near the the navel (N-zone) or near the groin (G-zone); where they were fixed to the skin.

Postoperative Management.   Ampicillin and kanamycin sulphate were injected (im) for 2 days and a topical antiseptics (povidon-iodine solution) was applied to the incision site. A quarternary ammonium disinfectant (benzetonium chloride) was used sterilise the metabolic cage. Oral electrolyte fluid (Bywater et al, 1980) was given 3 L/day to increase of the urinary volume.

Examination of Renal Function.   The patency of the ureter cannula and renal functions were examined by the phenolsulphonphthalein (PSP)-time test which was undertaken every 1 or 2 weeks. PSP (10 mg/kg) was injected

(iv) and urine collected every 10 min up to 180 min, the concentration of PSP excretion and urine volume was used to estimate the period required to excrete 50% of the injected dose. BUN (blood urea nitrogen) was assessed every week and Dipstick test for occult blood, ketone body, glucose, pH and protein was undertaken every day. Creatinine clearance could not be used as a means of assessing renal function because the renal tract of pig can reabsorb this molecule (Nielsen et al, 1965). Inulin was injected iv, at a priming dose of 100 mg/kg, followed by the additional injections of 50 mg/kg every 2 h.

Chemical analysis. The PSP concentration in the urine was determined by the spectrophotometric method (Finco, 1980), BUN was determined by urease indophenol method (BUN-S, Chugai Pharmaceutical Co. Ltd., Japan) and inulin clearance was determined from its concentration in blood and urine was determined by the spectrophotometric method (Vree et al., 1981).

RESULTS AND DISCUSSION

Clinical Condition of the Animal. Most animals were healthy and had a good appetite, and a large urinary flow from the cannula which was transparent or clean. On the other hand, some animals were inactive and lost their appetite, urinary flow from the cannula did not run well and urine was turbid or viscous. Some animals vomited or was febritic.

Examination of Renal Function. PSP urinary kinetics showed monoexponential decrease. PSP-time test was assessed 78 time in 22 pigs. Fifty-eight of the values were < 45 min, and always seen in pigs that looked healthy. urinary flow was large. It increased immediately after PSP injection. Twenty values had a PSP-time > 45 min, and were observed in animals that showed clinical disorders, and low urinary flow, which did not increase immediately after PSP injection. A PSP-time of < 45 min may be a useful criterion to show a functioning surgically prepared kidney.

BUN test: According to Pond et al (1978), the normal range of BUN in pig is 8-24 mg/dl. The 102 determinations were completed in 24 animals. Twenty of the values showed BUN > 20 mg/dl, in animals that showed serious disorder. Of the total BUN assays 82 were < 20 mg/dl, 7 were seen in pigs that showed serious or mild clinical disorders, while the remaining 75 were from pigs that looked healthy. The ranges of both groups (less than 20 mg/dl) overlapped, thus a BUN value of 20 mg/dl is a less useful criterion for assessing renal and cannulae functioning in these studies.

The urinary changes recorder by the Dipstick method was, with the exception of protein, an unreliable set of criteria for our purpose.

Correlation between PSP-time and BUN value: PSP-time and BUN value correlated (Fig. 1). Most data was within the range BUN, 5-20 mg/dl and PSP-time 10-45 min. Open circle represented data from animals that were 10 days postoperation, where they may have already recover from the surgical stress. Closed circles represented animals that were less than 10 days postoperative and include some animals that were reoperation. Some of these data show a disproportionately high PSP-time, which a degree of renal dysfunction that was not assessed by the BUN value.

Accordingly, PSP-time, less than 45 min and BUN value, 20 mg/dl, may be suitable for assessing the success of the chronic ureter cannulation, these criteria are supported by the clinical condition.

Table 1 shows the summary of these data where pigs are numbered in chronological order of investigation. In general the use of the thin silicone cannula in early studies gave a short period of functioning, and where the tube was brought out from F-zone urine flow did not run well. The thick silicone cannula, exteriorised at the N-zone run well, but were often kicked off; which reduced the period of function.

When the cannula was brought out at the G-zone, the metabolic cage rinsed with benzetonium chloride 3 times/day and the oral electrolyte fluid was given, the pigs drunk well and urinary volume increased extensively. The disinfection of the cage and much urine may prevent the bacterial infection of the ureter and kidney and the functional period was extended.

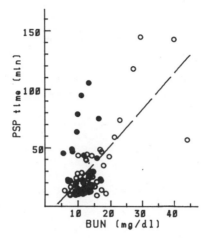

Fig. 1.   Correlation between PSP-time and BUN value.   Open circle represents postoperative more than 10 days. Closed circle represents postoperative less than 10 days. The regression coefficient was 0.68.

The renal autopsy with a histological examination was undertaken in all pigs. The pathological change, pyelectasa, pyelonephritis, infarction and haemorrhage etc, were observed in most kidneys with various severities. However only slight pathological change was observed in the kidney from the pig whose renal function was judged to be fully functional at the autopsy, ie pig no. 5, 10, 18 (Fig. 2-A), 21, 22, 23 (Fig. 2-B), 24 and 25.

The Inulin Clearance Value and Urinary Flow: Table 2 shows the result of inulin clearance test in 24 animals.   Twenty-three out of 58 determinations were done under an anaesthesia and 35 were done under a consciousness.   An apparent difference could be observed in inulin clearance value and urine flow rate between the anaesthetized and conscious groups. According to Pond et al (1978), the normal range of inulin clearance in pig is 30-138 ml/min/body.

Among the anaesthetized group, 5 pigs were studied immediately after the surgical operation. Eighteen determinations were undertaken after a postoperative period of > 10 days. Large difference were observed in urine volume between 2 groups, which could be caused by the surgical stress or the Ringers solution with mannitol which was infused (iv) at 1 ml/min in the anaesthetized animals. Almost the same volume could be recovered from

Table 1. Valid period, procedures and renal pathological change of the chronic ureter cannula.

Pig No.	flow days	survival days	cannula size	cannula outlet	renal* autopsy	cannula** validity
1	14	48	thin	F	PE+++,PN++(LR)	-
2	0	48	thin	F	PE+++,PN+++(LR)	-
3	0	35	thin	N	PE+++,PN++(LR)	-
4	18	40	thin	N	PE++,PN++,IF+(LR)	-
5	24	41	thick	N	PE+(LR),PN++,IF+(R)	*
6	5	27	thick	N	PE++(R),PN+(LR)	-
7#	0	16	thick	G	PE++,H++(LR)	nd
8	22	96	thick	G	PE+++(R),PN++,IF++(LR)	-
9	40	62	thick	G	PN++,IF+(LR)	-
10	32	42	thick	G	PE+,PN+,IF+4(LR)	+
11	33	43	thick	G	PE+++(R),PN++,IF4+(LR)	-
12	21	42	thick	G	PE4++,PN++,IF++(LR)	-
13	14	27	thick	G	PE+,PN+,IF++(LR),H+(L)	-
14	22	46	thick	G	PE+,PN++,IF++(LR)	-
15	17	49	thick	G	PE+,PE++,IF++(LR)	-
16	7	20	thick	G	PE++,IF+(LR)	-
17	7	30	thick	G	PE+,PN++,IF++(LR)	-
18	14	26	thick	G	PN+,IF+(LR)	+
19	6	20	thick	G	PE++(R),IF++(LR)	-
20##	0	9	thick	G	PE+,H+4(LR)	nd
21	10	20	thick	G	PE+,IF+(LR)	*
22	24	34	thick	G	PE4+(L),IF+(LR)	+
23	30	33	thick	G	PN+,PE+,IF+(L)	+
24	28	43	thick	G	PE+,PN+,IF+(L),PE+(R)	+
25	66	77	thick	G	PE+,IF4(LR)	+

* PE: pyelectasia, PN: pyelonephritis, IF: renal infarction, H: haemorrhage (+ slight, ++ mild, +++ severe)

(L): left kidney, (R): right kidney, (LR): both kidney

** the validity of the cannula at the autopsy (- invalid, * borderline, + valid, nd no data)

Goettingen minipig (died), ## died during surgery

Table 2. Urinary flow and inulin clearance under anaesthesia and consciousness

EXPERIMENT	TIME AFTER OPERATION	n	URINARY FLOW (ml/min)	INULIN CLEARANCE (ml/min/kg)
	immediately after	5	0.35±0.15**	1.2±0.99
anaesthesia*	>10 days	18	1,1±0.67	1.5±0.45
conscious	>10 days	35	3.1±1.1	5.9±2.7

* Ringer solution with mannitol was infused at 1 ml/min during experiment.

** mean±SD

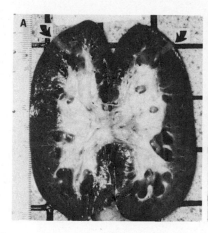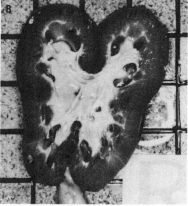

Fig. 2-A. The cut surface of kidney of pig no. 18, 26 days after the cannulation, showing infarction (arrows).

Fig. 2-B. The cut surface of right kidney of pig no. 24, 43 days after the cannulation, which shows pyelectesia.

ureter cannulae of the latter group. On the other hand, only about one third volume could be recovered from ureter cannula in the former group. The remaining part was accumulated in the abdominal cavity.

CONCLUSIONS

Several advantages of the chronic ureter cannula for pharmacokinetic study include:-

1) the collection of urine in any time, and blood at the same time.

2) investigations on conscious animals, where the large volume of urine reduces the dead space between kidney and test tube.

3) the use of the same animals repetitively, and the reduction in surgical and handling stress.

In summary the most successful approach to chronic ureter cannulation in the pig include the use of thick tube for cannula, which are exteriorised in the hypogastric zone near groin; to prevent the ascending type of bacteria infection by disinfection of animal housing and cannula outlet; and the ingestion of oral electrolyte fluid (about 3L/day or more) to maintain renal function and keep the anti-bacterial effect of urine at its highest levels.

REFERENCES

Bywater, R.J., and Woode, G.N., 1980, Use of an oral glucose-glycine electrolyte formulation for treatment of dehydration following diarrhoea in the piglet., In: "Proceedings of International Pig Veterinary Society (6th)", Copenhagen.

Finco, D.R., 1980, Kidney function, p.388, In: "Clinical Biochemistry of Domestic Animals", J.J. Kaneko, ed., Academic Press, inc., New York.

Nielsen, T.W., Maaske, C.A., and Booth, N.H., 1965, Some comparative aspects of porcine renal function., p.529, In: "Swine in Biomedical

Research, " L.K. Bustad, R.O. McClellan and M.P. Burns eds., United States
Atomic Energy Commission, Washington.

Pond, W.G., and Houpt, K.A., 1978, "The Biology of the Pig", p. 260,
Cornell University Press, Ithaca.

Shimoda, M., Aihara, E., Koyanagi, M., Kokue, E., and Hayama, T., 1986,
Possible active tubular secretion of sulfamonomethoxine and its
metabolites in pigs. J. Pharmacobio. Dyn., 9, 229-233.

Vree, T.B., Hekster, Y.A., Dansma, J.E., Tijhuis, M., and Friesen, W.T.,
1981, Pharmacokinetics and mechanism of renal excretion of short acting
sulfonamides and N-acetylsulfonamide derivatives in man. Euro. J.
Pharmacol. 20, 283-292.

EFFECTS OF GLYCEROL-INDUCED ACUTE RENAL FAILURE ON RENAL PHOSPHORUS HANDLING

Christos P. Carvounis and Peter Cushley

Department of Medicine, Section of Nephrology, Veterans Administration Medical Center and State University of New York, Syracuse, NY 13210

INTRODUCTION

Previous studies have shown that fractional excretion of phosphorus (FE_{pi}) is increased in rats that developed non-oliguric acute renal failure (ARF) close to 100% indicating that the bulk of filtered phosphorus was excreted in the urine. This finding differs significantly from the finding in rats with mercury chloride-induced oliguric ARF. In the latter, only about 1/4 of the filtered phosphorus reaches the urine, for an FE_{pi} of about 25% (1). A similar finding has been seen also in humans with variable types of ARF (Carvounis, unpublished data).

The importance of the findings of the rat study could be challenged on two different grounds. First, the glomerular filtration rate (GFR) of rats with non-oliguric ARF due to mercury chloride was excessively low (about 10% of the control values). This allows one to consider the possibility that the decreased phosphorus reabsorption may merely reflect a complete lack of function of the severely damaged tubules. Second, given the low GFR, even with a FE_{pi} of about 100%, phosphorus failed to be eliminated as needed and thus resulted in the development of a substantial hyperphosphatemia (1). It follows that in that study the increased FE_{pi} had little relevance to the overall phosphorus homeostasis.

METHODS

Sprague-Dawley rats (Taconic Farms, Germantown, NY) weighing 200-250 g were placed in metabolic cages and were fed either regular chow (Agway, Syracuse, NY) or chow devoid of phosphorus (ICN Biomedicals, Inc., Costa Mesa, CA). After 8 days of the baseline period the rats were injected with 3 ml of 50% glycerol as previously described (2). Blood was collected from the tail of rats one day prior to glycerol injection as well as in the middle of the day following the injection. Urine was collected during the 24 hr period that preceded glycerol injection as well as the 24 hr that followed it. Na, K, creatinine, phosphorus and urea nitrogen were measured in the serum and urines. Clearance of these substances were determined from the general formula:

$$C_x = U_x \cdot V / P_x$$

where C_x, U_x and P_x are the clearance, urine and plasma concentration of a given substance x.   V stands for urine flow.   Na and K were determined by flame photometry.   Creatinine was determined spectrophotometrically by a microassay as has been previously described (3).   Phosphorus was determined   spectrophotometrically (4).   GFR was determined from creatinine clearance. FE_x (fractional excretion of substance x) was found from:

$$FE_x = C_x.100 / GFR$$

RESULTS

Glycerol injection resulted in a decrease of about 50% in GFR in both the control and the phosphate deprived rats (Table I).   A significant increase in volume is also apparent in the normally fed rats.   Phosphate deprived rats started with an increased urine flow rate and an insignificant increase was seen following glycerol injection.   Both groups of rats had nevertheless significant urine output.

Table I - Urine Flow and GFR in Non-Oliguric Acute Renal Failure

	Baseline		Post-Glycerol	
	Urine Flow (ul/min)	GFR (ul/min)	Urine Flow (ul/min)	GFR (ul/min)
Regular Chow (n=36)	9.2±0.6	1976±143	16.7±1.1*	960±93*
Phosphorus-free (n=28)	15.3±1.8	1249±123	16.8±1.3	680±83*

Effects of glycerol injection on GFR and urine flow in normal and phosphorus-depleted rats. * $p < 0.001$

In the normal rats, glycerol-induced ARF resulted in a profound increase in FE_{pi} (79±6% vs 15±3% during baseline period).   More impressive is the increase in absolute phosphorus clearance that is shown in Figure 1.   As a result of this excessive phosphorus excretion we found a significant decrease in serum phosphorus from about 6 to about 4 mg/dl (Figure 2).

In the phosphate deprived rats FE_{pi} remained quite low and essentially not different from zero (0.7±0.4% vs 0.2±0.2 during baseline period).   The absolute phosphorus clearance also remained close to zero (Figure 3) and a minor, though statistically significant increase of about 0.2 mg/dl was 4 noted in the serum of these rats (Figure 4).   This probably reflects a degree of haemolysis that is common in glycerol-induced ARF (5) and signifies addition of cellular phosphorus to extracellular fluid when the kidneys quantitatively retain any filtered phosphorus.   The variable effects of glycerol injection on serum phosphorus in normal and phosphorus deprived rats is shown in Figure 5.

In the normally fed rats urine Na concentration decreased (34±1 vs 13±10 mEq/L, p < 0.001, at baseline).   A decrease of Na excretion was noted (1142±16 vs 1540±122 mEq/min at baseline p < 0.05).   An increase in FeNa was noted (1.18±0.12 vs 0.65±0.05%, p < 0.01).   Similar data were also found for the phosphorus deprived rats.

DISCUSSION

The present studies confirm the findings of the previous ones (1) regarding an increased FE_{pi} with non-oliguric ARF.   However, the relatively high GFR of our rats suggest that the increased phosphorus may not represent the result of excessively decreased renal function.

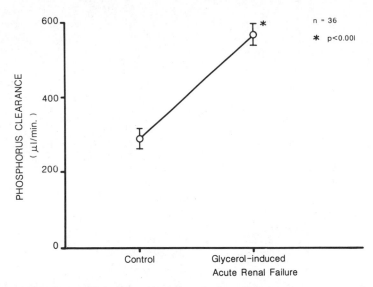

Figure 1.   Absolute clearance rates of phosphorus prior to and subsequent to glycerol-induced ARF in normally fed rats.

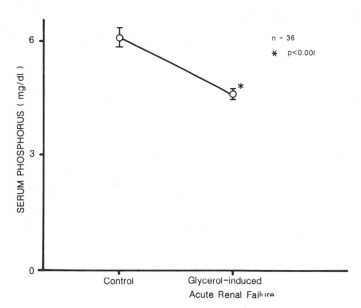

Figure 2.   Serum phosphorus prior to and subsequent to glycerol-induced ARF in normally fed rats.

Furthermore, the ability of tubules of kidneys that had glycerol-induced ARF to reabsorbed essentially all filtered phosphorus in Pi-deprived rats attests to their significant functional reserve.

It is of great interest that our findings in the normally fed rats indicate that phosphorus handling in non-oliguric ARF contributes to phosphorus homeostasis.   As shown in Figure 2, serum phosphorus decreases in the presence of significant phosphaturia, despite some increase in GFR.

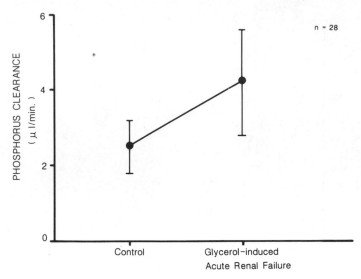

Figure 3.   Absolute clearance rates of phosphorus prior to and subsequent to glycerol-induced ARF in phosphorus depleted rats.   Note the scale is 100 times less than the one in Figure 1.

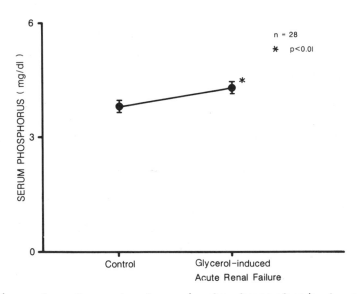

Figure 4.   Serum phosphorus in phosphorus deprived rats.

The close relationship between Na and phosphorus absorption by the proximal tubule (6) prompted us to evaluate renal Na handling during glycerol-induced ARF.   It is apparent from our findings that there is significant dissociation in the handling of the two substances in our present studies.   Actually absolute phosphorus excretion and clearance increased following glycerol injection while the exact opposite was shown for Na[+].   This favours some distinct tubular effect of glycerol to decrease phosphorus reabsorption which is independent of Na reabsorption and can be overcome by phosphorus deprivation.

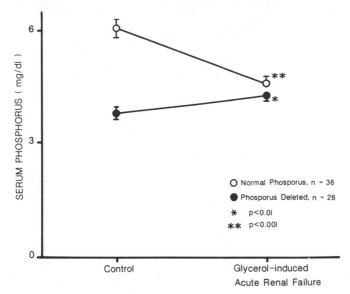

Figure 5.   Serum phosphorus prior to and subsequent to glycerol-induced ARF.

REFERENCES

1.   Popovtzer, M.M., Massry, S.G., Villamie, M., and Kleeman, C.R.: Renal handling of phosphorus in oliguric and non-oliguric mercury-induced acute renal failure in rats.   J. Clin. Invest. 50:2347-2354, 1971.

2.   Wilkes, B.M. and Hollenberg, N.K.: Saline- and glycerol-induced acute renal failure: "protection" occurs after insult.   Nephron. 30:352-356, 1982.

3.   Hewitt, S.: Method for the microassay of endogenous creatinine in blood and urine of small murid rodents. Lab. Anim. 16:201-203, 1982.

4.   Scheinman, S.J. and Coulson, R.: Effect of perfusate phosphate concentration on responses to PTH in isolated rat kidney. Am. J. Physiol. 246:F907-F915, 1984.

5.   Flamenbaum, W., Gehr, M., Gross, M., Kaufman, J., and Hamburger, R. In: Acute renal failure associated with myoglobinuria and hemoglobinuria; W.B. Saunders Co., Phila., 1983, pp 269-282.

6.   Agus, Z.S., Puschett, J.B., Senesky, D., and Goldberg, M.: Mode of action of parathyroid hormone and cyclic adenosine 3',5'-monophosphate on renal tubular phosphate reabsorption in the dog.   J. Clin. Invest. 50:617-626, 1971.

RENAL HAEMODYNAMICS AND RENIN RESPONSE DURING ACUTE HYPERCAPNEA IN DOGS

Hideo Fujii, Tetsuo Mitsuyama, Youji Nakashima and Reizo Kusukawa

Department of Internal Medicine, Yamaguchi University School of Medicine, Ube, Yamaguchi 755, Japan

INTRODUCTION

Renal haemodynamics are related to the amount of carbon dioxide inhaled. In respiratory acidosis 5% CO_2 inhalation increases renal blood flow (RBF) and renal plasma flow (RPF), whereas RBF and RPF decreased after inhalation of 15% CO_2. Recently, it was found that plasma renin activity (PRA) increased during acute respiratory acidosis. The PRA levels increased during both 5% CO_2 and 15% CO_2 inhalation [1]. An extensive literature has developed concerning renin-angiotensin control systems. Three major factors, the intrarenal baroreceptors, the macula densa and the sympathetic nervous system are capable of altering renin secretion under given experimental condition.

The purpose of this series of experiments was to determine the mechanisms of renin secretion and haemodynamic changes during acute hypercapnea.

MATERIALS AND METHODS

Experiment 1. Studies were conducted on 8 mongrel dogs anaesthetised using sodium methohexital (sodium brenital, 12 mg/kg, iv). Arterial blood samples for detemination of pH, $PaCO_2$ and PaO_2 were measured with Instruments Laboratories Model IL-213 Digital Blood Gas Analyser. To assure reliability of blood gas determinations, special care was taken to avoid air contamination and all samples were analysed within 2 min of collection. Arterial blood pressure was measured with a Statham p23DB strain gauge transducer. The pulsatile arterial pressure signal served as the input to a Beckman Instruments Type 9857B cardiotachometer for a moment-to-moment determination of heart rate. RBF was measured with a Zepeda model SW-3 square wave electromagnetic flow meter. Pulsatile pressure, mean pressure, mean RBF, heart rate and expiratory CO_2 were continuously recorded on a Beckman Instruments Type RM six-channel Dynograph. PRA was deterined in blood from the renal vein and was measured by radioimmunoassay.

Experimental protocol: The experimental protocol for these studies is depicted Figure 1. Data for all continuously recorded variables were analysed over the final one minute of a respective control or experimental period. Arterial samples for blood gases, pH and renin were also collected during the final minute. To insure that the proposed

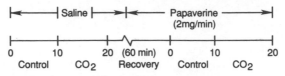

Fig. 1. Experimental time-line for the analysis of the effect of intrarenal papaverine on the renin response elicited during 10 minutes of 8% CO_2 inhalation.

intrarenal papaverine infusion did not elicit a "volume induced" response an intrarenal saline infusion was started after the 30 minute equilibration period. Two control observations were made 10 and 20 minutes after the infusion had begun. Immediately following the second control observation the dogs were ventilated with 8% CO_2 for 10 minutes. The dogs were then allowed to recover for 30 minutes. The entire experimental procedure was repeated following the recovery period, except that papaverine was substituted for the intrarenal saline infusion. This design permitted a comparison of the renin response to CO_2 in the same dog during saline infusion with that observed during intrarenal papaverine. The experimental protocol for these studies in depicted in Figure 1.

Experiment 2. The Experiments were conducted on 7 mongrel dogs under sodium pentobarbital anaesthetic. An abdominal aortic catheter was inserted via a femoral artery to record arterial blood pressure and to withdraw arterial samples for analysis of pH, $PaCO_2$ and PaO_2. Blood gases and pH were measured with an Instrument Laboratories Model 213-227 digital display blood gas analyser. An electric manometer measured arterial blood pressure which was continuously monitored on the dynography as both a pulsatile and an electronically averaged mean. Each dogs was suspended in a normal standing position to facilitate exposure of both kidneys. Both the left and right kidneys were approached via a retroperitoneal flank incision and the renal arteries and vein were carefully exposed to prevent any undesired damage to the nerves or vessels. The denervation procedure was completed by cutting all the visible renal nerves on or near the artery and vein of the kidney on one side. The ureter of the same kidney was then exposed and all three structures-artery, vein and ureter were painted with a solution of 10% phenol in absolute alcohol. The contralateral kidney remained innervated. Both ureters in all the dogs were cannulated for urine collection. The RPF and glomerular filtration rate (GFR) were measured by standard clearance methods, using 6ml of a mixed solution of p-aminohippurate (PAH) and thiosulphate (4 ml-10% PAH: 2 ml-10% thiosulphate) was injected intravenously. RBF was calculated by RPF x $(1-Het)^{-1}$ and renal vascular resistance (RVR) was calculated by mean blood pressure x RBF^{-1}.

Experimental protocol. After completion of surgical preparation, each dog was allowed to equibrate for a one hour period. The 90 min following equilibration were divided into three 30 min periods: the first 30 min served as the control period during which time the dog was ventilated with room air: during the second 30 min the dog was ventilated with 15% CO_2 in air: the third 30 min served as a recovery period during which the animal received room air. The 2 min of blood pressure recording just prior to the drawing of blood samples was used as data corresponding to that blood samples. Contamination of the arterial sample by room air was carefully avoided and the samples were analysed immediately.

Experiment 3. This experiments were conducted on 7 mongrel dogs with nonfiltering kidneys. This procedure consists of clamping the renal artery for two hours and ligating and sectioning the ureter. This procedure prevents filtration and thus renders tubular mechanism nonfunction. RBF was measured with electromagnetic flow meter. Blood gas, pH and PRA measured by the same method in experiment 1.

Experimental protocol. On the second day after the operation of non-filtering kidney, the effects of the intrarenal papaverine infusion were examined during acute hypercapnea in dogs with a denervated nonfiltering kidney in which the renal sympathetic nerves and the macula densa mechanism were nonfunctional, while the contralateral kidney was removed. Experimental time line for the analysis of effect on intrarenal papaverine infusion during 15% CO_2 inhalation was performed in dogs with a denervated nonfiltering kidney (Figure 1).

RESULT

Experiment 1. The role played by the renal vascula receptor in the renin response induced by ventilation with 8% CO_2 was studied in eight dogs. Data presented in Table I shows the cardiovascular responses, blood gas levels and PRA produced by respiratory acidosis during both the intrarenal saline and papaverine infusion periods. $PaCO_2$ increased and arterial pH decreased during 8% CO_2 inhalation in both saline and papaverine infusion. Hypercapnea produced a decreased in blood pressure and heart rate. RBF increased slightly during 8% CO_2 inhalation in both saline and papaverine infusion which is not significant. RVR had tended to decreased which is not significant in both saline and papaverine infusion during hypercapnea. The data in Table I shows that the respective renin responses to 10 minutes of 8% CO_2 inhalation during intrarenal saline and papaverine infusion. At the completion of experimental hypercapnea during intrarenal saline, PRA had increased ($p < 0.001$) by an average of 6.3 ng/ml/h from mean control levels of 4.2 ± 0.99 ng/ml/h to 10.5 ± 2.85 ng/ml/h. In contrast, during intrarenal papaverine administration, PRA increased ($p < 0.05$) by an average of 3.5 ng/ml/h from a mean control value of 3.2 ± 0.76 ng/ml/h to 6.7 ± 2.16 ng/ml/h. A student's paired t-test indicated that the difference between the renin response during acidosis with saline and with papaverine was statistically significant ($p < 0.05$).

Table I Effects of Intrarenal Papaverine (2 mg/min) Infusion During 10 Minutes 8% CO_2 Inhalation (n=8)

	Intrarenal Saline		Intrarenal Papaverine	
	Control	Exp.	Control	Exp.
Arterial pH	7.38 ± 0.22	7.13 ± 0.03***	7.37 ± 0.03	7.11 ± 0.03***
$PaCO_2$ (mmHg)	33.5 ± 1.7	65.6 ± 1.2***	34.2 ± 1.5	68.8 ± 1.6***
PaO_2 (mmHg)	97.4 ± 3.95	124.5 ± 5.3***	99.3 ± 4.2	128.4 ± 5.88***
Heart Rate (B/min)	130 ± 14.0	102 ± 12.7*	127 ± 17.4	104 ± 13.6**
Mean Blood Pressure (mmHg)	117 ± 8.9	112 ± 9.7	122 ± 5.6	101 ± 8.4**
Renal Blood Flow (ml/min)	126 ± 12.5	138 ± 16.2	140 ± 16.3	147 ± 25.5
Renal Vascular Resistance (mmHg/ml/min^{-1})	1.00 ± 0.14	0.95 ± 0.21	0.97 ± 0.16	0.86 ± 0.18
Plasma Renin Activity (ng/ml/h)	4.2 ± 0.99	10.5 ± 2.89**	3.2 ± 0.76	6.7 ± 2.16*

mean $\pm$ SE   * $P < 0.05$, ** $p < 0.01$, *** $p < 0.001$

Experiment 2. Table II shows that $PaCO_2$ and arterial pH were inversely related, with $PaCO_2$ increasing during 15% CO_2 inhalation and pH decreased during the same periods. Heart rate decreased significantly (p < 0.01) during hypercapnea. Mean blood pressure increased during 15% CO_2 inhalation, but this was not statistically significant. RBF (Table II) in both the denervated and innervated kidneys decreased significantly during hypercapnea. However, the reduction was greater in the innervated kidney. GFR decreased significantly during 15% CO_2 inhalation only in the innervated kidney, while in the denervated kidney GFR was not significantly changed during hypercapnea. RVR in the innervated kidney increased significantly during hypercapnea. The increase in RVR in the denervated kidney was not statistically significant (Table II). Table II shows plasma renin activity in the renal venous effluent drawn simultaneously from the two kidneys during control, 15% CO_2 inhalation and recovery conditions. In the innervated kidney, PRA of renal vein was significantly elevated from the control value of 4.85±2.01 ng/ml/h to 7.21±2.45 ng/ml/h during 15% CO_2 inhalation (p < 0.05). In the denervated kidney the small increase (4.73±2.15 ng/ml/h to 5.35±1.34 ng/ml/h) was not satistically significant.

Table II. Responses of a Parameters During 15% CO_2 Inhalation (n=7)

		Nerv. Control	15% CO_2	Recovery
Arterial pH		7.30±0.02	6.87±0.03***	7.29±0.03
$PaCO_2$ (mmHg)		34.7±3.3	107.7±4.9***	34.6±2.96
PaO_2 (mmHg)		96.0±3.81	108.0±4.32	101.2±4.25
Heart Rate (B/min)		146±11	105±6**	133±13
Mean Blood Pressure (mnHg)		129±6	134±5	125±7
Renal Blood Flow	+	73.1±6.6	33.3±5.9*	58.7±15.1
(ml/min)	−	82.2±13.6	56.2±12.2*	57.4±11.1
Renal Plasma Flow	+	45.6±3.9	17.4±6.3*	37.2±9.6
(ml/min)	−	51.8±9.4	37.0±6.3*	36.4±7.4
Glomerular Filtration Rate	+	28.0±4.7	6.6±2.1***	18.6±4.2
(p'l/min)	−	24.8±2.5	19.2±2.5	16.4±2.9
Renal V.iscular Resistance	+	1.88±0.22	6.02±1.85*	3.51±0.95
(mmHg/ml/min)	−	1.91±0.33	4.12±1.34	3.14±0.89
Plasma Renin Activity	+	4.85±2.01	7.21±2.45*	4.33±1.26
(ng/ml/h)	−	4.73±2.35	5.35±1.34	3.97±1.23

mean ± SE   * p < 0.05, ** p < 0.01, *** p < 0.001
+ = innervated kidney, − = denervated kidney

Experiment 3. $PaCO_2$ and PaO_2 increased significant and pH decreased significant in both intrarenal saline and papaverine infusion to denervated nonfiltering kidney during 15% CO_2 inhalation. Heart rate decreased significant during hypercapnea, but arterial blood pressure and RBF tendency to decreased and RVR tendency to increased in both saline and papaverine infusion during hypercapnea, these were not significant. During 15% CO_2 inhalation, PRA increased significantly in saline infusion, but the hypercapnic renin response was completely inhibited by intrarenal papaverine infusion in dogs with a denervated nonfiltering kidneys (Table III).

DISCUSSION

The purpose of this series of experiments was to determine the mechanism of renin secretion and renal haemodynamics during acute respiratory acidosis.

Table III.   Effects of Intrarenal Papaverine Infusion During 10 Minutes 15% CO_2 Inhalation   (n=7)

	Intrarenal Saline		Intrarenal Papaverine	
	Control	Exp.	Control	Exp.
Arterial pH	7.47+0.03	6.97±0.03**	7.44±0.02	6.96±0.05**
$PaCO_2$ (mmHg)	20.9±1.8	102.1±6.4**	26.9±1.4	107.6±8.7**
PaO_2 (mmHg)	111.8±10.9	145.7±14.5*	117.2±2.6	142.6±12.4*
Heart Rate (B/min)	126±7.4	90±8.5***	143±10.7	113±9.8***
Mean Blood Pressure (mmHg)	108±12.8	97±8.3	107±8.3	93±7.0
Renal Blood Flow (ml/min)	103±31 .3	77±17.7	81±16.3	77±20.1
Renal Vascular Resistance (mmHg/ml/min-1)	1.55±0.38	1.67±0.39	1.74±0.43	2.14±0.83
Plasma Renin Activity (ng/ml/h)	12.93±3.18	18.42±3.04*	14.44±20.6	14.23±1.09

mean±SE   * P < 0.05,   ** p < 0.01,   *** p < 0.001

The data of experiments 1 (Table I) clearly indicate that the vascular smooth muscle relaxant, papaverine, suppresses the renin response elicited during 10 minutes of 8% CO_2 inhalation.

Intrarenal papaverine infusions have been used to substantiate the existence of a renal vascular baroreceptor as well as the role of such a mechanism in regulating renin secretion during various physiological perturbation.   Gotshall   (2) reported that intrarenal papaverine administration in normal dogs did not significantly change renal vascular resistance; an observation consistent with the data in the present experiments (Table I).   They also noted a slight but insignificant reduction in renin secretion after 15 minutes of intrarenal papaverine infusion at an average dose of 4 mg/min The dose used in the present study was 2 mg/min and a small, insignificant decrease in renin activity was also noted.   The renin response produced by 10 minutes of 8% CO_2 inhalation was significantly blunted by papaverine.   It is possible that this decrease was the result of an inability of the renal vascular receptor to respond due to papaverine paralysis.   Blood pressure fell significantly (-21 mmHg, p < 0.01) while RBF did not change during hypercapnea and papaverine administration.   However, the renin output was reduced relative to hypercapnea alone.   This would indicate that the papaverine dose was adequate to at least partially block the vascular receptor,   especially since it has been reported that a pressure reduction of 10 to 15 mnHg with no change in RBF is adequate to stimulate renin secretion.

In view of the currently accepted renin control mechanisms, the major portion of papaverine action was to inhibit the renal vascular receptor. The most conservative interpretation of these data is that the renin response to 10 min of 8% CO_2 inhalation has a papaverine-sensitive component.   Based on reports in the literature, it seems feasible that papaverine had blocked the renal vascular receptor, presumably by causing arteriolar dilatation, and prevented a contributory role by this mechanism.   This data also indicated that the renin response during acute respiratory acidosis is papaverine sensitive and is mediated in part by the renal vascular baroreceptor mechanism.

In the experiment 2, indications are that inhalation of 15% CO_2 produces relatively severe respiratory acidosis.   It is evident that in the present study renovascular constriction was taking place during inhalation of 15% CO_2 because a decrease of RBF associated with elevated RVR is consistent with vasoconstriction both in the innervated and denervated kidneys. It was reported previously that the moderate hypercapnea increases RPF and RBF, while severe hypercapnea results in the reduction of these haemodynamic parameters. Renal vasodilatation resulting from increased arterial $PaCO_2$ may cause increased RPF and RBF in moderate respiratory acidosis, while in severe respiratory acidosis, renal vasoconstriction produced by catecholamine release through sympathoadrenal stimulation may result in decreased RPF and RBF. In this experiment, increased RVR and decreased RBF during 15% CO_2 inhalation indicated renal vasoconstriction in both the innervated and denervated kidneys. However, in both cases the response was two-fold greater in the kidney with nerves intact (Table II). It is clear from Table II that acute respiratory acidosis was produced in these animals because severe elevations in both hydrogen ion concentration and $PaCO_2$ were present. Since renin activity in the renal venous effluent was increased during CO_2 inhalation to a statistically significant degree in only the innervated kidney, there is a strong implication that the renal sympathetic nerves were at least partially involved, although other factors may also be present. The present data allow no more than speculation as to the contribution of such factors. For instance, during CO_2 inhalation RVR was increased while GFR was greatly reduced. In the first instance an increased RVR may induce renin release by an intrarenal baroreceptor mechanism and, while the precise signal which stimulates the baroreceptor to release renin is still unclear, it appears that some function of tension in the wall of the afferent arterioles of the renal vasculature is involved. In the present study, the local effects of CO_2 and pH may have altered afferent arteriolar tension and thereby influenced renin secretion. Indeed, the papaverine study suggests that the renin response during acute respiratory acidosis is papaverine-sensitive and implies that the baroreceptor may be involved. However, the fact that the kidneys with intact nerves (Table II) released renin to a much greater extent than denervated kidneys, clearly shows that a strong neural component is present. Furthermore, renin activity was increased during CO_2 inhalation only in the kidney with intact nerves.

A final possibility that must be considered is that the macula densa may have also contributed to the renin response during respiratory acidosis because of the major reduction in GFR in the innervated kidneys (Table II). The severely reduced GFR might be expected to result in substantial alterations in the filtered load and reabsorption of sodium and chloride, both of which may elicit changes in renin release by the mechanisms of the macula densa. Witty and his coworkers (3) demonstrated that papaverine completely blocked the usual increase in renin secretion which accompanies acute haemorrhage in dogs with a single, denervated, nonfiltering kidney. Therefore, in our experiment 3 the effects of intrarenal papaverine infusion were examined during acute respiratory acidosis in dogs with a denervated nonfiltering kidney in which the renal sympathetic nerves and the macula densa mechanism were nonfunctional. The model used in permits an observation of the role of the intrarenal baroreceptor, the macula densa mechanism and the renal sympathetic nerves during acute respiratory acidosis. The hypercapnic renin response was completely inhibited by intrarenal papaverine infusion in dogs with a denervated nonfiltering kidney. These results indicate that the hypercapnic renin response during acute respiratory acidosis in multifactorial and that the major factors which affect the renin secretion during acute respiratory acidosis are intrarenal baroreceptor, macula densa mechanism and the renal sympathetic nerves.

SUMMARY

The role of the renal vascular baroreceptor, macula densa mechanism and the renal sympathetic nerves system in the renin response elicited by acute respiratory acidosis was studied in anaesthetized dogs.

a) During acute respiratory acidosis, the response of renin is sensitive to papaverine and partially mediated by the renal vascular receptor mechanism.

b) The reductions in RBF and GFR and the increase in renin at the renal vein during hypercapnea are dependent, in part, on the presence of intact renal nerves.

c) The hypercapnic renin response was completely inhibited by intrarenal papaverine infusion in dogs with denervated, nonfiltering kidneys.

During acute respiratory acidosis, the plasma renin activity level would be affected by multiple factors, and intrarenal baroreceptor, macula densa and renal sympathetic nerve may play the important role in the regulation of the renin secretion.

REFERENCE

1.   H. Fujii and J.E.Zehr, The effects of respiratory acidosis on plasma renin activity in the dogs., Jpn. Cir. J. 39:1115-1121, (1975).

2.   R.W. Gotshall, J.O.Davis, E.W. Shade, W. Spielman, J.A. Johnson and B. Breverman, Effects of renal denervation on renin release in sodium-depleted dogs., Am. J. Physiol. 225:344-349, (1973).

3.   R.T. Witty, J.O. Davis, J.A. Johnson and R. Prewitt, Effects of papaverine and hemorrhage on renin secretion in the non-filtering kidney, Am. J. Physiol. 221:1666-1671, (1971).

THE ISOLATED PERFUSED RAT KIDNEY: FILTERING AND NON-FILTERING MODELS IN THE ASSESSMENT OF ALTERED RENAL VASCULAR RESISTANCE IN NEPHROTOXICITY

Peter Ratcliffe, Zoltan Endre, Lynn Nicholls, John Tange and John Ledingham

Nuffield Department of Clinical Medicine, John Radcliffe Hospital, Oxford, UK

INTRODUCTION

A reduction in renal blood flow arising from increased vascular resistance is observed in most models of nephrotoxic acute renal failure, and may exacerbate renal damage by compounding ischaemic with non-ischaemic injury (1). These changes in vascular resistance may arise from a direct vascular effect of the toxin or be secondary to tubular injury. We have used the isolated perfused rat kidney to address this issue in a model of mercuric chloride-induced acute renal failure. In the filtering isolated perfused kidney, a controlled exposure to a nephrotoxin can be made in a manner comparable to in vivo. To create a non-filtering preparation, the oncotic pressure of the perfusate was raised to stop glomerular filtration and hence luminal exposure to the nephrotoxin, whilst vascular and peri-tubular exposure were unchanged.

METHODS

Isolated kidneys from male Wistar rats (330-400g) were perfused using a blood-free recirculating medium (100 ml) consisting of dialysed bovine serum albumin in Krebs-Henseleit buffer gassed with O_2 + CO_2 (95:5 v/v); glucose (5 mmol/l) and all 20 physiological amino acids were added to the perfusate clearance.

Table 1. Baseline haemodynamic characteristics of filtering and non-filtering kidneys. Mean$\pm$1SD

	Perfusion pressure (mmHg)	Perfusate flow rate (ml/min/kidney)	Inulin clearance (ml/min/kidney)
Filtering kidney	92$\pm$9	53$\pm$8	0.76$\pm$0.17
Non-filtering kidney	61$\pm$3	31$\pm$5	0

Filtering kidneys were perfused at a cannula tip pressure of 80-100 mmHg using 6.7 g/dl bovine serum albumin. The non-filtering perfused kidney model was created by perfusing at a lower pressure with 10 g/dl bovine serum albumin. In this way filtration was stopped with a relatively minor reduction in the perfusate flow rate (Table 1). Cessation of filtration was demonstrated by a constant perfusate inulin concentration together with anuria.

In each experiment an equilibration period of 30 minutes was allowed at the start of perfusion. Baseline renal function was then measured for 30 minutes after which doses of mercuric chloride, 8 mg/dl was added to the perfusate and the effects observed for 90-120 minutes, before kidneys were fixed for morphological analysis by perfusion with 2.5% glutaraldehyde.

RESULTS

Addition of $HgCl_2$ (8 mg/dl) to the perfusate resulted in a profound decrease in inulin clearance (Fig. 1) and increase in fractional excretion of sodium. Urine flow rate first declined and then increased to a level greater than in the baseline period (Fig. 2). Urine sodium concentrations rose from 39 ± 11 (SD) mmol/l to 141 ± 9 mmol/l.

These changes were accompanied by a rapid increase in renal vascular resistance (RVR) of up to 1700% of baseline (Fig. 3). In this model, these responses add an ischaemic component to the non-ischaemic injury expected after exposure to mercuric chloride. Although a large increase in RVR persisted for the duration of the perfusion experiment, the immediate rise in RVR was poorly sustained. The time course was clearly different from that for changes in urine flow and sodium excretion.

In contrast, exposure of non-filtering kidneys even to this high dose of mercuric chloride had no immediate effect on vascular resistance. Only a very small increase in RVR was observed after continued exposure (Fig. 4).

Structural damage to proximal tubules was severe in filtering kidneys and was only partially attenuated in the non-filtering model.

DISCUSSION

The non-filtering perfused kidney model enables the effects of vascular and antiluminal exposure to a nephrotoxin to be observed in isolation from luminal exposure. Furthermore in the absence of filtration, action of a toxin on proximal tubular solute reabsorption can have no effect on distal solute delivery.

The large increases in vascular resistance observed after exposure of filtering isolated perfused kidneys to mercuric chloride, did not occur in non-filtering kidneys showing clearly that they are not due to a direct vascular action of mercuric chloride but arise as a secondary consequence of tubular exposure.

Possible mechanisms for this secondary increase in RVR include mechanical effects such as raised intrarenal pressure as a consequence of cell swelling as well as tubuloglomerular feedback mechanisms. The precise mechanism cannot be deduced from these experiments but the partial recovery of RVR suggests that it is not simply a reflection of structural cell damage. The time course in relation to that of changes in urine flow does not suggest a simple relationship to distal delivery of tubular fluid.

In other experiments captopril prevented the change in RVR only at doses greatly in excess of the concentration required to inhibit circulating angiotensin converting enzyme and enalaprilat was ineffective (3).

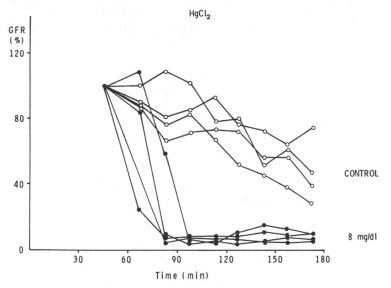

Fig. 1. Changes in inulin clearance of the isolated perfused rat kidney after addition of 8 mg $HgCl_2$ to 100 ml perfusate at t = 60 min.

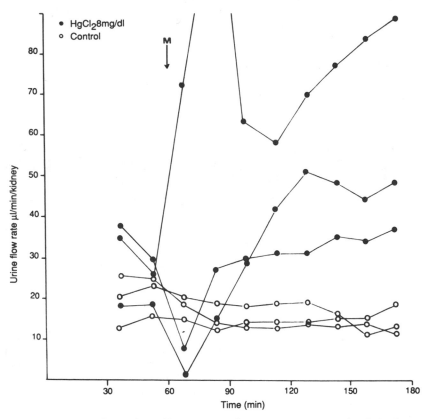

Fig. 2. Changes in urine flow rate after exposure as isolated perfused kidneys to $HgCl_2$. The response is variable and does not have the same time course as changes in renal vascular resistance.

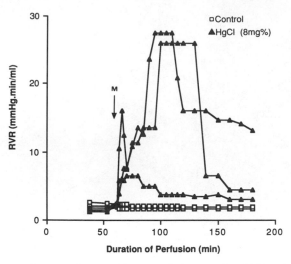

Fig. 3. Changes in renal vascular resistance in filtering kidneys after exposure to mercuric chloride (8 mg/dl)

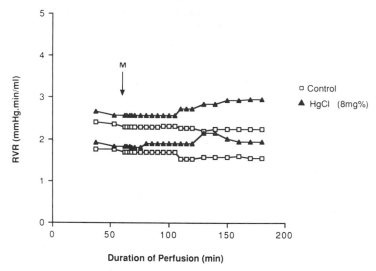

Fig. 4. Non-filtering kidneys. Changes in renal vascular resistance after exposure to mercuric chloride (8 mg/dl) are almost abolished.

In summary these experiments demonstrate that very large increases in RVR may arise as a secondary consequence of tubular exposure to a nephrotoxin. The mechanism remains unclear.

REFERENCES

1. T.H. Hostetter, B.M. Wilkes, and B.M. Brenner, Renal circulatory and nephron function in experimental acute renal failure, Chapter 4, In: "Acute Renal Failure", B.M. Brenner and J.M. Lazarus, ed., Publisher, W.R. Saunders (1983).

2. F.H. Epstein, J.T. Brosnan, J.D. Tange, and B.D. Ross, Improved function with amino acids in the isolated perfused kidney, Am. J. Physiol. 243:E284-F292 (1982).

3. Z.H. Endre, L.G. Nicholls, P.J. Ratcliffe, and J.G.G. Ledingham, Prevention and reversal of mercuric chloride-induced increases in renal vascular resistance by captopril (this Symposium).

ENDOTOXIN-HAEMOGLOBIN INDUCED NEPHROPATHY AND HAPTOGLOBIN ADMINISTRATION

Takeshi Ohshiro, Kiyoshi Mukai, and Takesada Mori

Department of Surgery II, Osaka University Medical School, 1-1-50, Fukushima, Fukushima-ku, Osaka 553, Japan

INTRODUCTION

Haemolytic renal failure means the renal insufficiency caused by severe haemolysis. This disease had been reported by Yorke (1) and Degowin (2) and recently attracted considerable attention because of the increase of cardiac surgery under extra-corporeal circulation. The pathogenesis is regarded as the nephrotoxic function of free haemoglobin (unbound haemoglobin). In 1975, we demonstrated that the administration of haptoglobin could prevent the morphological abnormalities in rabbits with haemoglobin induced nephropathy and proposed that the haptoglobin therapy could become the effective procedure to prevent haemolytic renal failure (3). Haptoglobin is a component of alpha-2-globulin, related to the metabolism of free haemoglobin by the formation of haptoglobin-haemoglobin complex.

As our previous experiment (3,4) in rabbits had failed to clarify the effects on the functional abnormalities, this experiment was carried out to investigate whether the administration of haptoglobin could prevent this in dogs which were pretreated with a small amount of endotoxin before the injection of haemolysate to produce endotoxin-haemolysate induced nephropathy.

MATERIALS AND METHODS

Materials

1) Experimental animals: Mature mongrel dogs, weighing 6.4-13.8 kg, were used.

2) Haemolysate (Hs): Erythrocytes, obtained from dogs, were washed and haemolysed with distilled water. After freezing and thawing, they were diluted in NaCl to yield the isotonic haemolysate.

3) Endotoxin (Ex): Lipopolysaccharide B (DIFCO) was dissolved in physiological saline.

4) Haptoglobin (Hp): Haptoglobin preparation, which was purified from human plasma and adjusted in 127.5 mg/ml with the binding capacity of 0.72, was employed.

Methods

1) Dogs were anaesthetized by intravenous injection of pentobarbital sodium (30 mg/kg).

2) After laparotomy, a catheter was inserted into each of the left and right ureters.

3) A catheter was inserted into femoral artery for intravenous injection of p-aminohippuric acid (PAH, 9 mg/kg) and creatinine (Cr, 160 mg/kg) dissolved in 50 ml of physiological saline (S), followed by serial infusion of physiological saline containing 3 mg PAH and 8 mg Cr per ml at a rate of 0.1 ml/min/kg.

4) One hr later, endotoxin (0.1 mg/kg) was intravenously injected.

5) Thirty min later, haemolysate (1 g/kg in haemoglobin content) was intravenously injected and haptoglobin (1.4 mg/kg with the binding amount of 1.0 g of haemoglobin) or physiological saline was simultaneously added.

Assay

1) Urine and blood were sampled in planned schedule for the following tests.

2) PAH was determined by the Brun's technique.

3) Cr was determined by the method of Folin-Wu.

4) Sodium (Na) and potassium (K) were determined by flame photometry.

Experiments

Dogs were divided into 4 groups each of which consisted of 5 animals.
Group Hs: injected with haemolysate alone.
Group Ex: injected with endotoxin alone.
Group Ex+Hs+S: injected with combination of endotoxin, haemolysate and physiological saline.
Group Ex+Hs+Hp: injected with combination of endotoxin, haemolysate and haptoglobin.

Statistical analysis.   Statistical significance of differences was tested with t-test.

RESULTS

These results were shown in Figure 1 and Figure 2.

Blood pressure.   Systolic blood pressure was kept at 130-140 mmHg in group Hs, but fell by 40-50 mmHg after 90-120 min of injection in group Ex, group EX+Hs+S, or group Ex+HS+Hp, although it gradually recovered thereafter. This result indicated that the hypotension caused by the combined injection of endotoxin and haemolysate could not be recovered by the administration of haptoglobin, suggesting that haptoglobin therapy was ineffective in these blood pressure changes.

Urinary volume.   In group Hs or group Ex, urinary volume transiently increased, although it easily returned to preinjection level. In group Ex+Hs+S, it began to decrease immediately and remarkably from 7.2 ± 2.3 to 0.5 ± 0.9 - 0.2 ± 0.3 ml/30 min after 60-90 min. However, in group EX+HS+Hp, it remained almost unchanged as 6.1 ± 3.8 - 5.4 ± 4.1 ml/30 min after 60-90 min, compared to 8.4±3.3 ml/30 min of preinjection level, presenting a significant difference (p < 0.01) from group Ex+Hs+S. Thus, the administration of haptoglobin was useful in the normalization of oliguria caused by the combined injection of endotoxin and haemolysate.

Creatinine clearance (Ccr). In group Hs, Ccr almost maintained the preinjection level. In group Ex, it decreased slowly and moderately from 3.8±1.2 ml/min/kg to 1.8±1.2 - 1.5±1.0 ml/min/kg more after 120 min and in group Ex+Hs+S, rapidly and deeply from 3.4±0.9 ml/min/kg to 0.8±1.2 - 0.2±0.3 ml/min/kg more after 30 min. while, in group Ex+HS+Hp, it decreased to the moderate degree, recording 1.8±1.0 - 1.2±0.7 ml/min/kg after 60-90 min, presenting a significant difference (p < 0.01) from group Ex+Hs+S. This decreased pattern remained within the variation range, recorded by group Ex. Thus, the administration of haptoglobin was useful in the prevention of low glomerular filtration rate caused by the combined injection of endotoxin and haemolysate.

p-Aminohippuric acid clearance (C_{PAH}). In group Hs, C_{PAH} almost maintained the preinjection level. In group Ex, it decreased slowly and moderately from 11.9±4.4 ml/min/kg to 6.2±4.0 - 4.9±1.2 ml/min/kg more after 120 min and in group Ex+Hs+S, rapidly and deeply from 10.0±3.3 ml/min/kg to 2.3±2.9 - 0.2±0.3 ml/min/kg more after 30 min. While, in group Ex+Hs+Hp, it decreased to the moderate degree, recording 1.4±4.2 - 5.9±4.1 ml/min/kg after 60-90 min, presenting a significant difference (p < 0.01-0.05) from group Ex+Hs+S. This decreased pattern remained within the variation range, recorded by group Ex. Thus, the administration of haptoglobin was useful in the prevention of low renal plasma flow caused by the combined injection of endotoxin and haemolysate.

Urinary electrolyte contents. In group Hs, urinary sodium and potassium contents slightly increased but in group Ex, gradually decreased. In group EX+Hs+Hp as well as in group EX+Hs+S, they began to decrease immediately and remarkably after 30 min. This result indicated that the hypotonic urine of sodium and potassium caused by the combined injection of endotoxin and haemolysate could not be normalized by the administration of haptoglobin.

Histological findings. Each dog was sacrificed 3 hr after the experiment, followed by histological examinations. In group Ex+Hs+S, iron deposit was noted in tubular epithelial cells, accompanied by vascular nephritis. While, in group Ex+Hs+Hp, these pathological findings were hardly detected. This result indicated that the administration of haptoglobin was useful in preventing or reducing the severity of iron deposit and vascular nephritis.

DISCUSSION

The effects of haptoglobin against haemolytic renal failure has been reported (5,6), where the influence of human haptoglobin in rats with the injection of overloaded methaemoglobin was demonstrated, and nephrotic changes were observed less frequently when an equivalent amount of haptoglobin to bind with methaemoglobin was simultaneously administered. We have undertaken similar experiment in rabbits (7), and clarified the following:

1) Haemoglobinuria can be prevented by the administration of haptoglobin.

2) Iron deposit in tubular epithelial cells can be prevented by the administration of haptoglobin.

3) Degeneration of tubular epithelial cells can be prevented by the administration of haptoglobin.

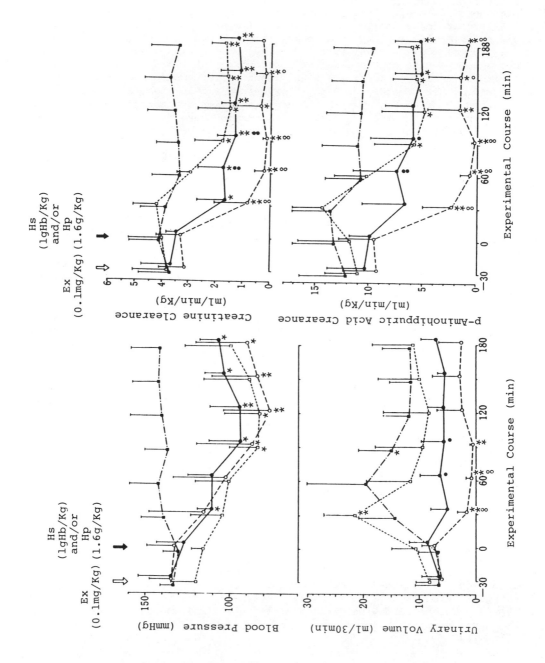

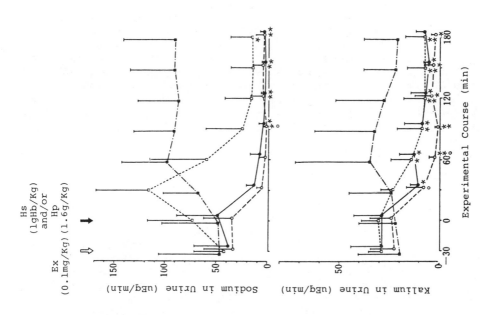

Figure 1. Serial changes of renal functions in dogs with endotoxin, haemolysate and/or haptoglobin.

In the experiment described above we investigated the effects of haptoglobin against endotoxin-haemolysate induced nephropathy in dogs and shown that it has the atleast three advantages:

Maintenance of urinary volume. Haemolysate is mainly made of stroma and haemoglobin, and there is still controversy over the question which of these two components is responsible for haemolytic renal failure. Assumed that haemoglobin is major contributing factor, we tried to detoxify free haemoglobin by the formation of haptoglobin-haemoglobin complex and shown the normalization of oliguria in dogs with the combined injection of endotoxin and haemolysate. The treatment of the complex formation proved to be effective as expected. Judging from this finding, we suggest that the main component of haemolysate for haemolytic renal failure is free haemoglobin.

Recovery of low clearance. Birndorf (8) reported that renal blood flow diminished in kidney perfused with haemoglobin solution. In this experiment, both Ccr and C_{PAH} decreased in dogs with the combined injection of endotoxin and haemolysate, but recovered moderately in dogs with additional injection of haptoglobin, although they remained below the normal level. This finding indicates that haptoglobin has the same ability of preventing the remarkable decrease of glomerular filtration rate and renal plasma flow which were caused by the synergism of endotoxin and haemolysate. We suppose that the ability is based on the function of haptoglobin to bind with free haemoglobin. Thus, it was clarified that the administration of haptoglobin could prevent the functional abnormalities in dogs with endotoxin-haemoglobin induced nephropathy.

Normal histological feature of kidney. The additional injection of haptoglobin was found to keep the normal histological feature of kidney in dogs. Iron deposit in tubular epithelial cells, which was detected in dogs with the combined injection of endotoxin and haemolysate, was less severe. This is associated with the fact that haptoglobin-haemoglobin complex can not pass through glomerulus and appear in urine.

Taken together these results indicate that the administration of haptoglobin is effective in preventing haemolytic renal failure.

We regard the clinical significance of haptoglobin therapy as follows: Free haemoglobin causes the functional disorder in glomerulus and the morphological disorder in tubules. However, haptoglobin-haemoglobin complex has none of these side effects. This is the reason why the complex can be normally metabolised in liver to produce bilirubin (9,10) the complex, were located on hepatic parenchymal cells and that haem-alpha-methenyl oxygenase, whose substrates were the complex, were presented in hepatic parenchyma cells.

CONCLUSION

In order to demonstrate the effect of haptoglobin against haemolytic renal failure, we studied how endotoxin-haemolysate induced nephropathy is prevented by the administration of haptoglobin. The following results were obtained.

1) In dogs injected with haemolysate alone, urinary volume transiently increased, although no change was observed in blood pressure, Ccr, C_{PAH}, urinary sodium and potassium levels.

2) In dogs injected with endotoxin alone, mild hypotension, transient

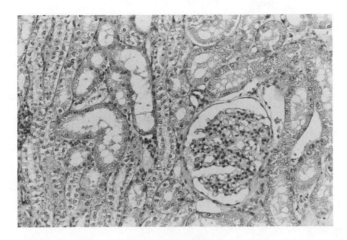

Group Ex+Hs+S

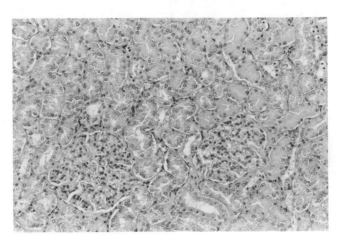

Group Ex+Hs+Hp

Figure 2.   Histological findings in dogs with and without the additional
injection of haptoglobin.

decrease of urinary volume, moderate decrease of Ccr and C_{PAH}, slow decrease of urinary sodium and potassium levels were noted.

3) In dogs injected with combination of endotoxin, haemolysate and physiological saline, mild hypotension, oliguria, remarkable decrease of Ccr and C_{PAH} hypotonic urine of sodium and potassium were noted. Moreover, they showed severe iron deposit in tubular epithelial cells and vascular nephritis. Liver and spleen were almost normal.

4) In dogs injected with combination of endotoxin, haemolysate and haptoglobin, urinary volume maintained within normal range and Ccr and C_{PAH} did not so seriously decrease and remained within the variation range, recorded by dogs injected with endotoxin alone, although hypotension and hypotonic urine of sodium and potassium were not recovered. In addition, they did not show any iron deposit in tubular epithelial cells and vascular nephritis.

5) Haptoglobin therapy was found to prevent both morphological and functional abnormalities of kidney, caused by the injection of haemolysate.

These results make us conclude that haptoglobin therapy is the effective procedure to prevent haemolytic renal failure.

REFERENCES

1. W. Yorke, and R. W. Nauss, The mechanism of the production of suppression of urine in blackwater fever, Ann. Trop. Med. Parasitol., 5:287 (1911).

2. E. L. Degowin, H. F. Osterhagen, and M. Andersch, Renal insufficiency from blood transfusion, Arch. Int. Med., 59:432 (1937).

3. T. Ohshiro, K. Mukai, S. D. Hong, A. Sugitachi, F. Murakami, D. Jinnai, S. Funakoshi, and T. Oomura, The prevention of hemolytic renal failure by haptoglobin-administration (No 1), Saishin Igaku (Japan), 30:656 (1975).

4. T. Ohshiro, and Y. Motoi, The prevention of hemolytic renal failure by haptoglobin-administration (No 2). Saishin Igaku (Japan), 30: 879 (1975).

5. J. Pintera, The protective influence of haptoglobin on hemoglobinuric kidney. I. Biochemical and macroscopic observations, Folia Haematol., 90:80 (1968).

6. J. Pintera, and V. Tomhsek, The protective influence of haptoglobin on hemoglobinuric kidney. II. Microscopic observations and clinical aspect, Inz. Z. Klin. Pharmakol. Ther. Toxikol., 34:371 (1970).

7. T. Ohshiro, K. Mukai, and G. Kosaki, Prevention of hemoglobinuria by administration of haptoglobin, Res. Exp. Med., 177:1 (1980).

8. N. I. Birrdorf, and H. Loapas, Effects of red cell stroma free hemoglobin solution on renal functions, J. Appl. Physiol., 29:573 (1970).

9. H. Nakajima, T. Takemura, O. Nakajima, and K. Yamaoka, Studies on heme alpha-methenyl oxygenase. I. The enzymatic conversion of pyridine-hemichromogen and hemoglobin-haptoglobin into a possible precursor of biliverdin, J. Biol. Chem., 238:3784 (1963).

10. K. Kino, H. Tsunoo, Y. Higa, M. Takami, H. Hamaguchi, and H. Nakajima, Hemoglobin-haptoglobin receptor in rat liver plasma membrane, J. Biol. Chem., 255:9616 (1980).

PARTIALLY PURIFIED BOVINE ATRIAL FRACTION ON ANIMAL KIDNEY,   SMOOTH MUSCLE AND SODIUM TRANSPORT IN TOAD SKIN

Beryl Norris, Juan Concha, Luciano Cuiang and Carmen Pantoja

Department of Physiology, University of Concepcion, Concepcion, Chile

INTRODUCTION

The potent diuretic, natriuretic, vasorelaxant and endocrine effects of atrial natriuretic peptides isolated from several mammals (rat, monkey, pig, man) have been extensively investigated (1-5) and this knowledge is being applied in the treatment of cardiorenal disease (6,7). The evidence as to the mechanisms underlying these effects is still incomplete (5). In an attempt to establish the existence and actions of a natriuretic factor we assayed the biological activity of a partially purified fraction isolated in our laboratory from bovine heart atria (AF) on diuresis and natriuresis in the anaesthetised dog, on mammalian vascular smooth muscle, small intestine, on the rate of active sodium transport in isolated toad skin, and on the response of the skin to aldosterone and to angiotensin II (Agt II). The action of synthetic atrial natriuretic peptide (Atriopeptin III, ANP) on the isolated toad skin was also examined.

MATERIALS AND METHODS

Preparation of Atrial Extracts. Atrial fractions were obtained as described in a previous paper (8). Homogenates of bovine atria were boiled 5 min, concentrated and dialyzed in distilled water. The dialysate was concentrated to a small volume and chromatographed on Sephadex G-25 and G-10 columns. The protein peak associated with maximal biological activity was used in these studies.

Experiments on Dogs. Mongrel dogs of either sex (15-25 kg) were anaesthetised with 30 mg/kg sodium pentobarbitone and hydrated with a saline solution at a rate of 2 ml/min throughout the experiments. Arterial pressure was monitored through a Statham pressure transducer. Blood samples were drawn from the left femoral artery catheter inserted above the origin of the renal artery and bolus injections of AF were made at this site. Ureters were cannulated distal to the renal pelvis and urine flow rate was monitored with a Grass PTT1 photoelectric drop counter. The electrocardiogram was monitored through intramuscular electrodes; glomerular filtration rate was measured by endogenous creatinine clearance and renal blood flow with Statham-Gould electromagnetic flow probes placed around the renal arteries. The general protocol was as follows: Two 10 min control clearance periods were

performed.   AF was administered as a bolus (40-120 ug/kg) into the aorta
just above the origin of the renal arteries.   One 10 min experimental
clearance period was started immediately, followed by two 30 min steady-
state experimental periods.   Arterial blood samples were collected at the
midpoint of each clearance period.   Creatinine was determined using a
Merck creatinine kit and a Beckman spectrophotometer; sodium and potassium
were determined by flame photometry and renal blood flow was directly
measured with the electromagnetic flowmeter.

Experiments on Vascular Smooth Muscle and on Small Intestine.   Helical
strips of the dog carotid artery were obtained under anaesthesia and
segments of the small intestine were taken from decapitated rats.   The
effect of AF was tested on noradrenaline and   carbachol-induced
contractions of the artery and small intestine respectively.   One unit of
activity was taken as the mg protein of partially purified AF necessary to
induce 50% relaxation of precontracted smooth muscae.

Experiments on Isolated Toad Skin.   The biological activity of the active
fraction was assayed on the abdominal skin of the Chilean toad Pleurodema
thaul (5-15 g) according to the method described by Ussing (9) z
Quantification was done by Isaacson's amiloride test (10); one unit of
activity was set to be equivalent to 1×10^{-6}M amiloride.   AF was added to
the inner (serosal) surface of the skin (25 uL, equivalent to 3.48 U
activity.   Net sodium fluxes across the skin were measured with ^{22}Na. The
effects of AF on the action of aldosterone and Agt II on the skin were
also examined.   The effect of pronase on the activity of AF was
investigated in all experimental groups.

RESULTS

In dogs, the intraarterial injection of 120 mg/kg AF induced a slight
transient decrease (15%) in arterial blood pressure, followed by a prompt
(2-10 min) 16-fold increase in natriuresis and a 14-fold increase in
diuresis and kaliuresis (Table 1).   Peak effects were observed at 60 min
and each parameter returned to near control values by 80 min (Fig. 1).
Preliminary studies of glomerular filtration rate and renal blood flow
showed an increase of about 20% and 11% respectively, which returned to
control values in less than 30 and 20 min.   Heart rate decreased by 50%,
T waves became low and biphasic and E-R intervals were slightly prolonged
after about 60 min.

AF (1.5 U) relaxed dog carotidhelical strips contracted by noradrenaline
and rat ileum contracted by carbachol and shifted the dose-response curves
to the right (Fig. 2).   The vasorelaxant effect of AF occurred within 2
min of the application of AF and after an observation period of 60 min the
preparation did not recover until the drug was washed out repeatedly.

AF produced a dose-dependent transient decrease in the PD and in the SCC
across the isolated toad skin when applied to the serosal surface as shown
by Norris (8).   Since the response to AF applied to the mucosal surface
was often irreversible, in most of the experiments the agent was applied
only to the serosal surface.   Amiloride analysis indicated a decrease in
sodium driving force (E_{Na}), sodium conductance (G_{Na}) and passive
conductance (G_{sh}), and the net Na^+ flux decreased by 33%.   AF also
decreased the skin response to aldosterone (Fig. 3) and to angiotensin II.
Mucosal atriopeptin III (ANP) reversibly decreased the PD, SCC and active
conductance across the isolated skin.

Serosal pronase (10 U) blocked the response to serosal AF (100-200 uL) in
all experiments: hypotensive and diuretic effects of AF were significantly

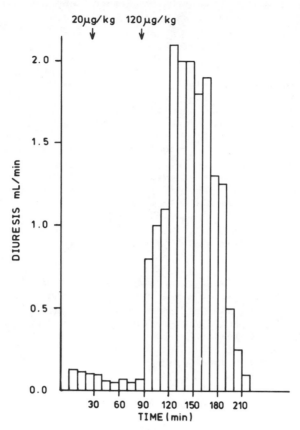

Fig. 1. Representative experiment showing the time course of the diuretic response to an intraarterial bolus injection of AF in an anaesthetised dog. Note that the effect of the larger concentration of AF was immediate.

Table I

Dose	$\Delta U_{Na} \dot{V}$ $\mu Eq/min/kg$	$\Delta U_K \dot{V}$ $\mu Eq/min/kg$	$\Delta \dot{V}$ $\mu L/kg/min$
40 μg	93.2 ± 15.8**	60.3 ± 13.9*	68.6 ± 7.8***
80 μg	650.9 ± 110.7**	530.0 ± 44.2***	297.1 ± 13.5***
120 μg	1294.9 ± 111.1***	869.8 ± 42.1***	1073.1 ± 120.7***

Net values were obtained by subtracting total sodium excretion, urine output and potassium excretion of control animals, from corresponding values of animals injected with AF.

In comparison with control values, p*< 0.02; **< 0.01; ***< 0.001

(P < 0.001) reduced in dogs, vasorelaxation was abolished and the inhibitory effect of AF on the toad skin was blocked.

DISCUSSION

The transient hypotension induced immediately after injection of a AF bolus might be related to relaxation of arterial or venous smooth muscle (11) or to suppression of renin secretion (4,12) and recovery may be due to compensatory reflexes in the animal (13). The relatively long duration of the diuretic effects, when compared to the shorter duration of the effects of the different atrial natriuretic peptides in the literature, could be due to endogenous ouabain-like activity in our experimental animals (14), or, as described by Tal (14) to the potentiation of AF by the appearance of non-specific Na,K-ATPase inhibitors. Since atrial peptides interfere with the synthesis of aldosterone (13) they could alter Na excretion and this mechanism could help to explain the fact that maximal Na excretion was found at 60 min. Furthermore, skin experiments showed that AF also inhibits the effect of aldosterone and of Agt II on this tissue.

Some observations suggests proximal site of action for rat atriopeptin III such as a decrease of sodium bicarbonate absorption (15). It has been shown that ANP reduces proximal tubular sodium reabsorption by antagonizing the effect of Agt II and passage of extra sodium into the distal tubule could increase distal sodium-potassium exchange to result in a significant potassium loss (16) which could be the result of incomplete inhibition of the synthesis and effect of aldosterone by AF in vivo, since potassium excretion in our dogs was high.

The considerable decrease in electric parameters and of net sodium flux in the isolated toad skin together with the decrease in the estimates of the equivalent electrical circuit of the skin show that bovine atrial fraction isolated in our laboratory inhibits sodium transport in this tissue. The amiloride test was compatible with inhibition of Na-H antiport in relation to sodium bicarbonate reabsorption since both E_{Na} and G_{Na} were reduced, and is in agreement with the findings of Hammond (17).

The inhibitory effects of mucosal ANP were found in preliminary experiments and were much weaker than the effects of serosal AF. AF induced strong inhibition on both surfaces of the skin whereas ANP decreased the electric parameters only when applied to the mucosal surface.

The rapid onset of the vasorelaxant effects of AF supports the hypothesis that decreases in arterial blood pressure after injection of AF may be due primarily to vasodilation (18) and the rapid recovery in the whole animal could be explained by compensatory reflexes as stated previously.

The destruction of peptide activity during the experiments (19) with pronase abolished the effect of AF showing that the active hormone is a peptide. This evidence shows that intraarterial injection of AF in the anaesthetised dog produces a potent natriuretic, diuretic and kaliuretic response associated with a transient decrease in arterial blood pressure, increase in glomerular filtration rate and renal blood flow, and relaxation of pre-contracted mammalian vascular smooth muscae. Furthermore, application of AF to the serosal surface of the isolated skin of the toad Pleurodema thaul decreases sodium transport and significantly decreased the skin response to aldosterone and Agt II.

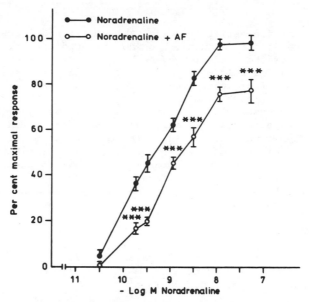

Fig. 2. The relaxation dose-response curve to AF 1.5 U in dog carotid helical strips. The carotid strips were contracted by noradrenaline and the concentration of AF was chosen to induce about 50% reduction of the response. Values±SEM; n = 6. ** p < 0.001; paired Student's t-test.

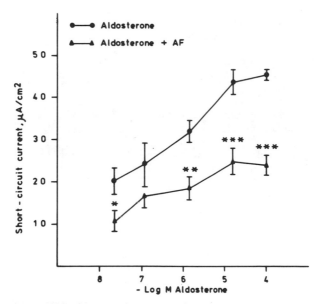

Fig. 3. Effect of bovine atrial fraction (AF 15 uL, serosal surface) on the short-circuit response to aldosterone to the isolated toad skin. The concentration of AF was chosen to induce about 50% reduction of the response. Means±SEM, n = 6. * p < 0.05; ** p < 0.01; *** p < 0.001; paired Student's t-test.

SUMMARY

The effect of bovine atrial fraction (AF) was investigated on canine diuresis, natriuresis and kaliuresis, on dog carotid artery, rat ileum and on isolated skin of the toad Pleurodema thaul. A 16-fold increase in natriuresis and a 14-fold increase in diuresis and kaliuresis were observed in the dog after intra-arterial injection of AF, an effect only partly due to an increase in glomerular filtration rate and renal blood flow. These increases were preceded by a transient (15%) hypotension. In smooth muscle experiments relaxation was observed; which might explain transient (15%) hypertension. In isolated skin net Na flux was reduced 33% and the amiloride test was compatible with inhibition of Na-H antiport: this could be due to proximal tubular decrease of sodium bicarbonate transport. AF significantly reduced the skin stimulatory response to aldosterone and to Agt II which suggests a similar mechanism of action in the kidney.

ACKNOWLEDGEMENTS

This work was supported by grants 20.33.32 and 20.33.33, University of Concepcion, Chile. We thank Mrs. Maria Cecilia Nova and Mr. Oscar Sepulveda for excellent technical assistance.

REFERENCES

1. A.J. DeBold, H.B. Borensteia, A.T. Veress and H. Sonnenberg, A rapid and potent natriuretic response to intravenous injection of atrial myocardial extract in rats, Life Sci 28:89 (1981).

2. U. Ackerman, Structure and function of atrial natriuretic peptides, Clin Chem 32:214 (1986).

3. H.D. Kleinert and T. Maack, Renal and cardiovascular effects of atrial natriuretic factor, Biochem Pharmacol 35:2057 (1986).

4. J.H. Laragh, The endocrine control of blood volume, blood pressure and sodium balance: atrial hormone and renin system interactions, Hypertension 4:S143 (1986).

5. R. Gerzer, J.M. Heim, B. Schutte and J. Weil, Cellular mechanism of action of atrial natriuretic factor, Klin Wochenschr 65:109 (1987).

6. J.H. Laragh, Endocrine mechanisms in congestive failure. Renin, aldosterone and atrial natriuretic hormone, Drugs 31:1 (1986).

7. G. Thibault, R. Garcia, J. Gutkowska, J. Genest and M. Cantin, Atrial natriuretic factor. A newly discovered hormone with Significant clinical implications, Drugs 31:369 (1986).

8. B.C. Norris, C. Pantoja, J.B. Concha and L.Ch. Chiang, Effect of bovine heart atrial natriuretic and diuretic fractions on sodium transport in isolated toad skin, Pharmacology 33:157 (1986).

9. H.H. Ussing and K. Zerahn, Active transport of sodium as the source of electric current in the short-circuited isolated frog skin,. Acta Physiol Scand 23:110 (1951).

10. L.C. Isaacson, Resolution of parameters in the equivalent electrical circuit of the sodium transport mechanism across toad skin, J. Membrane Biol 30:301 (1977).

11. B.A. Breuhaus, H.H. Saneil, M.A. Brandt and J.E. Chimoskey, Atriopeptin II lowers cardiac output in conscious sheep, <u>Am J Physiol</u> 249:R776 (1985).

12. J.C. Burnett, J.P. Granger and T.J. Opgenorth, Effects of synthetic atrial natriuretic factor on renal function and renin release, <u>Am J Physiol</u> 247:F863 (1984).

13. H. Sonnenberg, On the physiological role of atrial natriuretic factor, <u>Klin Wochenschr</u> 65 (Suppl VIII):8 (1987).

14. D.M. Tal, S. Katchalsky, D. Lichtstein and J.D. Karlish, Endogenous "Ouabain-like" activity in bovine plasma, <u>Biochem Biophys Res Commun</u> 135:1 (1986).

15. M. Hropot, E. Klaus, J. Knolle, W. Konig and W. Scholz, <u>Klin Wochenschr</u> 64 (Suppl VI):58 (1986).

16. B. Leckie, How the heart rules the kidneys, <u>Nature</u> 326:644 (1987).

17. P. Bolli, F.B. Muller, L. Linder, A.E.G. Raine, T.J. Resink, P. Erne, W. Kioski, R. Hitz and F.R. Buhler, The vasodilator potency of atrial natriuretic peptide in man, <u>Circulation</u> 75:221 (1987).

18. T.G. Hammond, A.N. Yusufi, F.G. Knox and T.P. Dousa, Administration of atrial natriuretic factor inhibits sodium-coupled transport in proximal tubules, <u>J Clin Invest</u> 75:1983 (1985).

19. C.V. Pantola, L.Ch. Chiang, B.C. Norris and J.B. Concha, Rapid method for the partial purification of atrial natriuretic factor, <u>IRCS Med Sci</u>, 14:611 (1986).

INVESTIGATIONS ON THE NEPHROTOXIC POTENTIAL OF RECOMBINANT HUMAN TUMOUR NECROSIS FACTOR

Ulrike Metz-Kurschel, Erhard Kurschel*, and Norbert Niederle*

Department of Renal and Hypertensive Diseases and * West German Tumour Centre, University Medical School, Hufelandstr.55, D-4300 Essen, FRG

INTRODUCTION

Tumour necrosis factor (TNF) is a protein produced by macrophages and monocytes after induction with endotoxin. It has the same primary structure as cachectin which is an important mediator of toxic shock and both substances are probably identical.

TNF exhibits in vitro and in vivo multiple biological activities. Application of TNF to tumour bearing mice leads to haemorrhagic necrosis of the tumours and of normal tissues as well. Haemoconcentration, shock, metabolic acidosis, pluging of the pulmonary arteries with thrombi composed primarily of polymorphonuclear granulocytes, severe interstitial pneumonitis and acute renal tubular necrosis are other important changes evoked by TNF (1). After synthesis of human TNF by recombinant DNA technique it was introduced into clinical oncology because of its cytotoxic or cytostatic properties in some tumours (2). During a phase-I study we made investigations in order to define the subclinical or clinical nephrotoxicity of this new substance.

PATIENTS AND METHODS

During a phase-I study 7 patients with metastatic colorectal cancers resistant to standard therapy were treated with TNF.

Patient characteristics were as follows:
 female: n = 5
 male: n = 2
 age: range 34 - 57 years, median 56 years

TNF was administered daily as a short time infusion over 5 days, dosage ranged from 0,08 - 0,16 mg/m^2. Before and during treatment we controlled the following parameters: serum creatinine, BUN, urinary sediment, protein excretion (Biuret-method). As particular sensitive parameters to detect even subclinical renal damage we used the determination of the following urinary enzymes:

Lactate dehydrogenase = LDH (EC 1.1.1.27)
Alanine aminopeptidase = AAP (EC 3.4.11.-)
gamma-Glutamyltransferase = GGT (EC 2.3.2.2)
ß-Galactosidase = GAL (EC 3.2.1.30)

N-acetyl-ß-D-Glucosaminidase = NAG (EC 3.2.1.23)

Urine for the enzyme and protein determination was collected in 3h morning periods from 6 to 9 a.m. to obviate any influence of the circadian variation of urinary enzyme excretion. Immediately after the collection periods urine samples were prepared by gel filtration on Sephadex-G50 fine. Urinary enzyme output was calculated as mU/3h, correcting for the average adult surface area of 1,73 m^2 (3). In two patients SDS-PAGE-electrophoresis was performed, additionally.

RESULTS

Two patients developed a deterioration of renal function, serum creatinine rose from 0,9 mg/dl to 1,4 mg/dl and from 1,1 mg/dl to 2,2 mg/dl. In all other patients renal function tests remained normal. Excretion of the brush border membrane enzymes AAP was increased in 4 patients (fig. 1) and GGT in 5 patients (fig. 2). Six patients had an increased excretion of the cytoplasm enzyme LDH (fig. 3). The lysosomal enzymes GAL and NAG were excreted in increased amounts in 3 and 5 patients (fig. 4 and 5). In 4 patients we observed a mild proteinuria of up to 2600 mg/24h (fig. 6). In these patients SDS-PAGE-electrophoresis showed complete tubular proteinuria. After cessation of therapy renal function tests normalized, proteinuria and enzymuria returned to the normal range.

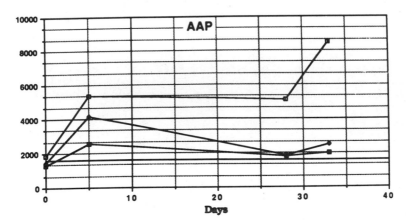

Fig. 1. Excretion of AAP in 4/7 patients following administration of TNF

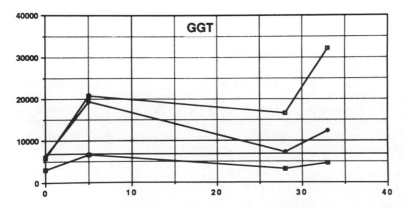

Fig. 2. Excretion of GGT in 5/7 patients following administration of TNF

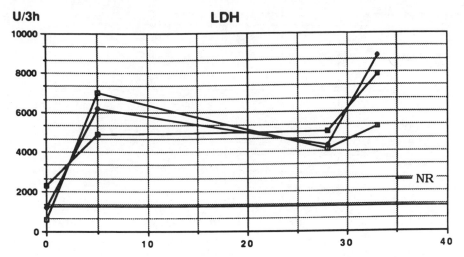

Fig. 3. Excretion of LDH in 6/7 patients following administration of TNF

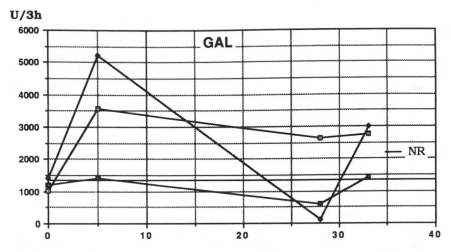

Fig. 4 . Excretion of GAL in 3/7 patients following administration of TNF

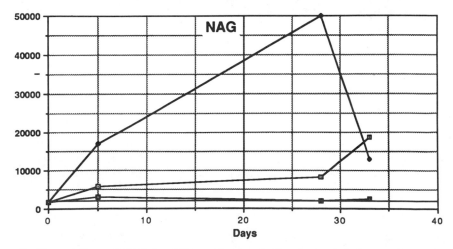

Fig. 5. Excretion of NAG in 5/7 patients following administration of TNF

683

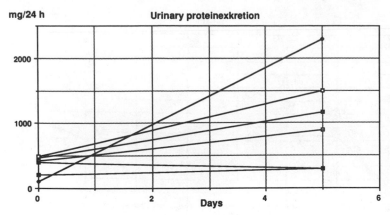

Fig. 6. Protein excretion in 6/7 patients following administration of TNF

DISCUSSION

In animals application of TNF leads to haemoconcentration, shock, metabolic acidosis and severe end-organ damage including acute renal tubular necrosis. Our results show that TNF seems to have a nephrotoxic potential in man, as well. In our study 6 out of 7 patients developed symptoms of renal injury after administration of recombinant human TNF. Impaired renal function was observed in 2 patients, 4 patients had proteinuria and 6 patients had enzymuria. Two patients showed an increase of serum creatinine despite sufficient hydration, there were no signs of haemoconcentration or hypotension. So the cause of deteriorated renal function is unlikely to be prerenal. In these 2 patients enzymuria preceeded renal function impairment for 4 days. All 5 enzymes determined have their highest activities in the tubular cells, so enzymuria, mild proteinuria and the results of SDS-PAGE-electrophoresis may reflect tubular lesions. Our data indicate that monitoring of renal function in patients treated with TNF may be warranted during TNF therapy. During treatment one should take care to maintain adequate hydration and avoid additional potential nephrotoxic agents. As enzymuria preceeded deterioration of renal function for 4 days determination of urinary enzymes seems to be a useful tool for early detection of nephrotoxicity of new drugs.

REFERENCES

1. B. Beutler, A. Cerami, Cachectin: More than a tumor necrosis factor, N Engl J Med. 316:379-384 (1987)

2. R. Munker, H.Ph. Koeffler, Tumor necrosis factor: Recent Adv Klin Wochenschr. 65:345-352 (1987)

3. D. Maruhn, I. Fuchs, G. Mues, K.D. Bock, Normal limits of urinary excretion of eleven enzymes, Clin Chem. 22:1567-1574 (1976)

CHARACTERISATION OF HUMAN RENAL EMBRYONIC ANTIGENS BY MONOCLONAL ANTIBODIES.

P. Eydoux, J.J. Candelier, P. Couillin, J.F. Oury and A. Boue

INSERM U 73, Chateau de Longchamps, 75016 Paris, France

INTRODUCTION

The importance of membrane and extra-membrane antigens as signals for growth, induction, morphogenesis and differentiation is now well documented. In the kidney, as in other organs, control of tissue differentiation can result in cell-cell interaction as well as interaction between cells and the extra-cellular matrix. Changes in extra cellular matrix protein are first seen, then conversion of undifferentiated mesenchymal-like cells into epithelial cells follows (Croisille, 1969; Ekblom et al., 1982; Ekblom et al., 1985).

The role of extra-cellular matrix in cell migration and cell adhesion has been demonstrated (Thiery et al., 1984). Basement membranes, because of their location between epithelia and connective tissue and their chemical composition, share an important role in exchange of information between epithelial and embryonic or adult connective tissue. Some of its components appear before overt morphogenesis, and may contribute to cell aggregation and to the organisation and maintenance of tissue in their definitive form.

Cell-cell interaction occurs according to various possibilities. These include transmission of molecules secreted by cell digitation (Saxen et al, 1978), membrane receptors (Ekblom et al., 1980; Yamada, 1983), gap junctions (Nicoas et al., 1981), electrical charge (Kanwar et al., 1981), or membranous adhesion molecules (Thiery et al., 1984). Membrane molecules seem to play an important role in the recognition of cells.

In the human embryo, renal antigens positioned during prenatal differentiation may have a role in prenatal renal function, and, if still present, throughout postnatal life.

Nephrotoxicity in the growing embryo includes impaired morphogenesis and histogenesis; one model of renal malformation could be by direct action on renal tissue. Many antigens in human organs are still to be discovered in order to understand normal mechanisms of growth, morphogenesis and differentiation, and their disturbances. Characterization of new antigens is now made possible by hybridoma technology. This immunological method allows discrimination of cell surface antigens, even when they are weakly expressed in the cell membrane. We have characterised new histologically epitopes on human kidney that have a possible role in renal differentiation and function.

MATERIAL AND METHODS

Production of monoclonal antibodies. Human embryos aged seven weeks were obtained from abortions performed independent of this study. Metanephros and mesonephros were dissected and cultivated using an explant technique and differentiated cells were selected on the basis of their epithelial morphology. After gentle trypsinization, cells were washed and then incubated for 2 hr at $37^{\circ}C$ in an atmosphere of 5% CO_2. Half of these cells were concentrated for booster injection, 10^6 cells were then injected into Balb/c mice aged 6 to 10 weeks, and after four weeks were given a second injection. Three days after the second inoculation, the mice were sacrificed and the spleen removed. Spleen cells were harvested and fused with 10^7 cells from the mouse myeloma cell line SP2/o-AG 14 using a 30% solution of polyethyleneglycol-1000. Hybrids were cultivated in MEM medium containing 15% heat-inactivated colt serum, then subcloned twice by limiting dilution and transferred into selective serum-free medium supplemented with 2% Ultroser KY-52 medium (Couillin et al., 1982). Preliminary screening was performed by indirect immunofluorescence (IIF) on frozen sections of human foeti aged 9 to 22 weeks; the same IIF technique was used for screening and histological studies.

Immuno-histological studies were made on human renal tissue (foetal mesonephros and/or metanephros aged 6 to 32 weeks; histologically normal parts of adult kidney with renal polar cancer) and vertebrate kidney. Species were selected to represent the principal classes and orders (Table 2. human and baboon for primates; cat for carnivores; pig, cow, sheep for artiodactylas; rabbit for lagomorphae; nutria, guinea-pig, hamster, rat, mouse for rodents; mole for insectivores; hen, quail for birds; Vipera aspic (snake), Lacerta vivipara (lizard), Trionix sinensis (tortoise) for reptiles; Rana exculenta, Xenopus laevis, Pleurodeles waltlii for batrachians; Salmo trutta fario, Salmo gairdneri, Carassiu carassiu for fish (Candelier et al., 1986). Tissues are frozen in liquid nitrogen within two hours after sampling, and 5 um sections cut immediately using a cryostat. Slides were air dried, stored at -20 or $-80^{\circ}C$ and used for IIF within one month. For this purpose, tissue sections were incubated with pure culture supernatant containing monoclonal antibody (MAB) for 30 to 60 min, then gently washed in phosphate buffer saline (PBS). The sections were then incubated for 30-60 min with goat anti-mouse immunoglobulins conjugated with fluorescein isothiocyanate. Slides were then washed and mounted in Mowiol solution (Oriol et al., 1983).

Electrophoretic analysis. Western blots were performed with MAB on the following antigens separated by sodium dodecyl sulphate polyacrylamide gel electrophoresis (Laemmli, 1970): type I, III, IV, V human collagens; human plasma fibronectin, human beta-2-microblogulin; human cellular fibronectin prepared by cyanogen bromide digestion of human placenta and kidney (Epstein et al., 1971). After separation, proteins were transferred to nitrocellulose and stained as described (Bellon, 1985).

Enzyme-Linked Immunosorbent Assays (ELISA). Tests with the above mentioned antigens were performed as follows (Bellon, 1985): wells of microtitre plates are coated with antigen solution, washed, and diluted MABs added to each well and incubated 2 hr at room temperature; goat anti-mouse immuno-globulins coupled to horseradish peroxidase are added to each well; the reaction is revealed with o-phenylenediamine, and optical density is measured at 492 nm.

Radioimmunoassays (RIA). All antibodies were tested for reactivity towards blood group related oligosaccharides by a solid phase RIA using artificial antigens as described (Le Pendu et al., 1985). The antigens tested included A, B, and H structures of types 1, 2, 3 and 4, Le^a, Le^D, X and Y antigen as well as type I and type II oligosaccharide precursors.

RESULTS

From 16 immunized Balb/C mice, 288 secreting hybridomas were obtained. We chose to present here 5 antibodies, which seemed of particular importance for differentiation because of their epithelium or mesenchyml-related location inside renal tissue. All antibodies are IgG, but one (EE 24-6) is an IgM.

Histological   Studies   and   Ontogeny.   Histological   repartition   of structures disclosed by our antibodies in foetal and adult kidney were studied by IIF (Table 1); two groups can be distinguished according to antigen location: epithelium-related and connective tissue antigens.

TABLE 1.   Histological pattern of monoclonal antibodies in Human

Mab Histology	EG 9-11	EG 14-1	EK 8-1	EK 17-1	EE 24-6
	(SSB)	(SSB)			UB
FOETUS	PCT	Glbm	Gl/M	Gl/M	CS
ADULT	PCT	Glbm	(Glms)/M	Glms/(M)	Ut

For legend, see table 2.

Epithelium-related antigens. Glomerulus antigen (EG 14-1) is located on adult glomerulus, outlining the basal part of glomerular epithelium; no labelling was seen on tubular basal membrane, nor in connective tissue. Staining appears weakly at S-shaped body stage into glomerular slit, to be then precisely located inside glomerular basal membrane.   Cells of distal S-shaped body surrounding glomerular slit are slightly stained, suggesting an epithelial origin of this antigen.

Tubular antigen (EG 9-11) binds to an intracellular proximal convoluted tubule (PCT) antigen, where fluorescence is intense on PCT cell membranes, but less intense in cytoplasm.   In 6 week old embryos, staining is observed on condensing blastema; it is then present with low intensity on the S-shaped body, and then on tubular cells in their first stages of differentiation. Slight fluorescence is present in mesenchyma surrounding glomeruli.

Urothelium antigen (EE 24-6) is seen in the basal layer of adult urothelium; staining covers heterogenously whole cytoplasm in some cells, and only membrane related cytoplasm in others.   Strong fluorescence is present on ureteral bud cells, and to some extent on inner wall of differentiating glomerulus.   At 22 weeks, basal layer of urothelium was stained as well as collecting tubule cells. Those are very heterogenously stained, and some display a weak membraneous fluorescence, others are more intensely stained, with fluorescence present in whole cytoplasm.

Connective tissue antigens. Extracellular matrix is stained with high intensity after exposure to EK 8-1, displaying a fibrillar pattern; basal membranes of renal tubuli are also fluorescent.   Inside glomerulus, mesangium shows light fluorescent spots. Antigen is present in 6 week old embryos, already very intensely stained in connective tissue, much lighter in mesangium and quickly evolving into adult pattern.   Fluorescence obtained with EK 17-1 in adult renal tissue is a little different from EK

8-1: the capsule is precisely outlined and mesangium very intensely stained, surrounding vascular tuft; fibrils in connective tissue are heterogeneous and with lighter staining; fluorescence intensity in basal membranes is lower. Labelling is light in 6th week embryo, rapidly becoming more intense in mesangium and lighter in extracellular matrix.

Phylogeny. Results are given in Table 2. The techniques used in human tissues could be employed in vertebrate tissues as well; fluorescence was similar, with some differences. staining intensity was greater in primates, cat, guinea-pig and sheep. Labelling was intense in snake and nutria. In other species tested, staining was weak when present. None of the five antigens studied are human specific as everyone of them is at least present in one other species. All are seen in mammals, and only EE 24-6 is present in non-mammalian species.

TABLE 2. Histological pattern of monoclonal antibodies in various species.

MAB SPECIES	EG 9-11	EG 14-1	EK 8-1	EK 17-1	EE 24-6
Human	PCT	Glbm	(Glms)/M	Glms/(M)	CS
Baboon	PCT/(CS)	Glbm	(Glms)/M	Glms/(M)	DT/M
Cat	PCT	Glbm	(Glms)/M		Glms/M
Pig					(DT/CS)
Cow			(M)	Glms/M	M
Sheep					Glms/(M)
Rabbit		(Glbm)			(DT/CS)
Nutria		Glbm	(M)		CS
Guinea-pig		Glbm			
Hamster			(M)		
Rat/Mouse					
Mole	PCT	Glbm	M	Glms/M	CS/M
Birds					(Gl)
Snake					Gl/PCT/CS
Lizard					PCT/M
Tortoise					Gl/PCT
Frog					Gl/CS/M
Xenopus					(CS)
Pleurodeles					
Fish					

Where data is absent species were tested but negative; structures in parenthesis display lighter staining.

CS: Collecting System DT: Distal Tubule GT: Glomerulus Glbm: Glomerular Basal Membrane Glms: Mesangium M: Extracellular Matrix PCT: Proximal Convoluted Tubule SSB: S-Shaped Body UB: Ureteral Bud Ut: Urothelium

Biochemical Studies. Based on the methods used only EK 17-1 was recognized to bind to an epitope common to plasma or cellular fibronectin; all other antigens tested were negative.

DISCUSSION

In order to obtain sufficient antigens for immunization, we augmented the quantity of renal tissue using cellular culture to improve immunization against renal specific antigens. Only cells with epithelial morphology were injected into Balb/C mice. Use of HY synthetic medium proved to be very useful to limit background fluorescence, thus improving the quality of IIF (Candelier et al., 1987). Fixation was not used, because all fixatives (eg. acetone, 5% formaldehyde or paraformaldehyde) resulted in loss of fluorescence. Time of incubation of MAB or antimouse immunoglobulin (30-60 min) did not seem to be important for quality of fluorescence. Mowiol is useful to stabilise tissue and limit fading when slides are exposed to ultra-violet light (Oriol et al., 1983).

All stages of nephron differentiation are seen in foetal metanephros. Thus the age of foeti used for screening was unimportant provided that all stages would be present. Nevertheless, we used very early embryos for histological studies in order to determine age of apparition of antigens in human. Fluorescence was present in every 6 weeks old embryo tested, showing the early appearance of these antigens in human development. MABs were tested on mesonephros aand each one of them was present on related structure of this organ: EG 14-1 in glomerulus, EG 9-1 in mesonephretic tubules, EE 24-6 in mesonephretic duct, EK 8-1 and EK 17-1 in mesenchyme. It can be concluded that mesonephros and metanephros share many common antigens. It is likely in this condition that a toxic effect mediated by one of those antigens - or any antigen common to both organs - during prenatal life would impair development or function of kidney as well as of mesonephros-derived organs.

Every antigen in foetal kidneys was also present on adult kidney, i.e. those identified by EG 14-1 and EG 9-1 are first seen in S-shaped body; ureteral bud antigen (EE 24-1) will later be detected on urothelium. The antigens studied display some degree of localization. As human renal differentiation carries on, their location seems to become specially restricted as intensity of staining gets stronger. for example, EG 9-1 is seen in proximal convoluted tubule in adult; EG 14-1 first binds to capsular epithelium and glomerular basal membrane in foetal kidney, but only to the later in adult kidney. Change in intensity is clearly illustrated with EK 17-1: staining intensity increase in mesangium as it decreased in connective tissue and basement membrane were it is first seen. The localization of antigens during development seems to be an important phenomenon, related to differentiation and morphogenesis.

The only identified antigen with the methods used in this study is fibronectin, recognized by EK 17-1. Histologic location is slightly different from other published data (Linder et al., 1980): one explanation could be that epitopes recognized are not identical.

Vertebrate species were chosen to represent the principal classes and order in evolution. In regard of phylogeny, two groups can be distinguised. Mammalian specific, histologically homogeneous antibodies (EG 9-11, EG 14-1, EK 8-1, EK 17-1) bind to antigens present only in mammals; the same histological structure is stained in the different species studied. Histologically heterogeneous antigen (EE 24-6) is present in mammalians, reptiles and batrachians; this earlier antigen in evolution was also seen in such different structures as glomerulus, neck segment, proximal convoluted tubule, distal tubule, collecting system and extra-cellular matrix, i.e. virtually every part of renal tissue. No positive reaction was seen with any of these antibodies with mouse or rat, as non-mouse antigens seem to have been selected by our methodology.

Antigens present in human renal epithelium or connective tissue have been described in glomerular basal membrane (Anand et al., 1978), tubular basement membrane (Michael, 1983), epithelial cell (Bander et al., 1985), extracellular matrix and podocytes (Ekblom et al., 1982; Mounier et al., 1986). To our knowledge, no antigen previously described displays the same histologic pattern as ours. They thus constitute new epitopes or antigens, which could provide a valuable tool for renal differentiation and physiology studies. Among these, EE 24-6 is associated with growing epithelium of ureteral bud origin. In the foetus ureteral bud and collecting tubules, where isolated cells showing fluorescence might be cells committed for division, whereas in adults they represent the germinative layer responsible for renewing of urothelium). This antigen might be related to cell-growth mechanisms. Other antibodies, as EG 9-1 or EG 14-1 are related to antigens set in the foetus and persisting in adult tissues; they constitute differentiation antigens.

Characterization of developmental antigens is aimed at having better understanding of cellular growth, differentiation, cancer or congenital nephropathies. They should provide valuable help for studies of toxic effects on renal development and function, as those antigens could be directly or indirectly involved in teratogenic or toxic processes.

BIBLIOGRAPHY

Anand SK, Landing BH, Heuser ET, Olson DL, Grushkin CM, Lieberman E, 1978, J Pediatr 92:952

Bander NH, Cordon-Caro C, Finstad CL, Whitmore WF, Daracott-Waughan JR, Oettgen HF, Melamed M, Old LJ, 1985, J Urology, 133:502

Bellon G, 1985, Anal Biochem, 150:188

Candelier JJ, Couillin P, Roturier M, Boue A, 1987, CR Acad Sc Paris, 303 III

Candelier JJ, Couillin P, Roturier M, Boue A, 1987, Ann Immunol (Inst Pasteur), 138 (In Press)

Couillin P, Carainic R, Cabau N, Horodniceanu F, Boue A, 1982, Ann Virol, 133E:315

Croisille Y, 1969, In: "Les interactions tissulaires au cours de l'organogenese", Dunod, Paris

Ekblom P, Mittinen A, Saxen L, 1980, Dev Biol, 74:263

Ekblom P, Saxen L, Timp R, 1982, In: "Membranes in growth and development", Hoffman, Giebisch, Bolis ed, AR Liss Inc, New-York

Epstein EH, Scott RD, Miller EJ, Piez KA, 1971, J Biol Chem, 246:1718

Kanwar YS, Hascall VC, Farquhar MG, 1981, J Cell Biol, 90:527

Laemmli UK, 1970, Nature, 227:680

Le Pendu J, Fredman P, Richter ND, Magnani JL, Willingham NC, Pastan I, Oriol R, Ginsburg V, 1985, Carbohydrate Res, 141:347

Linder E, Miettinen A, Toernroth R, 1980, Lab Invest, 42:70

Michael AF, Yang JY, Falk RJ, Bennington MJ, Scheinman JI, Vernier RL, Fish AJ, 1983, Kidney Int, 24:74

Mounier F, Foidart JM, Gubler MC, Beziau A, Lacoste M, 1986, Lab Invest, 54:394

Nicholas JF, Kemler, R, Jacob F, 1981, Dev Biol, 81:127

Oriol R, Mancilla-Jimenez R, 1983, *J Immunol Met*, 47:97

Saxen L, Lehtonen E, 1978, *J Embryol Exp Morphol*, 47:97

Thiery, JP, Delouvee A, Gallin WJ, Cunningham BA, Edelman GM, 1984, *Dev Biol*, 102:61

Yamada KM, 1983, *Ann Rev Biochem*, 52:761

SPECIES DIFFERENCES IN THE IMMUNOCYTOCHEMICAL DISTRIBUTION OF TAMM-HORSFALL GLYCOPROTEIN

C. J. Powell

The Robens Institute, Surrey University Guildford, Surrey GU2 5XH, UK
(Present address: DHSS Department of Toxicology, St Bartholomew's Hospital
Medical College, London EC1 7ED, UK.)

INTRODUCTION

Tamm-Horsfall glycoprotein was first described as a urinary inhibitor of
viral haemagglutination (Tamm and Horsfall, 1950). It is a 75,000 dalton
molecular weight glycoprotein, which is synthesised in the kidney and
excreted in urine. Normal individuals excrete approximately 100 mg per day
of this material, which has the ability to form massive aggregates of up
to 1.4×10^7 daltons. Tamm-Horsfall glycoprotein contains between 25 and
40% carbohydrate by weight and has a tertiary structure resembling a
spiralled string of beads (Wenk et al, 1981). It has a number of unusual
chemical and physical properties: such as a ready ability to transform
between sol and gel states in solution, according to pH, the ionic
environment, its osmotic concentration in solution, and/or the
concentration of other solutes (Hoyer and Seiler, 1979).

Even though excretion of Tamm-Horsfall glycoprotein may be increased in
certain experimental models of acute tubular necrosis (Schwartz et al,
1972), its normal physiological role is unresolved.

The functions most commonly proposed include:-

(i) an antibacterial agent, inhibiting fimbration in the distal nephron
and urinary tract (Orskov et al, 1980).

(ii) a modifier of crystal-formation, by virtue of its ability to alter
the zeta potential of calcium oxalate crystals and to chelate monovalent
cations in urine (Scurr and Robertson, 1986).

(iii) a waterproofing agent in the diluting segment of the distal nephron
(Hoyer and Sieler, 1979, Sikri et al, 1979)

(iv) a component of the chloride transport mechanism in the distal nephron
(Wirdnam and Milner, 1984).

Of these the waterproofing hypothesis has probably gained most ground,
primarily because the unusual ability of Tamm-Horsfall glycoprotein to
switch between aggregated (gel) and disaggregated (sol) forms would suit
such a function. Tamm-Horsfall glycoprotein has also been reported to be
absent specifically from the cells of the macula densa, which are thought

to sense the distal nephron luminal fluid as part of a tubulo-glomerular feed-back system. Furthermore, there is some evidence that loop diuretics may influence the concentration of Tamm-Horsfall glycoprotein in, and its excretion from, the kidney.

The object of this paper is to examine species differences in Tamm-Horsfall glycoprotein distribution, with a view to functional implications.

METHODS

Kidneys from the following 15 species: rat, mouse, syrian hamster, gerbil, guinea pig, rabbit, ferret, sheep, pig, dog, fox, baboon, man, fish (3-spined stickleback, Gasterosteus acculeatus) and hen were fixed in 10% neutral buffered formalin or Bouins fluid, embedded in paraffin wax and sectioned at 5um. Two different polyclonal antibodies raised against human Tamm-Horsfall glycoprotein, both of proven specificity (Dawnay et al, 1980), Dakopatts, Glostrup, Denmark), were used in the three layer PAP immunocytochemical method of Sternberger (1974). Endogenous peroxidase activity was blocked with methanol and hydrogen peroxide. The secondary antibody, affinity purified donkey anti-rabbit IgG, was obtained from Guildhay Antisera, Guildford. Antibody binding sites were revealed by incubation in the chromogen 3,3',4,4'-tetra-aminobiphenyl (Sigma, Poole, Dorset). Sections were lightly counterstained with Harris' Haematoxylin. Negative controls for immunocytochemical staining consisted of:-

(i) substituting normal rabbit serum for the primary antibody, (ii) absorbing out the primary antibody by addition of an equivalent amount of antigen.

Both of these procedures abolished staining.

RESULTS

In the rat, mouse, hamster, gerbil, pig and sheep immunostaining for Tamm-Horsfall glycoprotein was found in the thick ascending limbs of Henle in the outer medulla and cortex, and in the distal tubules. The staining intensity was strongest in the outer medulla/inner cortex and declined slightly towards the outer cortex (See Figs. 1 and 2). Intracellular staining was either homogenous or, in some instances, strongest at the apical face of the cell. In the rat, mouse and hamster the distal nephrons were randomly dispersed among the proximal tubules. But, in the two primate species examined: baboon and man, these segments traversed the inner cortex as discrete bundles, and only appeared to diverge in the region of their respective glomeruli (Fig. 3).

The patterns of Tamm-Horsfall glycoprotein immunostaining in the rabbit, ferret and guinea pig were similar to the rat, except that in these species certain regions of the distal tubule were particularly intensely stained, but then staining intensity declined conspicuously towards the terminal end of these nephron segments. The cells of the macula densa of the guinea pig were strongly stained (Fig. 4), in contrast to those of the baboon and most other species.

In both the dog and the fox the pattern of immunostaining was unusual. The innermost region of the outer medulla was scarcely stained at all, but most distinctively, the later distal tubule had a pattern of intermittent staining. Thorough examination of this nephron segment in both species revealed that positively stained cells were not randomly distributed, but were interspersed between non-staining cells. Thus two positively stained cells were never adjacent (Fig. 5). If the normal physiological function

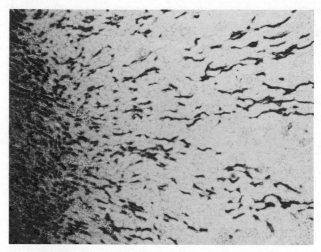

Figure 1. Immunostaining for Tamm-Horsfall glycoprotein in the rat kidney. Note a band of densely staining thick ascending limbs of Henle in the outer medulla (left), which then diverge as they pass through the proximal straight tubules or pars recta. Magnification x 48.

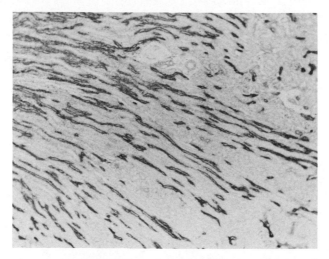

Figure 2. At the corticomedullary junction of the guinea pig kidney, (on left), the thick ascending limbs of Henle are clearly defined within medullary rays, and follow a more direct route to the outer cortex than do those of the rat. Magnification x 48.

of Tamm-Horsfall glycoprotein was a waterproofing agent, as many authors have suggested, then these tubules would leak like sieves!

CONCLUSIONS

Tamm-Horsfall glycoprotein was detected in all 13 mammalian species examined, but could not be demonstrated in the renal tissue of the hen or a teleost fish. With the exception of the dog and fox, the distribution described in this paper are similar to those previously noted in several species (Hoyer and Seiler, 1979, Sikri et al, 1979, Wenk et al, 1981). Shenk et al (1971) previously reported the distribution of Tamm-Horsfall glycoprotein in the dog (breed unspecified), but claimed a consistent

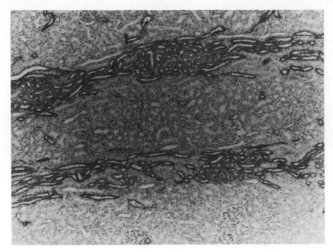

Figure 3. Tamm-Horsfall glycoprotein distribution in the kidney of the baboon. The corticomedullary junction is to the left. In this species the thick ascending limbs of Henle traverse the cortex in discrete bundles. Compare this pattern with the rat and guinea pig in Figures 1 and 2. Magnification x 48.

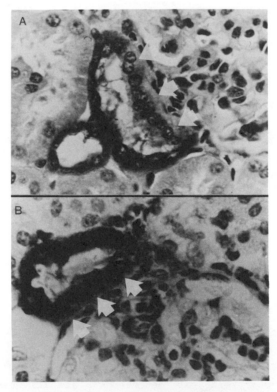

Figure 4. The macula densa of the baboon (A) and guinea pig (B) are shown by white arrows. In the baboon these cells are non-staining, as reported for most other species, whereas those of the guinea pig stained strongly with the rest of the tubule. Magnification x 788.

distribution throughout the ascending limb of Henle and distal tubule.

Their failure to recognize the unusual staining pattern in the distal nephron may have been related to limitations of the immunofluorescence method, such as autofluorescence; or may indicate that there are differences between breeds of dog.

These investigations demonstrate the utility of Tamm-Horsfall glycoprotein as a marker for illustrating species differences in renal micro-anatomy. The intermittent distribution of this glycoprotein in the dog and fox, and its presence in the macula densa cells of the guinea pig, are not

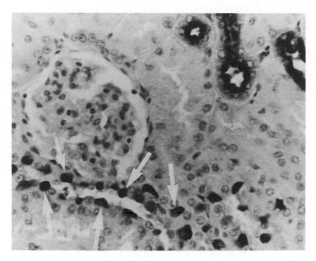

Figure 5. Immunostaining for Tamm-Horsfall glycoprotein in the cortex of Beagle dog kidney. Note strong staining towards the apical face of some tubules, but that late distal nephron segments have a pattern of positively stained cells (arrowed), interspersed with non-staining cells. Magnification x 500.

consistent with a role as a waterproofing agent. Further physiological studies, possibly on the unusual distal nephron segments of the dog or fox, may help to identify the normal function of this material.

REFERENCES

Chambers, R., Groufsky, A., Hunt, J.S., Lynn, K.L. and McGiven, A.R., 1986, Relationship of abnormal Tamm-Horsfall glycoprotein localisation to renal morphology, Clin. Nephrol., 26:21.

Dawnay, A.B. St J., McLean, C. and Cattell, W.R., 1980, The development of a radioimmunoassy for Tamm-Horsfall glycoprotein in serum, Biochem. J., 185:679.

Hoyer, J.R. and Seiler, M.W., 1979, Pathophysiology of Tamm-Horsfall protein, Kid. Int., 16:279.

Orskov, I., Ferencz, A. and Orskov, A., 1980, Tamm-Horsfall protein or uromucoid is the normal urinary slime that traps type-1 fimbrated Escherichia coli, Lancet, 1:887.

Schwartz, R.H., Lewis, R.A. and Schenk, E.A., 1972, Tamm-Horsfall mucoprotein III. Potassium dichromate induced renal tubular damage, Lab. Invest., 27:214.

Shenk, E.A., Schwartz, R.H. and Lewis, R.A., 1971, Tamm-Horsfall mucoprotein I. Localisation in the kidney, Lab. Invest., 25:92.

Sikri, K.L., Foster, C.L., Bloomfield, F.J. and Marshall, R.D., 1979, Localisation by immunofluorescence and by light and electron microscopic immunoperoxidase techniques of Tamm-Horsfall glycoprotein in adult hamster kidney, Biochem. J., 181:523.

Sternberger, L.A., 1974, Immunocytochemistry, 2nd edition, Raven Press, New York.

Tamm, I. and Horsfall, F.L., 1950, Characterisation and separation of an inhibitor of a viral haemagglutination present in urine, Proc. Soc. Exp. Bio. Med., 74:108.

Wenk, R.E., Bhagavan, B.S. and Rudert, J., 1981, Tamm-Horsfall uromuco-protein and the pathogenesis of casts, reflux nephropathy, and nephritides, In: "Pathology Annual", H.L. Ioachim, ed., Raven Press, New York, (1981).

Wirdnam, P.K. and Milner, R.D.G., 1984, Tamm-Horsfall glycoprotein release from rat kidney cortex slices in vitro, Clin. Sci., 67:529.

IMMUNOCYTOCHEMICAL LOCALIZATION OF GLUTATHIONE PEROXIDASE IN UREMIC RAT KIDNEY

S. Mizuiri, K. Hirata, S. Izumi*, N. Komatsu*, S. Yoshimura*, and K. Watanabe**

Dept. of Nephrology, Toho University School of Medicine, 6-11-1 Omori Nishi Ota-ku, Tokyo, *Cell. Biology Research Laboratory and **Department of Pathology, Tokai University, Isehara City, Kanagawa, Japan

INTRODUCTION

Lipid peroxidation is the oxidative deterioration of polyunsaturated lipid (1). Glutathione peroxidase (GSH-Po) is the enzlme which catalyzes the reduction of lipid peroxides with the concomitant oxidation of glutathione (2). Previously we reproted that the immunohistochemical localization of GSH-Po was mainly in the proximal tubules, there the proximal portions (S1+S2) were more intensely stained than the distal portion (S3), and the immunocytochemical localization of GSH-Po swas in cytosol, including the core of microvilli and lysosomes of the epithelial cells in proximai tubules (PT) in normal rat kidney (3). This study was designed to investigate the immunocytochemical localization of GSH-Po in the uremic rat kidney in order to clarify the pathophysiological significance of the enzyme.

MATERIALS AND METHODS

Animals and tissue preparation. Male Wistar rats weighing 150 g and fed standard laboratory chow were used in this experiment. Uremia was produced in 6 animals after a partial electrocoagulation on two-thirds of the left kidney and contralateral nephrectomy principally by the method of Boudet et al.(4). Another 6 animals underwent bilateral kidney decapsulization and were used as normal controls. six weeks after the operation, both groups of animals were sacrificed after blood samples were obtained. Subsequently, the middle one-third (which was not exposed to electrocoagulation) of the uremic kidneys of the experimental group, and the corresponding portions of kidneys of the normal control group were removed for the following procedures.

Biochemical study. Blood urea nitrogen (BUN) and serum creatinine were measured in experimental animals. GSH-Po activity was measured by the method described in our previous report (5) in both serum and kidney homoenate. Thiobarbituric acid values were measured by the method of Yagi (6) in both serum and kidney homogenate.

Statistical analysis. The results of blood chemistry and biochemical study of the kidneys are expressed as mean±SD. Student's t test was used to determine the significance of difference between groups.

Histopathological observations. Hematoxylin and eosin stained sections and oil red 0 stained sections were observed.

Antibodies. Rabbit anti-rat liver GSH-Po was prepared by immunization of rabbits with the purified protein. The method of purification of rat liver GSH-Po was described in our previous report (5). Rabbit anti-rat albumin and IgG were purchased from Cappel Company (U.S.A.). The specifity of antibody was assessed by Ouchterlony's immunodiffusion test in agarose gel and the immunoblotting (Western blotting) test. The Fab fragments of the gamma-globulin were labeled with horseradish peroxidase (HRP) (7). since the anti-GSH-pO antibody used in this experiment was raised in rabbits against rat liver GSH-Po, we examined the cross- reactivity of this antibody with rat kidney GSH-Po by immunochemical titration. The cross-reactivity was 92 percent.

Immunohistochemistry and immunocytochemistry. The dissected small pieces of kidney tissue were fixed in 4% periodate-lysin paraformaldehyde for 12 hrs at 40c, embedded in OCT compound, frozen, and sectioned into 6-um thick slices with a cryostat. GSH-Po, albumin and IgG of the rat kidney were localized by the direct enzyme (HRP)-labeled antibody method (7) and observed both light microscopically and ultrastructually.

RESULTS

The results of blood chemistry and biochemical study of the kidneys are summarized in Table I. Uremic rats showed significantly (P < 0.001) elevated BUN levels and serum creatinine levels compared with normal rats. In uremic rats, serum GSH-Po activity was significantly (P < 0.001) lower than that of normal controls and kidney GSH-Po activity of the uremic rats was significantly (P < 0.001) lower as well. In contrast, both serum thiobarbituric acid (P < 0.001) and kidney thiobarbituric acid values (P < 0.03) were significantly elevated in uremic rats as compared with those of normal controls.

Table I. Blood chemistry and biochemical study of the kidney

	Normal rats (n=6)	Uremic rats (n=6)
BUN (mg/dl)	19.7 $\pm$ 2.1	97.2 $\pm$ 19.5*
Serum creatinine (mg/dl)	0.7 $\pm$ 0.1	1.7 $\pm$ 0.3*
Serum GSH-Po (u/mg protein)	0.13 $\pm$ 0.01	0.06 $\pm$ 0.01*
Serum thiobarbituric acid (n moles/ml blood)	17.4 $\pm$ 3.1	25.6 $\pm$ 2.3*
Kidney GSH-Po (u/g kidney)	39.4 $\pm$ 3.9	26.4 $\pm$ 3.0*
Kidney thiobarbituric acid (n moles/g kidney)	143.3 $\pm$ 12.3	208.0 $\pm$ 45.3**

The values are expressed as mean$\pm$SD. *P < 0.001 compared with normal rats, **P < 0.03 compared with normal rats.

Histopathological observations. Uremic rat kidney showed very remarkable structural changes. Glomeruli were almost totally hyalinized. In the PT, the diameter of the lumen was dilated with loss of the brush border and flatness of the epithelial cells (Fig. 1). Atrophy of the distal tubules was also noted. Fatty degeneration was observed in the epithelial cells of PT in uremic rats by oil red 0 staining (Fig. 2).

Immunohistochemistry and immunocytochemistry.

A. GSH-Po localization in uremic rat kidneys under light microscopic

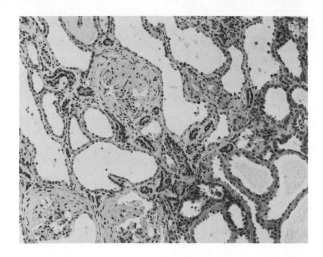

Fig. 1 Light micrograph of uremic rat kidney. Glomeruli are largely hyalinized. Many proximal tubules are extremely dilated. (hematoxilin and eosin x 150)

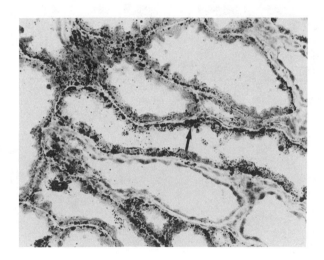

Fig. 2 Light micrograph of a uremic rat kidney section stained by oil red O. Arrow shows increased and enlarged lipid granules (x300)

observation diffuse immunohistochemical localization in the epithelial cells in PT was much less conspicuous than that in the normal rat kidneys. On the other hand, the localization in large granules of epithelial cells was very distinct. GSH-Po was also localized on the luminal surfaces (Fig. 3). Ultrastructurally the cytosolic GSH-Po in epithelial cells in PT was extremely decreased in all three segments, while markedly increased numbers of GSH-Po positive large phagosomes were observed (Fig. 4). GSH-Po was also observed in the increased tubulovesicular structures (Fig. 5).

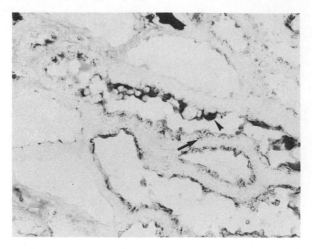

Fig. 3 Immunohistochemical localization of GSH-Po in uremic rat kidney. The arrow indicates localization in large granules of epithelial cells and the arrowhead shows localization in tubular lumen condensed upon the cellular surfaces (x300).

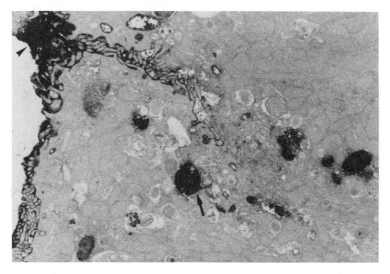

Fig. 4 Immunocytochemical localization of GSH-Po in uremic rat kidney. The arrow shows a GSH-Po positive large phagosome. The arrowhead shows the localization of GSH-Po in the lumen condensed in the areas adjacent to the cell surface (x10000).

B. Albumin and IgG localization in uremic rat kidney

Immunohistochemically albumin and IgG were localized in large granules but not diffusely in the epithelial cells of PT. Ultrastructural localizations of albumin and IgG were the same as that of GSH-Po except that weak cytosolic GSH-Po localization was not seen.

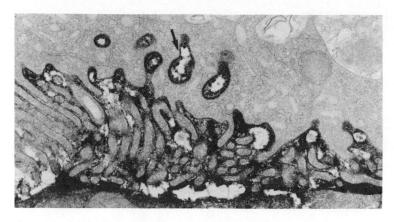

Fig. 5 Immunocytochemical localization of GSH-Po in uremic rat kidney. The arrow shows GSH-Po contained in the increased tubulovesicular structures (x126000).

DISCUSSION

In advanced chronic renal failure, besides a decrease in glomerular filtration rate, abnormal secretory and reabsorptive capacities are found in the nephron. This functional tubular insufficiency may be caused by tubular cell injury and necrosis. Our biochemical studies showed that elevated thiobarbituric acid values, namely enhanced in vitro lipid peroxidation, was found in both serum and kidney homogenate of uremic rats. Similar findings were reported in which malondialdehyde formation in the kidney was enhanced in nephrotoxic acute renal failure (8). Furthermore, the results of these biochemical studies substantiated reduced GSH-Po activity in both serum and kidney homogenate of uremic rats, indicating diminished capacity in eliminating lipid peroxides.

Histopathologically uremic rats showed fatty degeneration indicated by the intracellular accumulation of lipids in the epithelial cells of PT. This lipid accumulation may reflect the intracellular increase of lipid peroxides. This view was experimentally proved in fatty liver both by carbon tetrachloride and other lipoperoxidative cytotoxic agents (9).

Immunocytochemical studies in this experiment showed that, in uremic rat kidneys, cytosolic GSH-Po became far less conspicuous, while increased and enlarged phagosomes and luminal surfaces of PT were heavily loaded with GSH-Po. This immunocytochemical feature in the uremic rat kidneys, i.e., the marked increase of the enzyme in phagosomes, seems not to be compatible with the biochemically decreased activity of GSH-Po. A plausible explanation for this is that GSH-Po in phagolysosomes is segregated from the cytosol by the lysosomal membrane and does not function as an antilipoperoxidative agent. since it has been proved that both liver and adrenal GSH-Po in cytosol work as anti-lipoperoxidative agents (9,10) kidney GSH-Po in the cytosol of PT epithelial cells might play a similar role. Therefore it is conceivable that decreased cytosolic GSH-Po and impairment of the eliminative capacity of lipid peroxides seems to be partially responsible for fatty degeneration and the ensuing renal tubular cell damage. Although the cause of the decrease in cytosolic GSH-Po remains unclear, it may be a selenium deficiency in uremic rat kidney (11). The inmunostaining for albumin and IgG exhibited a localization similar to GSH-Po in phagolysosomes and luminal surfaces but not in the cytosol of PT epithelial cells in uremic rat kidneys. Accordingly, we postulated that GSH-Po in phagolysosomes and luminal surfaces could have been mostly derived from serum GSH-Po. Although this has not been ascertained, serum GSH-Po may be filtered through glomeruli and reabsorbed into the tubular epithelial cells. Localization of GSH-Po in the increased tubulovesicular structures may indicate increased endocytosis of the enzyme accumulated in the tubular lumen, while cytobolic GSH-Po in PT eithelial cells may be generated in situ, as we have previously reported.

REFERENCES

1. Tappel, A.L., Lipid peroxidation damage to cell components. Fed. Proc. 32:1870 (1973).

2. Mills, G.C. Randall, H.P., Hemoglobin catabolism. II. Protection of hemoglobin from oxidative breakdown in the intact erythrocyte. J. Biol. Chem. 232:589 (1958).

3. Mizuiri, S. Hirata, K. Izumi, S. Komatsu, N. Yoshimura, S. Watanabe, K., Immunocytochemical study of glutathione peroxidase in normal rat kidney. Renal Physiol. 9:249 (1986).

4. Boudet, J. Man, N.K. Sausse, A. Funk-Brentano, J.L., Experimental chronic renal failure in the rat by electrocoagulation of the renal cortex. Kidney Int.:82 (1978).

5. Yoshimura, S. Komatsu, N. Watanabe, K., Purification and immunohistochemical localization of rat liver glutathione peroxidase. Biochim. Biophys. Acta 621:130 (1980).

6. Yagi, K., A simple fluorimetric assay for lipoperoxide in blood plasma. Biochem. Med. 15:212 (1976).

7. Wilson, M.B. Nakane, P.K., Recent developments in the periodate method of conjugating horseradish peroxidase (HRPO) to antibodies; In: "Immunofluorescence and related staining techiques," W. Knapp ed., North-Holland Biochemical Press, Amsterdam (1978).

8. Gstraunthaler, G. Pfaller, W. Kotanko, P., Glutathione depletion and in vitro lipid peroxidation in mercury or maleate induced acute renal failure. Biochem. Pharmac. 32:2969 (1983).

9. Watanabe, K., Lipid peroxidation and cell injuries. Tr. Soc. Pathol. Jpn. 76:39 (1986).

10. Murakoshi, M. Osamura, Y. Yoshimura, S. Izumi, S. Komatsu, N., Watanabe, K., Biochemical and immunohistochemical studies of glutathione peroxidase in the rat adrenal cortex. Acta Histochem. 14:571 (1981).

11. Smythe, W.R. Alerey, A.C. Craswell, P.W. Crouch, C.A. Ibels, L.S. Kubo, H. Nunnelley, L.L. Rudolph, H., Trace element abnormalities in chronic uremia. Ann. Intern. Med. 96:302 (1982).

URINE GLUTATHIONE-S-TRANSFERASE ASSOCIATED WITH NEPHROTOXIC DRUGS

D.A. Feinfeld, R. Safirstein, H. Anderson, L. Johnson, M. Hardy, A. Benvenisty, V. D'Agati, and S.D. Levine

Albert Einstein College of Medicine, Mount Sinai School of Medicine, and Columbia University College of Physicians & Surgeons, New York, N.Y.

INTRODUCTION

Administration of a large number of therapeutic and diagnostic agents is associated with injury to the renal tubules. We have studied the appearance of glutathione-S-transferase (GST) in the urine as a marker of renal tubular injury. GST is a cytosolic enzyme found in kidney, liver, and small intestine (1). It binds many substances and catalyses the conjugation of some of its ligands to reduced glutathione (2,3). GST is abundant in cytosol (4) and is localized to the proximal nephron (5). Normally undetectable in urine or serum by enzymatic assay (6), GST appears in the urine in experimental tubular toxicity from substances such as mercury, chromium, and gentamicin (7,8). In this study we looked at urinary GST in rats and man following the administration of cisplatin, cyclosporin, and iodinated radiocontrast agents.

MATERIALS AND METHODS

Cisplatin. Sprague-Dawley rats were given a single dose of cisplatin, 5 mg/kg. Urine was collected serially for GST, and urine osmolality and plasma creatinine were followed.

Cyclosporin. Lewis rats were given daily intraperitoneal injections of cyclosporin, 10, 20, or 50 mg/kg. Urine GST and osmolality and plasma creatinine were studied. In addition, urine from patients given cyclosporin for renal transplantation was tested for GST, and the drug dosage was noted.

Iodinated Radiocontrast Agents. Patients receiving iodinated radiocontrast agents (diatrizoates) intravenously had their urines tested for GST before and 6-12 hr after injection of the agents. In the rat studies, the animals were housed in individual metabolic cages and allowed to reach a steady state. All studies were done at base-line and repeated after drug administration; hence all individuals served as their own controls.

GST activity was measured as the rate of catalysed conjugation of dinitro-chlorobenzene to reduced glutathione, as previously described (6).

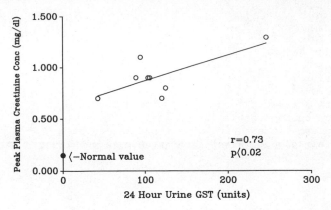

Fig. 1. Peak plasma creatinine and 24-hr urine GST in cisplatin toxicity.

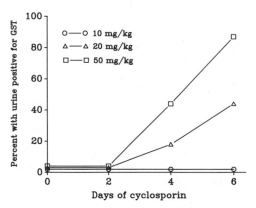

Fig. 2. Percent of rats' urines positive for GST on varying cyclosporin doses.

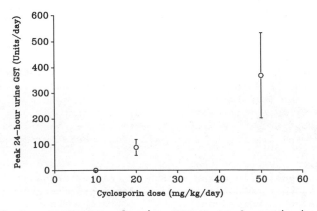

Fig. 3. Dose response of urine GST to cyclosporin in rats.

RESULTS

At baseline, before drug administration, urine from all rats and patients was negative for GST.

Cisplatin. Four to five days after a toxic dose of cisplatin, the rats' urine, previously negative for GST, became universally positive. This coincided with a rise in serum creatinine and a fall in urine osmolality, characteristic of nephrotoxicity in this model (9). Fig. 1 shows the rats' peak plasma creatinine as a function of their 24-hr urine GST. There was a fairly good correlation between these values, $r = .73$, $p < 0.02$. A similar degree of inverse correlation was found between minimum urine osmolality and 24-hr GST, $r = -.71$, $p < .05$.

Cyclosporin. All of the rats had normal plasma creatinine, high urine osmolality, and no detectable urine GST at baseline. After 6 days of cyclosporin, rats given 10 mg/kg had no biochemical evidence of renal injury and no urine GST. Rats given 20 mg/kg had no change in plasma creatinine, but had a significant drop in urine osmolality (1226 ± 106 to 841 ± 174 mOsm/kg, $p < .05$), and 44% had detectable urine GST. Those given 50 mg/kg had both a significant rise in plasma creatinine (0.2 ± 008 to 0.9 ± 03 mg%) and fall in urine osmolality (1460 ± 24 to 760 ± 181 mOsm/kg), $p < 0.05$ for both variables. Nearly all the rats in this group had GST-positive urine. As seen in Fig. 2, the percentage of rats with GST-positive urine increased with the number of days of cyclosporin and was higher in those receiving the higher dose. There was also a dose-response to cyclosporin in terms of the amount of GST in the final urine (Fig. 3). All rats had histologic evidence of cyclosporin-induced injury, with the mildest abnormalities (leukocyte margination) seen in the 10 mg/kg group and proximal tubular vacuolization and interstitial inflammation in the other groups, depending on the drug dose, as previously described (10).

Urine from renal transplant patients was also tested for GST before and after implantation. None of these patients had acute tubular necrosis or rejection at that time, and all urines were initially negative for GST. The patients whose urine became positive for GST (after 3 to 4 days of cyclosporin) were receiving a significantly higher daily dose of cyclosporin than those whose urines remained negative (Table 1).

Iodinated Radiocontrast Agents. We studied 20 consecutive patients who received iodinated radiocontrast agents intravenously for CT scanning. Six developed urinary GST between 6 and 12 hr after the injection. In the 6 patients whose urine became positive, there was a significant correlation between the iodine dose and the concentration of GST in the urine following injection, $r = .89$, $p < .01$. The mean dose of iodine per kg body weight was higher in the positive patients than in the others (0.58 ± 007 gm/kg compared to 0.48 ± 0.05 gm/kg), but this difference was not statistically significant. In another 6 patients given intravenous iodinated contrast agents for various studies (11), four had urinary ligandin, the major isoenzyme of GST, after receiving the dye. There was also a strong correlation in these patients between iodine dose and initial urinary enzyme levels, $r = .95$, $p < .001$ (Fig. 4). None of the patients developed clinical acute renal failure.

DISCUSSION

Previous studies have shown that the appearance of urinary GST, which is normally undetectable in urine except by radioimmunoassay, is a good indicator of tubular necrosis in the rat from proximal tubular toxins (7-10). The present studies confirm this for cisplatin and cyclosporin as well, in models with biochemical and histological evidence of acute renal injury.

Because GST is a cytosolic protein, its presence in urine in large quantities has generally been taken to indicate actual cellular disruption, with leakage of cellular contents into the urinary space (6). Unlike other markers of acute renal failure, some of which can become positive in urinary tract infection or renal ischaemia (12), GST is probably a more specific, if less sensitive indicator of cell injury. This has also been shown in chronic tubular toxicity, where the enzyme appears in the urine at the same time the cell damage occurs (13).

Table 1. Urine GST In Renal Transplant Patients

Oral Cyclosporin Dose (mg/kg)	Mean Urine GST (Units/ml)
0	0
10.2±0.2	0
14.5±0.5*	72.9±10.4**

* p < 0.05 compared to other groups
** p < 0.02 compared to other groups

GST has been shown to be confined to the proximal tubule in rat (4) and rabbit (5) and to the proximal tubule and the loop of Henle in man (14). Recently Bomhard et al. have used this localization of the enzyme as a marker of specific sites of renal tubular injury (15).

The present findings are compatible with the further concept that the amount of urinary GST may be a reflection of the actual amount of tissue injured. The degree of enzymuria was dose-related in all 3 drugs studied, both in rats and humans. In the cisplatin studies, the amount of urinary GST correlated with the peak plasma creatinine. A similar finding was noted in an earlier study of gentamicin-induced acute tubular necrosis in the rat (8). In both rats and patients given cyclosporin, urinary GST was highest in those individuals given the highest doses of the drug, while histological injury was most severe in the rats on the higher cyclosporin dosage. Finally, two groups of patients given intravenous radiocontrast media who had GST in their urine after receiving the agents showed a relationship between the level of urinary GST and the iodine dose. This suggests that the greater the number of tubular cells injured, the greater the amount of cytosolic proteins such as GST that will be released into the urine.

Still unclear is the relationship of the urinary GST in patients given iodinated radiocontrast agents to actual tubular necrosis. Goldstein et al. (16) reported that 35% of a group of patients undergoing renal arteriography developed detectable GST in their urine within 36 hr of injection of the agent. The present study found that 30% of a group of patients who received iodinated contrast media for CT scanning also developed enzymuria, a comparable incidence, even though the drug was not injected directly into the kidney. However, no patient in either study went into acute renal failure. The question arises then does the enzymuria represent subclinical injury to the renal tubule from the drug or is it merely the result of an interaction in the cell between enzyme and substrate? It has been shown that iodinated radiocontrast agents bind to ligandin, the major isoenzyme of GST, and may inhibit its ability to detoxify other substances (17). Further studies are needed on patients

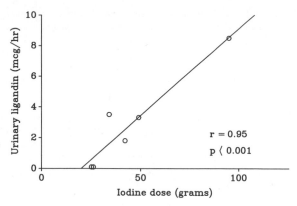

Fig. 4. Relationship of urinary ligandin (GST) to iodine dose in patients receiving iodinated radiocontrast agents.

with contrast agent-induced acute renal failure, as there is no good animal model of renal failure due to these substances.

Our findings, then, extend the concept of the use of urinary GST as an indicator of tubular cell injury following the administration of nephrotoxic drugs. The amount of enzyme appearing in the urine is often related to the dose of the drug and may reflect the actual degree of cellular necrosis as well as the severity of the renal failure.

REFERENCES

1. G. Fleischner, J. Robbins, and I.M. Arias, Immunological studies of Y protein: A major organic anion binding protein in rat liver. J. Clin. Invest. 51:677 (1972).

2. I.M. Arias, G. Fleischner, R. Kirsch, S. Mishking and Z. Gatmaitan, On the structure, regulation, and function of ligandin, In: "Glutathione: Metabolism and Function," I.M. Arias and W. Jakoby, eds., Raven Press, New York (1976).

3. W. Habig, M. Pabst, G. Fleischner, Z. Gatmaitan, and I.M. Arias, The identity of glutathione Transferase B and ligandin, the major organic anion binding protein of liver, Proc. Nat. Acad. Sci. 71:3879 (1974).

4. G. Fleischner, K. Kamisaka, Z. Gatmaitan, and I.M. Arias, Immunologic studies of rat and human ligandin, In: "Glutathione: Metabolism and function," I.M. Arias and W. Jakoby, eds., Raven Press, New York (1976).

5. L.G. Fine, E.J. Goldstein, and I.M. Arias, Localization of glutathione transferase activity in the rabbit nephron using isolated segments, Kidney Int. 8:474 (3975).

6. D.A. Feinfeld, G.M. Fleischner, E.J. Goldstein, R.D. Levine, S.D. Levine, M.M. Avram, and I.M. Arias, Ligandinuria: an indication of tubular cell necrosis, Curr. Prob. Clin. Biochem. 9:273 (1979).

7. D.A. Feinfeld, J.J. Bourgoignie, G.M. Fleischner, E.J. Goldstein, L. Biempica, and I.M. Arias, Ligandinuria in nephrotoxic acute tubular necrosis, Kidney Int. 12:387 (1977).

8. D.A. Feinfeld, G.M. Fleischner, and I.M. Arias, Urinary ligandin and glutathione-S-transferase in gentamicin-induced nephrotoxicity in the rat, Clin. Sci. 61:123 (1981).

9. D.A. Feinfeld, V.L. Fuh, and R. Safirstein, Urinary glutathione-S-transferase in cisplatin nephrotoxicity in the rat. J. Clin. Chem. Clin. Biochem. 24:529 (1986).

10. D.A. Feinfeld, A. Benvenisty, V. D'Agati, and M. Hardy, Cyclosporin A and urine glutathione-S-transferase. Proc. EDTA-ERA 22:561 (1985).

11. D.A. Feinfeld, R.A. Sherman, R. Safirstein, N. Ohmi, V.L. Fuh, I.M. Arias, and S. D. Levine, Urinary ligandin in renal tubular cell injury, Contr. Nephrol. 42:111 (1984).

12. R.G. Price, Urine N-acetyl-beta-D-glucosaminidase as an indicator of renal disease, Curr. Prob. Clin. Biochem. 9:150 (1979).

13. E. Bomhard, D. Maruhn, D. Paar, and K. Wehling, Urinary enzyme measurements as sensitive indicators of chronic cadmium nephrotoxicity. Contr. Nephrol. 42:142 (1984).

14. J.A.H. Campbell, N.M. Bass, and R.E. Kirsch, Immunohistochemical localization of ligandin in human tissues, Cancer 45:503 (1980).

15. E. Bomhard, D. Maruhn, and O. Vogel, Comparative investigations on the effects of acute intraperitoneal cadmium, chromium, and mercury exposure on the kidney, Uremia Invest. 9:131 (1985-86).

16. E.J. Goldstein, D.A. Feinfeld, G.M. Fleischner, and M. Elkin, Enzymatic evidence of renal tubular damage following renal angiography. Radiology 121:617 (1976).

17. E.J. Goldstein and I.M. Arias, Interaction of ligandin with radiographic contrast media, Invest. Radiol. 11:594 (1976).

AGE-RELATED CHANGES IN RENAL BRUSH BORDERS AND BRUSH BORDER ENZYMES

Masatoshi Nakano

Institute for Medical Science of Ageing, Aichi Medical University, Nagakute, Aichi-ken, Japan

INTRODUCTION

The ageing process leads to a deterioration of function in most body organs. Much attention has been paid to studying the effect of ageing on the kidney. These changes are both structural and functional. Thus far, the structural changes of kidney during ageing has been extensively studied (1,2), the number of glomeruli decreasing with age. The progressive thickening of the tubular and glomerular basement membrane occurs with the ageing process (1,2). Tauchi and his associates (2,3) have morphologically demonstrated that the number of tubular epithelial cells decrease with age.

Renal function in the aged has been extensively studied by Shock and his co-workers (4,5): Glomerular filtration rate and renal blood flow decline with advancing age. Transport maximum of glucose and tubular reabsorption of phosphate are reduced with age (5,6). While senescence is associated with a wide range of renal functional changes, those taking place in the renal brush borders and brush border enzymes during ageing will be presented.

AGE CHANGES IN RENAL BRUSH BORDERS

Renal brush borders play an important role in reabsorption of solutes at tubules. As shown in Fig. 1, renal tubular brush borders from 3 month-old rats showed tightly packed brush borders. On the other hand, tubular epithelial cells in the senescent rats had more loosely packed brush border projections than those in young rats (Fig. 1A). This loosely packed brush borders in senescent rats would be due to a progressive disappearance of brush borders during ageing process. It is interesting to know whether the brush border membrane components of the old are different from those of the young. Brush borders were prepared by calcium precipitation methods. Brush border membranes from senescent rat showed a change in the staining intensity of some protein bands as compared with young mature rats (7). Pratz and Corman (8) reported the similar results of SDS-polyacrylamide gel electrophoresis. Not so many proteins changed in the staining intensity (change in the contents of membrane protein components), but it is noteworthy that some of membrane proteins, even one kind of protein, change during ageing. Membrane fluidity decreases with age. Change in the membrane fluidity is due to a change in membrane lipid

711

during ageing. Thus, it is probable that change in renal brush border membrane protein components cause tubular functional changes.

AGE-CHANGES IN BRUSH BORDER ENZYMES

Leucine aminopeptidase: Activity of renal brush border enzymes such as leucine aminopeptidase and maltase was significantly decreased with age (Fig. 2). Leucine aminopeptidase (7) and maltase (9) activities were assayed as described previously. This decrease was also observed in brush border fraction expressed as specific activity (unit per mg protein). The activity showed a sharp declined from 20-24 months. Decrease in the specific activity would be due to an increase in "altered enzyme" (10,11) in the senescent animals. Thus, in order to examine biochemical properties of leucine aminopeptidase, we purified the enzyme from renal cortex of the young and senescent rats. Leucine aminopeptidase was purified as the followings: the enzyme was solubilized from the brush border membranes with 0.2% Na-deoxycholate, and the solubilized supernatant was applied on the column of Sephacryl S-300, DEAE-Sephacel, and then chromatofocusing on PBE-94. Finally, active fraction was passed through Sephacryl S-200 to remove poly-buffer. As shown in Fig. 3, maximum velocity (Vmax) and Km value for leucyl-beta-naphthylamide were declined with age and a decline in K_m and V_{max} was also observed in brush border fraction.

Renal leucine aminopeptidase from old rats was more heat labile than that from the young, and both 'old' and 'young' leucine aminopeptidase were biphasic pattern (Fig. 4) in the heat stability at 60° C (12). Molecular weight (230,000) and optimum pH (7.0-7.3) of leucine aminopeptidase were no significant difference between the senescent and young rats. Furthermore, the enzyme showed the same antigenicity between young and senescent rats.

Maltase: In the case of renal maltase, decrease in the specific activity was observed in both homogenate and brush border fractions. The decrease has been attributed to a lower Vmax of the old enzyme with no significant change in Km for maltose (9,13). Reiss and Sachtor (9) have purified renal maltase to homogeneity using Tris-Sepharose affinity chromatography from kidney cortex of Wistar-derived female rats. The decreased specific activity in the senescent rats is due to an increased inactive form of the enzyme. The old enzyme had more helical structure than did the young enzyme, suggesting a conformational alteration with age. Furthermore, maltase shows (Fig. 5) age-associated antigenic alterations (14). It has been proved by monoclonal antibody that enzymatically active and inactive

form of maltase is found mostly in enzyme preparations from aged rats. The increased prevalence of an inactive form of the enzyme in the old rat accounts for the decreased specific activity of maltase in the senescent rat.

Nutritional effects on brush border enzymes: Nutritional conditions affect the life span of animals. McCay et al. (15,16) have reported that dietary restriction increases the life span of rats. High protein diets cause severe chronic nephritis. As can be seen in Fig. 6, nutritional condition affected the decline of brush border enzymes during ageing (16). Namely, brush border leucine aminopeptidase activity in old rats fed high protein diet (51% casein) were significantly lower than that in low protein diet (8% casein). No significant difference in the homogenate, however, was observed in maltase activity between high and low protein diets (Fig. 6B).

As described above, both leucine aminopeptidase and maltase are decreased with age. The decreased maltase activity with age was not associated with an alteration in molecular weight, charge, amino acid composition or Km of

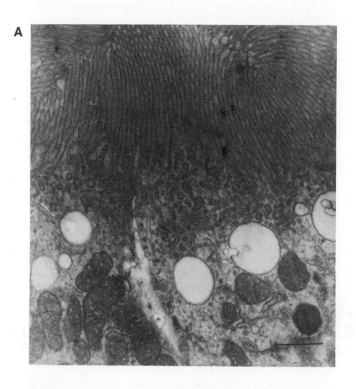

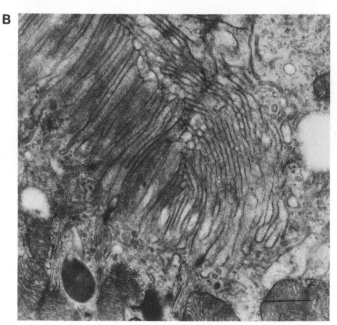

Fig. 1. Electron micrograph of brush borders of kidney cortex from young and senescent rats (Donryu strain; male). Original magnification x6000. Bar; 1.5 micrometer. A: 3-monthold rat, B: 28-month old rat.

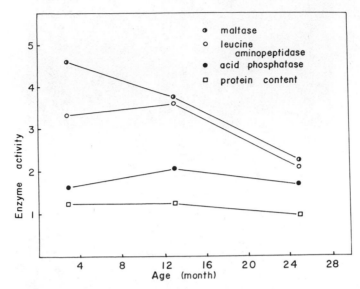

Fig. 2. Decrease in brush border enzyme activities in the homogenate of rat kidney cortex enzyme activities were expressed as ug/min/g fresh weight.

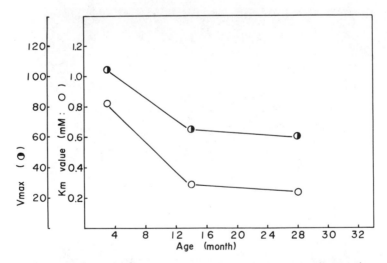

Fig. 3. Decrease in V_{max} and K_m values of purified leucine aminopeptidase.

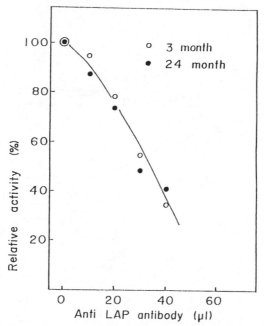

Fig. 4. Heat stability of leucine aminopeptidase from young and senescent rats.

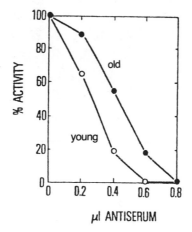

Fig. 5. Change in antigenicity of renal purified maltase.

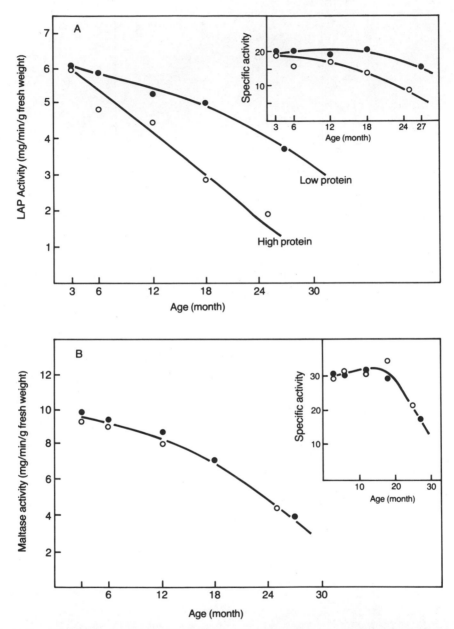

Fig. 6. Difference susceptibility of brush border enzymes to nutritional conditions. Inset shows specific activity of the enzymes. ●; low protein diet,○; high protein diet.

the enzyme. Circular dichroism (CD) spectra revealed conformational difference between renal maltase from young mature and aged animals. The configuration of the old enzyme had a higher proportion of beta-structure than did the young enzymes. Renal maltase shows age-related antigenic alterations, but not renal leucine aminopeptidase. Leucine aminopeptidase shows no difference in molecular weight, charge between young and old rats, and a decline in Km value for leucyl-beta-naphthylamide. From the data of Fig. 6, leucine aminopeptidase and maltase shows different susceptibility to nutritional conditions. From these results, it is inferred that each brush border enzyme (protein) shows a different process in age-related alterations.

In conclusion, renal brush borders progressively disappear with age, and the brush border membrane composition of senescent rats differ from the young. Brush border enzymes are significantly decreased with age. From the data of enzymatic, immunological and nutritional examination, it is inferred that each brush border enzyme shows different alterations with the ageing process.

REFERENCES

1. R. Goldman, Aging of the excretory system: kidney and bladder. In: "Handbook of the Biology of Aging", C.E. Hayflick, eds. Van Nostrand Reinhold Ltd., New York, pp 409-431 (1977).

2. H. Tauchi, "Morphology of Aging", Rikogakusha, Tokyo (1980)

3. H. Tauchi, K. Tsuboi, and J. Okutomi, Age changes in the human kidney of different races. Gerontologia, 17:87-97 (1971).

4. D.F. Davies and N.H. Shock, Age changes in glomerular filtration rate, effective renal plasma flow, and tubular excretory capacity in adult males. J. Clin. Invest. 29:496-507 (1950).

5. J.H. Miller, R.K. McDonald, and N.W. Shock, Age changes in the maximal rate of renal tubular reabsorption of glucose. J. Gerontol. 7:196-200 (1952).

6. C.M. Kiebzak and B. Sacktor, Effect of age on renal conservation of phosphate in the rat. Am. J. Physiol. 251:F399-F407 (1986)

7. M. Nakano, Y. Ito, K. Kohtani, T. Mizuno, and H. Tauchi, Age-related change in brush borders of rat kidney cortex. Mech. Aging Dev. 33:95-102 (1985).

8. J. Pratz and B. Corman, Age-related changes in enzyme activities, protein content and lipid composition of rat kidney brush border membrane. Biochim. Biophys. Acta, 814:265-273 (1985).

9. U. Reiss and B. Sacktor, Alteration of kidney brush border membrane maltase in aging rats. Biochim. Biophys. Acta, 704:422-426 (1982).

10. M. Rothstein, Age-related changes in enzyme levels and enzyme properties. In: "Review of Biological Research in Aging", M. Rothstein, ed. vol. 2, A.B. Liss, Inc., New York, pp 421-433 (1985).

11. D. Gershon, Current status of age-altered enzymes: Alternative mechanism, Mech. Ageing Dev., 9:189-196 (1979).

12. M. Nakano and H. Tauchi, Age-related alteration of renal brush border

leucine aminopeptidase in rat kidney cortex. <u>Mech. Ageing Dev.</u> , submitted for publication.

13. D. O'Bryan and L.M. Lowenstein, Effect of aging on renal membrane-bound enzyme activities. <u>Biochim. Biophys. Acta</u>, 339:1-9 (1974).

14. U. Reiss and B. Sacktor, Monoclonal antibodies to renal brush border membrane maltase: Age-associated antigenic alterations. <u>Proc. Natl. Acad. Sci., U.S</u>., 80:3255-3259 (1983).

15. C.M. McCay, L.A. Maynard, G. Sperling and L.L. Barnes, Retarded growth, life span, ultimate body size and age changes in the albino rat after feeding diets restricted in calories. <u>J. Nutr</u>., 18:1-18 (1939)

16.   M. Nakano, H. Taauchi, K. Kohtani, T. Mizuno, Y. Ito, and H. Tauchi, Age-related change of renal tubular brush border enzymes in different nutritional conditions. <u>Biomed. Gerontol</u>. 11:131-132 (1987).

CHARACTERIZATION OF ISOLATED RENAL PROXIMAL TUBULES FOR NEPHROTOXICITY STUDIES

Carol E. Green (1), Jack E. Dabbs (1), Katherine L. Allen (1), Charles A. Tyson (1), and Elmer J. Rauckman (2)

Target Organ Toxicity Department (1), SRI International, Menlo Park, CA, USA and National Institute of Environmental Health Sciences (2), Research Triangle Park, NC, USA.

INTRODUCTION

Isolated tubule or cell suspensions offer an important way of studying the mechanisms of nephrotoxicity in vitro, and screening novel compounds for their potential adverse affects on the kidney. The major drawback, however, appeared to be the short in vitro lifespan of isolated tubules prepared by any technique. In general, most investigators limit incubations to no more than 1 or 2 hr because of loss of viability and functional capabilities. Ormstad (1984) reported rapid loss of viability of isolated renal tubules and cells, where greater than 25% of the cellular lactate dehydrogenase (LDH) leaked to the medium in 1.5 to 2 hr of incubation. Obatomi and Plummer (1986) observed a 40% loss in tubule cell viability during 3-hr incubations of rat proximal tubules. Loss of renal functional capabilities, such as O_2 consumption, has also been reported for isolated tubules (Harris et al., 1981).

A number of fresh tubular systems have been prepared from collagenase digests of rat cortical tissue (Cunarro and Weiner, 1978; Jones et al., 1979; Bellemann et al., 1980; Vinay et al., 1981; Cojocel et al., 1983; Gstraunthaler et al., 1985; Obatomi and Plummer, 1986). These preparations exhibit high initial viability (>90% by trypan blue exclusion) and enrichment of 2-fold or greater in proximal tubule cells relative to cells from other areas of the nephron as indicated by the distribution of alkaline phosphatase (ALP) and hexokinase (HK) (Vinay et al., 1981).

We have approached the need to extend the lifespan of tubules using collagenase perfusion because it :-

a) produces high yields of viable tubule fragments, an absolute requirement for large scale cytotoxicity experiments;
b) has been successfully applied to the rat, the most commonly used laboratory species in nephrotoxicity research; and
c) is adaptable for use with kidney tissue from large species including humans for comparative studies.

MATERIALS AND METHODS

Young adult male F-344 rats (300-350g) were anaesthetized with sodium pentobarbital (65 mg/kg) and the kidneys were perfused in situ via a cannula inserted in the aorta below the renal arteries. Optimal yield and tubule quality were obtained when the kidneys were first flushed of blood with modified Hank's BSS containing 50 mM HEPES and 5 mM $CaCl_2$ for 5 min at a flow rate of 35 ml/min. The kidneys were excised and then perfused with the same buffer containing 180 U/ml collagenase (Type I, Sigma Chemical Co.) for approximately 15 min. After the tissue was soft to pressure, it was minced and disrupted by repeated pipetting. The tubule suspension was filtered through a sieve mesh of approximately 75 um. Tubules were purified by gravity sedimentation in buffer or culture medium containing 2% fatty acid poor BSA. Tubule viability was determined by measuring NADH penetration and LDH release (Moldeus et al., 1978; Tyson and Green, 1987) and yield was determined by measuring protein (Bradford, 1976).

Isolated tubules were incubated in Waymouth's 752/1 + 2% fatty acid poor BSA, 2 mg tubule protein/ml, at $37^{\circ}C$ with gentle shaking. Tubules were gassed with 95% air:5% CO_2 and incubated in gas-tight flasks with a side-arm for repeat sampling. LDH release and ALP stability were determined using semi-automated techniques (Tyson and Green, 1987). The method for total ALP was modified by extending the incubation time with Triton X100 to 60 min to ensure total release from the membrane. HK was determined by the method of Walker and Parry (1966). ATP and ADP were determined using a bioluminescence assay (Tyson and Green, 1987). Oxygen consumption was measured by direct transfer of the kidney tubules to an oxygen monitor chamber (YSI Model 53 Oxygen Monitor, Yellow Springs, OH).

RESULTS AND DISCUSSION

Initially, tubules were prepared by a modification of the two-step collagenase perfusion method developed by Jones et al. (1979) using the hepatocyte isolation perfusates (Green et al., 1983). Although tubule viability was high immediately after isolation, it decreased 30% or more during a 4-hr incubation, similar to the observations of others (Obatomi and Plummer, 1986). The procedure described above evolved through a series of experiments designed to optimize the isolation conditions. The omission of an initial perfusion step with an EGTA-containing buffer and the increase in the collagenase content of the perfusate from 90 U/ml to 180 U/ml resulted in shorter tubule preparation times and higher tubule yields (80.2 $\pm$ 23 mg protein vs 155 $\pm$ 46 mg protein per 2 kidneys). Although lower collagenase concentrations could be used, with the amount required dependent on the weight of the animal (as low as 45 U/ml with a 200 g rat), longer perfusion times and lower tubule yields resulted and no change in tubule quality was observed. These modifications combined with the use of a tubule wash medium supplemented with 2% BSA resulted in improved maintenance of tubule viability (Table 1).

Tubules isolated by the collagenase method exhibited greater than 95% viability based on qualitative observation of trypan blue stained cells and on quantitative measurement of released LDH. NADH penetration of tubules was found to be 2 to 3 times higher than initial LDH release, presumably because plasma membranes of some freshly isolated tubules are leaky to NADH, allowing retained LDH to be measured.

The ratios of ALP/HK, marker enzymes for proximal tubules and distal tubules, respectively, were uniformly high, averaging 75 $\pm$ 20 (n = 6). Light microscopic observation of periodic acid Schiff-stained preparations found that about 85% of the fragments were from proximal tubules. Immediately after isolation, the tubules have prominent brush borders, intact basement membranes and open lumens (Figure 1). In early studies, essentially all the lumens closed within 1 hr and the tubule brush borders

Table 1. Biochemical Characteristics of Isolated Renal Tubules [a]

Assay	Incubation Time (hr)		% Change during Incubation
	0	4	
Released LDH (% of total)	4.1 ± 1.9	25.0 ± 4.1	+21 ± 3.8
O_2 Consumption (nmol O_2/min mg protein)	32 ± 6.1	25 ± 4.2	-23 ± 4.6
Released ALP (% of total)	1.6 ± 0.5	6.7 ± 1.2	+5.1 ± 1.0
Total ALP (U/L)	412 ± 61	369 ± 62	-11 ± 5.3
ATP + ADP (nmol/mg protein)	8.3 ± 3.0	10.6 ± 4.0	+28 ± 13
ATP/ADP	2.8 ± 0.9	5.2 ± 1.6	+86 ± 13

[a] Values represent x ± SD of N = 3 to 6 experiments.

became less distinct with increasing incubation times. However, the modifications of the isolation procedure (inclusion of Ca^{2+} in all perfusion buffers and use of higher collagenase concentrations) have resulted in improved maintenance of lumen patency during incubation.

The biochemical characteristics of the tubules immediately after isolation and after a 4-hr incubation are listed in Table 1. The percentage LDH released to the medium increased and the rate of O_2 consumption decreased about 20% during a 4-hr incubation, suggesting a probable association between the loss in mitochondrial integrity and cell viability as noted previously by Obatomi and Plummer (1986). ALP release from isolated tubules was low (5% in 4 hr), but total ALP content decreased approximately 10%, confirming the microscopic observation of alterations in the brush border integrity during incubation of the tubules.

In contrast, adenine nucleotide levels and ATP/ADP ratios were somewhat depressed immediately after tubule isolation. Values for these parameters increased during a 4-hr incubation and in fact, recovered rapidly within 1 hr of incubation to 4.3 ± 0.7 for ATP/ADP and 10.6 ± 2.3 nmole ATP+ADP/mg protein, respectively. Another rapid change in the isolated tubules occurred in their ability to respond to nystatin, a polyene antibiotic that increases membrane permeability to Na^+, stimulating O_2 consumption to reveal maximum respiratory capacity. Figure 2 shows that initially nystatin addition caused only a slight change in the basal rate of O_2 consumption of the tubules (about 10%) but within 30 min it resulted in a peak value of greater than 50%. An incubation period as short as 10-15 min allowed the emergence of nystatin-stimulated O_2 consumption (data not shown). These data suggest that prior to beginning experiments, a short equilibration period at $37^{O}C$ in the incubation medium would be beneficial.

In conclusion, renal proximal tubules isolated by a single-step collagenase perfusion technique and incubated in a complex culture medium have been shown to exhibit more stable viability and functional properties

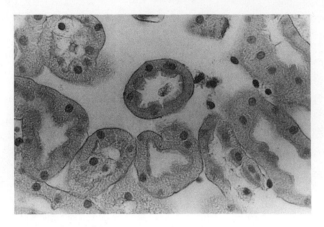

Fig. 1. Photomicrograph of freshly isolated rat renal tubule fragments. Tubules were stained with PAS and counterstained with haematoxylin.

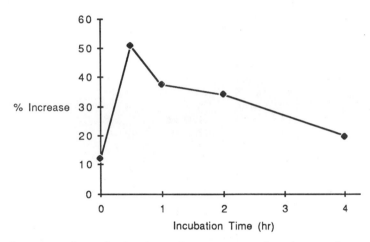

Fig. 2. Nystatin stimulation of O_2 consumption in renal proximal tubules. The basal rate was determined and nystatin (842 U/20 ul DMSO) was added to the tubule suspensions to stimulate O_2 consumption. Values represent the mean of 3 experiments.

than previous reports with these preparations. Tubules isolated by this method have open lumens initially and retain basement and brush border membranes. The isolation procedure requires technical mastery but are basically simple and expeditious, providing high yields of viable tubules suitable for large scale cytotoxicity experiments (40 or more flasks).

ACKNOWLEDGEMENTS

This research is supported by NIEHS contract ES-65145.

REFERENCES

Bradford, M.M., 1976, A rapid and sensitive method for quantitation of microgram quantities of protein utilizing the principle of protein dye binding, Anal. Biochem., 72:248.

Bellemann, P., 1980, Primary monolayer culture of liver parenchymal cells and kidney cortical tubules as a useful new model for biochemical pharmacology and experimental toxicology, Arch. Toxicol., 44:63.

Cojocel, C., Maita, K., Pasino, D.A., Kuo, C., and Hook, J.B., 1983, Metabolic heterogeneity of the proximal and distal kidney tubules, Life Sciences, 33:855.

Cunarro, J.A., and Weiner, M.W., 1978, Effects of ethacrynic acid and furosemide on respiration of isolated kidney tubules: the role of ion transport and the source of metabolic energy, J. Pharmacol. Exper. Therap., 206:198.

Green, C.E., Dabbs, J.E., and Tyson, C.A., 1983, Functional integrity of isolated rat hepatocytes prepared by whole liver vs biopsy perfusion, Anal. Biochem., 129:269.

Gstraunthaler, G., Pfaller, W., and Kotanko, P., 1985, Interrelation between oxygen consumption and Na-K-ATPase activity in rat renal proximal tubule suspension, Renal Physiol., 8:38.

Harris, S.I., Balaban, R.S., Barrett, L., and Mandel, L.J., 1981, Mitochondrial respiratory capacity and Na^+- and K^+-dependent adenosine triphosphatase-mediated ion transport in the intact renal cell, J. Biol. Chem., 256:10319.

Jones, D.P., Sundby, G., Ormstad, K., and Orrenius, S., 1979, Use of isolated kidney cells for study of drug metabolism, Biochem. Pharmacol., 28:929.

Moldeus, P., Hogberg, J., and Orrenius, S., 1978, Isolation and use of liver cells, In: "Methods in Enzymology, Vol. 52, Biomembranes", S. Fleisher and L. Packer, eds., Academic Press, New York.

Obatomi, D.K., and Plummer, D.T., 1986, Oxygen uptake and glutamate dehydrogenase release in isolated renal tubules from rat kidney, Biochem. Soc. Trans., 14:1281.

Ormstad, K., 1984, Preparation of isolated renal cells, Workshop presentation at Second International Symposium on Nephrotoxicity.

Tyson, C.A., and Green, C.E., 1987, Cytotoxicity measures: choices and methods, In: "The Isolated Hepatocyte: Use in Toxicology and Xenobiotic Biotransformations", E. J. Rauckman and G. Padilla, eds., Academic Press, New York.

Vinay, P., Gougoux, A., and Lemieux, G., 1981, Isolation of a pure suspension of rat proximal tubules. Amer. J. Physiol., 241:F403.

Walker, D.G., and Parry, M.J., 1966, Glucokinase, In: "Methods in Enzymology, Vol. 9, Carbohydrate Metabolism", W. A. Wood, ed., Academic Press, New York.

ISOLATED RAT RENAL PROXIMAL TUBULAR CELLS: A MODEL TO INVESTIGATE DRUG INDUCED NEPHROTOXICITY

E.M. Gordon [1,2,3], P.H. Whiting [2], J.G. Simpson [4] and G.M. Hawksworth [2,3]

Clinical Pharmacology Unit [1] and Departments of Chemical Pathology [2], Pharmacology [3] and Pathology [4], University of Aberdeen, Foresterhill, Aberdeen, U.K.

INTRODUCTION

The kidney shows marked functional, morphological and biochemical heterogeneity which may account for the site-specific toxicity of several drugs and xenobiotics. For example, the toxicity associated with cephaloridine and some aminoglycosides is confined to the proximal tubular cells (Kuo and Hook, 1982; Kaloyanides and Pastoriza-Munoz, 1980), whereas prolonged intake of paracetamol results in renal papillary necrosis (Mohandas et al., 1984). To investigate the mechanisms of toxicity using cell suspensions or primary cultures, it is therefore necessary to isolate the different cell types. Several approaches have been used to obtain preparations of proximal tubular cells or fragments. One approach uses existing cell lines of kidney origin (LLC-PK$_1$ or MDCK), the disadvantage being that the exact site of origin within the nephron is not known and, being a cell line, it may not be totally representative of the normal physiological state. A second approach is the digestion or explantation of kidney tissue in the presence of serum-free, hormonally defined culture media such that fibroblast proliferation is minimal and epithelial cell growth is encouraged (Chuman et al., 1982). Unfortunately both these cell preparations lack a brush border, which may be critical for the active uptake of drugs and chemicals.

The alternative approaches to obtain a preparation with an intact brush border include the use of different sized sieves to separate glomeruli and tubules (Bach et al., 1986), which may not result in a pure preparation of proximal tubular cells, or density gradient techniques to separate the different cell types. We have modified the technique of Vinay et al, (1981) using Percoll density gradient centrifugation to obtain a > 90% pure preparation of proximal tubular cells. In this paper we describe the characterization of these cells in terms of drug metabolizing enzymes, which may be responsible for the activation of drugs to reactive metabolites (mixed function oxidases) or the subsequent detoxification of chemicals in the kidney by conjugation reactions.

MATERIALS AND METHODS

Proximal tubular (PT) cell suspensions were prepared as previously described (Gordon et al., 1987). Kidney cortices were removed from Sprague

Dawley rats (250-300g) and chopped into 2-3mm fragments, washed in Hanks solution containing EGTA and then incubated for 20-30 min at 37°C in Hanks solution containing calcium (2.4mM) and collagenase (0.1% (w/v), Boehringer Mannheim). After filtering through 75u mesh and washing, the suspension was added to a Percoll solution (starting density 1.044g/ml, 300 mOsm/kg) and centrifuged at 20,000g for 30 min at 4°C. Three main bands were identified at densities of 1.040g/ml (A), 1.058g/ml (B) and 1.060g/ml (C), which were then characterised morphologically using light and electron microscopy. A and B bands contained single cells and a mixture of glomeruli, tubules and cells respectively. C, however, was found to contain mainly PT cells and fragments, with maintained intact brush border and tubular integrity. Hexokinase (HK; Schmidt et al., 1975) and fructose-1,6-bisphosphatase (FBP; Allen and Blair, 1972) were used as markers for distal and proximal tubules respectively (Guder and Ross, 1984). HK was found to have a higher specific activity in the medulla, while FBP was higher in the cortex. Band C showed a 6-fold enrichment in FBP activity when compared with cortical levels, confirming the histological data that this band contained mostly PT cells.

Further characterization included viability (as assessed by Trypan blue exclusion), cytochrome P450 content (Orrenius et al., 1973), reduced glutathione (GSH; Hissin and Hilf, 1976) and GSH conjugation with 1-chloro-2,4-dinitrobenzene (CDNB; Habig and Jakoby, 1981). GSH was measured during a 3 hr incubation period with or without the addition of amino acid precursors for GSH synthesis and also with serine borate (20 mM), an inhibitor of GGT activity. Cytochrome P450 mono-oxygenase activity (Burke and Mayer, 1974) was measured in cells obtained from rats pretreated with phenobarbitone (PB; 80mg/kg i.p. for 3 days) or with 3-methylcholanthrene (3MC; 80mg/kg i.p.) using a series of resorufin ethers. Ethoxyresorufin O-deethylase (EROD) activity was also measured in the presence and absence of alpha-naphthoflavone (ANF; Goujon et al., 1972).

RESULTS AND DISCUSSION

We have previously demonstrated that Percoll density centrifugation yields PT cells and fragments of > 90% viability (Table 1). Enzymatic markers have also been employed to further characterised the cell type present after centrifugation. FBP was found to be enriched in the cells in band C when compared to cortical values, which confirms the morphological data. In suspension, these cells maintained their tubular characteristics including intact luminal and basolateral membranes, as indicated by both the uptake into the cell of PAH (Gordon et al., this volume) and by light and electron microscopy. The maintenance of intact membranes is an essential prerequisite for transport and toxicity studies in these cells. This is an important observation as both size and number of microvilli have been shown to decline rapidly within 5 days in primary culture (Rosenberg and Michalopolous, 1987) so limiting the use of the primary culture method for this type of study.

The cells in suspension maintained their total P450 content (Table 1) when compared to a heterogeneous population (Jones et al., 1979) whereas GSH content and GSH-CDNB conjugation declined during the preparation. This may be due to the longer preparation time involved and to the high PT concentration of GGT. GSH is important in the detoxification of activated compounds (Kuo et al., 1983) and concentrations must be maintained at normal levels in untreated control cells in order to study the effect of toxins on intracellular GSH. In primary culture, GSH content in the cells decreases to 50% of their initial values by day 3, after an initial increase (Smith et al., 1986 and 1987), and therefore high initial levels are essential before the cells are cultured. The intracellular GSH in PT suspension

Table 1. Viability, cell number and drug metabolising activities in rat kidney cells

	Viability %	PT cell no x10^6	Cyt. P450 nmol	GSH nmol	CDNB-GSH nmol/min
Total kidney	88±5 (4)	23±1.2 (7)	N.P.	25.5±8.87 (6)	0.76
Cortex	83±14 (5)	19±8 (5)	0.04	9.3±5.0 (5)	0.64±0.07 (3)
A	91±3 (11)	4±2 (20)	0.03±0.02 (5)	11.2±6.9 (10)	0.34±0.15 (4)
C	93±5 (11)	8±2 (20)	0.06±0.04 (5)	11.9±8.1 (10)	0.44

Cell number is given per kidney.   Cytochrome P450 content, GSH and CDNB-GSH conjugation are expressed/10^6 cells. Results are expressed as mean±SD. N.p. = not performed

Preparations was found to decrease markedly at 37°C (Fig 1) in Hanks buffer containing calcium and this fall was not significantly improved by the addition of cysteine or methionine (0.2mM), which have previously been shown to maintain hepatocyte GSH levels. The addition of glycine (1 mM), glutamate (1 mM) and cystine (0.2mM) throughout the isolation and incubation period did however produce an intracellular GSH level which remained above 50% for 2 hr at 37° (Fig 1). The addition of serine borate, which resulted in a 70% reduction in GGT activity, did not significantly improve intracellular GSH concentrations. One explanation may be that the addition of the inhibitor was interfering with the uptake of amino acid precursors of GSH into the cells.

Cytochrome P450-dependent mono-oxygenase activity was observed with a series of resorufin ethers which had previously been studied in liver preparations (Burke et al., 1985). After pretreatment with PB (Table 2) no induction of activity was observed with any of the resorufin homologues. This confirmed the results of Endou et al. (1982) that no PB inducible activity is present in the kidney. The liver, however, does show induction following PB pretreatment, especially with pentoxyresorufin, indicating that different patterns of induction are produced in the liver and kidney. In contrast 3MC pretreatment (Tables 2 and 3) produced marked induction of O-dealkylation activity in PT cells, especially with EROD (150-fold). Similar results were also observed in renal cortical microsomes in this laboratory (results not shown). The magnitude of induction was greater than that found in the liver even thought the actual level of activity was lower in the kidney. That the induced activity with EROD was inhibited by 93% with ANF, a selective inhibitor of 3MC-induced enzyme activity, indicates the presence of P450c in the PT cells. Consequently it is this activity that may be important in the production of site specific nephro-toxicity in these cells. This also suggests that the 3MC induction can be used as a probe to investigate the maintenance of P450 activities in primary cultures of PT fragments.

The induction of mono-oxygenase activity by P450 inducers (Endou et al., 1982) and the effect of toxins on the kidney (Kuo and Hook, 1982) have been found to show interspecies variability. The rabbit, for example, demonstrates both PB and 3MC inducible activities (Endou et al., 1982) while, as shown here, rat kidney shows only the latter. We also hope to examine these induction profiles in human kidney in the near future.

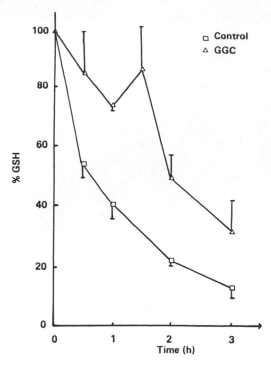

Fig. 1. GSH concentrations in PT cells isolated in the presence or absence of amino acid precursors. PT cells incubated for 3 hr at 37°C in Hanks solution containing 2.4mM calcium, with or without glycine (1 mM), glutamate (1 mM) and cystine (0.2mM). Results are shown as mean±SD (n = 4)

Table 2. Cytochrome P450-dependent mono-oxygenase activity in cells from band C after pretreatment of rats with 3MC, PB and appropriate controls.

	EROD	BROD	PROD
	pmol/ml/mg homogenate protein		
PB treatment	6.7±4.6	1.3±0.5	2.4±1.5
	(5)	(5)	(4)
PB control (Saline)	7.1±5.6	1.7±0.8	2.7±1.7
	(5)	(6)	(4)
3MC treatment	788.8±207.6	63.1±19.0	12.9±4.9
	(6)	(6)	(6)
3MC control (Olive oil)	5.7±2.8	0.7±0.4	2.2±2.0
	(3)	(3)	(3)
Control (No treatment)	6.8±4.8	2.3±1.0	1.9±1.1
	(8)	(6)	(6)

Results are expressed as the mean±S.D. Number of experiments are shown in parentheses. EROD, ethoxyresorufin O-deethylase; BROD, benzyloxyresorufin O-dealkylase; PROD, pentoxyresorufin O-dealkylase.

Table 3. Induction of monooxygenase activity with 3-methylcholanthrene

Carbon chain length	Control	3MC treated	Fold Induction
1	8.1±2.1	39.6±13.1	5
2	5.8±2.5	603.0±261.2	105
3	5.7±2.8	447.0±172.0	80
4	2.6±1.6	175.9±77.7	70
5	1.9±1.1	9.8±5.2	5
Benzyl	2.3±1.0	47.9±24.2	20

Induction of mono-oxygenase activity measured with a series of resorufin ethers of increasing chain length in PT cells obtained from 3MC pretreated rats and compared with that of control animals. Results are shown as mean±SD, n = 6 to 15.

The results presented here demonstrate that suspensions of PT fragments, prepared following Percoll density gradient centrifugation, retain their viability and maintain their GSH levels at > 50% for 2 hr at 37°C. Moreover they demonstrate cytochrome P450-dependent mono-oxygenase activity profiles which are inducible only by 3MC. Consequently this is an appropriate preparation to study the effects of various drugs and chemicals, in both rats and man, which following administration demonstrate nephrotoxicity to either the S1, S2 or S3 regions of the PT.

REFERENCES

Allen, M.B., Blair, J.McD., 1972, The regulation of rabbit liver fructose-1,6-diphosphatase activity by phospholipids in vivo, Biochem. J., 130:1167

Bach, P.H., Ketley, C.P., Ahmed, I., Dixit, M., 1986, The mechanisms of target cell injury by nephrotoxins, Fd. Chem. Toxic., 24:775

Burke, M.D., Mayer, R.T., 1974, Ethoxyresorufin: direct fluorimetric assay of a microsomal O-dealkylation which is preferentially inducible by 3-methylcholanthrene, Drug Metab. Dispos., 2:583

Burke, M.D., Thompson, S., Elcombe, C.R., Halpert, J., Haaparanta, T., Mayer, R.T., 1985, Ethoxy-, pentoxy- and benzyloxy-phenoxazones and 6 homologues. A series of substrates to distinguish between different induced cytochromes P450, Biochem. Pharm., 34:3337

Chuman, L., Fine, L.G., Cohen, A.H., Saier, M.H.Jr., 1982, Continuous growth of proximal tubular kidney epithelial cells in hormone-supplemented serum-free medium, J. Cell Biol., 94:506

Endou, H.,, Koseki, C., Haumara, S., Kakuno, K., Hojo, K., Sakai, F., 1982, Renal cytochrome P450; its localisation along a nephron and its induction, In: "Biochemistry of Kidney Functions", F. Morel, ed., Elsevier Biomedical Press

Gordon, E.M., McDougall, S.M., Whiting, P.H., Hawksworth, G.M., 1987, Gentamicin-stimulated increase in PAH uptake in renal slices and isolated proximal tubular cells, this volume.

Gordon, E.M., Whiting, P.H., Simpson, J.G., Hawksworth, G.M., 1987, Isolation and characterisation of rat renal proximal tubular cells, Biochem. Soc. Trans., 15:457

Goujon, F.M., Nebert, D.W., Gielen, J.E., 1972, Genetic expression of aryl hydrocarbon hydroxylase induction, Mol. Pharm., 8:667

Guder, W.G., Ross, B.D., 1984, Enzyme distribution along the nephron, Kid. Int., 26:101

Habig, W.H., Jakoby, W.B., 1981, Assays for determination of glutathione S-transferases, Meth. Enzymol., 77:398

Hissin, P.J., Hilf, R., 1976, A fluorimetric method for determination of oxidised and reduced glutathione in tissues, Analyt. Biochem., 74:214

Jones, D.P., Sundby, G., Ormstad, K., Orrenius, S., 1979, Use of isolated kidney cells for study of drug metabolism, Biochem. Pharm., 28:929

Kaloyanides, G.J. and Pastoriza-Munoz, E., 1980, Aminoglycoside nephrotoxicity, Kid. Int., 18:571

Kuo, C., Hook, J.B., 1982, Depletion of renal glutathione content and nephrotoxicity of cephaloridine in rabbits, rats and mice, Toxic Appl. Pharm., 63:292

Kuo, C., Maita, K., Sleight, S.D., Hook, J.B., 1983, Lipid peroxidation: A possible mechanism of cephaloridine-induced nephrotoxicity, Toxic. Appl. Pharm., 67:78

Mohandas, J., Marshall, J.J., Duggin, G.G., Horvarth, J.S., Tiller,. D.J., 1984, Differential distribution of glutathione and glutathione related enzymes in rabbit kidney: Possible implications in analgesic nephropathy, Biochem. Pharm., 33:1801

Orrenius, S., Ellin, A., Jakobson, S.V., Thor, H., Cinti, D.L., Schenkman, J.B., Estabrook, R.W., 1973, The cytochrome P450-containing mono-oxygenase system of rat kidney cortex microsomes, Drug Metab. Dispos., 1:350

Rosenberg, M.R., Michalopoulos, G., 1987, Kidney proximal tubular cells isolated by collagenase perfusion grow in defined media in the absence of growth factors, J. Cell Physiol., 131:107

Schmidt, U., Marosvari, I., Dubach, U.C., 1975, Renal metabolism of glucose: Anatomical sites of hexokinase activity in the rat nephron, FEBS Letts., 53:26

Smith, M.A., Acosta, D., Bruckner, J.V., 1986, Development of a primary culture system of rat kidney cortical cells to evaluate the nephrotoxicity of xenobiotics, Fd. Chem. Toxic., 24:551

Smith, M.A., Acosta, D., Bruckner, J.V., 1987, Cephaloridine toxicity in primary cultures of rat renal cortical epithelial cells, Toxicol. In Vitro, 1:23

Vinay, P., Gougoux, A., Lemieux, G., 1981, Isolation of a pure suspension of rat proximal tubules, Am. J. Physiol., 241:403

ION DEREGULATION IN INJURED PROXIMAL TUBULE EPITHELIAL CELLS

Benjamin F. Trump and Irene K. Berezesky

Department of Pathology, University of Maryland School of Medicine and the
Maryland Institute for Emergency Medical Services Systems, Baltimore,
Maryland 21201 USA

INTRODUCTION

The purpose of this paper is to reveal the importance of calcium in the
initiation and continuation of cell injury in kidney proximal tubule
epithelium (PTE). We have known, for some time, the association between
calcium and cell injury and, in fact, at this meeting, there have been
several papers involving chloroform, gasoline, and cisplatinum, that
relate cell calcium concentration to cell injury. However, this has long
been known by pathologists and other investigators who have related the
presence of calcium precipitates in tissues to the presence of necrosis.
At the same time, calcium has a beneficial effect in the extracellular
environment at all levels of organization, from the organism to the cell;
consider, for example, in the Chalk streams of England and, indeed, in the
streams of any country where calcium in the water is extremely beneficial
and leads to a much more rapid growth of both plants and animals,
vertebrates and invertebrates.

The role of cell injury and calcium in signal transduction (Berridge and
Irvine, 1984) is becoming increasingly important as the effects of
carcinogens on organs such as the kidney, liver, and lung lead to a
variety of preneoplastic and neoplastic changes. It has been shown, for
example, that A23187, a calcium ionophore, is a potent second stage
promoter (Slaga et al., 1983); however, at the same time, it is also known
that cell-cell communication and calcium movement between cells is
decreased in the case of tumour promoters (Wade et al., 1986). Most
complete carcinogens lead to acute and chronic cell injury as they produce
acute, sub-acute, and chronic cell injury accompanied by injury, repair,
and inflammation.

Until recently, it was impossible to examine the role of intracellular
ionized calcium ($[Ca^{2}+]_i$) in the cytosol except in certain cells, for
example, giant squid axons, using calcium-sensitive proteins such as
aequorin. However, with the development of the organic compounds, Quin 2
and Fura 2 (Grynkiewicz et al., 1985), coupled with the technology of
digital imaging fluorescence microscopy (DiGuiseppi et al., 1983) and
video microscopy (Inoue, 1986), we now have the necessary tools to
investigate the relationships of $[Ca^{2}+]_i$ in the processes of normal or
abnormal cell stimulation.

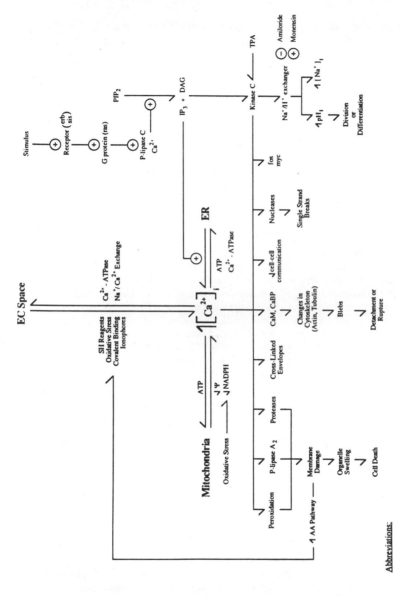

Figure 1. Flowchart illustrating the relationships between ion deregulation, cell injury, and carcinogensis (see text for discussion). Reprinted with permission from Trump and Berezesky, 1987.

Abbreviations:

PIP₂ = Phosphatidylinositol 4,5 - diphosphate
Ψ = Mitochondrial membrane potential
CaM = Calmodulin
CaBP = Other calcium-binding proteins.
TPA = 12 - O - Tetradecanoylphorbol - 13 - acetate

CALCIUM REGULATION IN THE NORMAL ANIMAL CELL

As shown in Fig. 1, $[Ca^{2}+]_i$ is regulated (at approximately 100 nM in the case of kidney epithelium) by three principal transport systems: the cell membrane, the mitochondria, and the endoplasmic reticulum (ER). Each of these membrane systems has high affinity sites for calcium and, therefore, can regulate $[Ca^{2}+]_i$ to very low concentrations, is ATP-dependent and quickly modified with ATP deficiency and, in addition, has particular agents that target at least initially on it. For example, inhibitors or uncouplers of respiration and phosphorylation, as well as depletion of NADPH, are associated with a rapid release of $Ca^{2}+$ from mitochondria; ouabain and other inhibitors of Na-K ATPase, direct mechanical damage, SH reagents, e.g., $HgCl_2$ and complement, oxidative stress and calcium ionophores are associated with deregulation at the cell membrane; and release of IP-3 from membrane inositol phospholipids and depletion of cell SH groups are among the classes of agents associated with release of $Ca^{2}+$ from the ER. There are thus many ways through which a variety of types of cell injury could potentially affect cellular calcium regulation. Some of these will be explored here as they apply to the kidney.

Cellular Changes Following Injury

The events or "stages" that occur following cell injury and lead to cell death (Ginn et al., 1968; Trump and Ginn, 1969; Trump and Arstila, 1975; Trump and Mergner, 1974; Trump et al., 1971; Trump and Berezesky, 1985b) are illustrated diagrammatically in Figs. 2 to 6, which are a series of diagrams illustrating the stages of cell injury (from Ginn et al., 1968). Briefly, early ultrastructural changes include dilatation of the ER, loss of mitochondrial granules, condensation of mitochondria, and blebs at the cell surface. At this time point, elevation of $[Ca^{2}+]_i$ has already occurred. All of these changes are clearly reversible but, later, mitochondrial condensation (possibly associated with loss of K^+ and $Ca^{2}+$) (Trump and Mergner, 1974) and then swelling of some mitochondria occurs, paralleled by changes in mitochondrial phospholipids, again reversible. Finally, as the cell injury passes from reversibility to irreversibility or the "point-of-no-return," the mitochondria become quite swollen and accumulate flocculent densities and/or calcium phosphate precipitates (Fig. 7). The latter, however, only occurs with certain types of injury: namely, those that follow primary injury in the cell membrane and which do not interfere with mitochondrial accumulation.

We have been investigating the possible relationships between ionized sodium, hydrogen, chloride, calcium, magnesium, and potassium in relation to the progress of cell injury and cell death. Our earlier studies, which clearly stated that accumulation of calcium correlated with cell death, has led us to formulate a hypothesis and to further investigate the role of calcium in this process (Trump and Berezesky, 1983,1985a,b,1987, 1988; Trump et al., 1988).

We had previously noted that during the process of cell injury and cell death, there was a modification of membrane lipids, i.e., the loss of cardiolipin and a modification of phosphatidyl-ethanolamine (Smith et al., 1980). We also noted that reducing the medium extracellular pH could inhibit the progress of cell injury and that, in the case of hypoxia in Ehrlich ascites tumour cells, kidney slices, and hepatocytes, this reduction in pH almost doubled the duration of cell life. Furthermore, the same effect occurred with other types of cell injury, e.g., the mercurials and thermal injury (Pentilla and Trump, 1974,1975; Pentilla et al., 1976). Although these studies were not understood at that time, we can now interpret them in the light of our recent data which suggests that pH and calcium are interdependent and, that as pH is raised, the $[Ca^{2}+]_i$

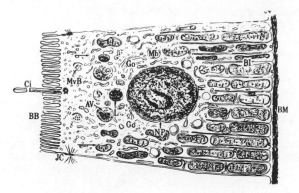

Fig. 2. Stage I represents the appearance of a normal kidney tubule cell.
Ci, cilium; BB, brush border; JC, junctional complex; MvB, multivesicular
bodies; L, secondary lysosomes; AV, autophagic vacuoles; Go, Golgi
apparatus; N, nucleus; Nc, nucleolus; NP, nuclear pore; Mb, microbodies;
free arrows, polysomes; BI, basilar invaginations of the plasma membrane;
BM, basement membrane.

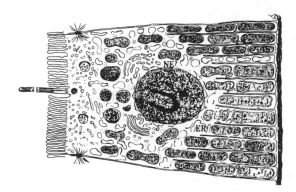

Fig. 3. Stage II illustrating changes consisting only of dilatation of the
endoplasmic reticulum (ER) and the nuclear envelope (NE).

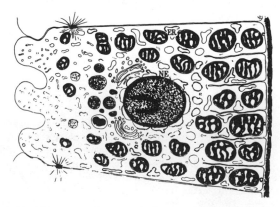

Fig. 4. Stage III illustrating additional changes including condensation
of mitochondrial inner compartments, enlargement of cell gap and
distortion of the brush border.

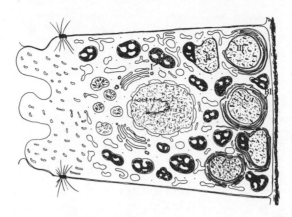

Fig. 5. Stage IV in which some mitochondria (I) are condensed, others are both condensed and swollen (II) and still others are swollen (III). Basilar infoldings (BI) often form circumferential wrappings around mitochondria and polysomes detach from the ER.

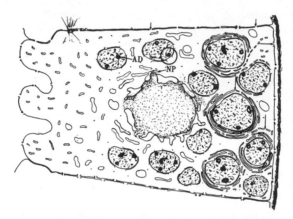

Fig. 6. In Stage V, all mitochondria exhibit marked swelling with most containing occasional calcifications (circled areas). The latter occurs only if mitochondrial function has not been inhibited. Karyolysis of the nucleus occurs with extrusion of nuclear contents through the nuclear pores (NP). Interruptions occur in the continuity of the plasma membrane and basilar infoldings (arrows).

concentration necessary to cause a given effect is reduced (Trump et al., 1988). As noted in Fig. 1, elevation of $[H^+]_i$ is at least one stimulus that can be associated with the initiation of cell division.

In rat PTE in vivo, one of the earliest changes following injury is the formation of blebs at the cell surface, separating the microvilli of the brush border and pushing out towards the tubular lumens (Glaumann and Trump, 1975) (Fig 8). Such blebs commonly detach without cell killing and result in tubular obstruction in the distal nephron. Recently, we have shown that we could reproduce the same effects using cultured rat or rabbit PTE in vitro (Trump et al., 1986; Phelps et al., 1988). The blebs are relatively organelle-free, perhaps due to a network of actin at the bleb base. With time, as the blebs form and pinch off, the actin pattern in the entire cell as seen by immunocytochemistry is greatly modified. Prior to and accompanying these continuing events, $[Ca^{2+}]_i$ increases. It

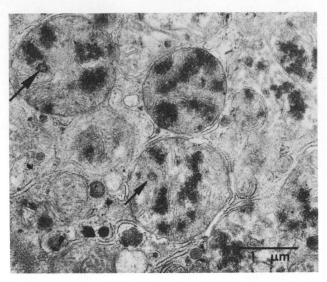

Fig. 7. TEM of a portion of a rat proximal tubule cell after 120 min of in vivo ischaemia followed by 24 hr of reflow. Mitochondria are swollen and certain large flocculent densities and occasional calcifications (arrows) indicative of Stage V. (From Trump et al., 1980.)

is our opinion that an increase in $[Ca^2+]_i$ above a threshold of approximately 300 nM may trigger bleb formation, possibly by directly affecting the cytoskeleton, including both actin filaments and microtubules and their membrane interactions.

Examples of Nephrotoxicity

Mercuric chloride. $HgCl_2$ is a classic example of a nephrotoxin that has similar effects in both humans and experimental animals (Gritzka and Trump, 1968; McDowell et al., 1976). These effects, depending on the dose, range from acute necrosis in the S3 segment to complete necrosis of the entire proximal tubule. Typically, this is accompanied in the necrotic stage by calcification of the cells which is visible even at the macroscopic level (Trump et al., 1971). This calcification, as mentioned above, is ordinarily confined to the mitochondria. The mechanism of action of $HgCl_2$ seems to involve interaction with membrane sulphydryl groups although interaction of SH groups within the cell cannot be totally excluded. Experiments with the penetrating organic mercurial PCMB, as compared with the non-penetrating charged PCMBS, suggest that interactions with the cell membrane alone are sufficient to produce cell injury and cell death, although requiring a higher dose than the lipid-soluble penetrating molecules.

When applied to cultured rabbit or rat PTE in vitro, $HgCl_2$ exhibits a good dose-response curve (Smith et al., 1987; Trump et al., 1988). We have explored doses between 10 uM and 50 uM and noted that cell death and necrosis occur within 10-30 min and are preceded by a variety of morphological changes, including cell blebbing and cell detachment (Fig. 9).

Studies using Fura 2 indicate that the morphological changes are preceded by changes in $[Ca^2+]_i$ which initially increase very rapidly, decrease through some type of intracellular buffering and then exhibit a further

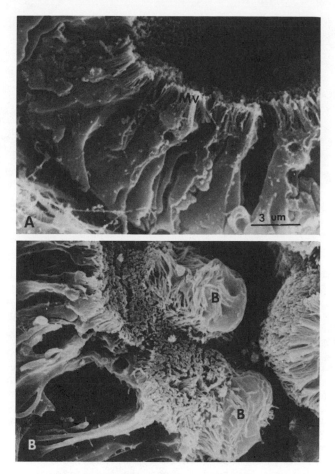

Figs. 8A and B. (A) SEM of a portion of control kidney proximal tubule illustrating a microvillous border (MB) projecting into a patent lumen. (B) SEM of a portion of a kidney proximal tubule following 15 min of in vivo ischaemia, illustrating distortion of the microvillous border to form large apical blebs (B). (From Trump et al., 1976.)

increase (Smith et al., 1987). The initial rapid increase is independent of extracellular calcium ($[Ca^2+]_e$) and independent of cell death for the first 30-60 min; however, the later increase which correlates with cell killing is dependent on $[Ca^2+]_e$. Reduction of $[Ca^2+]_e$ with low Ca^2+ media, especially with calcium chaelators such as EGTA, correlates with a significant delay of cell killing.

The initiation of bleb formation follows the increase of $[Ca^2+]_i$ and is correlated in time with modification of the actin patterns as seen with immunocytochemistry (Phelps et al., 1988). Although calcium-entry blockers do not modify the formation of blebs, the application of calmodulin inhibitors does modify their formation, suggesting a calmodulin/cytoskeletal interaction.

Inhibition of ATP Synthesis. This category includes ischaemia, anoxia, and inhibitors or uncouplers of ATP synthesis. In vivo, total ischaemia results in cell death and necrosis of rat PTE within 1-2 hr (Glaumann and Trump, 1975). This is preceded by marked diminution of ATP levels. During

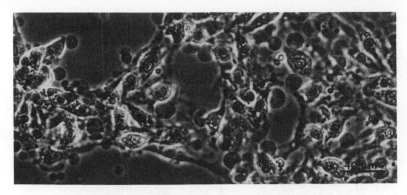

Fig. 9. Phase microscopy of cultured rabbit PTE cells treated with 50 uM HgCl$_2$ in the presence of 1.37 mM CaCl$_2$ at 37°C for 90 min. Note the presence of many blebs. (Courtesy of P.C. Phelps.)

the reversible phase, the formation of blebs occurs which, as mentioned above, detach and form casts in the distal nephron during Stages II-IV of cell injury (Fig. 10). After 1-2 hr, however, the cells pass the "point-of-no-return" and enter Stage V. In contrast to the effects of HgCl$_2$, calcification of the mitochondria is not observed unless reflow is permitted by releasing the clamp on the renal artery. This, we believe, is because mitochondrial calcium accumulation is ATP-dependent, which, in the totally ischaemic system, becomes impossible very rapidly.

We have attempted to simulate these conditions in vitro by using conditions such as the treatment of cultured PTE with potassium cyanide with or without the addition of iodoacetic acid. Under these conditions, again, there is rapid bleb formation, accompanied by the earlier reversible stages of cell injury. Blebs form as seen by light microscopy or scanning electron microscopy which are associated with alterations in actin patterns. Again, these changes are preceded and accompanied by increases in [Ca^{2}+]$_i$, although in contrast to plasma membrane active agents, such as HgCl$_2$ described above, the increases are significantly less.

The increase in [Ca^{2}+]$_i$ is independent of [Ca^{2}+]$_e$, indicating a redistribution within compartments within the cell, in this case, probably the mitochondria. Similar effects on [Ca^{2}+]$_i$ are seen following treatment with uncouplers of oxidative phosphorylation such as FCCP.

Hypothesis and Summary

Fig. 1 shows a flowchart depicting our current working hypothesis of the role of [Ca^{2}+]$_i$ in acute and chronic cell injury. Modifications of [Ca^{2}+]$_i$ based on influx from the extra-cellular space, the mitochondria, and the ER are illustrated. Also shown are the injurious agents that modify these three regulatory sites as well as compounds that modify each of these. Several important mediators are illustrated that can modify cell structure and function as well as the relationship between such deregulation and the signal transduction pathways.

In summary, our experiments indicate an important role for calcium deregulation in acute and chronic injury to the proximal tubule epithelium. Although current experiments suggest a pivotal role for [Ca^{2}+]$_i$, many more studies will be required to elucidate the mechanism(s)

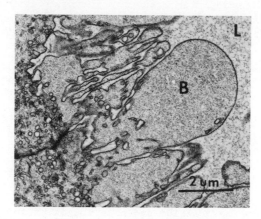

Fig. 10. TEM of a portion of an isolated flounder kidney tubule after addition of 10^{-3} M KCN for 5 min, illustrating several large apical blebs (B) projecting from the lumen (L). (From Trump and Arstila, 1975.)

of such calcium changes to the pathways leading to both acute and chronic cell injury.

ACKNOWLEDGEMENTS

This is Contribution No. 2516 from the Cellular Patholobiology Laboratory. Supported by NIH Grant AM15440.

REFERENCES

Berridge, M.J., and Irvine, R.F., 1984, Inositol triphosphate, a novel second messenger in cellular signal transduction, Nature, 312:315.

DiGuiseppi, J., Inman, R., Ishihara, A., Jacobsen, K., and Herman, B., 1985, Applications of digitized fluorescence microscopy to problems in cell biology, Biotechniques, 3:394.

Ginn, F.L., Shelburne, J.B., and Trump, B.F., 1968, Disorders of cell volume regulation. I. Effects of inhibition of plasma membrane ATPase with ouabain, Amer. J. Path., 53:1041.

Glaumann, B., and Trump, B.F., 1975, Studies on the pathogenesis of ischemic cell injury. III. Morphological changes of the proximal pars recta tubules (P-3) of the rat kidney made ischemic in vivo, Virchows Arch. B Cell Path., 19:303.

Gritzka, T.L., and Trump, B.F., 1968, Renal tubular lesions caused by mercuric chloride. Electron microscopic observations: Degeneration of the pars recta, Am. J. Pathol., 52:1225.

Grynkiewicz, G., Poenie, M., and Tsien, R.Y., 1985, A new generation of Ca^{2+} indicators with greatly improved fluorescence properties, J. Biol. Chem., 260:3440.

Inoue, S., 1986, "Video Microscopy," Plenum Press, New York.

McDowell, E.M., et al., 1976, Studies on the pathophysiology of acute renal failure. I. Correlation of ultrastructure and function in the proximal tubule of the rat following administration of mercuric chloride, Virchows Arch. B Cell Path., 22:173.

Pentilla, A., and Trump, B.F., 1974, Extracellular acidosis protects Ehrlich ascites tumor cells and rat renal cortex against anoxic injury, Science, 185:277.

Pentilla, A., and Trump, B.F., 1975, Studies on modification of the cellular response to injury. I. Protective effect of acidosis on p-chloromercuribenzene sulfonic acid-induced injury of Ehrlich ascites tumor cells, Lab. Invest., 32:690.

Pentilla, A., Glaumann, H., and Trump, B.F., 1976, Studies on the modification of cellular response to injury. IV. Protective effect of extracellular acidosis against anoxia, thermal, and p-chlorobenzene sulfonic acid treatment of isolated rat liver cells, Life Sci., 18:1419.

Phelps, P.C., Smith, M.W., Regec, A.L., Anthony, R.L., and Trump, B.F., 1988, Cytosolic ionized calcium and bleb formation following acute cell injury of cultured rabbit renal tubule cells, (in preparation.)

Slaga, T.J., 1983, Overview of tumor promotion in animals, Environ. Health Perspec., 50:3.

Smith, M.W., Collan, Y., Khang, M.W., and Trump, B.F., 1980, Changes in mitochondrial lipids of rat kidney during ischemia, Biochim. Biophys. Acta, 618:192.

Smith, M.W., Ambudkar, I.S., Phelps, P.C., Regec, A.L., and Trump, B.F., 1987, $HgCl_2$-induced changes in cytosolic Ca^2+ of cultured rabbit renal tubular cells, Biochim. Biophys. Acta, 931:130.

Trump, B.F., and Arstila, A.U., 1975, Cellular reaction to injury, In: "Principles of Pathology," Second Edition, M.F. LaVia and R.B. Hill, Jr., eds., Oxford University Press, London.

Trump, B.F., and Berezesky, I.K., 1983, The role of calcium deregulation in cell injury and cell death. Introduction, Surv. Synth. Path. Res., 2:165.

Trump, B.F., and Berezesky, I.K., 1985a, The role of calcium in cell injury and repair: a hypothesis, Surv. Synth. Path. Res., 4:248.

Trump, B.F., and Berezesky, I.K., 1985b, Cellular ion regulation and disease. A hypothesis, In: "Regulation of Calcium Transport in Muscle," A.E. Shamoo ed., Academic Press, New York.

Trump, B.F., and Berezesky, I.K., 1987, Ion regulation, cell injury and carcinogenesis, Carcinogenesis, 8:1027.

Trump, B.F., and Berezesky, I.K., 1988, The role of ion regulation in cell injury, cell death and carcinogenesis, In: "Cell Calcium Metabolism," C. Fiskum, ed., Plenum Press, New York (in press).

Trump, B.F., and Ginn, F.L., 1969, The pathogenesis of subcellular reaction to lethal injury, In: "Methods and Achievements in Experimental Pathology," E. Bajusz and G. Jasmin eds., Basel, Karger.

Trump, B.F., and Mergner, W.J., 1974, Cell injury, In: "The Inflammatory Process," Volume I, Second Edition, B.W. Zweifach, L. Grant, and R.T. McClusky, eds., Academic Press, New York.

Trump, B.F., Croker, B.P., and Mergner, W.J., 1971, The role of energy metabolism, ion and water shifts in the pathogenesis of cell injury, <u>In</u>: Cell Membranes: "Biological and Pathological Aspects," G.W. Richter and D.G. Scarpelli, eds., Academic Press, New York.

Trump, B.F., Berezesky, I.K., Collan, Y., Khang, M.W., Mergner, W.J., 1976, Recent studies on the pathophysiology of ischemic cell injury, <u>Beitr. Path</u>., 158:363.

Trump, B.F., Berezesky, I.K., Laiho, K.U., Osornio, A.R., Mergner, W.J., and Smith, M.W., 1980, The role of calcium in cell injury, <u>Scan. Electr</u>. <u>Microsc</u>., 2:437.

Trump, B.F., Berezesky, I.K., Sato, T., and Phelps, P.C., 1986, Ion regulation and bleb formation in epithelium of kidney and liver, <u>J. Cell</u> <u>Biol</u>. 103:452a.

Trump, B.F., Smith, M.W., Phelps, P.C., Regec, A.L., and Berezesky, I.K., 1988, The role of ionized cytosolic calcium ($[Ca^{2}+]_i$) in acute and chronic cell injury, <u>In</u>: "Integration of Mitochondrial Junction," J.J. Lemasters, C.R. Hackenbrook, R.G. Thurman, and H.V. Westerhoff, eds., Plenum Press, New York, in press.

Wade, M.H., Trosko, J.E., and Schindler, M., 1986, A fluorescence photobleaching assay of gap junction-mediated communication between human cells, <u>Science</u>, 232:525.

LIPOPHILIC CATIONS AS MEMBRANE PROBES IN CULTURED RENAL (LLC-PK$_1$) AND MUSCLE CELLS (L6)

R.T. Riley, D.E. Goeger, and W.P. Norred

Toxicology and Mycotoxins Research Unit,
Russel Research Center
U.S.D.A./A.R.S., Athens, Georgia 30613, U.S.A.

INTRODUCTION

Tetraphenylphosphonium (TPP) and triphenylmethylphosphonium (TPMP) are lipophilic cations which have been used to measure transmembrane potentials in vesicles, mitochondria, and plant and animal cells (Cafimo and Hubbell, 1978; Ritchie, 1984). The use of TPP and TPMP to estimate electrical potentials in animal cells has many sources of error. There is, however, a qualitative proportionality between their uptake and the transmembrane potential difference which can provide useful information about the biological activity of chemicals. Lipophilic cations have also been used as probes of charge alterations in both lipid and protein domains of biomembranes (Levitsky et al., 1986; Cafiso, 1984). The relationship between charge alterations on, or within, biomembranes and the manifestations of toxicity in animals is not well established. Nonetheless, in vitro studies indicate that such alterations can have profound effects on transport systems and receptors associated with cell membranes (Levitsby et al., 1986; Cafiso, 1984).

MATERIALS AND METHODS

Pig kidney epithelial cells (LLC-PK$_1$) were obtained from the American Type Tissue Collection (ATCC, CRL 1392) and were grown, subcultured as previously described (Riley et al., 1985; Riley et al., 1986). Rat skeletal muscle myoblasts (L6) (ATCC, CRL 1458) were grown, maintained and subcultured essentially the same as LLC-PK$_1$ cells, except that the growth medium (1:1 Dulbecco's modified Eagle's cells: Ham's F12), was supplemented with 10% foetal calf serum (instead of 5% in the LLC-PK$_1$ cells), and L6 seed stocks were always sub-cultured while at low cell density and prior to fusion.

The uptake and efflux of [^{3}H]TPP and [^{3}H]TPMP were determined using cultures grown in either 24-well culture plates or 35mm tissue culture dishes. One hour prior to an experiment the growth medium was aspirated and replaced with phosphate buffered saline 10 mM glucose (PBS). The cultures in PBS were transferred to a 37°C, > 70% relative humidity incubator. The assays were conducted directly in the plates or dishes as previously described (Riley et al.,1985; Riley et al., 1986). Unless specified otherwise, total TPP accumulation by cells was corrected for potential insensitive accumulation by subtracting TPP accumulation in the presence of the depolarizing agent, carbonylcyanide-m-chlorophenylhydrazone (CCCP, 5 uM).

Binding of TPP to lysed cells and cell fragments was determined using preparations of cells suspended in hypotonic buffer solutions (10 mM HEPES, pH7.2) and then lysed by freeze-thaw (-80°C for 10 min; thaw 10 min at room temperature). The cell lysate was centrifuged at 165,000g in a Beckman Airfuge for 10 min and radioactivity in the pellet was determined by liquid scintillation counting.

RESULTS AND DISCUSSION

TPP accumulation by LLC-PK$_1$ cells is nonsaturable (Fig. 1a) and efflux in the presence of depolarizing agents is rapid and complete (Fig. 1b). In LLC-PK$_1$ cells, TPMP is accumulated to a greater extent than either TPP or the natural quaternary cation, acetylcholine (ACH) (Fig. 1c), and the accumulation of TPP, TPMP and ACH is significantly inhibited by 5 uM CCCP. In L6 cells, neither TPMP nor ACH is appreciably accumulated.

Table 1 is a summary of chemicals which we have found to inhibit or potentiate TPP accumulation by LLC-PK$_1$ or L6 cells (Riley et al., 1985; Riley et al., 1986; unpublished result). Treatment of LLC-PK$_1$ or L6 cells with chemicals which dissipate transmembrane potentials (i.e. high [K+], ouabain, dinitrophenol, CCCP) inhibits intracellular TPP accumulation, while activation of the Na/H pump with monensin potentiates TPP accumulation. These observations are consistent with the hypothesis that TPP accumulation by animal cells is driven by the transmembrane potential. Alternatively, an endogenous lipophilic cation extrusion pump has been hypothesised to account for the apparent qualitative proportionality between lipophilic cation accumulation and the electrical potential gradients across membranes in animal cells (Ritchie, 1984). This latter hypothesis seems unlikely in LLC-PK$_1$ cells since choline, acetylcholine (endogenous quaternary compounds), and TPMP do not inhibit TPP accumulation (Riley et al., 1986). Inhibition of TPP accumulation by metabolic inhibitors, uncouplers and high potassium media is consistent with the hypothesis that TPP accumulation is proportional to the sum of the transmembrane potentials for all serially connected compartments within the cell.

Table 1. A partial listing of chemicals which inhibit or potentiate TPP accumulation by LLC-PK$_1$ cells or L6 cells and probable mechaniom ofaction.

    INHIBITORS

        Dinitrophenol (uncoupler)
        Carbonylcyanide-m-chlorophenylhydrazone (uncoupler)
        Tetrahexylammonium (uncoupler)
        Ouabain (inhibits Na/K pump)
        High potassium buffer (depolarizes cells)
        N,N-ethylmaleimide (sulphydryl reagent)

    POTENTIATORS

        Monensin (stimulates Na/K pump)
        Tetraphenylboron (surface charge alteration)
        Cyclopiazonic acid (intracellular charge alteration)
        Verapamil (weak charge alteration?)
        Dicyclohexylcarbodiimide (weak charge alteration?)

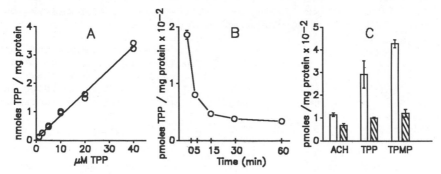

Fig. 1. a) Accumulation of TPP by LLC-PK$_1$ cells after 60 min at different TPP concentrations. b) cells after 60 min at cells allowed to accumulate TPP for 30 min and then depolarized with CCCP. c) Comparison of ACH, TPP: and TPMP accumulation (60 min) by LLC-PK$_1$ with (cross hatched bars) and without 5 uM CCCP (blank bars).

Increased accumulation of TPP can be explained by hyperpolarization of the plasma membrane potential aa is the case for monensin. Alternatively, dipole effects or change in surface charge can dramatically alter the zero potential partition coefficient for hydrophobic ions (Cafiso and Hubbell, 1978). Several chemicals that we have tested cause potentiated TPP uptake and reduced efflux kinetics, suggesting that the accumulated TPP is not in passive equilibrium across the plasma membrane (Fig. 2). For example, verapamil, dicyclohexylcarbodiimide (DCC), and the fungal metabolite, cyclopiazonic acid (CPA), all potentiate TPP accumulation by LLC-PK$_1$ cells (Riley et al, 1986). Three compounds exhibit efflux kinetics that suggest that the TPP may not be by passive equilibrium with the transmembrane potential difference. This is most apparent with CPA.

In LLC-PK$_1$ cells, TPP can be recovered bound in the plasma membrane and mitochondrial ractions (Table 2). However, the interaction between TPP and membranes, in CPA-treated cells, is weak as evidenced by the fact that TPP can be separated from the membranes by CHCl$_3$ extraction or by passage through a gel filtration column (Riley et al, 1986 and unpublished results).

Our studies with CPA and tetraphenylboron (TPB) suggest that these two chemicals induce electrical alterations at the inner and outer surfaces of cells, respectively. The CPA-potentiated TPP accumulation by intact LLC-PK$_1$ or L6 cells is totally inhibited by CCCP (Fig. 3a). The TPB-potentiated TPP accumulation, however, is not inhibited by CCCP (Fig. 3a). In CPA-treated L6 and LLC-PK$_1$ cells potentiated accumulation of TPP, in the presence of the uncoupler CCCP, is only observed in cells permeabilized by freeze-thaw (Fig. 3b). This suggests that the site of CPA interaction is intracellular. We hypothesize that access of TPP to the intracellular binding site in CFA-treated cells is prevented in de-energied cells because the membrane potential, which is the driving force for TPP to cross the membrane, has been eliminated.

Different cell types exhibit age and growth related difference in the extent of, TPP accumulation and in their sensitivity to toxin-induced alterations in TPP accumulation (Fig. 4a). For example, LLC-PK$_1$ and L6 cells show quite different effects of age on the potential menstire and CPA-potentiated TPP accumulation (Fig. 4b and 4c). Primary rat hepatocytes

Table 2. Distribution of TPP in subcellular fractions of LLC-PK$_1$ cells dosed with CCCP or test agents shown to potentiate accumulation of TPP (Riley et al., 1986).

	Picomoles TPP/mg protein (60 min)		
Additions [a]	Homogenate	25K x g pellet	105K x g supernatant
None	210	10	199
Monensin	502	22	470
Verapamil	315	10	313
DCC	399	18	370
CCCP	15	2	13
CPA	685	528	67

Percent of TPP in subcellular fractions of CPA-treated cells oompared to control cells (no additions)

	Additions	
	CPA	Control
Cytosolic	14%	88%
Microsomal	1%	2%
Nuclear	8%	7%
Plasma membrane	56%	1%
Mitochondrial	21%	1%

a Concentrations of additions = all were 2 uM TPP plus monensin = 20 uM, verapamil = 30 uM, DCC = 30 uM, CPA = 50 uM, CCCP = 5 uM.

do not exhibit CPA-potentiated TPP accumulation (results not shown), while LLC-PK$_1$ cells show potentiated accumulation at all ages even though the potential sensitive TPP uptake decreases with time (Fig. 4b). In L6 cells, potential sensitive TPP accumulation increases for several days after subculturing while CPA-potentiated TPP accumulation decreases with age (Fig. 4a and 4c). These differences in sensitivity to CPA by different cell types may be related to differences in the growth characteristics of the cells. Primary rat hepatocytes are incapable of proliferating in culture while LLC-PK$_1$ cells can be subcultured long after seeding. L6 cells can be subcultured for long periods, only if they are not allowed to undergo irreversible differentiation which in our test system, is first observed at 4 to 5 days after seeding. Thus, in the L6 cell the failure of older cells to respond to CPA is closely correlated with terminal differentiation. While in LLC-PK$_1$ cells the ability of the cells to proliferate, at all ages, confers sensitivity to CPA. We hypothesize that the susceptibility of cells to toxin-induced charge alterations in, on or across cell membranes may be related to age and growth dependent changes which are unique to each cell type.

CONCLUSIONS

Lipophilic cations such as TPP and TPMP can be used to detect toxicant induced alterations in transmembrane potentials differences and charge alterations in lipid or protein domains of biomembranes. The relationship between toxicant induced electrical alterations in cells and the expression of toxicity observed in vivo has not been determined. Nonetheless, we have found that with regards to these electrical alterations, different cell types exhibit different temporal patterns of responsiveness to toxicants. It is possible that these differences are due to basic biochemical properties of cell membranes which play an important role in the targeting of tissues by toxicants.

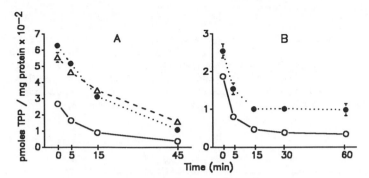

Figure 2. a) Efflux of TPP from depolarized LLC-PK$_1$ cells treated with DCC (●), verapamil (△), or untreated (○) were allowed to accumulate TPP for 60 min and then depolarized with CCCP. b) Efflux of TPP from CPA-treated (●) and untreated (○) LLC-PK$_1$ cells after accumulating TPF for 30 min and then depolarized with CCCP.

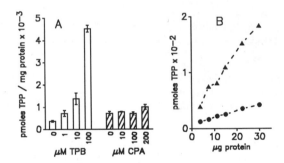

Figure 3. a) Effect of tetraphenyaboron (black bars) and cyclopiazonic acid (cross hatched bars) on TPP accumulation by intact L6 cells depolarized with CCCP. b) Accumulation of TPP by intact (●) and freeze-thaw permeabilized (▲) L6 cells with 50 uM CPA and 5 uM CCCP.

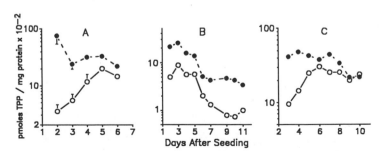

Figure 4. Effect of age of culture on the potential sensitive TPP accumulation (○) and CPA-potentiated TPP accumulation (●).

a) L6 cells with and without CPA (50 uM) and comparison of b) LLC-PK$_1$ cells and c) L6 cells seeded at cell densities which resulted in identical growth rate.

ABBREVIATIONS

ACH = acetylcholine, CCCP = carbonylcyanide-m-chlorophenylhydrazone, CPA = cyclopiazonic acid: DCC = dicyclohexylcarbodiimide, HEPES = N-2-hydroxsethylpiperamine-N'-2-ethanesulphonic acid. L6 cells = rat skeletal muscle myoblasts, LLC-PK$_1$ = pig kidney epithelial cells, PBS = phosphate buffered saline plus 10mM glucose, TPB = tetraphenylboron, TPMP = triphenylmethylphosphonium, TPP = tetraphenylphosphonium.

REFERENCES

Cafiso, D.S., 1984, Paramagnetic hydrophobic ions as probes for electrically active conformational transitions in ion channels, <u>Biophys. J.</u> 45:6.

Cafiso, D.S. and Hubbell, W.L., 1978, Estimation of transmembrane potentials from phase equilibria of hydrophobic paramagnetic ions, <u>Biochemistry</u>, 17:187.

Levitsky, D.O., Loginov, V.A. and Lebedev, A.V., 1986, Charge changes in sarcoplasmic reticulum and Ca^{2+}-ATPase induced by calcium binding and release: A study using lipophilic ions, <u>Membr. Biochem.</u>, 6:291.

Riley, R.T., Norred. W.P., Dorner, J.W. and Cole, R.J.: 1985, Increased accumulation of the lipophilic cation tetraphenylphosphonium by cyclopiazonic acid-treated renal epithelial cells, <u>Toxicol. Environ. Health</u>, 15:779.

Riley, R.T., Showker, J.L., Cole, R.J. and Dorner, J., 1986; The mechanism by which cyclopiazonic acid potentiates accumulation of tetraphenyl-phosphonium in cultured renal epithelial cells, <u>J. Biochem. Toxicol.</u>, 1:13.

Ritchie, R.J., 1984, A critical assessment of the use of lipophilic cations as membrane potential probes, <u>Prog. Biophys. Molec. Biol.</u>, 13:1.

CHARACTERIZATION OF AN UNSCHEDULED DNA SYNTHESIS ASSAY WITH A CULTURED LINE OF PORCINE KIDNEY CELLS (LLC-PK1)

S. Vamvakas, W. Dekant, D. Schiffmann and D. Henschler

Institute of Toxicology, University of Wurzburg, Versbacherstr. 9, 8700 Wurzburg, Federal Republic of Germany

INTRODUCTION

Proximal tubular cells are a primary site of tumour formation in the kidney probably due both to high exposure to absorbed chemicals and their multiple transport and bioactivation capacities (1). It is therefore important to develop appropriate short-term tests for investigating the organ specific genotoxicity of various chemicals. Since somatic mutations are considered as a crucial initiating step in chemical carcinogenesis (2), short-term tests detecting interactions of chemicals with DNA such as repair processes in damaged DNA sites are widely used for predicting potential carcinogenic properties of chemicals. The most appropriate method of estimating DNA repair is probably determination of unscheduled DNA synthesis (UDS) in exposed cells by monitoring the non-S-phase uptake of ^{3}H-thymidine (^{3}H-dThd) either by autoradiography of intact cells (3) or by liquid scintillation counting of the extracted DNA (4). UDS induction in renal tissue have already been undertaken using primary kidney cells exposed in vivo or in vitro to known or potential renal carcinogens and determining ^{3}H-dThd incorporation by autoradiography (5). This method is highly specific, but its disadvantages lie in the long duration and the relative high costs of the experiments as well as in the difficulty of obtaining cell preparations of reliable and reproducible quality.

LLC-PK1, a cell line derived from pig kidney, combines two important advantages. They are biochemically and morphologically similarity to the proximal tubular cells (6) and easy, inexpensive and reproducible to culture. We have used this cell line and the liquid scintillation technique to develop a UDS assay, as a tool for the preliminary evaluation of kidney specific genotoxic properties of chemicals.

MATERIALS AND METHODS

Chemicals. Streptozotocin (SZ), 4-nitroquinoline-1-oxide (NQ) and dimethylnitrosamine (DMN) were purchased from Sigma Chemical Co, St Louis U.S.A, S-(2-chloroethyl-L-cysteine (CEC) and S-(1,2-dichlorovinyl)gluta-thione (DCVG) were a present from Prof. Anders (Dept of Pharmacology, Rochester, U.S.A.), S-(1,2-dichlorovinyl)cysteine (DCVC) was synthesised as described previously (7).

Cells and growth conditions. LLC-PK1 cells (American Type Culture

Collection, passage 182 to 190) were grown in Dulbecco's modified Eagle's medium (DMEM) supplemented with 10% foetal calf serum (FCS), 3g/l glucose and antibiotics in a humidified atmosphere with 5% CO_2 in air at $37^{\circ}C$.

Inhibition of replicative DNA synthesis. Cells (3.5×10^5) in logarithmic growth were plated on 35mm tissue culture dishes, confluence and dome formation were observed after 72h cultivation which was continued for another 48h in medium containing 1 to 10% dialyzed FCS. Hydroxyurea (HU, 1-20mM) was added at the end of this incubation time for 1h. Rest replicative DNA synthesis was then estimated for 5h in absence of test substances as described below.

UDS assay. After replacement of the medium the cells were irradiated with UV-light or treated with the indicated chemicals for various times in DMEM containing 2.5% FCS, 10mM HU and 10uCi/ml ^{3}H-dThd. After treatment the cells were washed twice with buffer, removed from the dishes with 1ml 0.1% trypsin and solubilized with 1ml 2% sodium dodecylsulphate. 2ml 20% trichloroacetic acid (TCA) were then added to each sample, the resulting precipitate collected on Whatmann GF/C glass fibre filters and washed with TCA (10 and 5%) and ethanol. Finally the filters were treated with 0.5ml solubilizer for 5h followed by the addition of 20ul of glacial acetic acid and toluene scintillator for radioactivity determination.

The background levels of ^{3}H-dThd incorporation being less than 6,000cpm/culture well in untreated cells or in the present of methanol (0.1-0.5%) or DMSO (0.1-0.5%) were subtracted. All experiments were repeated at least twice and all determinations were made in triplicate.

Cytotoxicity assay. Per cent cell death was calculated after treatment of the cells (see UDS assay) as the per cent LDH released compared to Triton X-100 lysed control cells.

RESULTS AND DISCUSSION

Cultivation of confluent monolayers for 48h in medium containing 2.5% FCS instead of 10% and addition of 10mM HU for 1h at the end of this period resulted in a decrease in the rate of replicative DNA synthesis by 96% (Fig. 1 and 2) without exerting cytotoxicity to the cells according to LDH leakage (Table 1).

To examine whether the cells are able to repair DNA damage under our experimental conditions LLC-PK1 monolayers were exposed to UV, a well known DNA damaging agent. UV irradiation ($9-90J/m^2$) induced UDS in a dose

Table 1. Effect of various hydroxyurea concentrations (HU, 24h incubation time) and dialyzed foetal calf serum (FCS, 72h incubation time) on LDH release in confluent LLC-PK1 monolayers [a].

HU (mM)	FCS (%)	LDH release
---	10	5.2 ± 1.5
---	2.5	5.6 ± 1.8
10	10	5.3 ± 1.4
10	2.5	5.7 ± 1.6

[a] Per cent cell death was calculated as the per cent LDH released by treatment compared to Triton X-100 (0.2%) lysed control (10% FCS, 10mM HU) cells. Results are means of 6 determinations ± SD.

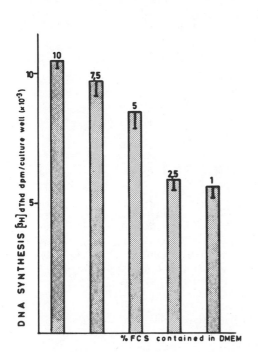

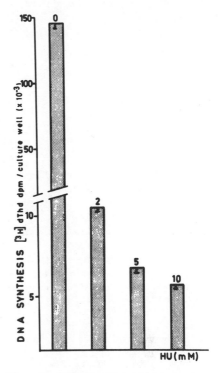

Fig. 1. Effect of decreased dialyzed
FCS concentration (expressed
as % in DMEM) in presence of
10 mM hydroxyurea on S-phase
DNA synthesis in LLC-PK1.[a]

Fig. 2. Effect of hydroxyurea
(HU) on S-phase DNA
synthesis in LLC-PK1
cultivated in DMEM/
2.5% FCS. [a]

[a] Results are means of 6 determinations ± SD.

dependent mode. There was no difference in the response between cells
treated with 1 or 10mM HU indicating that HU does not impair excision
repair (Fig 3).

When the cells were exposed to 5×10^{-5} of the known genotoxic agent NQ for
various times, the maximum rates of UDS were observed in cells treated for
10h (Fig. 4). Therefore this treatment time was chosen for the experiments
with the renal carcinogens SZ and DMN. The same protocol was used for
the genotoxic metabolite of 1,2-dichloroethane (CEC), and intermediates in
the bioactivation of trichoroethylene (DCVG) and dichloroacetylene
(DCVC), presumed to be involved in the nephrotoxic and nephrocarcinogenic
properties of these compounds. To ensure that the increased incorporation
of ^{3}H-dThd in exposed cells was not due to induction of the remaining weak
replicative capability of the cells as a result of cell death, LDH leakage
was monitored in all UDS experiments and clearly showed that the chemicals
tested were able to induce DNA repair without concomitantly killing cells
(Table 2).

While SZ and CEC interact directly with DNA, NQ must be reduced to the
ultimate genotoxic metabolite. Each of these compounds induced a strong,
dose dependent UDS response as shown in Fig. 5 (only the concentrations
producing the highest response are shown). The potent nephrotoxins and

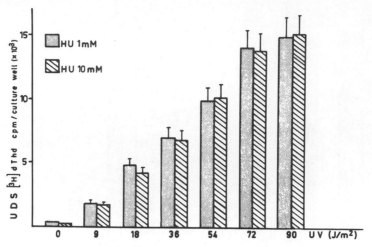

Fig. 3. Induction of UDS in LLC-PK1 by UV irradiation. Influence of hydroxyurea (HU) concentration on the repair capability of the cells. Residual S-phase DNA-synthesis has been subtracted. Results are means of 6 determinations ± SD

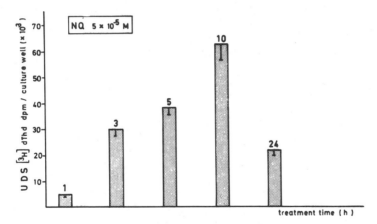

Fig. 4. Effect of treatment time with 4-nitroquinoline-1-oxide (NQ) on UDS induction in LLC-PK1. Residual S-phase DNA synthesis has been subtracted. Results are means of 6 determinations ± SD

bacterial mutagens DCVC and DCVG (8, 9) induced a lower dose dependent response, only when the exposure time was extended to 24h (Fig. 5). Gamma-glutamyl-transpeptidase and dipeptidases cleave DCVG to DCVC which is finally transformed to genotoxic intermediates by ß-lyase. High activities of these three enzymes are found both in the proximal tubule and in LLC-PK1 (10). The induction of UDS by DCVC and DCVG in LLC-PK1 is indicative of the capability of these cells to perform transport and bioactivation sequences which are characteristic for the proximal tubule in vivo.

No excision repair could be observed with DMN even when the incubation times were varied from 1 to 48h indicating that under the UDS cultivation procedure LLC-PK1 are not able to bioactivate this compound which also failed to induce UDS when tested in primary cells in vitro (11).

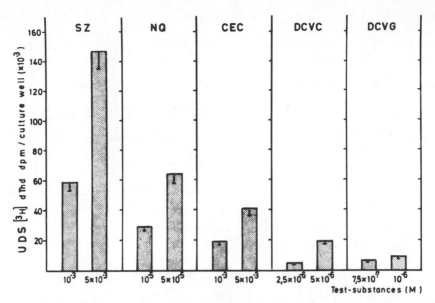

Fig. 5. Induction of UDS in LLC-PK1 by streptozotocin (SZ), 4-nitroquino-line-1-oxide (NQ), S-(2-chloroethyl)-L-cysteine (CEC), S-(1,2-dichloro-vinyl)cysteine (DCVC) and S-(1,2-dichlorovinyl)glutathione. CEC was dissolved in 0.5% methanol, NQ in 0.1% DMSO, SZ, DCVC and DCVG directly in the medium. Residual S-phase DNA synthesis has been subtracted. Results are means of 6 determinations ± SD

Table 2. Toxicity of NQ, CEC, SZ, DCVC, DCVG and DMN in LLC-PK1[a]

Test-subst.	Concentr. (M)	LDH release (%)	Test-subst.	Concentr. (M)	LDH release (%)
---		5.6 ± 1.5			
NQ	10^{-6}	5.4 ± 1.3	DCVC	10^{-6}	5.8 ± 1.6
	5×10^{-5}	5.6 ± 2.1		5×10^{-6}	6.2 ± 1.8
	10^{-4}	13.2 ± 1.8		10^{-5}	32.3 ± 4.6
CEC	10^{-4}	5.8 ± 1.8	DCVG	10^{-6}	6.2 ± 1.6
	5×10^{-3}	6.0 ± 1.6		5×10^{-6}	6.0 ± 1.6
				10^{-5}	31.2 ± 5.4
SZ	10^{-4}	5.6 ± 1.9	DMN	10^{-3}	5.4 ± 1.3
	5×10^{-3}	5.6 ± 1.7		10^{-2}	28.6 ± 1.5

[a] Confluent LLC-PK1 monolayers were incubated for 24h with the test compounds. Per cent cell death was calculated as the per cent LDH released ba treatment compared to Triton X-100 (0.2%) lysed control cells. Results are mean of 6 determinations ± SD.

Our results clearly demonstrate that LLC-PK1 possess the excision repair capability to determine the genotoxicity of mutagenic and some classes of promutagenic compounds and that the UDS assay developed with these cells may provide a valuable prescreening test in this area.

REFERENCES.

1. Robbin S.L., Cotran R.S. (1979). "Pathologic Basis of Disease", Philadelphia. WB Saunder Co

2. Bresnick E., Eastman A. (1982). <u>Drug Metab. Rev</u>. 13, 189-205

3. Stich H.F., San R.H.C. (1970). <u>Mutation Res</u>. 10, 389-404

4. Martin C.N., McDermid A.C., Garner R.C. (1977). <u>Cancer Lett</u> 2, 355-360

5. Tyson C.K., Mirsalis J.C. (1985). <u>Environm. Mutagen</u>. 7, 889-899

6. Gstraunthaler G., Pfaller W, Kotanko P. (1985). <u>Am. J. Physiol</u>. 171, F536-F544

7. Dekant W., Vamvakas S., Berthold K., Schmidt S., Wild D., Henschler D. (1986). <u>Chem.-Biol. Interact</u>. 60, 31-45

8. Lash L.H., Anders M.W. (1986). <u>Comments Toxicol</u>. 1, 2, 87-106

9. Vamvakas S., Elfarra A., Dekant W., Henschler D., Anders M.W. (1987). <u>Mutation Res</u>. (submitted)

10. Stevens J., Hayden P., Taylor G. (1986). <u>J. Biol. Chem</u>. 261, 7, 3325-3332

11. Loury D.J., Butterworth B.E. (1986). <u>CIIT Activities</u> 6, 4

MICROPUNCTURE STUDIES ON MECHANISMS OF PROTEINURIA IN EARLY ADRIAMYCIN-NEPHROSIS IN MWF-RATS

Uwe Haberstroh, Mechthild Soose, Gloria Rovira-Halbach, Reinhard Brunkhorst and Hilmar Stolte

Division of Nephrology, Hannover Medical School, Konstanty-Gutschow-Str. 8, 3000 Hannover, FRG

INTRODUCTION

The sensitivity of the kidney to many compounds is well recognized, and sequences of pathological events have been documented in detail. A model compound to induce nephrotic syndrome in rodents is adriamycin, an anthracyclin antitumour drug widely used in chemotherapy. As described by Bertani et al. (1982), pathological changes such as proteinuria, hyper-coagulability, and hyperlipemia occur with adriamycin use.

Most of the data available concerns chronic adriamycin-nephrosis. The actual cellular targets and molecular mechanisms responsible for the nephrotoxic activity of adriamycin are not clearly defined. Several studies support the involvement of adriamycin semiquinone radicals, which may be generated enzymatically by renal mixed-function oxidases. Subsequent reaction of the semiquinone with oxygen is suggested to produce reactive oxygen radicals which damage the cells by lipid peroxidation and cross-linking of cellular thiols (Bachur et al., 1977; Mimnaugh et al., 1986; Bakker et al., 1987; Scheulen et al., 1987).

To obtain more information on the mechanisms of adriamycin renal activity, our studies focused on the early changes responsible for proteinuria in rats. The questions were directed towards the influence of adriamycin on the glomerular barrier function with respect to albumin and high molecular weight (HMW)-proteins and the tubular uptake of these proteins. A first set of experiments was designed to consider overall proteinuria by analysis of final urines. In a second set of experiments, micropuncture techniques were applied to study adriamycin toxicity in more detail.

The rat strain of choice for these experiments were the Munich Wistar Fromter rats (MWF/Ztm), specially selected for their high number of super-ficial glomeruli. Rats in the F5 generation showed more than 50 superficial glomeruli per kidney (Hackbarth et al., 1980). As demonstrated in Fig. 1, a superficial glomerulus is in direct contact with the renal capsule and thus accessible to micropuncture. The aim of these studies was, to define the targets of adriamycin toxicity at the level of single nephrons. We further intended to reveal possible functional differences between nephrons situated in different zones of the kidney.

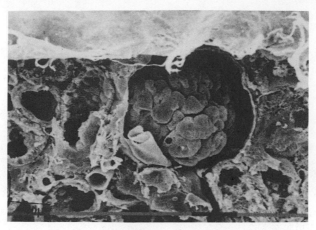

Fig. 1. Scanning electron micrograph of superficial glomerulus from MWF-rat (provided by B. Bartels and H. Hackbarth).

METHODS

Animals.   Female MWF/Ztm rats (100 ± 5 days old and 170-210g in weight) were treated with 5 mg/kg b.w. adriamycin, given as a single i.v. injection. An adriamycin incubation period of 7 days was chosen (see section "RESULTS"). Both control and experimental animals had free access to food and water, but were allowed only water 24 h before a micropuncture experiment. To collect final urine, animals were housed 24 h in individual metabolic cages.

Micropuncture Techniques.   Free-flow micropuncture was performed essentially as described by Rovira-Halbach et al. (1986). The puncture samples were defined by the following criteria:-

1. by the passage time of lissamine green solution (5 mg/100 ml), injected as a 0.05 ml bolus trough the jugular vein.

2. by the ratio of TF/P of inulin, given as a priming dose of 20 mg/100 g and subsequently infused with 45 mg/h x 100 g.

Analytical Methods.   Glomerular filtration rate (GFR) was determined by endogenous creatinine clearance, using a creatinine analyser. For measuring total protein in final urine, a microversion of the Biuret method according to Alt et al. (1975) was applied. Urinary albumin and high molecular weight (HMW)-proteins were separated by microdisc electro-phoresis using 2 ul capillaries. The gels were stained with amido black and scanned. Protein concentrations were determined using bovine serum albumin as a standard. The albumin concentrations in micropuncture samples were analysed by ultramicrodisc electrophoresis using 0.5 ul capillaries (Baldamus et al., 1975).

RESULTS

To get an overall picture of adriamycin-induced renal lesions, we observed the development of GFR and proteinuria in 12 MWF-rats over a period of 61 days after the administration of the drug. As is summarized in Fig. 2, the GFR was initially unchanged, but declined by approximately half after day 12. Proteinuria was detectable from day 5, reaching a maximum level of 630 mg/24 h by day 25. According to our definition of "early" renal lesions, early indicating the period of unchanged GFR, we chose an adriamycin incubation period of 7 days for further experiments.

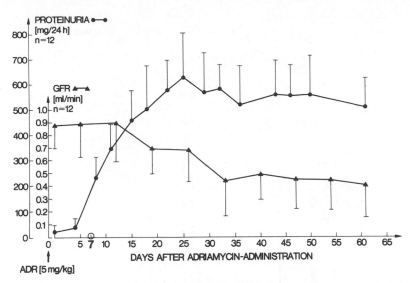

Fig. 2. GFR and development of proteinuria in MWF/Ztm rats (n=12) after administration of 5 mg/kg adriamycin. From this data an adriamycin incubation period of 7 days was chosen. All data presented as mean±SD.

Table 1. Protein excretion of MWF/Ztm rats after 7 days of single i.v. administration of 5 mg/kg. Adriamycin as compared to control rats.

	Total protein (mg/24 hr)	HMW-protein (mg/24 hr)	LMW-protein (mg/24 hr)	HMW:Albumin
CONTROL	25±20	3.5±2.5	9.6±8.6	0.365
(n)	41	13	33	
ADRIAMYCIN	253±91	58±26	158±67	0.367
(n)	8	8	8	

The protein contents in the final urine of control MWF-rats and of experimental animals are shown in Table 1. After 7 days of adriamycin-treatment total protein excretion was significantly higher as compared to controls (t-test, p < 0.001). This proteinuria was due to a leakage of both HMW-proteins and albumin. However, the ratio HMW-proteins/albumin in adriamycin-treated rats did not differ from control rats.

In order to determine the adriamycin-induced disturbances of barrier function and tubular uptake in more detail; free-flow micropunctures of superficial nephrons were performed. Samples were taken from the Bowman's capsular space (BCS) and from the early to mid-proximal tubule (MPT) of control and adriamycin-treated rats (Fig. 3). Superficial glomeruli of adriamycin-treated animals showed no significantly increased leakage of albumin (t-test, p > 0.05). Obviously, this represents a remarkable discrepancy to the overall albuminuria as albumin concentrations were clearly increased in final urine after the administration of adriamycin. In micropuncture samples of MPT only about 10% of the filtered protein load were detectable in both control and experimental groups.

757

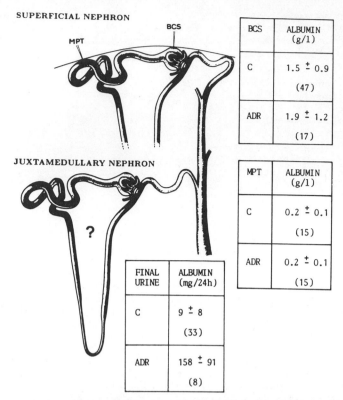

BCS	ALBUMIN (g/l)
C	1.5 $\pm$ 0.9 (47)
ADR	1.9 $\pm$ 1.2 (17)

MPT	ALBUMIN (g/l)
C	0.2 $\pm$ 0.1 (15)
ADR	0.2 $\pm$ 0.1 (15)

FINAL URINE	ALBUMIN (mg/24h)
C	9 $\pm$ 8 (33)
ADR	158 $\pm$ 91 (8)

SUPERFICIAL NEPHRON

JUXTAMEDULLARY NEPHRON

Fig. 3. Albumin concentrations in micropuncture samples and final urine of control (C) and adriamycin-treated (ADR) MWF-rats.

DISCUSSION

The administration of 5 mg/kg adriamycin to MWF/Ztm rats resulted in a heavy proteinuria and a moderately reduced GFR. In agreement with others (e.g. Calandra et al., 1983), these changes were delayed for 5 days, reached a maximum by 25, and were still present at day 61. The adriamycin-induced lesions are therefore assumed to be permanent. In treated animals, GFR was still approximately half that of the controls. In Wistar Furth rats, injected with 7.5 mg/kg adriamycin, only a 20% reduction of GFR was measured (Weening and Rennke, 1983). These findings suggest that overall renal function is not severely affected by the drug.

After 7 days of adriamycin treatment, that is, while the GFR is still unchanged, the total protein excretion was significantly increased in experimental animals due to a leakage of HMW-proteins and albumin. This pattern of urinary proteins indicates glomerular damage according to the classification of renal lesions by Alt et al. (1981). As the ratio of HMW-proteins/albumin does not differ from controls, the glomerular proteinuria is non selective. Several morphological studies on adriamycin-induced nephrotoxicity confirm an attack of the drug at the glomerular level. Severe ultrastructural changes in glomerular epithelium cells were detected, such as fusion and detachment of foot processes, vacuolization, focal dilatation of cisternae of the endoplasmic reticulum and invagination of plasma membrane. In progressing nephrosis, tubular dilatation, tubular casts, and interstitial fibrosis were reported (Fajardo et al., 1980; Van Vleet and Ferrans, 1980; Bertani et al., 1982; Weening and Rennke, 1983).

Remarkably, in contrast to the clearly increased protein excretion in final urine, the albumin concentrations in micropuncture samples taken from both BCS and MPT of adriamycin-treated animals did not differ significantly from control samples (Fig. 3). Also, preliminary studies on haemodynamic factors revealed no change in the single nephron GFR of superficial nephrons. Only after 4-5 weeks of persistent proteinuria, was there a 27% decline in SNGFR reported (O'Donnell et al., 1985).

Furthermore, in superficial nephrons the tubular uptake of filtered proteins presumably is not influenced by adriamycin. In micropuncture samples of early to mid-proximal tubules, only about 10% of the filtered albumin load was detectable (Fig. 3). This data suggests a very efficient tubular uptake of filtered proteins in superficial nephrons by both the control and experimental groups.

To summarize these results, it is obvious that the adriamycin-induced proteinuria in final urine is not corroborated by micropuncture studies of superficial nephrons. Neither glomerular barrier functions, nor tubular uptake by nephrons are markedly changed by the drug. We conclude that cortical (in contrast to juxtamedullary nephrons) might have a lower sensitivity to adriamycin. Possibly, difference in oxygen supply to both types of nephrons may occur in the kidney cortex. Thus, oxidative stress on membrane compounds, mediated by adriamycin semiquinone radicals may be enhanced in juxtamedullary nephrons. Our results are compatible with morphological studies of Fajardo et al. (1980) and Van Vleet and Ferrans (1980), who found that adriamycin-induced alterations in the rabbit kidney occurred almost exclusively in the inner cortex. Concerning the administration of potentially nephrotoxic drugs to man, it is important to be aware that certain nephron may not be adversely affected.

REFERENCES

Alt, J.M., Krisch, K., and Hirsch, K., 1975, Isolation of an inducible amidase from Pseudomonas acidovorans AE1, *J. Gen. Microbiol.*, 87:260.

Alt, J.M., von der Heyde, D., Assel, E., and Stolte, H., 1981, Characteristics of protein excretion in glomerular and tubular disease, *Contr. Nephrol.*, 24:115.

Bachur, N., Gordon, G.L., and Gee, M.V., 1977, Anthracyclin antibody augmentation of microsomal electron transport and free radical formation, *Mol. Pharmacol.*, 13:901.

Baldamus, C.A., Galaske, R., Eisenbach, G.M., Krause, H.P., and Stolte, H., 1975, Glomerular protein filtration in normal and nephritic rats. A micropuncture study, *Contr. Nephrol.*, 1:37.

Bakker, W.W., Kalicharan, D., Donga, J., Hulstaert, C.E., and Hardonk, M.J., 1987, Decreased ATPase activity in adriamycin nephrosis is independent of proteinuria, *Kidney Int.*, 31:704.

Bertani, T., Poggi, A., Pozzoni, R., Delaini, F., Sacchi, G., Thoua, Y., Mecca, G., Remuzzi, G., and Donati, M.B., 1982, Adriamycin-induced nephrotic syndrome in rats. Sequence of pathological events, *Lab. Invest.*, 46:16.

Calandra, S., Traugi, P., Ghisellini, M., Gherardi, L.E., 1983, Plasma and urine lipoproteins during development of nephrotic syndrome induced in the rat by adriamycin, *Exper. Molec. Path.*, 39:282.

Fajardo, L.F., Eltringham, J.R., Stewart, J.R., and Klauber, M. R., Adriamycin nephrotoxicity, Lab. Invest., 43:242.

Hackbarth, H., Gartner, K., Alt, J., and Stolte, H., 1980, A subline of the Munich Wistar (MW) strain, response to selection for surface glomeruli, Rat News Lett., 7:23.

Mimnaugh, E.G., Trush, M.A., and Gram, T.E., 1986, A possible role for membrane lipid peroxidation in anthracyclin nephrotoxicity, Biochem. Pharmac., 35:4327.

O'Donnell, M.P., Michels, L., Kasiske, B., Raij, L., and Keane, W. F., 1985, Adriamycin-induced chronic proteinuria: a structural and functional study, J. Lab. Clin. Med., 106:62.

Rovira-Halbach, G., Alt, J.M., Brtnkhorst, R., Frei, U., KUhn, K., and Stolte, H., 1986, Single nephron hyperfiltration and proteinuria in a newly selected rat strain with superficial glomeruli, Renal Physiol., 9:317.

Scheulen, M.E., Hoensch, H., Kappus, H., Seeber, S., and Schmidt, C.G., 1987, Positive correlation between decreased cellular uptake, NADPH-glutathione reductase activity and adriamycin resistance in Ehrlich ascites tumor lines, Arch. Toxicol., 60:154.

Van Vleet, J.F., and Ferrans, V.J., 1980, Clinical and pathologic features of chronic adriamycin toxicosis in rabbits, Am. J. Vet. Res., 41:1462.

Weening, J.J., and Rennke, H.G., 1983, Glomerular permeability and polyanion in adriamycin nephrosis in the rat, Kidney Int., 24:152.

INDEX

The page number refers to the first page of the chapter in which the topic is covered.

basement membrane 685
basolateral kidney membranes 247, 569
S-(2-benzothiazolyl)-cysteine 577
betaine 509
biliary ligation/cannulation 297, 423
biopsies 147
blood urea nitrogen levels 217, 267, 357, 371, 423, 447, 509, 569, 601, 623, 639, 681, 699
2-bromoethanamine (2-bromoethylamine) 383, 407, 411, 415
brush border 247, 711
brush border antigen 119
brush border membrane vesicles 247, 257, 303, 569, 633
buthionine sulphoxime 423
N-butyl-(4-hydroxylbutyl)-nitrosamine 411

cadmium 33, 37, 43, 51, 59, 65, 71, 75
cadmium-metallothionein 43
calcium 11, 65, 217, 247, 315, 607, 731
captopril 103, 207, 315, 627
carbon tetrachloride 451
carbonylcyanide-m-chlorophenyl-hydrazone 743
carboplatin 331
carcinogen(s) 93
carcinogenicity, carcinogenesis 93, 519
carcinomas 519, 557, 617
casts, hydrocarbon-induced 535
catalase levels/distribution 325, 331, 457
cathepsin 71
ceftaxime 377
ceftazidine 377
cell-cell interaction 685
cell culture 353, 595, 743, 749
celiphium 439
cephaloridine 457
cephalosporins 147
cephalothin 451
chelating agents 65
1-chloro-2,4-dinitrobenzene 725
S-(chloroethyl)-L-cysteine 749
chloroform 607
chlorofluoroacetic acid 595
chlorotrifluoroethylene 595
complement 59
chlorpromazine 607
chronic renal disease/failure 11, 307
cis-platinum 177, 331, 337, 343, 349, 353, 357, 361, 371, 383, 447, 497, 705

citrinin 569
cobalt 51
contrast media, radiographic (**see also** radiocontrast media) 337
copper 51, 133
copper-metallothioneins133
creatine phosphokinase 269
creatinine clearance 201, 233, 241, 267, 291, 307, 377, 383, 439, 469, 491, 497, 639, 645
culture(s) (**see also** cell culture) 99, 193
cyanidanol 343
cyclic AMP 193, 207
cyclohexanol/cyclohexanone 563
cyclophosphamide 139
cyclopiazonic acid 743
cyclosporin(e) A 147, 277, 285, 291, 297, 303, 307, 315, 325, 497, 705
cysteine 43, 107
cysteine-S-conjugates 439, 595, 595
cysteine conjugate ß-lyase 583, 595
cysteinylglycine dipeptidase 423
cytochrome-c 543
cytochrome P-450 725
cytosegrosomes 147

decalin 535
deferoxamine 457
dehydration 467, 491
diabetes mellitus 467
dialysis patients 389
diatrizoate (meglumine) 463, 491, 705
p-dichlorbenzene 93, 551, 557
N-(3,5-dichlorophenyl)succin-amide 601
dichlorovinyl-L-cysteine 577, 583, 749
S-(1,2-dichlorovinyl)glutathione 749
dichromate toxicity 569
diethyldithiocarbamate 353, 433
diethylmaleate 457, 569
di(2-ethylhexyl)phthalate 93
1,25-dihydroxyvitamin D 113
2,3-dimercapropane sulphonate 21
N,N'-diphenyl-p-phenylenediamine 343, 457
distal tubules 1, 113
dithiothreitol 457
diuresis 207, 233, 353 diuretics 357
DNA 85, 93, 557, 749
doxorubicin (**see** adriamycin)
dysplasia 411